KIDNEY TRANSPLANTATION – NEW PERSPECTIVES

Edited by **Magdalena Trzcińska**

Kidney Transplantation – New Perspectives
Edited by Magdalena Trzcińska

Published by InTech

Janeza Trdine 9, 51000 Rijeka, Croatia

Publishing Process Manager Davor Vidic

Technical Editor Teodora Smiljanic

Cover Designer InTech Design Team

Additional hard copies can be obtained from orders@intechopen.com

Kidney Transplantation – New Perspectives, Edited by Magdalena Trzcińska
p. cm.
ISBN 978-953-307-684-3

For EU product safety concerns:
IN TECH d.o.o., Prolaz Marije Krucifikse Kozulić 3, 51000 Rijeka, Croatia,
info@intechopen.com or visit our website at intechopen.com.

Meet the editor

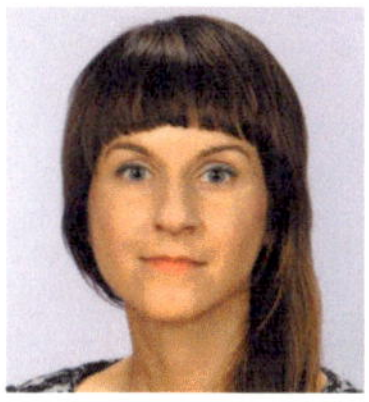

Dr. Magdalena Trzcińska , M.D., is a practicing, certified clinical psychologist, diplomate in clinical neuropsychology with more than 10 years experience. She received a MA from Warsaw University and a MD from Nicolaus Copernicus University. She works with patients (both children and adults) with neurological conditions, especially those who have cognitive deficits that result from the genetic or other somatic diseases (for example neurofibromatosis), who have developed progressive dementing disorders and who struggle with developmental neurobehavioral disorders. Beginning from the 2000 she is consultant psychologist in the Transplantology and Surgery Department in the University Hospital of Collegium Medicum in Bydgoszcz (Poland). Dr. Trzcińska is also a certified psychotherapist. She completed her postgraduate diploma in cognitive – behavioural therapy in Cognitive Behavioural Therapy Cenrtre in Warsaw in cooperation with the Oxford Cognitive Therapy Centre. She is a member of the Polish Association for Behavioral and Cognitive Therapies and the Polish Psychological Association.

Contents

Preface

To our Patients without whose effort, goodwill and trust no progress in medicine would be possible

The emergence of transplantology has definitely launched a new era in the history of medicine. And although the first attempts at transplanting organs would frequently end up with a failure, it is thanks to the determination and courage of pioneer doctors and sacrificial attitude of the patients that we can enjoy today's state of knowledge and potential in the field of organ transplantation. It should also not be forgotten that clinical transplantology owes its development and getting well-grounded to the development of such fields of medicine as nephrology or clinical immunology. A clear dynamic development has been observed over the last decades also in the field of immunosuppressant treatment. At present immunosuppressant drugs are more effective and safer, posing a lower risk for side-effects to the patients.

Many years have passed since the first successful kidney transplantation and the method, although no longer considered a medical experiment, is still perceived as controversial and, as such, it triggers many emotions. And even though family transplants attract more social understanding, unfortunately the same is still not true for recovering and transplanting organs from a dead donor. Much confusion concerns mostly the concept of brain death and its diagnostic procedures. Doubt is found even among medical doctors or heath-care related communities, most frequently due to a lack of knowledge or wrong understanding of the concept of brain death.

Many years and conscious educational efforts are still needed to make kidney transplantation, for many people the only chance for an active lifestyle and improved quality of life, win common social acceptance and stop triggering negative connotations. The need of mass transplantology education has been already effectively implemented in many EU countries, the United States and in Canada; it is spread not only by the medical community but also by the emerging and already active associations of organ transplant patients.

The statistics gathered by the World Health Organization (WHO) show that in 2009 in 27 EU countries 17886 thousand kidney transplants were performed, namely 668 (0.6%) transplantation cases more than in 2008. The statistics demonstrate that the number of transplantations performed has been regularly increasing for more than twenty years.

Apart from the transplantation controversies piling up over the years and transplantation not always winning social acceptance, transplantologists also face many other medical difficulties. Much research covers the phenomenon of graft rejection and algorithms of post-kidney-transplant procedure, and the effectiveness of new drugs is being tested. A growing potential of transplantology is also due to the advancement of research into the significance of gene polymorphism, the potential of the application of the achievements of proteomics in diagnostics (e.g. allowing for identifying urine proteins differentiating between active inflammatory changes in kidneys) or numerous research on various aspects of the immune system functioning.

The authors of chapters published herein are experts in their respective fields. The chapters selected are of high level of content, and the fact that their authors come from many different countries, and sometimes even cultures, has facilitated a comprehensive and interesting approach to the problem of kidney transplantation. The authors cover a wide spectrum of transplant-related topics: significance of research into gene polymorphism, possibilities of applying techniques offered by proteomics, the effect of ischemia or flow disturbances on the kidney graft, monitoring its function after transplantation as well as multi-aspect research and analyses of immunologic mechanisms. The book does not disregard the problem of mental aspects, essential especially from the patient's perspective.

As the editor, I wish to thank all the authors for their cooperation, research efforts, literature reviews and their precious clinical observations as well as for their desire to share with the medical community their precious experience without which this book would not be possible.

Finally, on behalf of all the authors I wish to express hope that our publication will not only facilitate access to the latest scientific achievements in the field but also enhance a further progress in transplantology and propagating the idea all across the world.

Magdalena Trzcińska, MD.
University Hospital of Collegium Medicum in Bydgoszcz,
Psychiatry Department, Nicolaus Copernicus University in Torun,
Poland

1

Mechanisms of T Lymphocytes in the Damage and Repair Long Term after Renal Ischemia Reperfusion Injury

Dolores Ascon and Miguel Ascon
Cell Therapy Unit. BriJen Biotech, LLC. The BioInnovation Center, University of Maryland BioPark, Baltimore, MD 21201, U.S.A.

1. Introduction

Acute kidney injury (AKI) is a frequent event associated with decreased allograft survival in patients with transplanted kidneys and high mortality in patients with native kidneys (1,2). AKI is a common complication in hospitalized patients, and its incidence has risen substantially over the past 15 years (1-3). As a conservative estimate, roughly 17 million admissions annually in the United States are complicated by AKI, resulting in over $10 billion in costs to the health care system (4). Kidney transplants from living unrelated donors (not well HLA matched) with minimal ischemic injury have improved allograft survival, compared with grafts from well matched cadaveric donors with significant ischemia (5, 6). This implies that renal ischemia reperfusion injury (IRI) can have important consequences on long-term graft survival and native kidneys.

IRI is a highly complex cascade of events that includes interactions between vascular endothelium, interstitial compartments, circulating cells, and numerous mediator molecules (7). Renal ischemic injury has been found to permanently damage peritubular capillaries causing hypoxia, which may be involved in the progression of chronic renal disease after AKI (7, 8). Tubulointerstitial influx of inflammatory cells is found in many forms of chronic renal diseases, including 'nonimmune' diseases such as diabetes and hypertension (9). T-lymphocyte infiltration has also been observed early after moderate ischemia injury (10,11) however, the dynamics of infiltrating lymphocyte populations long term after moderate or severe ischemic injury is not very clear.

It has been demonstrated that T and B lymphocytes are important mediators in the pathogenesis of renal IRI (10, 12) however, the mechanisms by which these cells induce kidney injury is largely unknown. The trafficking of pathogenic lymphocytes into kidneys after moderate and severe ischemic injury has been postulated to contribute to kidney damage (11, 13, 14) however the physiologic state and the dynamics of trafficking of these populations long term after ischemia have not been rigorously studied. Furthermore, the activation and expression of the effector-memory phenotype by infiltrated lymphocytes suggests the possibility that these lymphocytes are responding to an injury-associated antigen (15, 16). In addition, these lymphocytes are responsible to produce inflammatory mediators not only causing local kidney structure damage, but also the severe effects on the other long distance organs, including lung, hearth, intestine, brain, liver, bone medulla.

Here we describe the trafficking of T lymphocytes into the mice (male C57BL/6J) kidneys both, in normal mice, earlier (3 to 24 h), and long term (1 to 11 weeks) after the renal injury was performed as previously described (17, 18, 19). The different T cell phenotypes and cytokine/chemokines raised at different times are compared with the baseline level cells maintained in normal kidneys (17). In the long term studies, to make our observations clinically relevant for both allograft and native kidneys, we have studied these phenomena in both a moderate bilateral ischemia (a kin to ischemia in native kidneys) and a severe unilateral ischemia (a kin to IRI in an allograft). The different kidney infiltrating T cell phenotypes and its effector molecules raised at different times after ischemia injury are presented and discussed.

2. Overview of experimental acute kidney injury

The mechanisms involved in renal ischemia-reperfusion injury (IRI) are complex (20, 21), invoking both innate and adaptive immunity (22, 23). Following IR, the cascade of events leading to endothelial cell dysfunction, tubular epithelial cell injury and activation of tissue-resident and infiltrating leukocytes consists of the coordinated action of cytokines/chemokines, reactive oxygen intermediates and adhesion molecules (21, 23). The early phase of innate immune response to IR begins within minutes of reperfusion, whereas the late phase adaptive response requires days to manifest. For our experiments, a well-established model of renal IRI in mice was used (17, 18, and 19).

3. Early trafficking of T lymphocytes into kidneys after IRI

Trafficking of CD4$^+$ and CD8$^+$ T lymphocytes

We have examined the trafficking of CD4$^+$ and CD8$^+$ T cell subsets into kidneys after ischemic injury (18). After 3 h of renal IRI, the percentages of CD4$^+$ and CD4$^+$NK1.1$^+$ cells increased similarly in both sham-operated and IRI mice as compared with normal mice. However, 24 h after renal IRI, while the percentage of CD4$^+$ T cells in the IRI mice was similar to that of control groups, the percentage of CD4$^+$NK1.1$^+$ cells increased (3.2%) when compared with normal (1.2%) and sham-operated (1.6%) mice. The percentage of CD8$^+$ T cells was similar in all groups 3 and 24 h after renal IRI and no expression of NK1.1 Ag was observed on these cells. However, the increased percentage of the CD4$^+$NK1.1$^+$ cells in the IRI group 24 h after renal IRI could be related to renal ischemic injury because at this time point serum creatinine was increasing and visible kidney structure damage was observed. Table 1 shows summarized results.

Expression of CD69 on CD4$^+$ and CD8$^+$ T lymphocytes

We have investigated the activation state of the intrarenal CD4$^+$ and CD8$^+$ T cell subsets analyzing the expression of activation markers CD69 and CD25 (18). After 3 h of renal IRI, we observed increased expression of CD69 on CD4$^+$ T cells in sham-operated (14.7%) and IRI (14.2%) compared with normal mice (7.1%). CD69 expression on CD8$^+$ T cells tended to increase at 3 h, but was not statistically significant. After 24 h of renal IRI, the expression of CD69 on CD4$^+$ and CD8$^+$ T cells declined to lower levels than normal mice. Moreover, no increased expression of CD25 Ag on CD4$^+$ and CD8$^+$ T cells in any of the studied groups was found. Results demonstrated that CD4+ and CD8+ T lymphocytes infiltrating kidneys of sham-operated and IRI mice display some features of activated T lymphocytes. We hypothesized that T cells might be activated after renal IRI; however, we found a similarly increased expression of CD69 on the CD4+ and CD8+ T cells in both sham-operated and IRI mice 3 h after renal IRI. Results are summarized in Table 1.

Kidney assessment and histology changes earlier after ischemia injury

We evaluated the Ischemic kidneys following the serum creatinine levels 3 and 24 h after renal IRI (18). After 3 h of renal IRI, a significant increase in serum creatinine of IRI mice (n = 8, 1.18 mg/dl) when compared with normal (n = 8, 0.50 mg/dl) and sham-operated (n = 8, 0.70 mg/dl) mice was observed. After 24 h of renal IRI, serum creatinine significantly increased in the IRI mice (n = 8, 2.83 mg/dl) as compared with control groups. In the sham-operated mice, serum creatinine was slightly increased compared with normal mice 3 h after surgery (Fig. 1). The kidney structural injury in the cortex and the medulla of IRI mice was evaluated. Compared with kidneys of normal mice (Fig. 1*A*) and sham-operated mice, 3 (Fig. 1*B*) and 24 h (Fig. 1*C*) after surgery, IRI mice show slightly tubular epithelial necrosis 3 h after renal IRI (Fig. 1*D*) and significant tubular injury with loss of tubular structure 24 h after renal IRI (Fig. 1*E*).

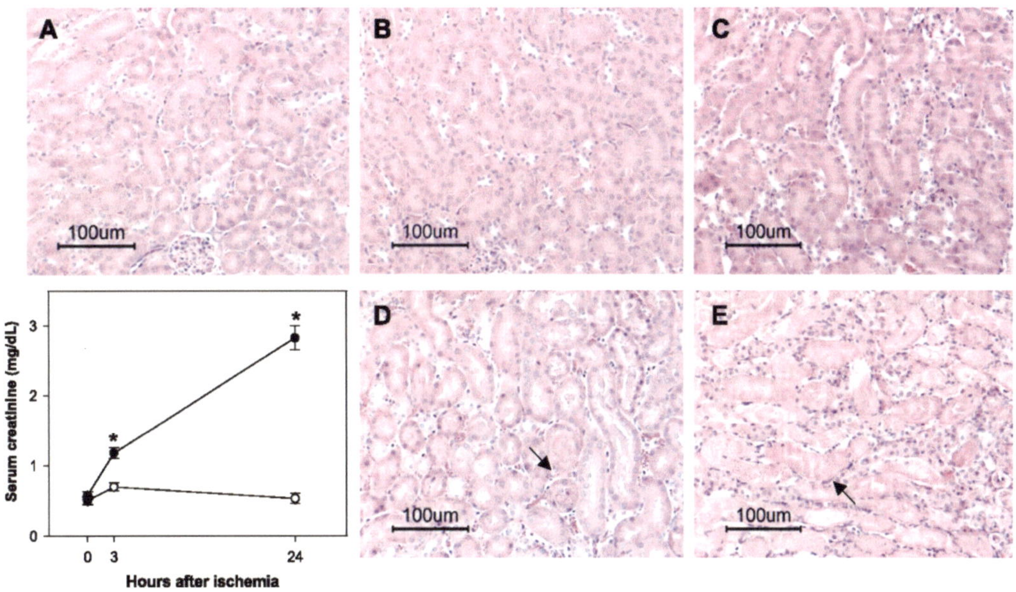

Fig. 1. Kidney injury after 30-min bilateral ischemia. Serum creatinine of IRI mice (•) compared with normal (▴) and sham-operated (○) mice 3 and 24 h after renal IRI. *A*, Normal mouse kidney (no IRI). *B* and *C*, Sham-operated mice kidneys showing normal histology 3 and 24 h after surgery, respectively. *D*, IRI mouse kidney showing same proteinaceous casts in tubules 3 h after renal IRI. *E*, IRI kidney showing severe damage 24 h after renal IRI. (Pictures used with permission and courtesy of the original authors [18]).

Lymphocyte Phenotypes	Normal mice	Early trafficking		Long term trafficking		
	0h	3h	24h	2w	6w	11w
$CD4^+$	18.6	24.8	18.5	29	51[a](48)[b]	48
$CD8^+$	8.2	10.1	9.1	16	30(21)	27
$CD4^+CD69^+$	7.1	14.2	5.5	17	22(29)	28
$CD8^+CD69^+$	2.3	4.3	0.4	9	18(15)	16
$CD4^+CD44^+CD62L^-$	57	ND	ND	77	ND(96)	93
$CD8^+CD44^+CD62L^-$	49	ND	ND	ND	90ND	ND
$CD4^+$NK1.1 (NKT)	1.2	1.3	3.2	1.1	2.0(0.2)	0.4
$CD4^+CD25^+$ (FOXP3+)	1.8	ND	1.8[c]	2.6[d]	ND	ND

[a] After 6 weeks of bilateral ischemia
[b] After 6 weeks of unilateral ischemia
[c] After 3 days of unilateral ischemia
[d] After 10 days of unilateral ischemia

Table 1. T lymphocytes phenotypic trafficking into mouse kidney after IRI, expressed as cells percentages.

4. Trafficking of T lymphocytes into kidneys long term after IRI

Trafficking of $CD4^+$ and $CD8^+$ T cells

Analysis of infiltrating lymphocytes long term after renal IRI (19, 24) revealed increased percentages of $CD4^+$ (29%) and $CD8^+$ (16%) T lymphocytes in IRI kidneys compared with kidneys of sham mice ($CD4^+$: 11% and $CD8^+$: 6%) after 2 weeks of bilateral renal IRI. However, similar percentage of $CD4^+$ and $CD8^+$ T cells was observed in sham and IRI kidneys 6 weeks after bilateral renal IRI. 6 weeks after unilateral renal IRI, we observed a significantly increased percentage of $CD4^+$ (48%) and $CD8^+$ (21%) T lymphocytes compared with kidneys from sham mice ($CD4^+$: 16% and $CD8^+$: 7%) and contralateral kidneys ($CD4^+$: 11% and $CD8^+$: 5%). No changes in $CD4^+$ and $CD8^+$ T-cell populations were observed in any of the groups 11 weeks after unilateral renal IRI. Results are summarized in Table 1. The higher levels of $CD4^+$ and $CD8^+$ T cells 6 and 11 weeks after ischemia as well as the return to normal levels of some populations as $CD69^+$ and $CD44^+$ markers after 6 weeks, demonstrate the possible limit and suppression of the immune response after long-term renal IRI. Potential modulators of this immunosuppresion could be the regulatory T cells $CD4^+CD25^+$ or $CD4^+CD25^+$ FoxP3 (25, 26) as increased populations of these regulatory T cells have been observed in long-term allogenic transplants (27).

Infiltrating of CD4+ and CD8+ T lymphocytes expressing CD69

After 2 weeks of bilateral renal IRI (19), we observed an increased expression of CD69 on $CD4^+$ (17%) and $CD8^+$ (9%) T cells in IRI mice when compared with sham mice ($CD4^+$: 6% and $CD8^+$: 2%). Similarly, increased expression of CD69 on $CD4^+$ (22%) and $CD8^+$ (18%) T cells in IRI mice compared with sham mice ($CD4^+$: 15% and $CD8^+$: 11%) was observed after 6 weeks of bilateral renal IRI. Six weeks after unilateral ischemia, we observed a significantly increased expression of CD69 on $CD4^+$ (29%) and $CD8^+$ (15%) T cells compared with kidneys from sham mice ($CD4^+$: 7% and $CD8^+$: 2%) and contralateral kidneys ($CD4^+$: 4% and $CD8^+$: 2%). However, 11 weeks after renal IRI, only $CD4^+$ T cells from IRI kidneys showed increased expression of CD69 (28%) when compared with sham (13%) and contralateral (12%) kidneys. Results are summarized in Table 1. The increased infiltration of the activated $CD69^+$ marker T lymphocytes in both unilateral and bilateral IRI kidneys, is consistent with upregulation of the early activation marker CD69 antigen observed in allograft rejections and some autoimmune diseases (28–31). Activated cells produce inflammatory factors which can participate in tissue damage including fibrosis, as observed in patients with systemic sclerosis and pulmonary fibrosis (32, 33).

Infiltrating of $CD4^+$ and $CD8^+$ T cells displaying effector-memory phenotype

Two weeks after bilateral renal IRI (19), significantly increased percentage of effector-memory $CD4^+CD44^{hi}CD62L^-$ T cells in IRI kidneys (77%) was observed when compared with kidneys from sham mice (54%). Six weeks after bilateral renal IRI, a significantly increased percentage of $CD8^+$ $CD44^{hi}CD62L^-$ T cells in IRI kidneys (90%) compared with sham mice (79%) was observed. Similarly, 6 weeks after unilateral renal IRI, the IRI kidneys showed significantly increased percentage of $CD4^+CD44^{hi}CD62L^-$ T cells (96%) when compared with kidneys from sham mice (71%) and contralateral kidneys (65%). A significant increase in percentage of $CD4^+CD44^{hi}CD62L^-$ T cells was observed in IRI kidneys (93%) when compared with sham (80%) and contralateral kidneys (75%) 11 weeks after renal IRI. Results are summarized in Table 1. The high levels of effector-memory $CD4^+CD44^{hi}CD62L^-$ T cells, the 'footprints' of an immune response to antigens, in both unilateral and bilateral IRI kidneys, are consistent with the response to self-antigens involved in the pathogenesis of skeletal and intestinal ischemia induced by hypoxic stress (34), indicating that immune response to renal IRI could be also initiated by specific antigens.

Decreasing of NKT lymphocytes

Similar percentage of NKT cells ($CD4^+NK1.1^+$) was observed after 2 weeks of bilateral renal IRI (19). However, 6 weeks after bilateral renal IRI, we found a significantly decreased percentage of NKT cells in IRI kidneys (2%) when compared with kidneys of sham mice (4%). Eleven weeks after unilateral renal IRI, decreased percentage of NKT cells was observed in IRI kidneys (0.4%) when compared to sham (1.91%) and contralateral kidneys (3.1%; Figure 4a). However, no changes were observed in mice that underwent bilateral renal IRI with reduced ischemia times. In Table 1 are summarized the results. The decreased number of NKT cells 6 and 11 weeks after bilateral and unilateral renal IRI, respectively, are similar to that in liver injury (35) and rheumatoid arthritis (36).

Effect of CD^+ and $CD8^+$ T-cell depletion on kidney-cell infiltration

To determine the pathophysiologic role of infiltrating $CD4^+$ and $CD8^+$ T cells long term after ischemia, we depleted these cells before and after unilateral ischemia during the 6-week experiments (19). Depletion started 24 h preischemia and 3 days postischemia and cell analysis by flow cytometry was performed weekly in blood and after 6 weeks in kidney samples. Blood was 98% depleted of $CD4^+$ and $CD8^+$ T cells during the 6 weeks after renal IRI. In kidneys, the $CD4^+CD69^+$, $CD8^+CD69^+$, $CD4^+CD44^{hi}CD62L^-$, and $CD4^+NK1.1^+$ cells were also depleted by approximately 98%, in relationship with the cell profiles of nondepleted control mice (data are not showed).

Histology of structural damage after long term ischemia

To observe the degree of structural damage of ischemic kidneys after 6 weeks of renal IRI in depleted mice, the kidney histology of depleted and control mice were compared. The damage in the cortex (Figure 2a) was similar in control and both depleted mice, however, medullary damage (Figure 2b) was more extensive in control and post-ischemia depleted mice (Figure 2c) than in preischemia depleted mice. Therefore, the reduced damage observed in the kidney medulla of preischemia depleted mice when compared to control mice could be related to the low expression of IFN-γ (Table 2). The IFN-γ produced by $CD4^+$ and $CD8^+$ T lymphocytes is involved early after renal ischemia (37, 38), and has been detected in acute and chronic kidney rejections (39). However, the increased expression of IL-1β in postischemia depleted mice could be related to the increased structural damage of kidney observed and could have distant organ affects (40).

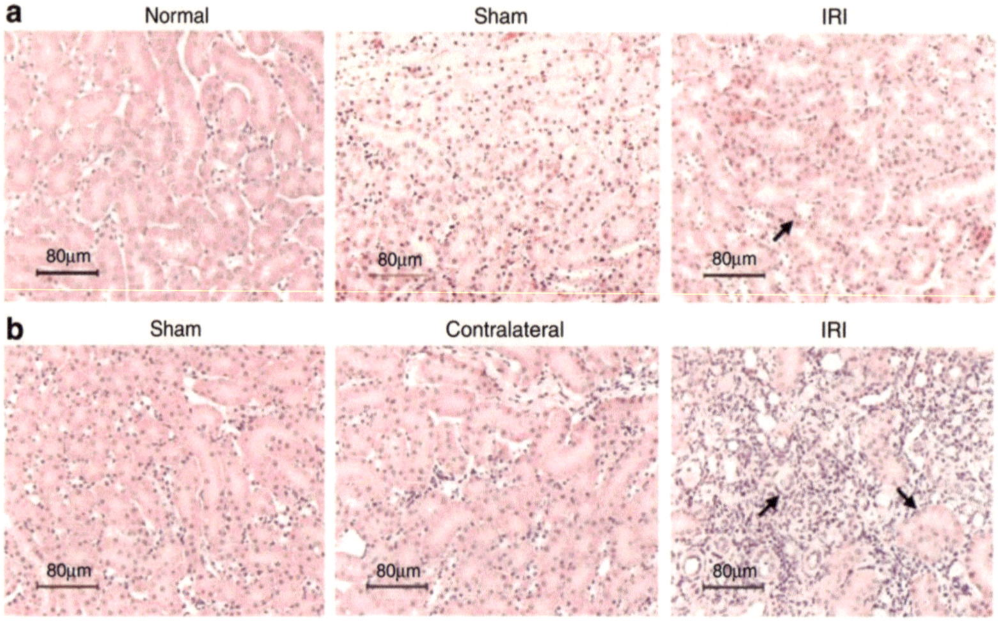

Fig. 2. Kidney tissue from IRI mice after 2 weeks of 25 min of bilateral ischemia (**a**, upper panel) shows some proteinaceous casts in tubules compared with normal histology of normal and sham mouse kidneys. Kidney structure 6 weeks after unilateral renal IRI (**b**, lower panel) shows normal histology of sham and contralateral kidneys compared with severe kidney damage, loss of structure, and cyst formation in IRI kidneys. (Pictures used with permission and courtesy of the original authors [19]).

Regulatory T (Treg) cells involved in damage inhibition and reparative phase

Treg cells are lymphocytes with immunosuppressive properties. One important subset of Treg cells express CD4 and CD25 on the cell surface and the transcription factor, FoxP3 (41). The mechanisms of suppression by Treg cells are diverse and include: production of antiinflammatory cytokines such as IL-10 or TGF-β, direct cell-cell contact or CTLA-4 mediated inhibition and production of extracellular adenosine (42). Recently, Treg cells have been identified in normal mouse kidneys (17, 43). In WT mice, treatment with an anti-CD25 monoclonal antibody (PC61) selectively decreased kidney, spleen and blood $CD4^+$ $FoxP3^+$ Treg cell numbers by approximately 50%, five days after PC61 treatment (44). At that time point, Treg cell deficiency potentiated kidney IRI, measured by plasma creatinine, acute tubular necrosis (ATN), neutrophil and macrophage accumulation and pro-inflammatory cytokine transcription in the kidney after 24 hr of reperfusion (43). In lymphocyte-deficient Rag-1 KO mice, adoptive transfer of WT, but not IL-10 KO, Treg cells blocked IR-induced inflammation and kidney injury (43). These findings demonstrate that Treg cells can directly suppress the early innate inflammation, induced by IR, in an IL-10 dependent manner. In a different study, PC61 was administered 1 day prior to IRI, and while BUN levels and ATN scores were no different than control antibody-treated mice at 24 hr of reperfusion, the necrosis failed to resolve by 72 hr in the PC61-treated mice (45). In other study, using a murine model of ischemic acute kidney injury it was found that the percentage of the $CD25^+Foxp3^+$ Treg subset in the total kidney-infiltrating $TCR\beta^+CD4^+$ T lymphocyte compartment was increased from 1.8 to 2.6% in IR kidneys at 3 and 10 days (46). This infiltration was accompanied of an enhanced pro-inflammatory cytokine production. These results strongly support an important role of regulatory T cells during IRI and in kidney repair after IRI.

Cytokines chemokines	Normal mice	Early trafficking		Long term trafficking		
	0 h[a]	3h[b]	24 h[ab]	1w[c]	6w (no-deple)[c]	6w (deple)[c]
IFN-ɣ (CD4)	6.0	ND	18	ND	16.0	7-8
IFN-ɣ (CD8)	7.1	ND	19			
TNF- α (CD4)	5.0	ND	19	ND	38	37-39
TNF- α (CD8)	2.2	ND	4.9			
IL-1β	ND	ND	ND	ND	18	28-45
IL-6	ND	ND	ND	ND	3.0	3-6
MIP-2	ND	4.2	30.0	147.4	18	20-28
MCP-1	ND	ND	13.8	24.6	ND	ND
KC	ND	ND	14.9	14.0	ND	ND
IP-10	ND	3.9	8.9	14.2	ND	ND
RANTES	1.0[d]	2.0[d]	ND	50[d]	38	35-37

[a]IFN-ɣ and TNF-α at 0 and 24h were determined by flow cytometry as internal cell cytokines.
[b]MIP-2, MCP-1, KC, and IP-10 at 3 and 24 h were determined using qPCR
[c]All cytokines and chemokines during the long term trafficking (at 1 and 6 weeks) were determined using qPCR.
[d]Protein levels of CCL5 (RANTES) were detected by ELISA values in pg/mg.

Table 2. Cytokines and chemokines expressed after IRI in kidney.

5. Upregulation of cytokines and chemokines long term after IRI

Expression of cytokines

Cytokine and chemokines are known to modulate lymphocyte and kidney cell interactions to mediate kidney injury and fibrosis. We found (19) an increased intracellular cytokine production of TNF-α and IFN-γ by CD3T+ cells infiltrating kidneys after 24 hours of IRI in mice. This observation suggests that lymphocytes infiltrating into the postischemic kidneys could have a major downstream effect on later inflammation and organ dysfunction. Thus, not only the trafficking of T cells postischemia is a potential mechanism, but what those infiltrating cells are doing at the site of injury could be crucial for pathogenesis. Given that infiltrating T cells are activated and selectively expanded in kidney long term after IRI, we hypothesized that there would be a different upregulation of these molecules postischemia in depleted and nondepleted mice. Using real-time RT-PCR, a significant upregulation of IL-1β, IL-6, tumor necrosis factor (TNF)-α, IFN-γ, MIP-2, and RANTES was seen 6 weeks after 60 min of unilateral renal IRI in normal (nondepleted T cells), compared to sham and contralateral kidneys. Depletion of CD4 and CD8 T cells starting preischemia led to significant decrease in kidney IFN-γ levels. In contrast, depletion starting 3 days after ischemia led to significant increase in IL-1β. However, the IRI kidneys of both depleted and nondepleted groups had prominent expression levels of TNF-α and RANTES. As demonstrated in both depleted and nondepleted mice 6 weeks after unilateral ischemia, the cytokines and chemokines including IL-1β, IL-6, TNF-α, MIP-2, and RANTES were significantly upregulated. The results are summarized in the Table 2. It has been reported that in moderate ischemia a modest upregulation of TNF-α and RANTES and strong upregulation of IL-1β, IL-6, IFN-γ, and MIP-2 exist (47), whereas after severe ischemia strong upregulation of TNF-α and RANTES and to a lesser extent IL-1β, IL-6, IFN-γ, and MIP-2 occur (48, 49). Similarly, in patients with acute rejection and chronic allograft nephropathy significant expression of TNF-α and RANTES were reported (49).

Expression of CXC and CC chemokines

Chemokines are mainly known for their ability to attract inflammatory cells to sites of injury. Recently, the highest levels of chemokine expression at the stage of active repair (i.e. 7 days after ischemic injury) was observed, and temporal chemokines expression pattern in more detail was examinated (50). The expression of the CC and CXC chemokines at additional reperfusion periods after ischemic injury was evaluated to determine if there is a biphasic expression coinciding with the inflammatory and reparative response after ischemic injury. Some chemokine results are summarized in the Table 2. The four CC chemokines were expressed in a monophasic fashion with a clear peak 7 days after ischemic injury. In contrast, the CXC chemokines had a biphasic expression after ischemic injury with the first peak in the early (i.e. inflammatory) phase and the second peak during the reparative phase. The CXC chemokines Cxcl1/KC, Cxcl2/MIP-2a and Cxcl10/IP-10 had the highest expression during the inflammatory phase.

6. Effect of renal ischemic injury on distant organs

Acute kidney injury (AKI) in native kidneys is a major clinical problem with high mortality and morbidity in the intensive care unit. This problem remains unchanged for the past 50 years in part because AKI is associated with extra-renal complications (51, 52, 53). Much of the increased risk of death associated with AKI is usually related to multi-organ dysfunction including brain, heart, lungs, liver and small intestine. After kidney IRI, inflammatory cytokines and chemokines in plasma IL-1β, IL-6, KC (IL-8), TNF-α, TNF-β, INF-γ, IL-17A, C5a, and MCP-1 increased significantly which eventually could lead to develop multi-organ failure. (54, 55, 56). In particular, AKI caused by IRI increased pulmonary vascular permeability with capillary leak (57) and change of fluid absorption in alveolar epithelial cells (58). Inflammation and apoptosis could be important mechanisms connecting the effect of AKI on lung and distant organs as show in changes of inflammatory transcriptome identified in lung after kidney IRI (59). Studies using gene microarrays analysis found marked changes in immune, inflammatory, and apoptotic processes (60). Caspase-dependent pulmonary apoptosis concurrent with activated T cell trafficking was also demonstrated in kidney after IRI (61). Altered gene expression associated with inflammation, apoptosis, and cytoskeletal structure in pulmonary endothelial cells after kidney IRI suggested possible mechanisms underlying the increased pulmonary microvascular permeability (62). Increase of IL-1β, IL-6, TNFα, MCP-1, KC (IL-8) and ICAM-1 may act as mediators in the crosstalk between kidney and lung (55, 60, 63). AKI following

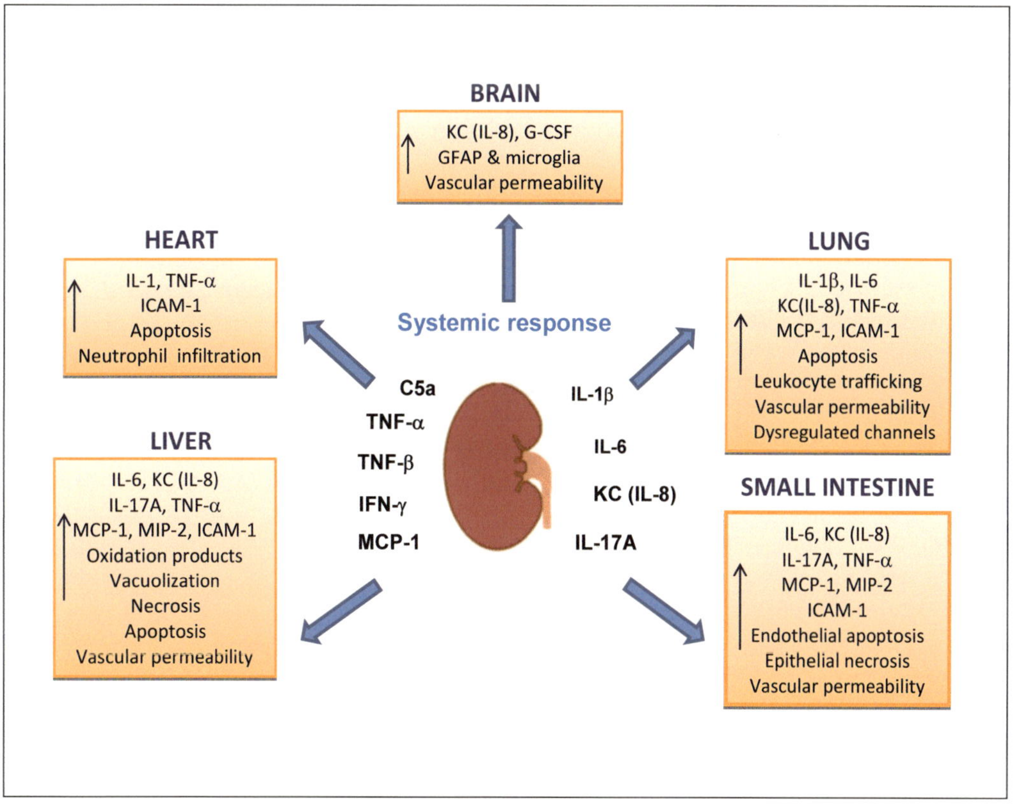

Fig. 3. AKI induce distant organ effects. AKI leads to changes in distant organs, including brain, lungs, heart, liver, and small intestine, involving multiple inflammatory pathways, including increased expression of soluble pro-inflammatory mediators, innate and adaptive immunity, cellular apoptosis, microvascular inflammation and dysregulation of transport activity, oxidative stress, transcriptional responses, etc.

IRI has been reported to increase apoptosis and production of IL-1, TNF-α, and ICAM-1 in cardiac tissue (56). Changes in the microvasculature after kidney IRI were also demonstrated in brain and conferred susceptibility to stroke (64). In brain has been found increased expression of KC (IL-8), granulocyte colony-stimulating factor (G-CSF), and glial fibrillary acidic protein, an inflammatory marker (65). More recently, hepatic and small intestine dysfunction has been observed in patients suffering from AKI. Liver injury after ischemic shows peri-portal hepatocyte vacuolization, necrosis and apoptosis with inflammatory changes. Small intestinal injury after ischemic was characterized by villous lacteal capillary endothelial apoptosis, epithelial necrosis and increased leukocyte (neutrophils, macrophages and lymphocytes) infiltration. Vascular permeability was severely impaired in both liver and small intestine. After ischemic insult TNF-α, IL-17A and IL-6 levels in plasma, liver and small intestine increased significantly. Furthermore, up-regulation of KC (IL-8), MCP-1, MIP-2, ICAM-1 has been found in liver and small intestine (54). The Figure 3, shows a summarized picture of the cross talking between AKI and several long distance organs.

7. References

[1] Tilney NL, Guttmann RD. Effects of initial ischemia/reperfusion injury on the transplanted kidney. Transplantation 1997; 64: 945–947.

[2] Bonventre JV, Zuk A: Ischemic acute renal failure: An inflammatory disease? *Kidney Int* 66: 480–485, 2004.

[3] Terasaki PI, Cecka JM, Gjertson DW et al. survival rates of kidney transplants from spousal and living unrelated donors. N Engl J Med 1995; 333: 333–336.

[4] Chertow GM, Burdick E, Honour M, Bonventre JV, Bates DW. Acute kidney injury, mortality, length of stay, and costs in hospitalized patients. *JAmSoc Nephrol.* 2005;16(11):3365-3370.

[5] Sanfilippo F, Vaughn WK, Spees EK et al. The detrimental effects of delayed graft function in cadaver donor renal transplantation. Transplantation 1984; 38: 643–648.

[6] Halloran PF, Aprile MA, Farewell V et al. Early function as the principal correlate of graft survival. A multivariate analysis of 200 cadaveric renal transplants treated with a protocol incorporating antilymphocyte globulin and cyclosporine. Transplantation 1988; 46: 223–228.

[7] Basile DP, Donohoe D, Roethe K et al. Renal ischemia injury results in permanent damage to peritubular capillaries and influences long-term function. Am J Physiol Renal Physiol 2001; 281: F887–F899.

[8] Basile DP, Donohoe DL, Roethe K et al. Chronic renal hypoxia after acute ischemic injury: effects of L-arginine on hypoxia and secondary damage. Am J Physiol Renal Physiol 2003; 284: F338–F348.

[9] Remuzzi G, Bertani T. Pathophysiology of progressive nephropathies. N Engl J Med 1998; 339: 1448–1456.

[10] Burne MJ, Daniels F, El Ghandour A et al. Identification of the CD4(+) T cell as a major pathogenic factor in ischemic acute renal failure. J Clin Invest 2001; 108: 1283–1290.

[11] Pinheiro HS, Camara NO, Noronha IL, Maugeri IL, Franco MF, Medina JO, Pacheco-Silva A. Contribution of CD4+ T cells to the early mechanisms of ischemia-reperfusion injury in a mouse model of acute renal failure. Braz J Med Biol Res. 2007 40:557-68.

[12] Burne-Taney MJ, Ascon DB, Daniels F et al. B cell deficiency confers protection from renal ischemia reperfusion injury. J Immunol 2003; 171: 3210–3215.

[13] Burne-Taney M, Yokota N, Rabb H. Persistent renal and extra renal changes long term after severe renal ischemia reperfusion injury. Kidney Int 2005; 67: 1002–1009.

[14] Ibrahim S, Jacobs F, Zukin Y et al. Immunohistochemical manifestations of unilateral kidney ischemia. Clin Transplant 1996; 10: 646–652.

[15] Briscoe DM, Sayegh MH. A rendezvous before rejection: where do T cells meet transplant antigens? Nat Med 2002; 8: 220–222.

[16] Zhang M, Austen Jr WG, Chiu I et al. Identification of a specific self-reactive IgM antibody that initiates intestinal ischemia/reperfusion injury. Proc Natl Acad Sci USA 2004; 101: 3886–3891.

[17] Ascon DB, Ascon M, Satpute S, Lopez-Briones S, Racusen L, Colvin RB, Soloski MJ, Rabb H. Normal mouse kidneys contain activated and CD3+CD4- CD8- double-negative T lymphocytes with a distinct TCR repertoire. J Leukoc Biol. 2008; 84:1400-1409.

[18] Ascon DB, Lopez-Briones S, Liu M et al. Phenotypic and functional characterization of kidney-infiltrating lymphocytes in renal ischemia reperfusion injury. J Immunol 2006; 177: 3380–3387.

[19] Ascon M, Ascon DB, Liu M, Cheadle C, Sarkar C, Racusen L, Hassoun HT, Rabb H. Renal ischemia-reperfusion leads to long term infiltration of activated and effector-memory T lymphocytes. Kidney Int. 2009;75:526-535

[20] Schrier RW, Wang W, Poole B, Mitra A. Acute renal failure: definitions, diagnosis, pathogenesis, and therapy. J Clin Invest 2004;114:5–14.

[21] Bonventre JV, Weinberg JM. Recent advances in the pathophysiology of ischemic acute renal failure. J Am Soc Nephrol 2003;14:2199–210.

[22] Rabb H. The T cell as a bridge between innate and adaptive immune systems: implications for the kidney. Kidney Int 2002;61:1935–46.

[23] Li L, Okusa MD. Blocking the Immune respone in ischemic acute kidney injury: the role of adenosine 2A agonists. Nat Clin Pract Nephrology 2006;2:432–44.

[24] Ibrahim S, Jacobs F, Zukin Y et al. Immunohistochemical manifestations of unilateral kidney ischemia. Clin Transplant 1996; 10: 646–652.

[25] Sarween N, Chodos A, Raykundalia C et al. CD4+CD25+ cells controlling a pathogenic CD4 response inhibit cytokine differentiation, CXCR-3 expression, and tissue invasion. J Immunol 2004; 173: 2942–2951.

[26] Murphy TJ, Ni Choileain N, Zang Y et al. CD4+CD25+ regulatory T cells control innate immune reactivity after injury. J Immunol 2005; 174: 2957–2963.

[27] Braudeau C, Racape M, Giral M et al. Variation in numbers of CD4+CD25highFOXP3+ T cells with normal immuno-regulatory properties in long-term graft outcome. Transpl Int 2007; 20: 845–855.

[28] Afeltra AM, Galeazzi GD, Sebastiani GM et al. Coexpression of CD69 and HLADR activation markers on synovial fluid T lymphocytes of patients affected by rheumatoid arthritis: a three-colour cytometric analysis. Int J Exp Pathol 1997; 78: 331–336.

[29] Santamaria M, Marubayashi M, Arizon JM et al. The activation antigen CD69 is selectively expressed on CD8+ endomyocardium infiltrating T lymphocytes in human rejecting heart allografts. Hum Immunol 1992; 33: 1–4.

[30] Crispin JC, Martinez A, de Pablo P et al. Participation of the CD69 antigen in the T-cell activation process of patients with systemic lupus erythematosus. Scand J Immunol 1998; 48: 196–200.
[31] Posselt AM, Vincenti F, Bedolli M et al. CD69 expression on peripheral CD8 T cells correlates with acute rejection in renal transplant recipients. Transplantation 2003; 76: 190–195.
[32] Bresser P, Jansen HM, Weller FR et al. T-cell activation in the lungs of patients with systemic sclerosis and its relation with pulmonary fibrosis. Chest 2001; 120: 66S–68S.
[33] Luzina IG, Atamas SP, Wise R et al. Occurrence of an activated, profibrotic pattern of gene expression in lung CD8+ T cells from scleroderma patients. Arthritis Rheum 2003; 48: 2262–2274.
[34] Zhang M, Alicot EM, Chiu I et al. Identification of the target self-antigens in reperfusion injury. J Exp Med 2006; 203: 141–152.
[35] Shimamura K, Kawamura H, Nagura T et al. Association of NKT cells and granulocytes with liver injury after reperfusion of the portal vein. Cell Immunol 2005; 234: 31–38.
[36] Yanagihara Y, Shiozawa K, Takai M et al. Natural killer (NK) T cells are significantly decreased in the peripheral blood of patients with rheumatoid arthritis (RA). Clin Exp Immunol 1999; 118: 131–136.
[37] Li L, Huang L, Sung SS et al. NKT cell activation mediates neutrophil IFN-gamma production and renal ischemia-reperfusion injury. J Immunol 2007; 178: 5899–5911.
[38] Day YJ, Huang L, Ye H et al. Renal ischemia-reperfusion injury and adenosine 2A receptor-mediated tissue protection: the role of CD4+ T cells and IFN-gamma. J Immunol 2006; 176: 3108–3114.
[39] Obata F, Yoshida K, Ohkubo M et al. Contribution of CD4+ and CD8+ T cells and interferon-gamma to the progress of chronic rejection of kidney allografts: the Th1 response mediates both acute and chronic rejection. Transpl Immunol 2005; 14: 21–25.
[40] Kelly KJ. Distant effects of experimental renal ischemia/reperfusion injury. J Am Soc Nephrol 2003; 14: 1549–1558.
[41] Fontenot JD, Gavin MA, Rudensky AY. Foxp3 programs the development and function of CD4 +CD25+ regulatory T cells. Nat Immunol 2003;4:330–6.
[42] Shevach EM. Mechanisms of foxp3+ T regulatory cell-mediated suppression. Immunity 2009;30:636–45.
[43] Kinsey GR, Sharma R, Huang L, Li L, Vergis AL, Ye H, et al. Regulatory T Cells Suppress Innate Immunity in Kidney Ischemia-Reperfusion Injury. J Am Soc Nephrol 2009;20:1744–53.
[44] Kinsey GR, Huang L, Vergis AL, Li L, Okusa MD. Regulatory T cells contribute to the protective effect of ischemic preconditioning in the kidney. Kidney Int. 2010; 77:771-80.
[45] Monteiro RM, Camara NO, Rodrigues MM, Tzelepis F, Damiao MJ, Cenedeze MA, et al. A role for regulatory T cells in renal acute kidney injury. Transpl Immunol 2009;21:50–55.
[46] Gandolfo MT, Jang HR, Bagnasco SM, Ko GJ, Agreda P, Satpute SR, Crow MT, King LS, Rabb H. Foxp3+ regulatory T cells participate in repair of ischemic acute kidney injury. Kidney Int. 2009; 76:717-729.

[47] Hribova P, Kotsch K, Brabcova I et al. Cytokines and chemokine gene expression in human kidney transplantation. Transplant Proc 2005; 37: 760–763.
[48] Atamas SP. Complex cytokine regulation of tissue fibrosis. Life Sci 2002; 72: 631 643.
[49] Lemay S, Rabb H, Postler G et al. Prominent and sustained up-regulation of gp130-signaling cytokines and the chemokine MIP-2 in murine renal ischemia-reperfusion injury. Transplantation 2000; 69: 959–963.
[50] Stroo I, Stokman G, Teske GJ, Raven A, Butter LM, Florquin S, Leemans JC. Chemokine expression in renal ischemia/reperfusion injury is most profound during the reparative phase. Int Immunol. 2010; 22:433-42.
[51] Chertow GM, Levy EM, Hammermeister KE, Grover F, Daley J. Independent association between acute renal failure and mortality following cardiac surgery. Am J Med. 1998;104:343–8.
[52] Palevsky PM, Zhang JH, O'Connor TZ, Chertow GM, Crowley ST, Choudhury D, et al. Intensity of renal support in critically ill patients with acute kidney injury. N Engl J Med. 2008;359:7–20.
[53] Jones DR, Lee HT. Perioperative renal protection. Best Pract Res Clin Anaesthesiol 2008;22:193–208.
[54] Park SW, Chen SWC, Kim M, Brown KM, Kolls JK, D'Agati VD and Lee HT. Cytokines induce small intestine and liver injury after renal ischemia or nephrectomy. Laboratory Investigation (2011) 91, 63–84.
[55] Campanholle G, Landgraf RG, Gonçalves GM, Paiva VN, Martins JO, Wang PH, Monteiro RM, Silva RC, Cenedeze MA, Teixeira VP, Reis MA, Pacheco-Silva A, Jancar S, Camara NO. Lung inflammation is induced by renal ischemia and reperfusion injury as part of the systemic inflammatory syndrome. Inflamm Res. 2010 Oct;59(10):861-9. Epub 2010.
[56] Kelly KJ. Distant effects of experimental renal ischemia/reperfusion injury. J Am Soc Nephrol. 2003;14:1549–58.
[57] Kramer AA, Postler G, Salhab KF, Mendez C, Carey LC, Rabb H. Renal ischemia/reperfusion leads to macrophage-mediated increase in pulmonary vascular permeability. Kidney Int. 1999;55:2362–7.
[58] Rabb H, Wang Z, Nemoto T, Hotchkiss J, Yokota N, Soleimani M. Acute renal failure leads to dysregulation of lung salt and water channels. Kidney Int. 2003;63:600–6.
[59] Hassoun HT, Grigoryev DN, Lie ML, Liu M, Cheadle C, Tuder RM, et al. Ischemic acute kidney injury induces a distant organ functional and genomic response distinguishable from bilateral nephrectomy. Am J Physiol Renal Physiol. 2007;293:F30–40.
[60] Grigoryev DN, Liu M, Hassoun HT, Cheadle C, Barnes KC, Rabb H. The local and systemic inflammatory transcriptome after acute kidney injury. J Am Soc Nephrol. 2008;19:547–58.
[61] Hassoun HT, Lie ML, Grigoryev DN, Liu M, Tuder RM, Rabb H. Kidney ischemia-reperfusion injury induces caspase-dependent pulmonary apoptosis. Am J Physiol Renal Physiol. 2009;297:F125–37.
[62] Feltes C, Rabb H: Acute kidney injury leads to pulmonary endothelial cell transcriptional, cytoskeletal and apoptotic changes. ASN renal week 2009, San Diego; 2009.

[63] Hoke TS, Douglas IS, Klein CL, He Z, Fang W, Thurman JM, Tao Y, et al. Acute renal failure after bilateral nephrectomy is associated with cytokine-mediated pulmonary injury. *J Am Soc Nephrol* 18: 155–164, 2007.
[64] Liu M, Stins M, Saleem S, Dore S, Rabb H: Acute kidney injury disrupts blood brain barrier and increases susceptibility to stroke. ASN renal week 2009, San Diego; 2009.
[65] Liu M, Liang Y, Chigurupati S, Lathia JD, Pletnikov M, Sun Z, et al. Acute kidney injury leads to inflammation and functional changes in the brain. J Am Soc Nephrol. 2008;19:1360–70.

2

Characteristics, Detection, and Clinical Relevance of Alloantibodies in Kidney Transplantation

Andrew Lobashevsky
Indiana University
USA

1. Introduction

Almost four decades ago, Porter (Porter, 1970) and Edelman (Edelman, 1970) established the structure of antibodies (immunoglobulins). This discovery dramatically improved the understanding that antibodies function as both receptor and effector molecules. Humoral or antibody-mediated immunity requires noncovalent contact between antigens (ligands) and antibodies (receptors). Hypervariable regions of immunoglobulin light and heavy chains 1, 2, and 3, which are termed complementarity-determining regions (CDR), are primarily involved in the interaction with antigens (Figure 1).

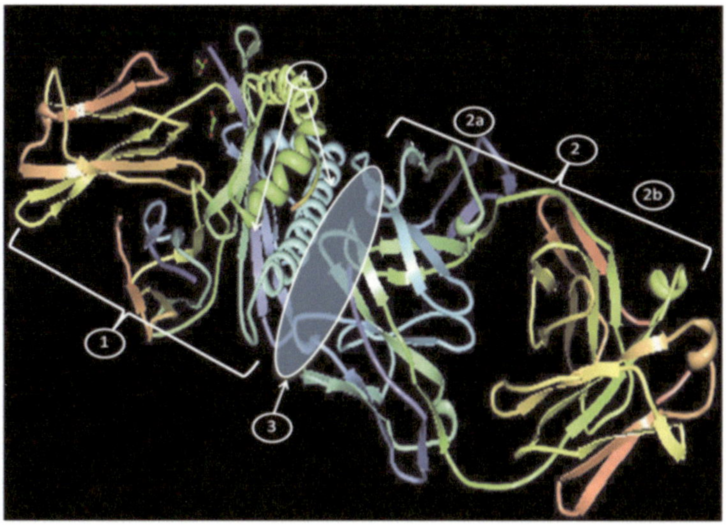

Fig. 1. Three-dimensional structure of HLA-I and alloantibody IgG complex.
1. HLA class I protein
2. IgG molecule.
   a. Variable regions of light and heavy chains
   b. Constant region of heavy chains
3. CDRs 1, 2, and 3 of heavy and light chains

The contact region of the antigen that the antibody binds to is called the epitope, or antigenic determinant. The portion of antibody that makes this contact is referred to as the paratope. Antibody effector functions are specified by the constant domains of heavy chains. Their most important function is the activation of the complement cascade, which is triggered by conformational changes in the hinge area after antigen binding. Complement activation results in the destruction of the cell membrane. An additional important effector function of immunoglobulins is their binding to pathogens, including bacteria and viruses. Pathogens that are coated with antibodies are recognized by Fc (constant fragment) receptors that are expressed on the surfaces of reticuloendothelial cells, including macrophages, monocytes, neutrophils, and dendritic cells. This event not only results in the elimination of the pathogen from the circulation and the tissues but also triggers additional functions of these cells, such as phagocytosis and degranulation. The latter ultimately results in the destruction of the invading pathogen. In contrast to strong and irreversible covalent bonds, antibody-antigen interactions are noncovalent. They strictly depend on temperature, pH, ionic strength, van der Waal's forces, hydrogen bonds and hydrophobic interactions. These weak bonds are formed by the interactions of many groups of biological molecules, including IgG, nominal protein antigens, and major histocompatibility complex (MHC) class I and class II proteins. In humans, the latter are called human leukocyte antigens (HLAs). A unique characteristic of genes that code HLAs is the extremely high occurrence of polymorphisms.

2. Role of alloantibodies in kidney transplantation

In kidney transplantation, graft outcomes critically depend on the degree of HLA matching between the donor and recipient (Abe et al., 1997; Akalin & Pascual, 2006; Balan et al., 2008; Bas et al., 1998; Claas et al., 2005; Scornik et al., 1992; Takemoto et al., 2004; Terasaki 2003; Terasaki & Cai, 2005, 2008;). Although the cellular component of the allogenic immune response to the transplanted tissue plays a key role in this matching, the contribution of antibodies should not be underestimated (Arnold et al., 2005; Bartel et al., 2007; Stegall et al., 2009; Sumitran-Holgersson, 2001; Vasilescu et al., 2004; Zeevi et al., 2009). Transplant candidates (TCs) with preexisting antibodies against HLA are called sensitized patients. The percent of reactive antibodies (PRA) is a major characteristic that defines the level of sensitization. Essentially, greater PRA values indicate greater numbers of anti-HLA antibodies in the patient, indicating a lower probability of receiving a kidney transplant. Indeed, donor-specific antibodies (DSAs) undeniably participate in hyperacute rejection (HAR), humoral acute rejection [also called accelerated antibody-mediated rejection (AMR)], and chronic rejection (CR) (Claas & Doxiadis, 2009; Gebel et al., 2003; Georgescu et al., 2007; Grandtnerova et al., 2008; Kerman et al., 1997; Lefaucheur et al., 2009; Poli et al., 2009; Scornik et al., 1989, 1992; Supon et al., 2001; Takemoto, 1995; Terasaki & Cai, 2008; Vasilescu et al., 2004; Ferry et al., 1997; Martin et al., 2003). HAR is frequently caused by preexisting DSAs that are directed at mismatched HLAs or by high concentrations of isohemagglutinins against major blood group antigens. Graft loss due to HAR has been shown to take place within hours after transplantation; however, in particular cases, wherein the recipient is exposed to multiple cycles of plasmapheresis (PP), post-transplant HAR may develop days later, and this condition is termed delayed HAR (DHAR). The pathological findings in both scenarios appear to be the same (Sugiyama, 2005). Today, HAR is a rare event owing to development of highly sensitive flow cytometry (FC) cross match (CM) technology, which enables the prospective detection of low concentrations of DSAs (Bray, 1994; Shenton et al., 1995; Wang-Rodriguez & Rearden, 1995). Relatively low concentrations of preexisting DSAs are generally not a contraindication for transplantation (Bray, 1994, 2001; Gebel & Bray, 2000; Graff et al., 2009; Reinsmoen et al., 2008).

2.1 The development of alloantibodies against HLAs

In more than 30% of transplant cases, DSAs develop post-transplant, increasing the risk of AMR (Christiaans et al., 1998; Haririan et al., 2009; Martin et al., 2003; McKenna et al., 2000; Zachary et al., 2005). The development of these antibodies depends on multiple factors, including the immunogenicity of mismatched HLAs, HLA class II typing of the responder, immunosuppressive protocols, cytokine and chemokine production, and the hormonal background of the recipient (Adeyi et al., 2005; Claas et al., 2005; Fuller et al., 1999; Fuller & Fuller, 1999; Lachmann et al., 2008; Laux et al., 2003; Lobashevsky et al., 2002). Regulatory immune cells, such as NKT cells, T regs (CD4+/CD25+) (Tsang et al., 2007; Stasi et al., 2008 ; Bas et al., 1998; Jiang & Lechler, 2003; Levings & Thomson, 2009; Toyofuku et al., 2006) and B regs (so-called CD1d/CD5 B10 cells) (Amu et al., 2007), substantially contribute to the development of antibody-mediated immunity. Anti-HLA antibodies have been demonstrated in patients with a history of blood transfusion(s), pregnancy and previous transplant(s). In addition, serological cross-reactivity between HLA-B27 and the 60.0-80.0 kD protein of *Klebsiella pneumoniae* has been demonstrated (Husby et al., 1989; Ogasawara et al., 1986). Considerable effects on antibody profiles of pre-sensitized TCs may also be produced by vaccinations, including Hepatitis B/C and influenza. Indeed, Danziger-Isakov and R. Kennedy have reported bystander effects of vaccine immunization on humoral alloreactivity (Danziger-Isakov et al., 2010; Kennedy et al., 2010). The mechanism of vaccination-mediated sensitization in TCs has been described as follows. Antigen-specific CD4+ T helper cells are central components in naturally acquired and vaccine-induced immunity. These cells control the differentiation of HLA-specific B cells into plasma (antibody producing) cells and memory cells through the production of cytokines, such as interleukin (IL)-4, IL-5, IL-6, IL-2, IL-13, and IFNγ. Subsequent vaccination or infection triggers distinct groups of T helper cells to begin producing the cytokines mentioned above. These cytokines activate quiescent B memory and long-living plasma cells that reside in the bone marrow. These HLA-specific plasma cells then begin vigorously producing antibodies, resulting in changes in the PRA (Benson et al., 2009; Di Genova et al., 2010; Di Genova et al., 2006). Recently, the development of so-called "natural" anti-HLA antibodies has been reported by P. Terasaki's group. These investigators discovered that natural immunizing events, such as infection, protein ingestion and allergen exposure, result in the formation of HLA-A, - B, -C, and DQ loci-specific alloantibodies in non-alloimmunized healthy males. The "natural" antibodies are directed against rare HLA specificities, such as A80, B76, A82, and C17, and should not be ignored in clinical decisions for organ allocation (Morales-Buenrostro et al., 2008).

2.2 B lymphocytes and alloantibody production

After naïve CD20+/CD138-/CD38-/CD27- B cells interact with the HLA protein antigen, two key events occur. First, the naïve B cells become activated in lymphoid tissue, differentiate into short-lived CD20-/CD138-/CD38+/CD27- plasma cells (PCs), and secrete low-affinity antibodies. Second, another group of activated B cells rapidly divides and differentiates into long-term, high-affinity antibody-secreting CD20-

/CD138+/CD38+/CD27- PCs upon interaction with follicular dendritic cells after receiving signals, such as IL-4 and IL-5, that are produced by T helper cells (Stegall et al., 2009; Higgins et al., 2009). These cells often migrate back to the bone marrow, where they may continuously secrete antibodies for years. An additional important event in the process of alloantibody production is the formation of B memory CD20+/CD27+ CD138-/CD38- cells, which are able to transform into long-lived PCs after secondary stimulation by antigens or bystander T cells (Stegall et al., 2009; Bohmig et al., 2008; Cai & Terasaki, 2005; Armitage & Alderson, 1995) (Figure 2).

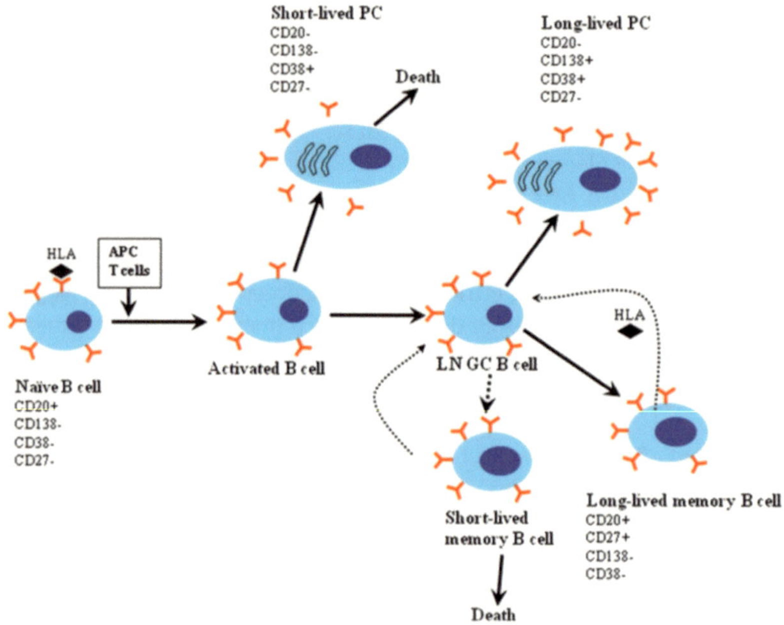

Fig. 2. Model for the generation of long-lived alloantibody-secreting plasma cells (PC) after recognition of HLA. APC, antigen presenting cells; LN, lymph node; GC, germinal center;

3. Some immunological factors determining alloantibody production

As mentioned above, the risk of AMR and kidney graft survival strictly depends on HLA matching between donor and recipient tissues. Highly sensitized TCs, i.e., those having a high PRA, have the highest risk of AMR-mediated graft failure. In addition, these patients are disadvantaged in comparison to those with a low PRA. They typically experience longer times on the waiting list (until a cross-match-negative donor is found) and dialysis. Numerous clinical studies since the 1990s have demonstrated various strategies for identifying donors for high PRA patients. Rodey's and Takemoto's groups have reported successful kidney graft outcomes and negative cross-matching when HLA matching was performed using cross-reactive groups (CREG) and/or public epitopes (Rodey & Fuller, 1987; Takemoto, 1995, 2004). Terasaki's method for analyzing donor and recipient compatibility applies the amino acid sequencing of HLA alleles (Cai et al., 2006; Deng, 2008; El-Awar et al., 2005, 2006a, 2006b, 2007; El-Awar & Terasaki, 2007).

3.1 Amino acids and the triplet/eplet concept of HLA matching

In 2002, Duquesnoy described a molecularly-based algorithm for histocompatibility determination called HLAMatchmaker (Duquesnoy, 2002). This approach considers a comparison of linear amino acid residue (AAR) sequences (or triplets) between donors and recipients to be elements of potential epitopes. Therefore, each HLA protein represents a linear sequence of triplets, and the degree of mismatch is assessed by the number of triplets that are not shared between the donor and recipient. There are two important points in this approach. First, the location of the particular triplet in the HLA protein is carefully examined. Only those AARs that are accessible to antibodies, i.e., triplets residing on α-helical coils and β-loops, are considered. In contrast, those triplets that are located on the β - pleated floor and beneath the α-chains are not available for antibody binding (Figure 3).

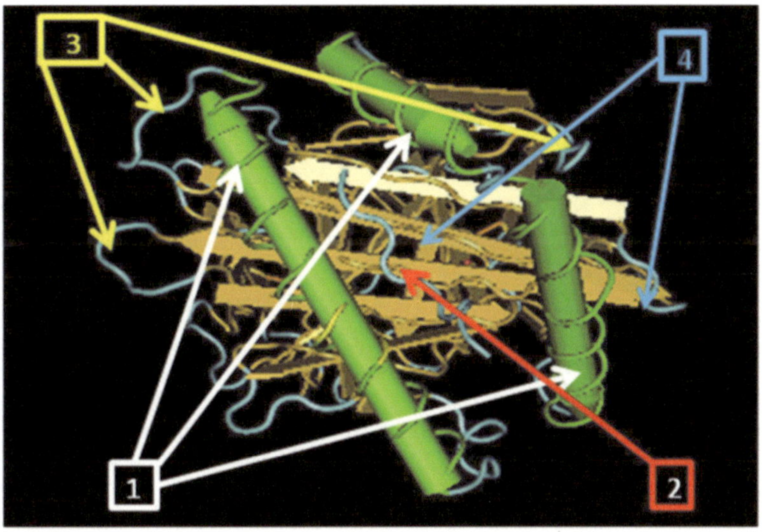

Fig. 3. Three-dimensional structure of HLA-I molecule (top view).
1. α helical coils
2. oligopeptide located in the antigen presenting groove
3. β loops
4. β pleated floor of antigen presenting groove

For this reason, the mismatched triplets residing on the bottom of the antigen-presenting groove of the HLA proteins are often not critical to antibody production and are not immunogenic. Secondly, alloantibodies can be produced only against non-self mismatched triplets. Subsequent clinical studies have proven the validity of the HLAMatchmaker algorithm as a method for finding cross-match compatible donors for TCs with PRA values above 80% (Claas et al. 2005; Claas et al. 2004; 2005; Doxiadis et al. 2005; Duquesnoy 2007, 2008a, 2008b; Duquesnoy & Claas, 2005; Lobashevsky et al., 2002). Furthermore, AAR triplet analysis has appeared to be capable of explaining or predicting the development of non-DSAs in kidney allograft recipients (Lobashevsky et al., 2002; Adeyi et al., 2005); however, subsequent clinical studies of alloantibody profiles in post-transplant nephrectomized TCs have demonstrated that the HLAMatchmaker computer algorithm provides an incomplete HLA epitope repertoire. Indeed, an inconsistency between mismatched triplets and the pattern of antibody reactivity has been reported. In 2005, Duquesnoy's group, using human monoclonal antibodies, demonstrated reactivity against HLA-A3 (triplotype 62Qe, 142mI, 144tKr, and 163dT) owing to a unique 163dT triplet; however, other monoclonal antibodies also reacted with 62Qe, 142mI, or 144tKr triplets, although these triplets were present on different HLA-A locus antigens. Furthermore, the 62Qe triplet that is carried by A30 and A31; the 142mI triplet that is carried by A23, A24, A25, and A32; and the 144tKr triplet that is carried by A80 did not react with the monoclonal antibodies that were directed against the triplets mentioned above (Duquesnoy et al., 2005). Similar results were summarized in a report on the structural basis of HLA compatibility at the 14th International HLA and Immunogenetics Workshop (Duquesnoy & Claas, 2007). Further investigations of the three-dimensional structure of antibody-antigen complexes showed that functional HLA epitopes could be presented by a group of AARs that are not located beside one another, but rather represent a 3-Å to 5-Å radius patch. These patches have been defined as "eplets." Some of eplets include short sequences of AARs, which are equivalent to triplets, whereas, others contain residues that are located distally (apart). For instance, the presence of glycine in position 56 is required for reactivity of monoclonal antibodies specific for 62Qe triplet. The AARs of each eplet are clustered together on the surface of the HLA protein molecule that represents a functional immunogenic epitope (Marrari et al., 2010; Marrari & Duquesnoy, 2010; Duquesnoy et al., 2005; Duquesnoy & Askar, 2007) (Figure 4). Therefore, the eplet concept of the HLAMatchmaker algorithm appears to more accurately define functional HLA-A, -B, -C, -DR, -DQ (α andβ chains) and DP (α andβ chains) epitopes (Claas et al., 2005; Claas & Duquesnoy, 2008; Duquesnoy, and Marrari, 2010; Duquesnoy, 2006, 2008a, 2008b; Duquesnoy & Askar, 2007; Marrari et al., 2010; Lomago et al., 2010). Thus, HLA epitope- (eplet) matching using the HLAMatchmaker computer algorithm represents a robust and valid approach to finding compatible donors for highly sensitized TCs. It may also be used to analyze antibody reactivity patterns in sensitized patients by defining the mismatched eplets the patient has been exposed to. This information, in turn, facilitates the interpretation of antibody profiles in TCs. In addition, a comparative analysis of the HLA epitopes that were defined by Terasaki's group (amino acids that are unique to a group of alleles that react with mouse monoclonal antibodies) and HLA epitopes that are defined by eplets showed more than a 90% correlation (Marrari & Duquesnoy, 2010; Duquesnoy & Marrari, 2010).

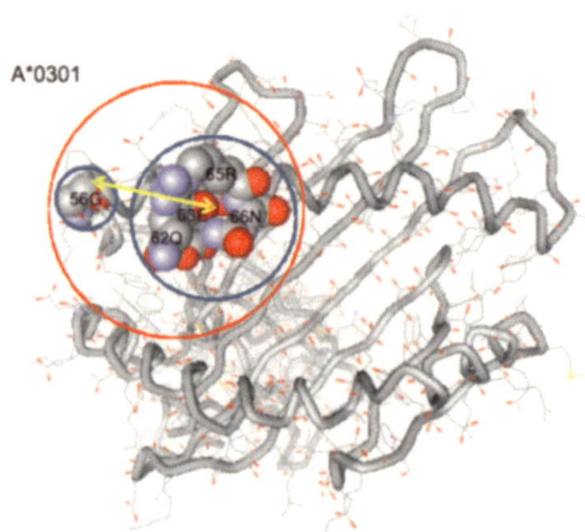

Fig. 4. Topography of 62Q eplet (red circle) of HLA-A*03:01 allele consisting of two patches (blue circles) 56G and 62, 63, 65, 66QERN. These patches are approximately 11Å apart (yellow arrow).

3.2 HLA class II typing of the responder

It is generally accepted that mismatched allogenic HLAs can be recognized by the immune system both directly and indirectly. In kidney transplantation, both of these processes take place simultaneously. The immunological response to non-self HLAs is MHC restricted. The phenomenon of MHC restriction postulates that non-self proteins, including HLAs, are recognized by the immune system after being processed and presented by host antigen presenting cells, in the context of self-MHC I and/or MHC II, to the responder's (host) T cells (Doherty and Zinkernagel, 2005). Although many factors influence the strength of the immune response, the affinity between the members of the tri-molecular complex, including self-HLA II, peptide, and T cell receptors (TCRs), is believed to be the most important. HLA class II proteins have six regions or pockets that participate in peptide binding. These pockets contain highly polymorphic amino acids, which interact with the motifs of the peptides that are being presented to the TCRs. The stronger the affinity between the peptide, HLA and TCRs, the stronger the stimulation signal the T cell receives. Anderson and colleagues have demonstrated that antibody production against tumor HEP-2 peptide was considerably stronger in an HLA-DR11 patient than in an HLA-DR14 individual (Anderson et al., 2000). Furthermore, a report by Fuller demonstrated increased antibody synthesis against HLA-Bw4 antigenic inclusions in HLA-DRB1*01 or HLA-DRB1*03 positive individuals in comparison to HLA-DRB1*04 recipients (Fuller & Fuller, 1999).

4. Role of alloantibodies directed against other than HLA determinants

4.1 Antibodies against A and B blood groups

The compatibility of HLA and the ABO blood groups, which are two antigenic systems in the human body, have a significant effect on graft outcome. Historically, ABO incompatibility has been considered to be an absolute contraindication for renal transplantation due to the high risk of HAR development that is caused by preexisting anti-A or anti-B antibodies. Unlike HLA, the A, B and O (H) blood group antigens are oligosaccharides that structurally differ via α-galactose (α-Gal) and N-acetyllactosamine (NAc). Adding these sugars to precursor backbones requires catalyzation by a group of enzymes that are called glycosyltransferases. The A blood group has two common subgroups, A1 and A2. There are quantitative and qualitative differences between A1 and A2; the A1 phenotype has 4 glycolipids, whereas the A2 phenotype contains very low levels or none at all. Immunological cross-reactivity between them has been reported (Gloor et al., 2006; Gloor & Stegall, 2007; Tyden et al., 2010). Furthermore, 8% of A2 individuals produce antibodies against A1. The ABO system also plays an important role in kidney allocation; donors and recipients must be either ABO identical or compatible (Futagawa & Terasaki, 2006). A/B antigens are known to be passively absorbed by different tissues of the kidney, including the glomerular endothelium and the tubular epithelium (Rivera & Scornik, 1986, Aikawa et al., 2003; Fidler et al., 2004; Rydberg et al., 2007). Endothelial and epithelial cell surface densities of A/B antigens are also different. For example, the A blood group antigen has higher expression levels than the B blood group antigen. Interestingly, immunohistochemical analysis has revealed that the A2 blood group has the lowest cell surface expression (Pober et al., 1997; Shimmura et al., 2004; Yung et al., 2007); however, data analysis of kidney transplants that has been performed across ABO barriers has not revealed statistically significant differences between the A (donor) →B (recipient) or B (donor) →A (recipient) groups (Squifflet et al., 2004; Sugiyama et al., 2005; Valli et al., 2009).

Anti-A/B blood group antibodies belong to the IgM and IgG isotypes, and their titers, which are determined by the direct agglutination test, vary from 1:2 to 1:256 (Issitt & Issitt, 1979). These titer differences are particularly meaningful in cases of ABO-incompatible kidney transplantation (see below).

4.2 Antiphospholipid antibodies

Phospholipids (PLs) are known to play an important role in regulating coagulation. They form complexes with plasma proteins, such as prothrombin, protein S, protein C, annexin, and β_2-glycoprotein (Forman et al., 2004; Wagenknecht et al., 2000). These proteins are known to be natural anticoagulants (Vaidya et al., 1998). Anti-PL antibodies (APLAs) are autologous antibodies, which can cause venous and arterial thrombosis. The binding of APLAs to PLs or plasma proteins results in the inhibition of natural anticlotting effects, which triggers thrombosis and subsequent fibrin deposition (Knight et al., 1995, Pierangeli, 2003). There are several groups of APLAs, including anti-cardiolipin antibodies (ACA), anti-β_2-glycoprotein and the lupus anticoagulant (Forman et al., 2004; Vella, 2004). High concentrations of APLAs, (as determined by ELISA) and particularly ACAs in association with vascular thrombosis or thrombocytopenia result in a clinical disorder that is called antiphospholipid syndrome (APLS) (Pierangeli, 2003, Harris & Pierangeli, 2000). An analysis of APLA levels in kidney transplant recipients has demonstrated that high titers could cause vascular thrombosis and subsequent graft loss. Tolkoff-Rubin's group, in a study that included 337 renal TCs, reported a 25% reduction in the glomerular filtration rate in post-transplant patients with low to medium ACA titers. Graft losses were observed in two cases where high concentrations of ACA were detected (Forman et al., 2004). Furthermore, Knight reported kidney transplant losses on the second day after transplantation due to vascular thrombosis that was caused by high concentrations of ACA (Knight et al., 1995; Vaidya et al., 1998). Similar results have been reported by Wagenknecht, who showed that of 56 failed renal transplant recipients who were maintained on hemodialysis prior to transplantation, 32 were positive for APLAs (Wagenknecht et al., 2000). In summary, preoperative testing for APLAs should be considered for renal TCs with a history of maintenance hemodialysis, particularly if the patients have a history of thrombotic events. If high concentrations of APLA are detected, the risk of post-transplant thrombosis is increased and anticoagulation therapy is a concern. In contrast, no significant difference in graft outcomes have been detected between TCs that tested positive or negative for APLA if the ACA titers were low (Forman et al., 2004). Anti- β_2-glycoprotein antibodies were shown to activate endothelial cells (ECs) by affecting NFκB. EC activation is accompanied by the upregulation of adhesion molecules, such as vascular cell adhesion molecules (VCAM)-1, which represents a potential pathogenic mechanism for cellular rejection and accelerated arteriosclerosis (Meroni et al., 2002).

4.3 Cold agglutinins

Cold agglutinins (CAs) are autologous antibodies that are usually of the IgMκ subtype but are occasionally of the IgG and IgA subtypes. CAs are specific to the Ii (N-acetyllactoseamine) red blood cells antigenic system. The components of this system present on the surfaces of adult human erythrocytes (Diaz et al., 1984; Roelcke, 1974). CA typically found at low titers in the peripheral blood of healthy individuals; however, their titers increase following infections by *Mycoplasma pneumoniae,* Epstein-Barr virus, and

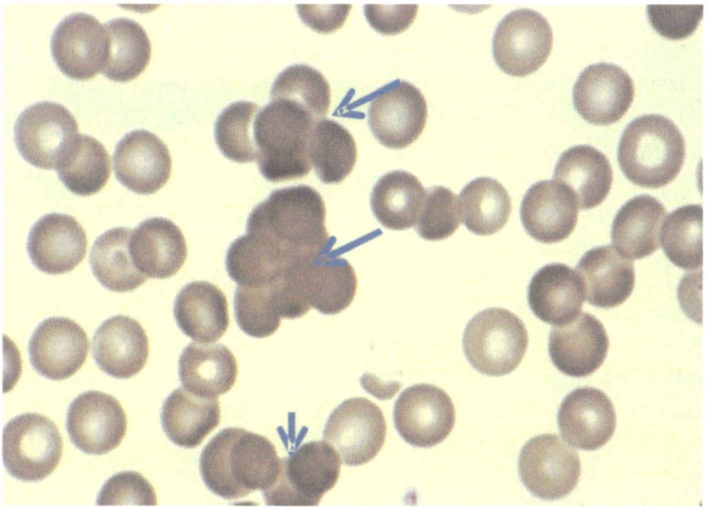

Fig. 5. Human blood smear. Blue arrows indicate agglutinated red blood cells

cytomegalovirus. These antibodies are termed CAs because they have a range of thermally-mediated activities, with the temperature of 0°C being the best (Zilow et al., 1994). CAs may also react with red blood cells at higher temperatures. The range of their reactivity is called the thermal amplitude. It has been demonstrated that the maximum thermal amplitude temperature is always less than the normal body temperature (37°C) because their activity ceases above this temperature (Diaz et al., 1984; Roelcke, 1989) (Figure 5). CAs destroy erythrocytes and can cause autoimmune hemolytic anemia through complement activation. In addition, they cause red blood cell aggregation, which, in turn, can lead to microcirculation failures (Izzat et al., 1993; Roelcke, 1974, 1989). Activation of the complement system at low temperatures can initiate the formation of microemboli and microthrombi, which may obstruct capillaries and cause organ ischemia (Roelcke, 1989; Diaz et al., 1984; Lobo et al., 1984). Carloss and Tavassoni have reported CA-mediated hyperacute kidney failure. They described a patient who developed oliguria and showed increased creatinine levels following stomach surgery. The autopsy revealed glomerulonephritis that was caused by immune complex deposition. In addition, high levels of CAs of the IgM isotype that reacted at 32°C were also detected (Carloss & Tavassoli, 1980). Sturgill and coworkers have reported hyperacute allograft failure in two diseased donor-kidney recipients. Both recipients did not have preexisting donor-specific HLA antibodies, and tissue typing indicated a six-antigen match. Kidney failure occurred immediately after the establishment of vascular anastomosis, and biopsies were performed. Marked red blood cell aggregation and fibrin thrombi in capillaries and small arteries were observed in both TCs. Elevated CA levels of the IgM isotype were also demonstrated in the serum from the recipients. The kidney from one of the recipients was removed 23 days after transplantation despite therapeutic intervention (Sturgill et al., 1984). Thus, CAs can cause irreversible changes after renal transplantation that may lead to graft loss. High concentrations of CAs in the serum may represent a potential explanation for hyperacute graft injury in non-HLA sensitized patients.

4.4 Anti-endothelial cells (EC) antibodies

The importance of DSAs for kidney allograft outcomes was documented many years ago. A strong correlation between the development of alloantibodies to mismatched HLAs and poor graft outcomes has been reported by many investigators (Adeyi et al. 2005; Baid-Agrawal & Frei, 2007; Bray & Gebel, 2008; Cai & Terasaki, 2005; Mujtaba et al., 2010; Terasaki & Cai, 2005). Recipients of perfectly matched kidney transplants generally survive longer and do not frequently develop rejection; however, 2-5% of zero HLA-mismatched kidney recipients lose their grafts due to HAR or AMR (Rodriguez et al., 2000). These graft failures can be caused by HLA allele-specific antibodies and/or non-HLA antibodies (Ferry et al., 1997; Grandtnerova et al., 2008; Lomago et al., 2010; Lucchiari et al., 2000; Perrey et al., 1998; Sumitran-Karuppan et al., 1997). In 1976, Moraes and Stastny described eight groups of non-HLA antigens that are expressed on monocytes and EC (Moraes & Stastny, 1976). Subsequent studies have demonstrated that anti-endothelial cell antibodies (AECAs) were directed against adhesion molecules, such as ICAM, VCAM, ELAM, PECAM, and vimentin (Le Bas-Bernardet et al., 2003; Lucchiari et al., 2000). Antibodies against the protein Tie2, which is one of tyrosine kinase receptors that is expressed on vascular endothelium, have also been described (Peters et al., 2004). Unlike MHC, the genes coding non-HLAs are not located on the 6th chromosome (Kalil et al., 1989). This fact offers an explanation for the rejection of HLA-identical grafts. Indeed, transplant recipients from HLA-identical siblings with no PRA had considerably longer graft survival times in comparison to those who had anti-HLA antibodies (Opelz, 2005). The vascular endothelium of transplanted kidneys and other organs is the first line of defense between the allograft and the host immune system. Similar to classical MHC antigens, the non-HLAs represent immune system targets, and AECAs appear to be clinically important as a potential risk factor for AMR (Han et al., 2009; Pober et al., 1996; Rodriguez et al., 2000; Vasilescu et al., 2004; Yard et al., 1993; Vanderwoude et al., 1995). FCCM analysis using peripheral blood EC for the detection of AECAs has been recently described. This method was shown to be reliable for identifying patients at risk for AMR that is mediated by non-HLA antibodies (Alheim et al., 2010; Breimer et al., 2009).

4.5 Antibodies against MHC class I chain-related antigens (MIC)

Another group of non-HLAs are represented by non-classical MIC antigens A (MICA) and B (MICB). These proteins are expressed on endothelial cells, fibroblasts, keratinocytes, and monocytes (Zwirner et al., 2006). In contrast to the non-HLAs described above, MICs are polymorphic (MICA has 40 alleles, MICB has 23 alleles), and their gene family is located on the 6th chromosome close to the HLA-B locus. The presence of antibodies against these antigens has been demonstrated to be associated with inferior kidney graft outcomes (Rebellato et al., 2006). Relatively high frequencies (26%) of anti-MICA antibodies have been reported in recipients with anti-HLA antibodies who lost their kidney grafts because of AMR (Mizutani et al., 2005; Mizutani et al., 2006). In summary, non-HLA antigens are expressed on graft EC but not on lymphocytes, which are routinely used for CM. Antibodies that are directed against these antigens, produce different types of rejection, including HAR, AMR, and chronic allograft nephropathy (CAN). Therefore, the detection of AECAs and anti-MIC antibodies in TCs may provide insight into unexplained graft rejection, particularly in recipients without DSAs and those who have received zero HLA-mismatched kidneys.

5. The significance of alloantibody concentration, isotype and subtype

When the initial work up of a potential renal TC is performed, the following important questions regarding humoral immunity must be answered. Does this recipient have anti-HLA antibodies? If so, what is the PRA? Are these antibodies donor-specific (DSAs)? What is the isotype of the DSAs? How much DSAs does this particular TC have? The rationale for obtaining this information is related to clinical studies, which have universally demonstrated that pre-existing DSAs can cause HAR, accelerated or AMR, and CAN (Al-Lamki, 2008; Bartel et al., 2007; Bishay et al., 2000; Bohmig et al., 2008; Cornell LD et al., 2008; Ghasemian et al., 1998; Grandtnerova et al., 1995; Lefaucheur et al., 2009; Lobo et al., 1995; Terasaki & Cai, 2008; Racusen et al., 1998). The earliest method that was used to routinely detect anti-HLA antibodies was the complement-dependent cytotoxicity assay (CDC). This technology has a relatively low sensitivity (see below), wherein it identifies anti-HLA class I antibodies using a panel of HLA-typed lymphocytes or DSA class I and class II antibodies, which are obtained from patient serum and donor lymphocytes at high concentrations. Transplanting kidneys to recipients that have been found to have DSAs by CDC generally results in irreversible HAR. The CDC assay is able to detect anti-HLA antibodies of both the IgG and IgM isotypes. Discrimination between the two isotypes is accomplished by using heating or reducing agents, such as dithiothreitol (DDT) or dithioerythritol (DTE). These compounds destroy disulfide bonds between heavy chains of IgMs and abolish their reactivity. The identification of the isotypes of DSAs is important because they differentially influence graft survival (Schonemann et al., 1998; Stastny et al., 2009). Indeed, DSAs of the IgM isotype are generally not believed to be detrimental to renal allografts (McCalmon et al., 1997; Schonemann et al., 1998; Fredrich et al., 1999); however, there have been reports of DSAs of the IgM isotype that mediate HAR and decrease the survival of kidney transplants (Demirhan et al., 1998; Stastny et al., 2009). Many investigators have reported the distribution of DSA isotypes/subclasses in kidney TCs. Arnold and colleagues have demonstrated the usefulness of ELISA in the detection of the IgG (IgG1, IgG2, IgG3, and IgG4) and IgA (IgA1 and IgA2) subtypes in kidney TCs (Arnold et al., 2005, 2008). These investigators have observed considerably higher frequencies of IgA1 and IgA2 alloantibodies in retransplant patients than in first-transplant recipients (Arnold et al., 2008). Kerman (Kerman et al., 1996) and Koka (Koka et al., 1993) have reported the non-complement fixing of IgG2/IgG4 and IgA antibodies to have a beneficial effect on kidney graft survival. Results from our transplant center have shown uneventful kidney graft outcomes in three recipients with high levels of pre-existing DSAs. Subsequent IgG subtype analysis revealed that more than 50% of these antibodies were of the IgG2/IgG4 isotype (Lobashevsky et al., 2010). It is generally accepted that low (CDC assay-negative) concentrations of DSAs of the IgG isotype are not a contraindication for transplantation, provided that pre- and post-transplantation desensitization (DS) (see below) and proper DSA monitoring are used (Bohmig et al., 2008; Bray, 1994; Christiaans et al., 1998, 2000; Graff et al., 2009; Martin et al., 2003; Patel et al., 2007; Reinsmoen et al., 2008; Vaidya et al., 2001). TCs with low DSA concentrations are considered to be medium risk patients due to higher AMR frequencies over a long-term (>5 years) follow up period in comparison to negative-DSA recipients (Gebel et al., 2009; Jordan et al., 2004, 2006; Reinsmoen et al., 2008; Vo et al., 2008).

6. Alloantibodies against HLA specificities and their impact on kidney graft outcomes

Because the deleterious effects of DSAs, which are directed against HLA-A, -B, -DRB1, and DQB1 molecules, on kidney transplant outcomes have been well documented (Abe et al., 1997; Adeyi et al., 2005; Baid-Agrawal & Frei, 2007; Billen et al., 2009a, 2009b; Bohmig et al., 2008; Cai et al., 2006a, 2006b; Christiaans et al., 1998; Dunn et al., 2010; Gebel et al., 2009; Ghasemian et al., 1998; Kerman et al., 1997; Lederer et al., 1996; Lefaucheur et al., 2009; McKenna et al., 2000; Schonemann et al., 1998; Scornik et al., 1992; Terasaki, 2003; Terasaki & Cai, 2005; 2008), this section of the review is focused on the role of antibodies against additional HLAs, such as C, non-DRB1 (DRB3, DRB4, and DRB5), DQA1, DPB1, and DPA1. This group of molecules are classical MHC antigens, meaning that, by definition, they are able to elicit cellular and humoral immune responses and present non-self antigens to CD8 (cytotoxic T lymphocytes) and CD4 (helper) T cells. In comparison to other classical HLAs, these proteins are less polymorphic (Marsh et al., 2000).

6.1 Anti-HLA-C locus alloantibodies

The immunobiology of the HLA-C locus is not well defined. One of the features of this MHC antigen is its low (~10%) cell membrane expression in comparison to HLA-A and HLA-B proteins. In addition, the products of HLA-C locus genes are not expressed on platelets (Zemmour & Parham, 1992). During the last decade, several reports have addressed their role in clinical transplantation. Kidney transplant failures and graft losses due to DSAs that are directed against mismatched HLA-C have been reported by Worthington (Worthington et al., 2003) and Qasi (Qasi et al., 2006). T cell-positive FCCM due to anti-HLA-C antibodies that have been detected by solid phase Luminex technology (see below) has been reported by Stastny (Stastny et al., 2006). These investigators have also discovered that, to produce a positive FCCM, the median fluorescence intensity (MFI) values of anti-HLA-C antibodies must be significantly higher that those produced by antibodies against HLA-A and –B. The considerable influence of anti-HLA-C antibodies on kidney allocation and graft outcomes has been noted in a recent review of Gebel and Bray (Gebel and Bray, 2010).

6.2 Anti-HLA-DRB3, -DRB4, -DRB5, -DQA1, and -DP loci alloantibodies

The immunological role of mismatches at HLA-non-DRB1, HLA-DQA, and HLA-DP loci in renal transplantation is currently under investigation. The impact of these mismatches on graft survival depends on the level of expression, immunogenicity and distribution within renal tissue. Kidney glomerular epithelium and mesangium constitutively express HLA-DRB determinants (Hart et al., 1981; Williams et al., 1980). Using an immunofluorescence technique, Fuggle and colleagues were able to detect the aforementioned antigens on glomerular endothelium, tubular capillaries and cortical and medullary tubules (Fuggle et al., 1983). They also found considerable variation in the expression of HLA-DR by proximal tubular cells. Interestingly, as was later reported by Müller, these cells lack HLA-DQ and HLA-DP antigens (Müller et al., 1989). Muczynski and colleagues, using three-laser multicolor FC analysis, have demonstrated the co-expression of HLA-DR, -DQ, and –DP proteins in renal microvascular cells (Muczynski et al., 2003). Subsequent studies have shown that all class II genes are expressed, whether constitutively or upon induction, at the following levels in decreasing order: DR>DP>DQ (Guardiola & Maffei, 1993). In addition, the degree of cell surface expression largely depends on the cytokine milieu, particularly TNFα and IFNγ as well as the activity of the CIITA (class II, major histocompatibility complex, transactivator) transcription factor (Guardiola & Maffei, 1993; Muczynski et al., 2003). The impact of promoter activity on the haplotype expression of HLA class II DRB1-DRB3, DRB1-DRB4, and DRB1-DRB5 has been investigated by Vincent and colleagues. These investigators, using a competitive PCR methodology, analyzed the transcriptional levels of these genes and have shown that DRB1-DRB3 (serologically DR52) haplotypes have the highest levels of promoter activity, followed by DRB1-DRB4 (serologically DR53) and DRB1-DRB5 (serologically DR51) (Vincent et al., 1996). It is necessary to mention that the α chains of HLA-DQ and -DP heterodimers are polymorphic, which is unlike the α chain of DR (only two alleles have been reported thus far). This may have a significant impact on graft outcomes due to potential antibody production in cases where the donor and recipient are HLA-DQA and/or HLA-DPA mismatched. Johnson and colleagues have described the first case of anti-HLA-DP single-allele antibody development. These investigators have reported an increase in HLA-DP-specific alloantiserum in a recipient who received multiple immunizations of intradermal injections of mononuclear cells from a healthy donor (Johnson et al., 1986). Subsequent studies have not shown a significant effect of HLA-DP mismatches on graft outcomes in first transplant recipients; however, a considerable reduction in graft survival time was observed in retransplant patients (Arnold et al., 2005; Laux et al., 2003; Mytilineos et al., 1997; Qiu et al., 2005; Rosenberg et al., 1992). In kidney transplantation from deceased donors, a B cell-positive FCCM due to HLA-DP DSA was observed to result in adverse graft outcomes (Goral et al., 2008; Piazza et al., 2006; Vaidya et al., 2007). Kamoun and coworkers have reported successful kidney transplantation in a regraft patient, who showed positive FCCM due to HLA-DP DSAs, by using intensive immunosuppressive therapy (Kamoun et al., 2006). The role of pre-existing anti-HLA-DQA1 antibodies in kidney transplantation is still uncertain. Results from our transplant center have demonstrated uneventful graft outcomes in retransplant kidney recipients who had high concentrations of HLA-DQA1*05 DSAs (Lobashevsky et al., 2010). Paul Terasaki's group reported a rejection episode in a kidney transplant recipient due to HLA-DQA1*02:01 DSAs (Deng, 2008). These investigators used homozygous lymphoblastoid B cell lines for antibody absorption to demonstrate reactivity to a single DQA1/DQB1 epitope that is shared by multiple DQ determinants. Similar results were obtained by Tambur and coworkers, who reported the presence of antibodies in the pre-transplant serum of kidney TCs that were directed toward conformational changes that had been generated by a combination of DQα and DQβ-chains (Barabanova et al., 2009). In summary, the immunogenicity of HLA-non-DRB1, HLA-DQA, and HLA-DP antigens has been demonstrated by many investigators (Lobashevsky et al., 2011; Arnold et al., 2005a, 2005b; Barabanova et al., 2009; Duquesnoy et al., 2008; Duquesnoy & Askar, 2007; El-Awar et al., 2009; Laux et al., 2003; Qiu et al., 2005; Rosenberg et al., 1992). DSAs against these determinants have appeared to be less clinically significant in comparison to anti-class I and anti-DRB1 antibodies. They cause graft failure at significantly lower rates, and transplantation in individuals with a positive CM that was caused by antibodies against the aforementioned HLA determinants is less deleterious than that when a positive CM that is caused by anti-DRB1 antibodies is involved. One potential explanation for this is a lower complement binding activity in comparison to anti-DRB1 or anti-class I DSAs (Bartel et al., 2007; Fuller et al., 1999; Scornik et al., 1992); however, anti-HLA-non-DRB1, HLA-DQA, and

HLA-DP antibodies may need to be evaluated in retransplant recipients for matching and graft outcomes.

7. Methodological considerations of anti-HLA antibody detection

Antibodies against HLA can be detected by many techniques, which differ in sensitivity. This section of the review is devoted to highly sensitive FC and solid-phase methods, which employ live cells or purified HLA proteins, respectively. These methods are currently used worldwide for pre- and post-transplant alloantibody monitoring. Due to their high sensitivities, these techniques allow investigators to detect low concentrations of anti-HLA antibodies, which may be missed by low-sensitivity methods, such as CDC (Aubert et al., 2009; Fuggle & Martin, 2008; Fujita et al., 1997; Gebel & Halloran, 2010; Grandtnerova et al., 1995; Haririan et al., 2009; Jordan et al., 2006; Kerman et al., 1996; Lobo et al., 1995; Lucchiari et al., 2000; Susal & Opelz, 2002; Terasaki & Cai, J 2005, 2008; Yard et al., 1993).

7.1 Flow cytometry cell based alloantibody analysis

FC cell-based technology has been introduced in two variations: donor-specific CM (Garovoy et al., 1983) and anti-HLA antibody screening using a pool of Epstein-Barr virus (EBV)-transformed B lymphoblastoid cells or peripheral blood lymphocytes (Harmer et al., 1993; Shroyer et al., 1995). This assay uses a laser beam to detect alloantibodies. The intensity of the signal that is produced by secondary anti-human antibodies that have been conjugated to fluorochrome is proportional to the amount of bound anti-HLA antibodies and can be interpreted as the percent of reactive antibodies or PRA. The FCCM assay is the most important immunological test that is performed in transplantation because it allows for both the detection and quantification of DSAs (Bray, 1994, 2001, 2004; Bray et al., 1989; Christiaans et al., 1998; Dunn et al., 2010); however, the presence of autologous antibodies, non-HLA antibodies, or mono- and poly-clonal IgG antibodies that are used for immunosuppressive therapy in the recipient serum have significantly hampered the interpretation of the FCCM results (Lobashevsky et al., 2000; Rodriguez et al., 2000; Scornik et al., 1997). These problems were eliminated with the introduction of solid-phase assays.

7.2 Solid-phase alloantibody analysis

Solid-phase technology uses purified HLA class I and/or class II proteins that are attached to an artificial substrate or matrix. These assays offer significantly higher sensitivities and specificities than cellular methods (Fuggle & Martin, 2008; McKenna et al., 2000; Smith & Rose, 2009). The enzyme-linked immunosorbent assay (ELISA) was the first solid-phase analysis that was developed for antibody screening and specificity determination (Buelow et al., 1995). In this assay, HLA molecules are bound to the wells of plastic trays, and positive reactions are measured by the color signal intensity, which is produced by enzymes that have been conjugated to anti-human antibodies followed by the addition of substrate to the wells. Subsequent studies have shown that the ELISA methodology was less sensitive than FC methods (Arnold et al., 2004; Christiaans et al., 2000; Kerman et al., 1996; Lefaucheur et al., 2009; Schonemann et al., 1998; Smith & Rose, 2009). FC solid-phase assays use microspheres that have been coated with soluble HLA proteins, which can be extracted from a single cell line for specificity analysis or mixed for PRA analysis (Flow PRASpecific, FlowPRA, One Lambda) (Pei et al., 2003). LUMINEX bead technology incorporates microparticles that have been conjugated to varying amounts of two dyes, which enables the identification of 100 sets of beads. HLA-specific alloantibodies are detected via addition to a reaction mixture of secondary PE-conjugated anti-human antibodies. Because each group of beads can be identified by the amount of conjugated fluorochrome, it is possible to identify which HLAs have bound antibodies. The original assay was introduced as a combination of beads that were coated with HLA proteins that had been extracted from individual cells. More recently, with the development of recombinant HLA proteins, LUMINEX technology produced microparticles that were covered with a single class I or class II HLA. This methodological approach revolutionized antibody specificity analyses, particularly in highly sensitized patients (Billen et al., 2009; El-Awar et al., 2005, 2006; Lobashevsky & Higgins, 2009; Mujtaba et al., 2010; Pei et al., 2003; Zeevi et al., 2009). The considerably higher surface density of HLAs on the microbeads in comparison to that achieved on lymphocytes (Jar How Lee, personal communication, 2010) makes the LUMINEX single-antigen (SA) methodology extremely specific and highly sensitive, enabling investigators to detect very low concentrations of HLA-directed antibodies. The latter is particularly important from a clinical point of view. Yet, how strong must the DSA signal that is produced by a SA Luminex assay be to generate a positive FCCM? In order to address this question, correlation analyses between MFI values that are detected by SA beads and signals that are detected by lymphocyte FCCM must be performed (Lobashevsky & Higgins, 2009; Martin et al., 2003; Mizutani et al., 2006; Ozawa et al., 2006; Poli et al., 2009; Qasi Y et al., 2006; Stegall et al., 2009; Terasaki & Cai, 2005; Zachary et al., 2005, 2009). At our transplant center, the positive MFI thresholds for anti-HLA class I and class II antibodies, which are detected via SA technology and produce positive FCCMs, are 2800 and 3500, respectively (predictive value >95%) (Figure 6).

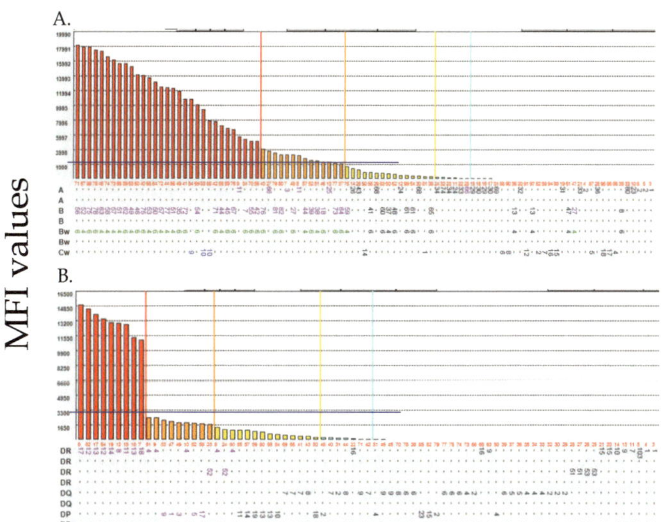

Fig. 6. HLA class I (A) and class II (B) antibody specificity determination using Luminex platform solid phase methodology. Vertical axis indicates mean fluorescence intensity (MFI), horizontal axis indicates single HLA class I and class II proteins conjugated to the beads. Blue lines determine positive cut-offs (i.e. MFI value levels producing positive FC CM results when donor lymphocytes are used) established by our laboratory.

This effect is cumulative when multiple DSAs are being considered (Lobashevsky & Higgins, 2009). There are a few caveats regarding the SA LUMINEX analysis. First, as mentioned above, the density of HLA molecules on the bead is significantly higher than that on lymphocyte (5 x 10^4 - 10^5 molecules per cell) or endothelial cells. Therefore, even a minor admixture of anti-HLA antibodies of the IgM isotype may cause false negative results. To overcome this obstacle, serum DTT-treatment is recommended (Zachary et al., 2009). More recently, discrepant results between negative FCCMs and highly reactive DSAs that have been determined by SA Luminex have been reported. In this study, strong DSA anti-B44 (high-resolution donor HLA-B locus typing confirmed DSAs) reactivity was determined in the recipient serum by SA beads; however, negative T- and B- cell FCCM was observed when donor lymphocytes were used. Biochemical modification (denaturing) of HLA proteins during the bead conjugation process can account for this discrepancy. In comparison to unmodified HLAs, denatured HLAs have a higher affinity for DSAs and, when present in large amounts, they produce strong false positive signals. To rule out antibodies against denatured HLAs, an acid treatment is used. Antibodies against denatured HLA proteins are likely present when no difference in MFI values is observed between treated and untreated beads (Gandhi et al., 2011). Several years ago, solid-phase bead-based CM assays were developed at the Tepnel Lifecodes Corporation. This technique utilizes synthetic micro-particles that have been labeled with different fluorochromes and coated with capturing antibodies that are directed to non-polymorphic domains of class I (α3) and class II (β2) HLA molecules. Donor HLAs (lysate) are extracted from lymphocytes and incubated with the beads. Recipient serum and anti-human antibodies are then added. Fluorescent signals identify each set of microparticles as well as the reporter dye that is linked to the secondary antibodies. In this way, it can be determined if the potential recipient has class I or/and class II DSAs. A comparative analysis of solid-phase and lymphocyte CM assays, which have been performed by our group, have demonstrated a 100% agreement when sera with anti-HLA-A, -B, and -DR antibodies were used (Lobashevsky et al., 2009).

Complement activation following antibody/HLA interactions is clinically important in two ways. First, the classical pathway of complement activation causes C4d deposition in peritubular capillaries and is usually associated with graft cell damage and poor graft outcomes. Second, high concentrations of pre-existing IgG DSAs (positive CDC CM) are a risk factor for HAR. Over the course of the last decade, the implementation of various DS protocols (see below) for highly sensitized patients has resulted in successful kidney transplantation in patients with positive FCCMs that have been caused by DSAs; however, the graft outcome and survival times appear to depend on several parameters, e.g., the amount of DSAs that are producing a positive FCCM, their isotype, the cytokine profile of the recipient and others (Akalin & Bromberg, 2005; Bray 1994; Christiaans et al., 1998; Graff et al., 2009; Horsburgh et al., 2000; Lobashevsky et al., 2010; Martin et al., 2003; Mujtaba et al., 2010; Qasi et al., 2006; Scornik et al., 1997; Worthington et al., 2003; Zachary et al., 2005). It has recently been demonstrated that some DSAs that are detected by FC, but not by CDC (FC pos/CDC neg), are able to activate complement. Bartel and colleagues demonstrated, using SA bead technology and antibodies against C4d, C1q and C3b, that inferior graft outcomes were observed more frequently in recipients whose DSAs were able to bind the complement (Bartel et al., 2007). Similar findings have been reported by others (Bohmig et al., 2008; Yabu et al., 2010). Saw and coworkers have developed a comprehensive procedure that determines cell death and antibody binding in a single assay by using TOPRO-3 staining for apoptotic cells (Saw et al., 2008). In summary, solid-phase analysis represents a powerful tool for anti-HLA antibody analysis and has several advantages over other assays. First, due to its superior sensitivity and specificity, low concentrations of DSAs pre- and post-transplant can be detected. Second, this technology does not require viable cells. Third, it detects only anti-HLA antibodies.

8. Desensitization is a method for the removal of pre-existing anti-HLA antibodies

The development of anti-HLA antibodies represents a significant barrier to transplantation for many patients because of the high risk of AMR-mediated graft failure (Adeyi et al., 2005; Zachary, 2009; Bray, 1994, 2001; Haririan et al., 2009; Yard et al., 1993; Zeevi et al., 2009). Historically, transplantation for such patients was possible only when a donor could be found whose tissues did not express any HLA that the recipient produced antibodies against.

8.1 Intravenous immunoglobulin (IVIG)

During the last two decades, however, protocols using pooled human IVIG and/or plasmapheresis (PP) have been shown to eliminate some or all DSAs (Jordan et al., 2004, 2006; Reinsmoen et al., 2008; Rogers et al., 2011; Thielke et al., - 2005; Claas et al., 2004; Gloor et al., 2004; Stegall et al., 2009; Leong et al., 2008). Furthermore, a beneficial effect of IVIG/PP treatment for AMR has been reported by many transplant centers (Akalin et al., 2008; Furth et al., 1999; Lehrich et al., 2005; Rifle & Mousson, 2003; Toyoda et al., 2004; Vo et al., 2010). More recently, it was reported that sensitized TCs require different DS regimens to reduce DSA levels, including varying the IVIG dose and the number of PP cycles (Cai & Terasaki, 2005; Thielke et al., 2005; Ferrari-Lacraz et al., 2006; Glotz et al., 2004; Rogers et al., 2011). Subsequent studies have demonstrated that susceptibility to IVIG/PP DS depends on immunoregulatory mechanisms, such as polymorphisms in cytokine genes, the frequency of regulatory cells, and hormonal backgrounds (Figure 7) (Glotz et al., 2004; Lobashevsky et al., 2009; Rogers et al., 2011; Zachary et al., 2003; Bas et al., 1998; Di Genova et al., 2006, 2010; Jiang & Lechler, 2003, Amu et al., 2007; Anderson et al., 2000; Hill & Sarvetnick, 2002; Kalil et al., 1989; Stasi et al., 2008; Stastny P et al., 2006; Yoo et al., 1995).

Furthermore, the efficacy of DS has been reported to be different for DSAs and third-party HLA antibodies. For example, Andrea Zachary's group reported a considerable reduction in DSAs in a TC that had been subjected to IVIG DS in comparison to the level of alloantibodies against a third party (Zachary et al., 2003). Higgins et al. observed similar results (Higgins et al., 2009). Our data are also in agreement with these findings; however, they did not reach statistical significance (Lobashevsky et al., 2009). IVIGs are commercially prepared products that contain IgGs (>90%) that are derived from human plasma that has been pooled from tens of thousands of healthy individuals. In addition, IVIGs contain antibodies against CMV, T cell receptor idiotypes, and some cytokines, including GM-CSF and IL-1β (Jordan et al., 2003). The primary mechanisms of IVIG-mediated immunomodulation are summarized as the following: first, the inhibition of complement binding through blockage of C3 convertase (Kazatchkine & Kaveri, 2001; Lutz et al., 2004; Watanabe & Scornik, 2005); second, the neutralization of circulating antibodies through idiotype-anti-idiotype interactions (Glotz et al., 2004; Jordan et al., 2004, 2006; Watanabe & Scornik, 2005); third, the inhibition of IL-2 and IFN-γ secretion (Glotz et al., 2004;

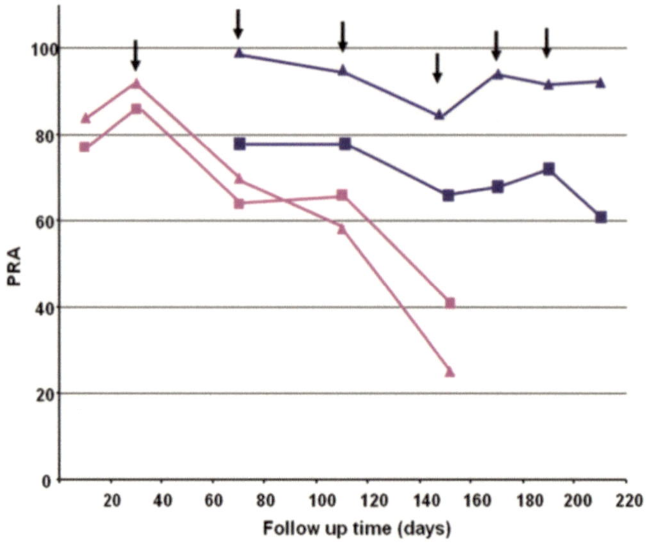

Fig. 7. PRA changes (—■— class I, —▲— class II) in susceptible (pink line) and resistant (blue line) to DS TCs after sequential courses of IVIG/PP. Black arrows indicate IVIG administration.

Kazatchkine & Kaveri, 2001); forth, the inhibition of T cell proliferation through anti-T cell receptor activity (Jordan et al., 2006; Klaesson et al., 1993); and fifth, the downregulation of antigen that presents cell (APC) activity, which causes the inhibition of T cell activation through Fc receptor-mediated interactions (Bayry et al., 2003). Clinically, IVIG are known to be well tolerated; however, adverse events, such as osmotic nephropathy and hemolytic anemia in non-O blood type patients, have been reported (Banerjee et al., 2003). Commercial preparations of IVIG contain different concentrations of anti-A and anti-B isohemagglutinins. The highest concentrations have been found in Privigen (1:64 and 1:32 titers of IgG anti-A and anti-B, respectively). In contrast, Carimune contains the lowest titers of anti-A and anti-B isohemagglutinins; however, this preparation is hyperosmolar, which limits its use in patients who are not on dialysis or present with an increased risk of thrombosis (Kahwaji et al., 2009). IVIG immunomodulation should be considered for treatment in non-O blood type TCs due to the increased risk of IVIG-induced hemolytic anemia. Anti-A and/or anti-B isohemagglutinin titers in IVIG preparations are particularly meaningful when AB blood type-incompatible kidney transplantation is an option due to the increased risk of anti-A/B antibody-mediated graft failure.

8.2 Rituximab

A combination of IVIG and Rituximab (Rituxan) (chimeric humanized monoclonal antibodies against the CD20 marker for B lymphocytes) DS has been shown to effectively reduce DSAs. The rates of the conversions of positive to negative CDC CMs and reductions of MCS in FCCMs were higher in comparison to cases where DS was used without Rituxan (Lefaucheur et al., 2009; Rogers et al., 2011; Vo et al., 2008; Vo et al., 2010). Rituxan affects mature B-cells (CD20+, IgG-, CD19+) and at lesser degree memory B cells (CD20+, CD27+, IgG+) and prevents the formation of plasma cells (CD20-, CD19- IgG-, CD38+, CD138+) *de novo*. A beneficial effect of Rituxan and IVIG for AMR treatment in kidney transplantation was reported by Vo et al. (Vo et al., 2010) and Lefaucheur et al. (Lefaucheur et al., 2009). The IVIG/Rituxan treatment resulted in more effective DSA removal, likely by blocking the indirect pathway of mismatched HLA protein recognition. In this case, mature B cells function as APCs and present donor HLA-processed peptides to the host T helper cells. The latter become activated and stimulate the differentiation of B memory and mature B cells into antibody-producing short- and long-living plasma cells by secreting IL-4, IL-6, IL-1β, GM-CSF, and IL-17 (Yoo et al., 1995).

8.3 Plasmapheresis (PP) or therapeutic plasma exchange (TPE)

As mentioned above, PP [or therapeutic plasma exchange (TPE)] is a necessary component of immunomodulation/DS or AMR therapy because it physically removes anti-HLA antibodies from the circulation. This function can also be applied to paraproteins, polyclonal autoantibodies, or antibodies in immune complexes. Although PP implementation results in a considerable reduction of anti-HLA antibodies, the effect can only be achieved after multiple cycles of treatment in highly sensitized TCs. This is presumably because of IgG equilibration between the intravascular and extravascular spaces. For example, depleting the total body IgGs by 85% was observed to require five exchanges of 1.25 times the plasma volume (Weinstein 2003). In addition, the removal of immunoglobulins by PP may be followed by an increase in specific antibody titers (the rebound effect) to levels that are even higher than those at baseline. The mechanism of this phenomenon is through biofeedback stimulation to increase IgG synthesis (Dau P 1995).

8.4 The removal of anti-AB blood group antibodies

Historically, ABO incompatibility (ABOi) is considered to be a contraindication for kidney transplantation due to irreversible HAR of the graft. The shortage of kidney donors has led to an increasing gap between the number of patients who are waiting for kidney transplantation and the number of available kidney donors. An expansion of the kidney donor pool can be achieved by performing transplantations despite the immunological barrier of ABOi. Successful kidney transplantation from A2 (A2B or A2O) donors to B or O recipients was reported (Alkhunaizi, 2006; Bryan et al., 1998; Nelson et al., 1998). Bryan and colleagues demonstrated that the graft outcomes in A2 donor (deceased and living) kidney recipients were comparable to ABO-compatible transplants (Bryan et al., 1998). Subsequent investigations have shown that the success of A2 donor transplantation depends on anti-A1 and anti-A2 IgG isohemagglutinin titers in the recipient serum prior to transplantation. A1 and A2 blood group antigens differ qualitatively and quantitatively (see above). Indeed, for transplantation from A2 donors into B or O recipients, anti-A1 IgG titers that were above 1:128 have been shown to represent a significant risk factor for AMR (Squifflet et al., 2004; Tyden et al., 2010; Valli et al., 2009; Warren et al., 2004). In addition, Alkhunaizi reports that up to 8% of A2 individuals have anti-A1 IgG antibodies in their sera (Alkhunaizi, 2006). Anti-A1 IgG antibody titers of less than or equal to 1:8 have been considered to be a cut-off for assuming a low risk of AMR (Gloor & Stegall, 2007; Jordan et al., 2009; Rydberg et al., 2007; Warren et al., 2004). Additional therapeutic measures are required when titers of anti-A1 IgG antibodies are high, such as plasma exchange that is accompanied by a bimonthly monitoring of anti-A1 titers (Montgomery & Locke, 2007; Tobian et al., 2009; Tyden et al., 2010; Winters et al., 2004).

About a decade ago, more A1 to B, B to A1, and A1 or B to O ABOi kidney transplants were initiated to increase the potential donor pool. Reports from Europe, Japan and the United States have demonstrated successful ABOi kidney transplantation from both living and deceased donors. Tanabe reported a relatively high percentage of 1- and 2-year graft survivals (96% and 94%, respectively) after using 3-4 pre-transplant PPs along with splenectomy and/or Rituximab (Tanabe, 2007; Beimler & Zeier, 2007). A new protocol for ABOi kidney transplantation was introduced in Sweden in 2001. In this method, immunoabsorption columns that were filled with A/B oligosaccharides (Glycosorb, Glycorex Transplantation AB, Lund, Sweden) were used instead of PP in order to remove anti-A or anti-B antibodies. In addition, Rituximab was used instead of splenectomy in order to prevent rebound effects (Tyden 2007; Valli et al., 2009). These investigators demonstrated that anti-AB IgG antibody titers were reduced from 1:2 – 1:128 to 1:1-1:2 after 4-8 cycles of immunoabsorption. A rebound effect was observed in only one of eleven recipients after 36 months post-transplantation. Notably, no differences in graft survival time between ABOi and ABO-compatible transplantations were observed (Rydberg et al., 2007; Tyden et al., 2005). Five years ago, the John Hopkins Transplant Center established a DS protocol for ABOi transplantation, which consisted of PP, IVIG and Rituxan administration (Sonnenday et al., 2004; Tobian et al., 2009). This immunomodulating strategy included multiple cycles of pre-transplant PP so as to reduce anti-A/B antibody titers to <1:16 followed by a single dose of Rituximab. The post-transplantation treatment included an additional 3-4 PP/IVIG cycles. An analysis of graft outcomes in six ABOi donor/recipient combinations did not demonstrate any differences in either creatinine levels or the rate of humoral rejection (Sonnenday et al., 2004). More recently, several groups have reported successful implementations of the drug Bortezomib ($C_{19}H_{25}BN_4O_4$) (Velcade) for DS and AMR treatment in kidney transplantation (Everly et al., 2009; Raghavan et al., 2010; Walsh et al., 2010). Originally, Bortezomib was used for the treatment of multiple myeloma, which is a tumor consisting of plasma cells (PCs) (Cavo 2006; Mitchell 2003). The mechanism of action for this drug involves proteosome inhibition, which is accomplished by the binding of the 26S subunit and subsequent apoptosis, through caspase 3/7, in antibody-producing PCs (Diwan et al., 2011; Perry et al., 2009; Ruschak et al., 2010). The use of Bortezomib in clinical transplantation is advantageous for the specific targeting of long-living CD38+/CD138+/CD20- PCs in the bone marrow and secondary lymphoid tissue. Subsequent studies have shown that Bortezomib alone had little or no impact on DSA levels (Sberro-Soussan et al., 2010); however, when used in combination with PP, IVIG or Rituximab, a prominent reduction in class I and class II DSA concentrations were demonstrated (Diwan et al., 2011; Everly et al., 2009; Perry et al., 2009). In summary, removing DSAs or anti-A/B blood group antibodies expands the donor pool for highly sensitized or ABOi kidney TCs; however, these methods introduce several concerning issues. First, in the majority of cases, DS does not completely eliminate DSAs. Second, the DSA rebound effect presents considerable concern. The rate and intensity of alloantibody return depends on multiple factors, including the production of cytokines, hormones, frequency immunoregulatory cells, and infection. Third, desensitized patients require regular post-transplant DSA monitoring so as to determine if additional immunomodulating therapy is necessary. Finally, long-term kidney graft outcomes in desensitized recipients are beset with frequent humoral rejection episodes and graft loss when compared to DSA-negative TCs.

9. The association between post-transplant alloantibody production and rejection

9.1 Antibody-mediated rejection (AMR) or humoral rejection

AMR is a frequent complication in renal transplant recipients and may develop any time after transplantation (Abe et al., 1997; Christiaans et al., 1998; Cornell et al., 2008; Gloor et al., 2004; Lefaucheur et al., 2009; Matas et al., 2000; Patel et al., 2007; Perrey et al., 1998; Supon et al., 2001; Zeevi et al., 2009). Alloantibodies that are produced against donor tissues are usually directed against mismatched HLA class I and/or class II antigens, in addition to non-HLAs, including MIC and EC antigens (reviewed in Cornell et al., 2008; Smith & Rose, 2009; Smith, 2007). It is generally accepted that complement-mediated cytolysis is the major mechanism of kidney vascular endothelial and parenchymal cell damage. The clinicopathological presentation of AMR is characterized by peritubular capillary C4d deposition, which is characterized by a rapid rise in serum creatinine and the appearance of DSAs in the circulation. C4d is a component of the classical pathway of complement activation, which remains in the tissue for several days (Cornell et al., 2008; Haririan et al., 2009). Peritubular capillary C4d deposition has been demonstrated in 88%-95% of kidney transplant recipients who developed class I and class II DSAs (Colvin, 2007); however, AMR can occur even without detectable concentrations of DSAs in the circulation, which is likely due to their absorption by the kidney graft. The subsequent nephrectomy is usually accompanied by a rise in DSAs within several days (Cornell et al., 2008; Duquesnoy, 2008; Duquesnoy & Claas, 2007). The detrimental effects of non-HLA antibodies are also associated with complement fixing but at a lower degree; however, in the absence of complement, anti-MIC antibodies and AECA can activate graft ECs to proliferate, resulting in the upregulation of adhesion molecules, such as ELAM, ECAM, and neuropilin-2 receptor, as well as the production of TGF-β, which stimulates the growth of connective tissue fibroblasts [reviewed in (Smith & Rose, 2009)]. Recently, graft accommodation in experimental models was described (Aikawa et al., 2003; Jin, 2002; Tabata, 2003). The state of accommodation is defined as normal graft function and appearance, which is evaluated by light microscopy, in the presence of circulating DSAs (Cornell, et al., 2008). The mechanism of accommodation was found to be associated with the upregulation of anti-apoptotic genes, such as bcl-2, bcl-xL, and A20. The precise mechanism of accommodation is still under thorough investigation.

9.2 The role of aloantibodies in chronic rejection or chronic allograft nephropathy (CAN)

DSAs also participate in the development of chronic allograft changes, which can be seen in glomeruli, vessels, tubules and the interstitium (Cornell et al., 2008; Racusen et al., 1998). Their pathological effects therein are mediated by two major processes. First, DSAs cause EC damage by complement-dependent cytotoxicity, which is also a mechanism of humoral rejection; however, unlike AMR, C4d deposition has been reported in approximately 30% - 50% of cases (Colvin 2007). Second, the upregulation of fibroblast growth factor receptors has been demonstrated in elegant studies that were conducted by E. Reed's group (Jin, 2002). These investigators found that the antibody-mediated ligation of class I HLAs triggers an activation signal in ECs, resulting in arterial smooth muscle cell and basement membrane fibroblast proliferation. As a consequence, the lumen of glomerular arteries is decreased and subsequent fibrosis and tissue/organ ischemia develop.

10. Conclusions

1. HLA and non-HLA-specific DSAs play a critical role in the pre- and post-transplant monitoring of renal patients. High levels of anti-HLA (high PRA) antibodies are generally associated with longer periods of time on dialysis and/or on the transplant waiting list until a CM-compatible donor can be found. Post-transplant DSA development often leads to AMR, graft deterioration, or eventual loss.
2. AMR or humoral rejection is mediated by a multi-component mechanism that is associated with anti-HLA class I and class II alloantibodies, complement, and T cells whose primary targets are graft endothelial and tubular cells. Although complement-dependent cytotoxicity is the chief mechanism of antibody-mediated graft damage, additional biological processes result in EC proliferation, pro-inflammatory cytokine production, and apoptosis. Post-transplant DSA development depends on multiple factors, including donor-recipient HLA mismatches (epitope levels), recipient HLA-class II typing, and immunoregulatory mechanisms. Careful analysis of mismatched epitopes can predict, with some degree of accuracy, the profile of antibodies that will develop post-transplant. The latter is particularly meaningful for subsequent donor searches.
3. The pre-transplant deletion of anti-HLA antibodies, or DS, considerably expands the pool of donors for highly sensitized TCs. This therapeutic approach (or immunomodulation) often includes combinations of different protocols, including the use of PP, IVIG, Rituximab and Bortezomib; however, DS is not a panacea for patients with high PRAs, and not all recipients are susceptible to this treatment. In addition, the rebound effect is a frequent consequence of this type of immunomodulation. Furthermore, all of the aforementioned DS protocols are not free from adverse effects. Although the majority of cases show considerable decreases in DSA antibody levels, they are not completely eliminated (the rate of antibody production is 1000 molecule/PC cell/second). These remaining DSAs represent a risk factor for humoral graft rejection in long-term follow up.
4. The development of DSAs is a major obstacle to long-term graft survival. Because of this, individual immunosuppression/DS is one of the most hopeful future directions for progress in kidney transplantation. This therapeutic approach must incorporate the analysis of the genes that are involved in cytokine (IL-12, TNFα, IFNγ) and chemokine production, the frequency of T regs and NKT cell production, as well as detailed analysis of the alloantibody profiles.

11. References

Abe, M.; Kawai, T. & Futatsuyama, K. (1997). Postoperative production of anti-donor antibody and chronic rejection in renal transplantation, *Transplantation,* Vol.63, No.11, (n.d.), pp.1616-1619.

Adeyi, O.; Girnita, A. & Howe, J. (2005). Serum analysis after transplant nephrectomy reveals restricted antibody specificity patterns against structurally defined HLA class I mismatches. *Transplant Immunolology,* Vol.14, No.1, (n.d.), pp.53-62.

Aikawa, A.; Yamashita, M. & Hadano, T. (2003).ABO incompatible kidney transplantation -- immunological aspects, *Exp Clin Transplant,* Vol.1, No.2, (n.d.), pp. 112-118.

Akalin, E. & Bromberg, J. (2005). Intravenous immunoglobulin induction treatment in flow cytometry cross-match-positive kidney transplant recipients. *Human Immunology,* Vol.66, No.4, (n.d.), pp.359-363.

Akalin, E.; Dinavahi, R. & Friedlander, R. (2008). Addition of plasmapheresis decreases the incidence of acute antibody-mediated rejection in sensitized patients with strong donor-specific antibodies. *Clinical Journal of American Society of Nephrology,* Vol.3, No.4, (n.d.), pp.1160-1167.

Akalin, E. & Pascual, M. (2006). Sensitization after kidney transplantation. *Clinical Journal of American Society of Nephrology,* Vol.1, No.3, (n.d.), pp.433-440.

Al-Lamki, R.; Bradley, J. & Pober, J. (2008). Endothelial cells in allograft rejection. *Transplantation,* Vol.86, No.10, (November 27), (n.d.), pp.1340-1348.Alheim, M. et al. (2010). A flow cytometric crossmatch test for simultaneous detection of antibodies against donor lymphocytes and endothelial precursor cells. *Tissue Antigens,* Vol.75, No.3, (n.d.), pp.269-277.

Alkhunaizi, A. (2006). Renal transplantation across the ABO barrier. *Saudi Journal of Kidney Disease Transplantation,* Vol.17, No.3, (n.d.), pp.311-315.

Amu, S. (2007). The human immunomodulatory CD25(+) B cell population belongs to the memory B cell pool. *Scandinavian Journal of Immunology,* Vol.66, No.1, (n.d.), pp.77-86, ISSN 0300-9475

Anderson, B. et al. (2000). Induction of determinant spreading and of Th1 responses by in vitro stimulation with HER-2 peptides. *Cancer Immunology and Immunotherapy,* Vol.49, No.9, (November 2007), pp.459-468.

Armitage, R. & Alderson, M. (1995). B-Cell Stimulation. *Current Opinion in Immunology,* Vol.7, No.2, (April 1995), pp.243-247.

Arnold, M. et al. (2004). Detection and specification of noncomplement binding anti-HLA alloantibodies. *Human Immunology,* Vol.65, No.11, (November 2004), pp.1288-1296, ISSN 0198-8859

Arnold, M. et al. (2005).HLA DQ antibodies in patients awaiting kidney re-transplantation. *Genes and Immunity,* Vol.6, No.6, (n.d.), p.6, ISSN 81466-4879

Arnold, M. et al. (2005). Anti-HLA class II antibodies in kidney retransplant patients. *Tissue Antigens,* Vol.65, No. 4, (April 2005), (n.d.), pp.370-378, ISSN 0001-2815Arnold, M. et al. (2008). Prevalence and specificity of IgG and IgA non-complement binding anti-HLA alloantibodies in retransplant candidates. *Tissue Antigens,* Vol.72, No.1, (July 2008), pp.60-66.

Aubert V. et al. (2009). Low levels of human leukocyte antigen donor-specific antibodies detected by solid phase assay before transplantation are frequently clinically irrelevant. *Human Immunology,* Vol.70, No.8, (n.d.), pp.580-583.

Baid-Agrawal, S. & Frei, U. (2007). Living donor renal transplantation: recent developments and perspectives. *Nature Clinical Practice. Nephrology,* Vol.3, No.1, (January 2007), pp. 31-41, ISSN 1745-8323

Balan, V. (2008). Long-term outcome of human leukocyte antigen mismatching in liver transplantation: results of the National Institute of Diabetes and Digestive and Kidney Diseases Liver Transplantation Database. Hepatology. Vol. 48, No.3, (September 2008), pp.878-888.

Banerjee, D.; Kupin, W. & Roth, D. (2003). Hemolytic uremic syndrome after multivisceral transplantation treated with intravenous immunoglobulin. *Juornal of Nephrology,* Vol.16, No.5, (October 2003), pp.733-735, ISSN 1121-8428

Barabanova Y.; Ramon, D. & Tambur, A. (2009). Antibodies against HLA-DQ alpha-chain and their role in organ transplantation. *Human Immunology,* Vol.70, No.6, (n.d.), pp.410-412.

Bartel, G. et al. (2007). Determinants of the complement-fixing ability of recipient presensitization against HLA antigens. *Transplantation,* Vol.83, No.6, (n.d.), pp.727-733.

Bas, J. et al. (1998). Peripheral blood lymphoid subsets and long-term clinical course of kidney recipients: A longitudinal study. *Cytometry,* Vol.34, No.2, (April 1998), pp.103-112,0196-4763

Bayry, J. et al. (2003). Inhibition of maturation and function of dendritic cells by intravenous immunoglobulin. *Blood,* Vol.101, No. 2, (January 2003), pp.758-765, ISSN 0006-4971

Beimler J. & Zeier, M. 2007ABO-incompatible transplantation - a safe way to perform renal transplantation?, *Nephrology, Dialysis, Transplantation*, Vol.22, No.1, (January 2007), pp.25-27, ISSN 0931-0509

Benson, M. et al. (2009). Distinction of the memory B cell response to cognate antigen versus bystander inflammatory signals. *Journal of Experimental Medicine,* Vol.206, No.9, (n.d.), pp.2013-2025.

Billen, E. et al. (2009). Donor-directed HLA antibodies before and after transplantectomy detected by the luminex single antigen assay. *Transplantation,* Vol.87, No.4, (February 2009), pp.563-569.

Billen, E.; Christiaans, M. & van den Berg-Loonen, M. (2009). Clinical relevance of Luminex donor-specific crossmatches: data from 165 renal transplants. *Tissue Antigens,* Vol.74, No.3, (September 2009), pp. 205-212.

Bishay, E. et al. (2000). The clinical significance of flow cytometry crossmatching in heart transplantation. *European Journal of Cardiothorac Surgery,* Vol.17, No.4, (n.d.), pp.362-369.

Bohmig, G.; Bartel, G. & Wahrmann, M. (2008). Antibodies, isotypes and complement in allograft rejection. *Curr Opin Organ Transplant,* Vol.13, No.4, (n.d.), pp.411-418, ISSN 1087-2418

Bray, R.; Lebeck, L. & Gebel, H. (1989). The flow cytometric crossmatch. Dual-color analysis of T cell and B cell reactivities. *Transplantation,* Vol.48, No.5, (November 1989), pp.834-840

Bray, R. (1994). Flow cytometry crossmatching for solid organ transplantation. *Methods in Cellular Biology,* Vol.41, (n.d.), pp.103-119

Bray, R. (2001). Flow cytometry in human leukocyte antigen testing. *Seminars in Hematology,* Vol.38, No.2, (April 2001), pp.194-200.

Bray, R. et al. (2004). Evolution of HLA antibody detection: technology emulating biology. *Immunological Research,* Vol.29, No.1-3, (n.d.), pp.41-54,

Bray, R. & Gebel, H. (2008). Monitoring after renal transplantation: recommendations and caveats. *Nature Clinical Practice. Nephrology,* Vol.4, No.12, (December 2008), pp.658-659.

Breimer, M. et al. (2009). Multicenter evaluation of a novel endothelial cell crossmatch test in kidney transplantation. *Transplantation,* Vol.87, No.4, (n.d.), pp.549-556.

Bryan, C.; Shield, C. & Nelson, P. (1998). Transplantation rate of the blood group B waiting list is increased by using A2 and A2B kidneys. *Transplantation,* Vol.66, No.12, (n.d.), pp.1714-1717.

Buelow, R. et al. (1995). Soluble HLA antigens and ELISA - A new technology for crossmatch testing. *Transplantation,* Vol.60, No.12, (December 1995), pp.1594-1599, ISSN 0041-1337

Cai, J. & Terasaki, P. (2005). Humoral theory of transplantation: mechanism, prevention, and treatment. *Human Immunology,* Vol.66, No.4, (April 2005), pp.334-342.

Cai, J.; Kohanof, S. & Terasaki, P. (2006). HLA-DR antibody epitopes. *Clinical Transplantation,* Vol.20, No.1, (n.d.), pp.103-114.

Cai, J.; et al. (2006). Development of nondonor-specific HLA-DR antibodies in allograft recipients is associated with shared epitopes with mismatched donor DR antigens. *American Journal of Transplantation,* Vol.6, No.12, (December 2006),pp.2947-2954, ISSN 1600-6135

Carloss, H. & Tavassoli, M. (1980). Acute renal failure from precipitation of cryoglobulins in a cool operating room. *Journal of American Medical Association,* Vol.244, No.13, (September 1980), pp.1472-1473,

Cavo, M. (2006). Proteasome inhibitor bortezomib for the treatment of multiple myeloma. *Leukemia,* , Vol.20, No.8, (August 2006), (n.d.), pp.1341-1352, ISSN 0887-6924

Christiaans, M. (2000). Detection of HLA class I and II antibodies by ELISA and complement-dependent cytotoxicity before and after transplantation. *Transplantation,* Vol.69, No.5, (March 2000), pp.917-927, ISSN 0041-1337

Christiaans, M. et al. (1998). Donor-specific antibodies after transplantation by flow cytometry - Relative change in fluorescence ratio most sensitive risk factor for graft survival. *Transplantation,* Vol.65, No.3, (n.d.), pp.427-433, ISSN 0041-1337

Claas, F. et al. (2005). Differential immunogenicity of HLA mismatches in clinical transplantation. *Transplant Immunology,* Vol.14, No.3, (n.d.), pp.187-191.

Claas, F. & Doxiadis, I. (2009). Human leukocyte antigen antibody detection and kidney allocation within Eurotransplant. *Human Immunology,* Vol.70, No.8, (n.d.), pp.636-639.

Claas, F. & Duquesnoy, R. (2008).The polymorphic alloimmune response in clinical transplantation.
Current Opinions in Immunology, Vol.20, No.5, (n.d.), pp.566-567.

Claas, F. (2004). The acceptable mismatch program as a fast tool for highly sensitized patients awaiting cadaveric kidney transplantation: short waiting time and excellent graft outcome. *Transplantation,* Vol.78, No.2, (n.d.), pp.1046-1056, ISSN 1046-6673

Cornell, L.; Smith, R & Colvin, R. (2008). Kidney Transplantation: Mechanisms of Rejection and Acceptance. *Annual Review of Pathology: Mechanism of Disease,* Vol.3, No.12, (n.d.), pp.189-220.

Colvin, R. (2007). Antibody-mediated renal allograft rejection: Diagnosis and pathogenesis. *Journal of the American Society of Nephrology,* Vol.18, No.4, (n.d.), pp.1046-1056.

Danziger-Isakov, L. et al. (2010). Effects of influenza immunization on humoral and cellular alloreactivity in humans- *Transplantation,* Vol.89, No.7, (n.d.), pp.838-844.

Dau, P. (1995). Immunologic rebound. *Journal of clinical apheresis,* Vol.10, No.4, (n.d.), pp.210-217.

Demirhan, B. et al. (1998). Hyperacute allograft rejection mediated by IgM antibodies and a negative lymphocyte crossmatch: Report of two cases. *Transplantation Proceedings*, Vol.30, No.3, (n.d.), pp.732-733, ISSN 0041-1345

Deng, C. et al. (2008). Human leukocyte antigen class II DQ alpha and beta epitopes identified from sera of kidney allograft recipients. *Transplantation,* Vol.86, No.3, (n.d.), pp.452-459.

Di Genova, G. et al. (2006). Vaccination of human subjects expands both specific and bystander memory T cells but antibody production remains vaccine specific. *Blood,* Vol.107, No.7, (n.d.), pp.2806-2813.

Di Genova, G. et al. (2010). Bystander stimulation of activated CD4+ T cells of unrelated specificity following a booster vaccination with tetanus toxoid. *European Journal of Immunology,* Vol. 40, No.4, (n.d.), pp.976-985.

Diaz, J. Cooper, E. & Ochsner, J. (1984). Cold hemagglutination pathophysiology. Evaluation and management of patients undergoing cardiac surgery with induced hypothermia. *Archive of Internal Medicine,* Vol.144, No.8, (n.d.), pp.1639-1641,

Diwan, T. et al. (2011). The impact of proteosome inhibition on alloantibody-producing plasma cells in Vivo. *Transplantation,* Vol.9, No.15, (n.d.), pp.536-541.

Doherty, P. & Zinkernagel, R. (1997). Rules of engagement: the discovery of MHC restriction. *Immunology Today,* Vol.18, No. 1, (n.d.), pp.14-17.

Doxiadis, I.; Duquesnoy, R. & Claas, F. (2005). Extending options for highly sensitized patients to receive a suitable kidney graft. *Curr Opin Immunol,* Vol.17, No.5, (n.d.), pp.536-540.

Dunn, T. et al. (2010). Impact of Flow XM Results on Kidney Transplant Outcomes for Recipients with Donor Specific Antibody (DSA). *Lancet,* Vol. 339, No.8809, (n.d.), pp.1566-1570, ISSN 102361600-6135

Duquesnoy, R. (2002). HLAMatchmaker: A molecularly based algorithm for histocompatibility determination. I. Description of the algorithm. *Human Immunology,* Vol.63, No.5, (n.d.), pp.339-352, ISSN 0198-8859

Duquesnoy, R. & Claas, F. (2005). Is the application of HLAMatchmaker relevant in kidney transplantation? *Transplantation,* Vol.79, No.2, (n.d.), pp. 250-251

Duquesnoy, R. et al. (2005). HLAMatchmaker-based analysis of human monoclonal antibody reactivity demonstrates the importance of an additional contact site for specific recognition of triplet-defined epitopes. Human Immunology, Vol.66, No.7, (n.d.), pp.749-761

Duquesnoy, R. (2006). A structurally based approach to determine HLA compatibility at the humoral immune level. *Human Immunology,* Vol.67, No.11, (n.d.), pp. 847-862

Duquesnoy, R. (2007). "Match and treat": an effective strategy for transplanting highly sensitized pediatric transplant candidates? *Pediatric Transplantation,* Vol.11, No.1, (n.d.), pp.3-4,

Duquesnoy, R. & Claas, F. (2007). 14th International HLA and Immunogenetics Workshop: report on the structural basis of HLA compatibility. *Tissue Antigens,* Vol.69, Suppl. 1, (n.d.), pp.180-184,

Duquesnoy, R. & Askar, M. (2007). HLAMatchmaker: a molecularly based algorithm for histocompatibility determination. V. Eplet matching for HLA-DR, HLA-DQ, and HLA-DP. *Human Immunology,* Vol.68, No.1, (n.d.), pp.12-25.

Duquesnoy, R. (2008). Clinical usefulness of HLAMatchmaker in HLA epitope matching for organ transplantation. *Current Opinions in Immunology,* Vol.20, No.5, (n.d.), pp.594-601.

Duquesnoy, R. (2008). Human leukocyte antigen class II antibodies and transplant outcome. *Transplantation,* Vol.86, No.5, (n.d.), pp.638-640,

Duquesnoy, R. (2008). Structural epitope matching for HLA-alloimmunized thrombocytopenic patients: a new strategy to provide more effective platelet transfusion support? *Transfusion,* Vol.48, No.2, (n.d.), pp.221-227

Duquesnoy, R. (2008). Retransplant candidates have donor-specific antibodies that react with structurally defined HLA-DR, DQ, DP epitopes. *Transplant Immunology,* Vol.18, No.4, (n.d.), pp.352-360

Duquesnoy, R. (2008). Structurally based epitope analysis of major histocompatibility complex class I-related chain A (MICA) antibody specificity patterns. *Human Immunology,* Vol.69, No.12, (n.d.), pp. 826-832

Duquesnoy, R. & Marrari, M. (2009). Correlations between Terasaki's HLA class I epitopes and HLAMatchmaker-defined eplets on HLA-A, -B and -C antigens. *Tissue Antigens,* Vol.74, No.2, (August 2009), pp.117-133

Duquesnoy, R. & Marrari, M. (2010). Detection of antibodies against HLA-C Epitopes in Patients with Rejected Kidney Transplants. *Tissue Antigens,* Vol.74, No.2, (n.d.), pp.23-35.

Edelman, G. (1970). The covalent structure of a human gamma G-immunoglobulin. XI. Functional implications. *Biochemistry,* Vol.9, No.16, (n.d.), pp.3197-3205.

El-Awar, N.; Lee, J. & Terasaki, P. (2005). HLA antibody identification with single antigen beads compared to conventional methods. *Human Immunology,* Vol.68, No.3, (n.d.), pp.989-999, ISSN 0198-8859

El-Awar, N.; Cook, D. & Terasaki, P. (2006). HLA class I epitopes: A and B loci. *Clinical Transplantation,* Vol.20, No.1, (n.d.), pp.79-94.

El-Awar, N.; Lee, J. & Terasaki, P. (2006). HLA class I epitopes I: Detection by eluted antibodies from recombinant single-antigen cell lines. *Human Immunology,* Vol.67, No.10, (n.d.), p.105, ISSN 0198-8859

El-Awar, N. & Terasaki, P. (2007). HLA Class I epitopes: 103 total epitopes to-date including the C locus. *Human Immunology,*Vol.68, Suppl. 1, (n.d.), p.45, ISSN 0198-8859

El-Awar, N. (2007). Human leukocyte antigen class I epitopes: Update to 103 total epitopes, including the C locus. *Transplantation,* Vol.84, No.4, (n.d.), pp.532-540, ISSN 0041-1337

El-Awar, N. et al. (2009). Epitopes of HLA-A, B, C, DR, DQ, DP and MICA antigens, *Clinical Transplantation,*

Vol.23, No.3, (n.d.), pp.295-321.

Everly, J. et al. (2009). Proteasome inhibition for antibody-mediated rejection. *Current Opinion in Organ Transplantation,* Vol.14, No.6, (August 2009), pp.662-666, 1087-2418

Ferrari-Lacraz, S.; Aubert, V. & Buhler L. (2006). Anti-HLA antibody repertoire after IVIg infusion in highly sensitized patients waiting for kidney transplantation. *Swiss Med Wkly,* Vol.136, No.44, (n.d.), pp.696-702.

Ferry, B. et al. (1997). Anti-cell surface endothelial antibodies in sera from cardiac and kidney transplant recipients: association with chronic rejection. *Transplant Immunology,* Vol.5, No.1, (n.d.), pp.17-24.

Fidler, M. et al. (2004). Histologic findings of antibody-mediated rejection in ABO blood-group-incompatible living-donor kidney transplantation. *American Journal of Transplantation,* Vol.4, No.1, (n.d.), pp.101-107.

Forman, J. et al. (2004). Significance of anticardiolipin antibodies on short and long term allograft survival and function following kidney transplantation. *American Journal of Transplantation,* Vol.4, No.11, (n.d.), pp.1786-1791, ISSN 1600-6135

Fredrich, R. et al. (1999). The clinical significance of antibodies to human vascular endothelial cells after cardiac transplantation. *Transplantation,* Vol.67, No.3, (n.d.), pp.385-391.

Fuggle, S. et al. (1983). Localization of major histocompatibility complex (HLA-ABC and DR) antigens in 46 kidneys. *Transplantation,* Vol.35, No.4, (n.d.), pp.385-390

Fuggle, S. & Martin, S. (2008). Tools for human leukocyte antigen antibody detection and their application to transplanting sensitized patients. *Transplantation,* Vol.86, No.3, (n.d.), pp. 384-390

Fujita S.; Rosen, C.; Reed, A. 1997Significance of preformed anti-donor antibodies in liver transplantation. *Transplantation,* Vol.63, No.1, (n.d.), pp. 84-88

Fuller, A. et al. (1999). Repeat donor HLA-DR mismatches in renal transplantation: is the increased failure rate caused by noncytotoxic HLA-DR alloantibodies? *Transplantation,* Vol.68, No.4, (n.d.), pp.589-591.

Fuller, T. & Fuller, A. (1999). The humoral immune response against an HLA class I allodeterminant correlates with the HLA-DR phenotype of the responder. *Transplantation,* Vol.68, No.2, (n.d.), pp.173-182.

Furth, S. et al. (1999). Plasmapheresis, intravenous cytomegalovirus-specific immunoglobulin and reversal of antibody-mediated rejection in a pediatric renal transplant recipient: a case report. *Pediatrics Transplantation,* Vol.3, No.2, (n.d.), pp. 146-149.

Futagawa, Y. & Terasaki, P. (2006). ABO incompatible kidney transplantation - an analysis of UNOS Registry data. *Clinical Transplantation,* Vol.20, No.1, (n.d.), pp.122-126, ISSN 0902-0063

Gandhi, M.; Ploeger, N. & DeGoey, S. (2010). Positive virtual crossmatch (VXM), negative flow crossmatch (FXM): a case of antibody (Abs) to denatured antige (dAg). *Human Immunology,* Vol.71, No.10, Suppl. 1, (n.d.), p. 4

Garovoy, M.; Rheinschmidt, M. & Bigos M. (1983). Flow cytometry analysis: A high technology crossmatch technique facilitating transplantation. *Transplantation Proceedings,* Vol.15, No.5, (n.d.), pp.1939-1941

Gebel, H. & Bray, R. (2000). Sensitization and sensitivity: defining the unsensitized patient. *Transplantation,* Vol.69, No.7, pp.1370-1374.

Gebel, H. et al. (2002). Conundrums with FlowPRA beads. *Clinical Transplantation,* Vol.16, Suppl. 7, (n.d.), pp.24-29,

Gebel, H.; Bray, R. & Nickerson, P. (2003). Pre-transplant assessment of donor-reactive, HLA-specific antibodies in renal transplantation: contraindication vs. risk. *American Journal of Transplantation,* Vol.3, No.12, (n.d.), pp.1488-1500

Gebel, H. et al. (2009). Donor-reactive HLA antibodies in renal allograft recipients: considerations, complications, and conundrums. *Human Immunology,* Vol.70, No.8, (n.d.), pp.610-617.

Gebel, H. & Bray, R. (2010). The evolution and clinical impact of Human Leukocyte Antigen technology. *Current Opinions in Nephrology and Hypertension,* Vol.19, No.6, (n.d.), pp.598-602, ISSN 1062-4821

Gebel H. & Halloran, P. (2010). Making Sense of Desensitization. *American Journal of Transplantation,* Vol.10, No.3, (n.d.), pp.443-444, ISSN 1600-6135

Georgescu, D.; Ferrari-Lacraz, S. & Villard, J. (2007). Anti-HLA antibody detection and rejection in kidney transplantation: impact of the new technologies. *Reviews Medicale Suisse,* Vol.25, No.3, (n.d.), pp.1064-1069.

Ghasemian, S. et al. (1998). Dec- Hyperacute rejection from antibody against class II HLA antigens- 12- 6, *Clinical Transplantation,* Vol.12, No.6, (n.d.), pp.569-571.

Gloor, J. et al. (2004). Persistence of low levels of alloantibody after desensitization in crossmatch-positive living-donor kidney transplantation. *Transplantation,* Vol.78, No.2, (n.d.), pp.221-227, ISSN 0041-1337

Gloor, J. et al. (2004). Kidney transplantation following administration of high dose intravenous immunoglobulin in patients with positive flow cytometric/negative enhanced cytotoxicity crossmatch. *American Journal of Transplantation,* Vol.4, Suppl. 8, (n.d.), p.256, ISSN 1600-6135

Gloor, J. (2006). Histologic findings one year after positive crossmatch or ABO blood group incompatible living donor kidney transplantation. *American Journal of Transplantation,* Vol.6, No.8, (n.d.), pp.1841-1847, ISSN 1600-6135

Gloor, J. & Stegall, M. (2007).ABO incompatible kidney transplantation. *Current Opinions in Nephrology and Hypertension,* Vol.16, No.6, (November 2007), (n.d.), pp.529-534

Glotz, D. (2004). Intravenous immunoglobulins and transplantation for patients with anti-HLA antibodies. *Transplant International,* Vol.17, No.1, (n.d.), pp.1-8, ISSN 0934-0874

Goral, S. et al. (2008). Preformed donor-directed anti-HLA-DP antibodies may be an impediment to successful kidney transplantation. *Nephrology Dialysis and Transplantation,* Vol.23, No.1, (n.d.), pp.390-392, ISSN 0931-0509

Graff, R. et al. (2009). The role of positive flow cytometry crossmatch in late renal allograft loss. *Human Immunology,* Vol.70, No.7, (n.d.), pp.502-505.

Grandtnerova, B. et al. (1995). Treatment of Acute Humoral Rejection in Kidney-Transplantation with Plasmapheresis. *Transplantation Proceedings,* Vol.27, No.1, (n.d.), pp.934-935.

Grandtnerova, B. (2008). Hyperacute rejection of living related kidney grafts caused by endothelial cell-specific antibodies: Case reports. *Transplantation Proceedings,* Vol.40, No.7, (n.d.), pp.2422-2424.

Guardiola, J. & Maffei, A. (1993). Control of MHC class II gene expression in autoimmune, infectious, and neoplastic diseases. *Critical Reviews in Immunology,* Vol.13, No.4, (n.d.), pp.247-268.

Han, F. et al. (2009). Pre-transplant serum concentrations of anti-endothelial cell antibody in panel reactive antibody negative renal recipients and its impact on acute rejection. *Clinical Chemistry and Laboratory Medicine,* Vol.47, No.10, (n.d.), pp.1265-1269.

Haririan, A. et al. (2009). The Impact of C4d Pattern and Donor-Specific Antibody on Graft Survival in Recipients Requiring Indication Renal Allograft Biopsy. *American Journal of Transplantation*, Vol.9, No.12, (n.d.), pp.2758-2767, ISSN 1600-6135

Haririan, A. et al.(2009). Positive Cross-Match Living Donor Kidney Transplantation: Longer-Term Outcomes Editorial Comment. *Journal of Urology*, Vol.182, No.3, (n.d.), p.1138, ISSN 0022-5347

Harmer, A. et al. (1993). Highly Sensitive, Rapid Screening Method for the Detection of Antibodies Directed Against Hla Class-I and Class-Ii Antigens. *Transplant International*, Vol. 6, No.5, (n.d.), pp.277-280, ISSN 0934-0874.

Harris, E. & Pierangeli, S. (2000). Equivocal' antiphospholipid syndrome. *Journal of Autoimmunity*, Vol. 15, No.2, (n.d.), pp. 81-85, ISSN 0896-8411

Hart, D. (1981). Localization of HLA-ABC and DR antigens in human kidney. *Transplantation*, Vol.31, No.6, (n.d.), pp.428-433,

Higgins, R. (2009). Rises and falls in donor-specific and third-party HLA antibody levels after antibody incompatible transplantation. *Transplantation*, Vol.87, No.6, (n.d.), pp.882-888.

Hill, N. & Sarvetnick, N. (2002). Cytokines: promoters and dampeners of autoimmunity. *Current Opinion in Immunology*, Vol.14, No.6, (n.d.), pp.791-797, ISSN 0952-7915

Horsburgh, T.; Martin, S. & Robson, A. (2000). The application of flow cytometry to histocompatibility testing. *Transplant Immunology*, Vol.8, No.1, (n.d.), pp.3-15, ISSN 0966-3274

Husby, G. et al. (1989). Cross-reactive epitope with Klebsiella pneumoniae nitrogenase in articular tissue of HLA-B27+ patients with ankylosing spondylitis. *Arthritis Rheum*, Vol.32, No.4, (n. d.), pp.437-445.

Issitt, P. & Issitt, C. (1979). *Applied Blood Group Serology* (2 nd edition), Spectra Biologicals, ISBN 7434546, Oxnard, CA.

Izzat, M.; Rajesh, P. & Smith, G. (1993). Use of retrograde cold crystalloid cardioplegia in a patient with unexpected cold agglutination. *Annals of Thoracic Surgery*, Vol.56, No.6, (n.d.), pp.1395-1397

Jiang, S. & Lechler, R. (2003). Regulatory T cells in the control of transplantation tolerance and autoimmunity. *American Journal of Transplantation*, Vol.3, No.5, (n.d.), pp.516-524.

Jin, Y. et al. (2002). Ligation of HLA class I molecules on endothelial cells induces phosphorylation of Src, paxillin, and focal adhesion kinase in an actin-dependent manner. *Journal of Immunology*, Vol.168, No.11, (n.d.), pp.5415-5423,

Johnson, A. et al. (1986). Recognition of an HLA-DPw1 specific alloantiserum raised by planned Immunization. *Human Immunology*, Vol.17, No.2, pp.21-29.

Jordan, S.; Cunningham-Rundles, C. & McEwan R. (2003). Utility of Intravenous immune globulin in Kidney Transplantatio: Efficacy, Safety, and Cost Implications. *American Journal of Transplantation*, Vol.3, No.12, (n.d.), pp.653-664.

Jordan, S. et al. (2004). Evaluation of intravenous immunoglobulin as are agent to lower allosensitization and improve transplantation in highly sensitized adult patients with end-stage renal disease: Report of the NIHIG02 trial. *Journal of the American Society of Nephrology*, Vol.15, No.12, (n.d.), pp.3256-3262, ISSN 1046-6673.

Jordan, S. et al. (2006). Desensitization therapy with intravenous immunoglobulin (IVIG): applications in solid organ transplantation. *Transactions of the American clinical and climatological association,* Vol.117, No.8, (n.d.), pp.199-211

Jordan, S.; Peng, A. & Vo A. (2009). Therapeutiv Strategies in Management of the Highly HLA-Sensitized and ABO-incompatible Transplant Recipients, In: *Humoral Immunity in Kidney Transplanation. What clinicians Need to know,* G. Remuzzi, S. Chiaramonte, N. Perico, C. Ronco, (Eds), pp. 13-26, Karger, ISBN 1021-9749, Basel.

Kahwaji, J. et al. (2009). Acute Hemolysis After High-Dose Intravenous Immunoglobulin Therapy in Highly HLA Sensitized Patients. *Clinical Journal of the American Society of Nephrology,* Vol.4, No.12, (n.d.), pp.1993-1997, ISSN 1555-9041

Kalil, J. (1989). Humoral Rejection in 2 HLA Identical Living Related Donor Kidney-Transplants. *Transplantation Proceedings,* Vol.21, No.1, (n.d.), pp.711-713, ISSN 0041-1345

Kamoun M. et al. (2006). A successful kidney transplant in a patient re-grafted across an incompatible crossmatch secondary to anti-HLA-DP antibodies using intensive immunosuppression. *Transplantation,* Vol.82, No.1, (n.d.), pp.779-1018,

Kazatchkine, M. & Kaveri, S. (2001). Advances in immunology: Immunomodulation of autoimmune and inflammatory diseases with intravenous immune globulin. *New England Journal of Medicine,* Vol.345, No.10, (n.d.), pp.747-755, ISSN 0028-4793

Kennedy, R. et al. (2010). Effect of human leukocyte antigen homozygosity on rubella vaccine-induced humoral and cell-mediated immune responses. Human Immunology, Vol.71, No.2, (n.d.), pp.128-135.

Kerman, R. et al. (1996). Correlation of ELISA-detected IgG and IgA anti-HLA antibodies in pretransplant sera with renal allograft rejection. *Clinical Transplantation,* Vol. 62, No.2, (n.d.), pp.201-205, ISSN 0041-1337

Kerman, R.; Orosz, C. & Lorber, M. (1997). Clinical relevance of anti-HLA antibodies pre and post transplant. *American Journal of Medical Science,* Vol.13, No.5, (n.d.), pp.275-278, ISSN 0002-9629

Klaesson, S. et al. (1993). Immune modulatory effects of immunoglobulins on cell-mediated immune responses in vitro. *Scandinavian Journal of Immunology,* Vol.38, No.5, (n.d.), pp.477-484.

Knight, R. et al. (1995). Renal allograft thrombosis associated with the antiphospholipid antibody syndrome. *Transplantation,* Vol.60, No.6, (n.d.), pp.614-615.

Koka, P. et al. (1993).The Role of IgA Anti-HLA Class-I Antibodies in Kidney-Transplant Survival. *Transplantation,* Vol.56, No.1, (n.d.), pp.207-211, ISSN 0041-1337

Lachmann, N. (2008). Single amino acid mismatches determine immunogenic HLA epitopes. *Tissue Antigens,* Vol.72, No.3, p.253, ISSN 0001-2815

Laux G.; Mansmann, U.; Deufel, A. 2003A new epitope-based HLA-DPB matching approach for cadaver kidney retransplants. *Transplantation,* Vol.75, No.9, (n.d.), pp.1527-1532, ISSN 0041-1337

Le Bas-Bernardet, S. et al. (2003). Non-HLA-type endothelial cell reactive alloantibodies in pre-transplant sera of kidney recipients trigger apoptosis. *American Journal of Transplantation,* Vol.3, No.2, (n.d.), pp.167-177, ISSN 1600-6135

Lederer, S. et al. (1996). Early renal graft dysfunction - The role of preformed antibodies to DR-typed lymphoblastoid cell lines. *Transplantation,* Vol.61, No.2, (n.d.), pp.313-319, ISSN 0041-1337

Lefaucheur, C. et al. (2009). Clinical relevance of preformed HLA donor-specific antibodies in kidney transplantation. *Contributive Nephrology,* Vol.162, No.1, (n.d.), pp.1-12.

Lehrich, R. et al. (2005). Intravenous immunoglobulin and plasmapheresis in acute humoral rejection: experience in renal allograft transplantation. *Human Immunology,* Vol.66, No.4, pp.350-358.

Leong H.; Stachnik, J.; Bonk, M.E. (2008). Unlabeled uses of intravenous immune globulin. *American Journal of Health-System Pharmacy,* Vol. 65, No.19, (n.d.), pp.1815-1824, ISSN 1079-2082

Levings, M. & Thomson, A. (2009). Mastering Treg function to promote tolerance. *American Journal of Transplantation,* Vol.9, No.10, (n.d.), pp.2209-2210.

Lobashevsky, A. et al. (2000). Specificity of preformed alloantibodies causing B cell positive flow crossmatch (FCXM) in renal transplantation. *Clinical Transplantation,* Vol.14, No.6, (n.d.), pp.533-542, ISSN 0902-0063

Lobashevsky, A. et al. (2002). The number of amino acid residues mismatches correlates with flow cytometry crossmatching results in high PRA renal patients. *Human Immunology,* Vol.63, No.5, pp.364-374, ISSN 0198-8859

Lobashevsky, A. et al. (2009). Comparative evaluation of tepnel lifecodes solid phase and lymphocyte cross match assay. *Tissue Antigens,* Vol.73, No.5, (n.d.), p.119

Lobashevsky, A. et al. (2009). Effect of desensitization in solid organ transplant recipients depends on some cytokines genes polymorphism. *Transplant Immunology,* Vol.21, No.3, (n.d.), pp.169-178.

Lobashevsky, A. & Higgins N. (2009). Predictive values (PV) of class I and class II antibodies (Ab) detected by luminex. *Human Immunology,* Vol.70, Suppl. 1, (n.d.), p.32.

Lobashevsky, A. et al. (2010). Subtypes of immunoglobulin (Ig)-G antibodies against donor Class II HLA and cross-match results in three kidney transplant candidates. Vol.23, No.77, (n.d.), pp.81-85, ISSN 0966-3274

Lobashevsky, A. et al. (2011). Allelic mismatch at HLA-DRB3 locus resulted in production of broad specrtrum of alloantibodies. *Tissue antigens,*Vol.77, No.5, (May 2011), p.377.

Lobo, P. et al. (1995).Evidence Demonstrating Poor Kidney Graft-Survival When Acute Rejections Are Associated with IgG Donor-Specific Lymphocytotoxin. *Transplantation,* Vol.59, No.3, (n.d.), pp.357-360, 0041-1337

Lobo, P.; Sturgill, B. & Bolton, W. (1984). Cold-reactive alloantibodies and allograft malfunction occurring immediately posttransplant. *Transplantation,* Vol.37, No.1, (n.d.), pp.76-81.

Lomago, J. et al. (2010). How did a patient who types for HLA-B*4403 develop antibodies that react with HLA-B*4402? *Human Immunology,* Vol.71, No.2, (n.d.), pp.176-178.

Lucchiari, N. et al. (2000). Antibodies fluted from acutely rejected renal allografts bind to and activate human endothelial cells *Human Immunology,* Vol.61, No.5, (n.d.), pp.518-527, 0198-8859

Lutz, H. et al. (2004). Intravenously applied IgG stimulates complement attenuation in a complement-dependent auto-immune disease at the amplifying C3 convertase level. *Blood,* Vol. 103, No.11, (n.d.), pp.465-472.

Marrari, M. & Duquesnoy, R. (2009). Correlations between Terasaki's HLA class II epitopes and HLAMatchmaker-defined eplets on HLA-DR and -DQ antigens. *Tissue Antigens,* Vol.74, No.2, (August 2009), pp.34-46

Marrari, M. & Duquesnoy, R. (2009). Why can sensitization by an HLA-DR2 mismatch lead to antibodies that react also with HLA-DR1? *Human Immunology,* Vol.70, No.6, (n.d.), pp.403-409.

Marrari, M. & Duquesnoy, R.J. (2010). Detection of donor-specific HLA antibodies before and after removal of a rejected kidney transplant. *Transplant Immunology,* Vol.22, No.3-4, (n.d.), pp.105-109, ISSN 0966-3274

Marrari, M. et al. (2010). Human Monoclonal Antibody Reactivity With Human Leukocyte Antigen Class I Epitopes Defined by Pairs of Mismatched Eplets and Self-Eplets. *Transplantation,* Vol.90, No.12, (December 2010), pp.1468-1472, ISSN 0041-1337

Marsh, S.; Parham, P. & Barber L. (2000). *The HLA Facts Book,* Academic Press, ISBN 0125450257, San Diego, CA

Martin, L. et al. (2003). Detection of donor-specific anti-HLA antibodies with flow cytometry in eluates and sera from renal transplant recipients with chronic allograft nephropathy. *Transplantation,* Vol. 76, No.2, (July 2003), pp.395-400, ISSN 0041-1337

Matas, A. et al. (2000). Immunologic and nonimmunologic factors - Different risks for cadaver and living donor transplantation. *Transplantation,* Vol.69, No.1, (n.d.), pp.54-58, ISSN 0041-1337

McCalmon, R. et al. (1997). IgM antibodies in renal transplantation. *Clinical Transplantation,* Vol.11, No.6, pp.558-564, ISSN 0902-0063

McKenna, R. Takemoto, S. & Terasaki, P. (2000). Anti-HLA antibodies after solid organ transplantation. *Transplantation,* Vol.69, No.3, (n.d.), pp.319-326, ISSN 0041-1337

Meroni, P.; Raschi, E. & Testoni, C. (2002). Endothelium as a target for anti-phospholipid antibodies and for therapeutic intervention. *Autoimmunity Reviews,* Vol.1, No.1, (n.d.), pp.55-60,

Mitchell, B. (2003). The proteasome - An emerging therapeutic target in cancer. *New England Journal of Medicine,* Vol.348, No.26, (n.d.), pp.2597-2598, ISSN 0028-4793

Mizutani, K. et al. (2005).Identical kidney transplant recipients who reject grafts have high incidences of antibodies to endothelial cells and MICA. *Human Immunology,* Vol.6, No.6, (n.d.), p86, ISSN 0198-8859.

Mizutani, K. et al. (2006). Frequency of MIC antibody in rejected renal transplant patients without HLA antibody. *Human Immunology,* Vol.67, No.3, (n.d.), pp.223-229, ISSN 0198-8859

Montgomery, R. & Locke, J. (2007). ABO-incompatible transplantation: less may be more. *Transplantation,* Vol.84, No.12, (Supp.l), (n.d.), pp.8-9.

Moraes, J. & Stastny P. (1976). Eight groups of human endothelial cell alloantigens. *Tissue Antigens,* Vol.8, No.4, (n.d.), pp.273-276.

Morales-Buenrostro, L. et al. (2008). "Natural" human leukocyte antigen antibodies found in nonalloimmunized healthy males. *Transplantation,* Vol.86, No. 8, (October 2007), pp.1111-1115,

Muczynski, K. et al. (2003). Normal human kidney HLA-DR-expressing renal microvascular endothelial cells: characterization, isolation, and regulation of MHC class II expression. *Journal of American Society for Nephrology,* Vol.14, No.5, (n.d.), pp.1336-1348.

Mujtaba, M. et al. (2011). The strength of donor-specific antibody is a more reliable predictor of antibody-mediated rejection than flow cytometry crossmatch analysis in desensitized kidney recipients. *Clinical Transplantation,* Vol. 25, No.1, (n.d.), pp.96-102.

Müller, C. et al.(1989).Expression of HLA-DQ, -DR, and -DP antigens in normal kidney and glomerunephritis. *Kidney International,* Vol.35, No.1, pp.116-124

Mytilineos, J.; Deufel, A. & Opelz, G. (1997). Clinical relevance of HLA-DPB locus matching for cadaver kidney retransplants - A report of the Collaborative Transplant Study. *Transplantation,* Vol.63, No.9, (n.d.), pp.1351-1354, ISSN 0041-1337

Nelson, P. (1998). Ten-year experience in transplantation of A2 kidneys into B and O recipients. *Transplantation,* Vol.65, No.2, (n.d.), pp.55-60.

Ogasawara, M.; Kono, D. & Yu, D. (1986). Mimicry of human histocompatibility HLA-B27 antigens by *Klebsiella pneumoniae. Infectious Immunology,* Vol.51, No.3, (n.d.), pp.901-908.

Opelz, G. (2005). Non-HLA transplantation immunity revealed by lymphocytotoxic antibodies. *Lancet,*

Vol.365, No.9470, (n.d.), pp.1570-1576, ISSN 0140-6736

Ozawa, M. et al. (2006). Detection of MICA antibodies and epitope analysis using Luminex MICA single antigen bead. *Human Immunology,* Vol.67, No.10, (n.d.), p.52, ISSN 0198-8859

Patel, A. et al. (2007). Renal transplantation in patients with pre-transplant donor-specificantibodies and negative flow cytometry crossmatches. *American Journal of Transplantation,* Vol. 7, No.10, (n.d.), pp.2371-2377.

Pei, R. et al. (2003). Single human leukocyte antigen flow cytometry beads for accurate identification of human leukocyte antigen antibody specificities. *Transplantation,* Vol.75, No.1, (n.d.), pp.43-49, ISSN 0041-1337

Perrey, C. et al. (1998). An association between antibodies specific for endothelial cells and renal transplant failure. *Transplant Immunology,* Vol.6, No.2, (n.d.), pp.101-106, ISSN 0966-3274

Perry, D. et al. (2009). Proteasome Inhibition Causes Apoptosis of Normal Human Plasma Cells Preventing Alloantibody Production. *American Journal of Transplantation,* Vol.9, No.1, (n.d.), pp.201-209, ISSN 1600-6135

Peters, K. et al. (2004). Functional significance of Tie2 signaling in the adult vasculature. *Recent Progress in Hormone Research,* Vol.59, No. 6, (n.d.), pp.51-71,

Piazza, A. et al. (2006). Anti-DP antibodies and graft failure in kidney transplantation. *American Journal of Transplantation,* Vol.6, No.7, (n.d.), pp.473-476

Pierangeli, S. & Harris, N. (2003). Diagnosis of Antiphopholipid Syndrome. *Clinical Immunology,* Vol.3, No.1, (n.d.), pp.13-17.

Pober, J. et al. (1997). Vascular cells have limited capacities to activate and differentiate T cells: implications for transplant vascular sclerosis. *Transplant Immunology,* Vol.5, No.4, (n.d.), pp.251-254.

Pober, J. et al. (1996). Can graft endothelial, cells initiate a host anti-graft immune response? *Transplantation,*Vol.61, No.3, (n.d.), pp.343-349, ISSN 0041-1337

Poli, F.; Cardillo, M. & Scalamogna, M. (2009). Clinical relevance of human leukocyte antigen antibodies in kidney transplantation from deceased donors: the North Italy Transplant program approach. *Human Immunology,* Vol.70, No.8, (n.d.), pp.631-635.

Porter, R. (1970). The structure and combining specificity of antibodies. *Biochemical Society Symposia,* Vol.30, (n.d.), pp.89-98.

Qasi, Y.; Hermes, M. & Cicciarelli, J. (2006). Graft loss in three patients with donor-specific antibody (DSA). In: *Clinical transplants,* Terasaki, P., pp.541-543, Terasaki foundation Laboratory, ISBN 978-1-880318-15-7, Los Angeles, CA.

Qiu, J. et al. (2005). Detection of antibodies to HLA-DP in renal transplant recipients using single antigen beads. *Transplantation,* Vol.80, No.10, (n.d.), pp.1511-1513, ISSN 0041-1337

Racusen, L.; Solwz, K. & Burdick J. (1998). *Kidney transplant rejection. Diagnosis and treatment,* Dekker Inc., 3d edition, ISBN 1260-8247-0139-9, Marcel, New York, Bazel, Hong Kong.

Raghavan, R. et al. (2010). Bortezomib in Kidney transplantation. *Journal of Transplantation,* Vol.2010, No.11, (n.d.), pp.1-6

Rebellato, L. et al. (2006). Antibodies against HLA class I/II and MICA in rejection and at graft failure. *Human Immunology,* Vol.67, No. 10, (n.d.), p.86, ISSN 0198-8859

Reinsmoen, N. et al. (2008). Acceptable donor-specific antibody levels allowing for successful deceased and living donor kidney transplantation after desensitization therapy. *Transplantation,* 866, (n.d.), pp.820-825, ISSN 0041-1337

Rifle, G. & Mousson, C. (2003). Donor-derived hematopoietic cells in organ transplantation: A major step toward allograft tolerance? *Transplantation,* Vol.75, No.9, (n.d.), pp.3-7, ISSN 0041-1337

Rivera, R. & Scornik, J. (1986). HLA antigens on red cells. Implications for achieving low HLA antigen content in blood transfusions. *Transfusion,* Vol.26, No.4, (n.d.), pp.375-381

Rodey, G. & Fuller, T. (1987). Public epitopes and the antigenic structure of the HLA molecules. *Critical Reviews in Immunology,* Vol.7, No.3, (n.d.), pp.229-267.

Rodriguez, P. (2000). Detection of alloantibodies against non-HLA antigens in kidney transplantation by flow cytometry. *Clinical Transplantation,* Vol.14, No.5, (n.d.), pp.472-478, ISSN 0902-0063

Roelcke, D. (1974). Cold agglutination. Antibodies and antigens. *Clinical Immunology and Immunopathology,* Vol.2, No.2, (n.d.), pp.266-280,

Roelcke, D. (1989). Cold agglutination. *Transfusion Medicine Reviews,* Vol.3, No.2, (n.d.), pp.140-166,

Rogers, N. et al. (2011). Desensitization for renal transplantation: depletion of donor-specific anti-HLA antibodies, preservation of memory antibodies, and clinical risks. *Transplant International,* Vol.24, No.1, (n.d.), pp.21-29, ISSN 0934-0874

Rosenberg WMC; Bushell A; Higgins R. 1992Isolated HLA-DP mismatches between donors and recipients Do Not Influence the function or outcome of renal transplants. *Human Immunology,* Vol.35, No.9, (n.d.), pp.5-9,

Ruschak, A. et al. (2010). The proteasome antechamber maintains substrates in an unfolded state. *Nature,* Vol.467, No.7317, (n.d.), pp. 868-872, ISSN 0028-0836

Rydberg, L.; Skogsberg, U. & Molne, J. (2007). ABO antigen expression in graft tissue: is titration against donor erythrocytes relevant? *Transplantation,* Vol.84, No.12, (Supp. l), (n.d.), pp. 10-12.

Saw, C.; Bray, R. & Gebel, H. (2008). Cytotoxicity and antibody binding by flow cytometry: a single assay to simultaneously assess two parameters. *Cytometry B. Clinical Cytometry,* Vol.74, No.5, (n.d.), pp.287-294.

Sberro-Soussan, R. et al. (2010). Bortezomib as the Sole Post-Renal Transplantation Desensitization Agent Does Not Decrease Donor-Specific Anti-HLA Antibodies. *American Journal of Transplantation,* Vol.10, No.3, (n.d.), pp.681-686, ISSN 1600-6135

Schonemann, C. et al. (1998). HLA class I and class II antibodies - Monitoring before and after kidney transplantation and their clinical relevance. *Transplantation,* Vol.65, No.11, (n.d.), pp.1519-1523, ISSN 0041-1337

Scornik, J. et al. (1989). Role of anti-donor antibodies in bone marrow transplant rejection: evaluation by flow cytometry and effect of plasma exchanges. *Transplant Proc,* Vol.21, No.1, Pt. 3, (n.d.), pp.2974-2975, ISSN 0041-1345

Scornik, J. et al. (1992). Hyperacute and acute kidney graft rejection due to antibodies against B cells. *Transplantation,* Vol.54, No.1, (n.d.), pp.61-64.

Scornik, J. et al. (1997). Multicenter evaluation of the flow cytometry T-cell crossmatch: results from the American Society of Histocompatibility and Immunogenetics-College of American Pathologists proficiency testing program. *Transplantation,* Vol.63, No.10, (n.d.), pp.1440-1445,

Shenton, B. et al. (1995). The value of flow cytometric crossmatching in lung transplantation: relevance of pretransplant antibodies to lung epithelial cells. *Transplant Proc,* Vol.27, No.1, (n.d.), pp.1295-1297, ISSN 0041-1345.

Shimmura, H. et al. (2004). Impact of positive PRA on the results of ABO-incompatible kidney transplantation. *Transplant Proceedings,* Vol.36, No. 7, (September 2004), (n.d.), pp.2169-2171

Shroyer, T. et al. (1995). A Rapid Flow-Cytometry Assay for HLA Antibody Detection Using A Pooled Cell Panel Covering 14 Serological Cross-Reacting Groups. *Transplantation,* Vol.59, No.4, (n.d.), pp.626-630, ISSN 0041-1337

Smith, J. et al. (2007). C4d fixing, luminex binding antibodies - a new tool for prediction of graft failure after heart transplantation. *American Journal of Transplantation,* Vol.7, No.12, pp.2809-2815.

Smith, J. & Rose M. (2009). Transplantation Immunology: methods and Protocols. In: *Detection and Clinical Relevance of Antibodies After Transplantation,* Hornick, P. & Rose, M., pp.227-245, Humana Press Inc., Totowa, NJ

Sonnenday, C. et al. (2004). Plasmapheresis, CMV hyperimmune globulin, and anti-CD20 allow ABO-incompatible renal transplantation without splenectomy. *American Journal of Transplantation,* Vol.4, No.8, (n.d.), pp.1315-1322, ISSN 1600-6135

Squifflet, J. et al. (2004). Lessons learned from ABO-incompatible living donor kidney transplantation: 20 years later. *Experimental Clinical Transplantation,* Vol.2, No.1, (n.d.), pp.208-213.

Stasi, R. et al. (2008). Analysis of regulatory T-cell changes in patients with idiopathic thrombocytopenic purpura receiving B cell-depleting therapy with rituximab. *Blood,* Vol.112, No.4, (n.d.), pp.1147-1150, ISSN 0006-4971

Stastny, P. et al. (2006). Four short projects about antibodies, soluble CD30, and organ transplant rejection. In: *Clinical transplants 2006,* Terasaki, P., pp.337-342, Terasaki foundation Laboratory, ISBN 978-1-880318-15-7,Los Angeles, CA

Stastny, P. et al. (2009). Role of immunoglobulin (Ig)-G and IgM antibodies against donor human leukocyte antigens in organ transplant recipients. *Human Immunology,* Vol.70, No.8, (n.d.), pp.600-604.

Stegall, M.; Dean, P. & Gloor, J. (2009). Mechanisms of alloantibody production in sensitized renal allograft recipients- Am J *Transplantation,* Vol.9, No.5, (n.d.), pp.998-1005.

Sturgill, B.; Lobo, P. & Bolton, W. (1984).Cold-reacting IgM antibody-induced renal allograft failure. Similarity to hyperacute rejection. *Nephron*, Vol.36, No.2, (n.d.), pp.125-127

Sugiyama, K. et al. (2005). Reversibility from delayed hyperacute rejection in ABO-incompatible renal transplantation: histopathological findings of renal allograft biopsy. *Transplantation Proceedings,* Vol.37, No.2, (n.d.), pp.701-704.

Sumitran-Holgersson, S. (2001). HLA-specific alloantibodies and renal graft outcome. *Nephrology Dialysis and Transplantation,* Vol.16, No.5, (n.d.), pp.897-904.

Sumitran-Karuppan, S. et al. (1997). Hyperacute rejections of two consecutive renal allografts and early loss of the third transplant caused by non-HLA antibodies specific for endothelial cells. *Transplant Immunology,* Vol.5, No.4, (n.d.), pp.321-327, ISSN 0966-3274

Supon P. et al. (2001). Prevalence of donor-specific anti-HLA antibodies during episodes of renal allograft rejection. *Transplantation,* Vol.7, No.14, (n.d.), pp.577-580, ISSN 0041-1337

Susal, C. & Opelz, G. (2002). Kidney graft failure and presensitization against HLA class I and class II antigens. *Transplantation,* Vol.73, No.8, (n.d.), pp.1269-1273.

Tabata, T. et al. (2003). Accommodation after lung xenografting from hamster to rat. *Transplantation,* Vol.75, No.5, (n.d.), pp.607-612

Takemoto, S. (1995). Sensitization and Crossmatch. In: *Clinical Transplants,* Terasaki, P., pp.417-432. Astellas Pharma US, Inc., ISBN 0890-9016, Los Angeles, CA

Takemoto, S. et al. (2004). HLA matching for kidney transplantation. *Human Immunology,* Vol.65, No.12, (n.d.), pp.1489-1505,

Tanabe, K. (2007). Japanese experience of ABO-incompatible living kidney transplantation. *Transplantation,* Vol.84, No.12, (Suppl. 1), (n.d.), pp. 4-7.

Terasaki, P. (2003). Humoral theory of transplantation. *American Journal of Transplantation,* Vol.3, No.6, (n.d.), pp.665-673.

Terasaki, P. & Cai, J. (2008). Human leukocyte antigen antibodies and chronic rejection: from association to causation. *Transplantation,* Vol.86, No.3, (n.d.), pp.377-383.

Terasaki, P. & Cai, J. (2005). Humoral theory of transplantation: further evidence. *Current Opinions in Immunology,*

Vol.17, No.5, (n.d.), pp.541-545, ISSN 0952-7915

Thielke, J. et al. (2005). Highly successful living donor kidney transplantation after conversion to negative of a previously positive flow-cytometry cross-match by pretransplant plasmapheresis. *Transplantation Proceedings,* Vol.37, No.2, (n.d.), pp.643-644.

Tobian, A. et al. (2009). Therapeutic plasma exchange reduces ABO titers to permit ABO-incompatible renal transplantation. *Transfusion,* Vol.49, No.6, (n.d.), pp.1248-1254, ISSN 0041-1132

Toyoda, M. (2004). Modulation of anti-class I, anti-class II and anti-endothelial cell antibodies by intravenous gammaglobulin (IVIG) improves transplant rates and reduces allograft rejection in highly-sensitized patients. *American Journal of Transplantation,* Vol.4, No.10, (n.d.), pp.550-556, ISSN 1600-6135

Toyofuku, A. et al. (2006). Natural killer T-cells participate in rejection of islet allografts in the liver of mice. *Diabetes,* Vol.55, No.1, (n.d.), pp.34-39.

Tsang J. et al. (2007). Generation of CD4+CD25+ regulatory T cells with indirect alloresponses by T cell receptor gene transfer: A novel therapeutic agent for the induction of transplantation tolerance. *American Journal of Transplantation*, Vol.7, No.9, (n.d.), pp.172-180. ISSN 1600-6135

Tyden, G. et al. (2005). ABO incompatible kidney transplantations without splenectomy, using antigen-specific immunoadsorption and rituximab. *Transplantation Proceedings*, Vol.37, No.8, (n.d.), pp.145-148, ISSN 1600-6135

Tyden, G. (2007). The European experience. *Transplantation*, Vol.84, No.12, (n.d.), pp.1-3.

Tyden, G. (2010). ABO-incompatible kidney transplantation and rituximab. *Transplantation*, Vol.74, No.8, pp.11-7

Vaidya, S. et al. (1998). Relative risk of post-transplant renal thrombosis in patients with antiphospholipid antibodies. *Clinical Transplantation*, Vol.12, No.5, (n.d.), pp.439-444.

Vaidya, S. et al. (2001). Pronase improves detection of HLA antibodies in flow crossmatches. *Transplantation Proceedings*, Vol.33, No.1-2, (n.d.), pp.473-474, ISSN 0041-1345

Vaidya, S. et al. (2007). DP reactive antibody in a zero mismatch renal transplant pair. *Human Immunology*,

Vol.68, No.11, (n.d.), pp.947-949

Valli, P. et al. (2009). Changes of circulating antibody levels induced by ABO antibody adsorption for ABO-incompatible kidney transplantation. *American Journal of Transplantation*, Vol.9, No.5, (n.d.), pp.1072-1080.

Vanderwoude, F. et al. (1995). Tissue Antigens in Tubulointerstitial and Vascular Rejection. *Kidney International*, Vol.48, No. 4, (n.d.), pp.11-13, ISSN 0085-2538

Vasilescu, E. et al. (2004). Anti-HLA antibodies in heart transplantation. *Transplant Immunology*, Vol.12, No.2, (n.d.), pp.177-183.

Vella, J. (2004). Significance of anticardiolipin antibodies on short- and long-term allograft survival and function following kidney transplantation. *American Journal of Transplantation*, Vol.4, No.11, (n.d.), pp.1731-1732, ISSN 1600-6135

Vincent, R. et al. (1996). Quantitative analysis of the expression of the HLA-DRB genes at the transcriptional level by competitive polymerase chain reaction. *Journal of Immunology*, Vol.156, No.2, (n.d.), pp.603-610, ISSN 0022-1767

Vo, A. et al. (2008). Rituximab and intravenous immune globulin for desensitization during renal transplantation. *New England Journal of Medicine*, Vol.359, No.3, pp.242-251, ISSN 0028-4793

Vo, A. et al. (2010). Use of Intravenous Immune Globulin and Rituximab for Desensitization of Highly HLA-Sensitized Patients Awaiting Kidney Transplantation. *Transplantation*, Vol.89, No.9, (n.d.), pp.1095-1102, ISSN 0041-1337

Wagenknecht, D. et al. (2000). Risk of early renal allograft failure is increased for patients with antiphospholipid antibodies- *Transplant International*, Vol.13, Suppl. 1, (n.d.), pp.78-81.

Walsh, R. et al. (2010). Proteasome Inhibitor-Based Primary Therapy for Antibody-Mediated Renal Allograft Rejection. *Transplantation*, 893, (n.d.), pp.277-284, ISSN 0041-1337

Wang-Rodriguez, J. & Rearden, A. (1995). Effect of crossmatching on outcome in organ transplantation. *Critical Reviews in Clinical and Laboratory Science*,Vol.32, No.4, (n.d.), pp.345-376.

Warren, D.; Zachary, A. & Sonnenday, C. (2004). Successful renal transplantation across simultaneous ABO incompatible and positive crossmatch barriers. *American Journal of Transplantation,* Vol.4, No.4, (April 2004), pp.561-568, ISSN 1600-6135

Watanabe, J. & Scornik, J. (2005). IVIG and HLA antibodies. Evidence for inhibition of complement activation but not for anti-idiotypic activity. *American Journal of Transplantation,* Vol.5, No.11, (n.d.), pp.2786-2790.

Weinstein, R. (2003). Basic Principles of Therapeutic Blood Exchange. In: *Apheresis: principles and practice,* McLeod, B. & Weinstein, R., pp.295-320, AABB Press, ISBN 1563951703, Bethesda, MD

Williams KA; Hart, D.N.; Fabre, J.W. 1980Distrinution and quantitation of HLA-ABC and DR (Ia) antigens on human kidney and other tissues. *Transplantation,* Vol.29, No. 4, (n.d.), pp.274-279.

Winters, J. et al. (2004). Plasma exchange conditioning for ABO-incompatible renal transplantation. *Journal of clinical apheresis,* Vol.19, No.2, (April 2004), pp.79-85, ISSN 0733-2459

Worthington, J. et al. (2003). Posttransplantation production of donor HLA-specific antibodies as a predictor of renal transplant outcome. *Transplantation,* Vol.75, No.7, (n.d.), pp.1034-1040, ISSN 0041-1337

Yabu, J. et al. (2011). C1q-Fixing Human Leukocyte Antigen Antibodies Are Specific for Predicting Transplant Glomerulopathy and Late Graft Failure After Kidney Transplantation. *Transplantation,* Vol.91, No.3, (February 2011), pp.342-347

Yard, B. et al. (1993). The Clinical Significance of Allospecific Antibodies Against Endothelial Cells Detected with An Antibody Dependent Cellular Cytotoxicity Assay for Vascular Rejection and Graft Loss After Renal Transplantation. *Transplantation,* Vol.55, No.6, (June 1993), pp.1287-1293, ISSN 0041-1337

Yoo, Z. et al. (1995). Human IL-17 - A Novel Cytokine Derived from T-Cells. *Journal of Immunology,* Vol.155, No.12, (December 1995), pp.5483-5486.

Yung, G. et al. (2007). Flow cytometric measurement of ABO antibodies in ABO-incompatible living donor kidney transplantation. *Transplantation,* Vol.84, No.12, Suppl. 3, (n.d.), pp.20-31.

Zachary, A. et al. (2003). Specific and durable elimination of antibody to donor HLA antigens in renal-transplant patients. *Transplantation,* Vol.76, No.10, (November 2003), pp.1519-1525

Zachary, A.; Montgomery, R. & Leffell, M. (2005). Factors associated with and predictive of persistence of donor-specific antibody after treatment with plasmapheresis and intravenous immunoglobulin. *Human Immunology,* Vol.66, No.4, (n.d.), pp.364-370.

Zachary, A. et al. (2009).Naturally occurring interference in Luminex assays for HLA-specific antibodies: characteristics and resolution. *Human Immunology,* Vol.70, No.7, (April 2009) pp.496-501

Zachary, A. et al. (2009). Using real data for a virtual crossmatch. *Human Immunology,* Vol.70, No.8, (n.d.), pp.574-579.Zeevi, A. et al. (2009). Emerging role of donor-specific anti-human leukocyte antigen antibody determination for clinical management after solid organ transplantation. *Human Immunology,* Vol.70, No.8, (n.d.), pp.645-650.

Zemmour, J. & Parham, P. (1992). Distinctive Polymorphism at the HLA-C Locus - Implications for the Expression of HLA-C. *Journal of Experimental Medicine,* Vol.176, No.4, (November 1992), pp.937-950, ISSN 0022-1007

Zilow, G.; Kirschfink, M. & Roelcke, D. (1994). Red-Cell Destruction in Cold Agglutinin Disease. *Infusiontherapy and Transfusionmedicine,* Vol.21, No.6, (December 1994), pp.410-415, ISSN 1019-8466

Zwirner, N. et al. (2006). Immunobiology of the human MHC class I chain-related gene A (MICA): from transplant immunology to tumor immune escape. *Immunologia,* Vol.25, No.1, (n.d.), pp.25-38.

3

Urothelial Carcinoma in Renal Transplant Recipients

Ming-Kuen Lai[1], Shuo-Meng Wang[2] and Huai-Ching Tai[2]
[1]*Department of Surgery/Division of Urology, Chang Gung University/Chang Gung Memorial Hospital, Taoyuan,*
[2]*Department of Urology, National Taiwan University Hospital , Taipei, Taiwan*

1. Introduction

The risk of renal transplant recipients to develope malignant disease is significantly higher than these in general population. The incidence of malignancy is estimated to be around 15-20% of renal recipients 10 years after renal transplantation and increases as high as 49.6% after 20 years.(Alberu, 2010; Kapoor, 2008; Penn, 2000; Gaya, et al, 1995). The most common malignancies are skin carcinomas and lymphomas (Lutz & Heemann, 2003). The immunosuppressive agents play an important role in contributing to such happenings. United Network for Organ Sharing (UNOS) registry data demonstrated that mammalian target of rapamycin (mTOR) inhibitors is associated with a reduced incidence of tumors compared to regimens that do not utilize mTOR-inhibitor (Rama & Grinyo, 2010). In UK transplant registry (UKTR) database, 1.9% of patients were reported to have a subsequent urological malignancy after renal transplantation (Besarani & Cranston, 2007).

2. Urothelial carcinoma after kidney transplantation

2.1 Urologic cancer after kidney transplantation

With increasing age of donor and recipient, the risk of post-transplant malignancy including genitourinary cancers is increasing. Urologists have an increasing likelihood of treating these cases. Melchior et al reported 29 urological de novo malignancies [12 renal cell carcinoma, 8 urothelial carcinoma (6 bladder, 2 renal pelvis), 7 carcinoma of the prostate, 2 seminoma] developed in a series of 802 patients after renal transplantation (Melchior et al, 2011). The overall incidence of urological neoplasms varied from 0.38% to 3.1% (Ravaud et al, 2010). Urothelial carcinoma (UC) of the bladder is not common in Western countries (Master et al, 2004) while it is the most common genitourinary tumor following kidney transplantation in China, Iran, Taiwan and Thailand (Einollahi et al, 2009; Ativitavas et al, 2008). Among the Chinese population, urological malignancies, especially UC, are an important complication after renal transplanatation (Zhou et al, 2006). In some areas around the world, the incidence of UC (or "transitional cell carcinoma, TCC") of the urinary tract in renal transplant recipients is singificantly higher than other parts of world. Majority of previous studies showing increased incidence of UC in renal transplant recipients came from Taiwan where it was attributed to environmental and occupational factors (Husain et

al, 2009). Urinary tract UC is the leading de novo malignancy following renal transplantation in Taiwan followed by hepatoma (Wang et al, 2010; Hung et al, 2007; Liao et al, 2004; Kang et al, 2004; Kao et al, 2003; Wang et al, 2002; Yang et al, 1998). This is very different from the Western countries or other Asian countries such as Japan, Korea.
Wu at al from Taiwan reported that as high as 17.5% of renal transplanta recipients developed urinary tract UC at 10 years after transplantation. Compared with the general population in Taiwan, the standardized mortality ratio (SMR) was 398.4 among renal transplant recipients and the SMR was much higher among female patients (875.6). Painless gross hematuria was the cardinal initial symptom in 73.3% of patients (Wu et al, 2004). The male to female ratio is reported to be 1:1.7~3.5. Female predominance among these patients is uniformly found in the reports from Taiwan and China (Liao et al, 2004; Wu et al, 2004; Li et al, 2009; Wang et al, 2010). However, in our early report, although uremic patients were at greater risk of developing urologic cancer, UC was uncommon among the renal transplant recipients (Chen et al, 1995).

2.2 Carcinogenesis of urothelial carcinoma in renal transplant recipients

Among the general population, only 5% of UC arise in the upper urinary tract (UUT) and only 2.5% involved bilaterally. UUT-UC is restricted to the renal pelvis in 58% of cases, 35% in the ureter, especially in the distal ureter. Many environmental factors have been reported to contribute to the development of these cancers. Some are quite similar to bladder cancer-associated factors related to occupational and environmental exposure such as tobacco, industrial dye and certain aromatic amines, etc, while others are more specific to the carcinogenesis of the UC such as analgesic, Balkan endemic nephropathy (BEN), Chinese herb nephropathy (CHN) or association with Blackfoot disease (BFD) (Hall et al, 1998; Colin et al, 2009). In Western countries, analgesic nephropathy (AN) is implicated to contribute to development of UC following renal transplantation. UC occurred more frequently in the AN group (2.8%) than these in the control group (0.49%) (Swindle et al, 1998). In Taiwan, older age at kidney transplantation, female recipient, compound analgesics usage, Chinese herb usage, underground water intake and low educational status were the significant risk factors for the development of de novo UC (Wang et al, 2010; Liao et al, 2004).

2.2.1 Chinese herb nephropathy (Aristolochic acid nephropathy)

Chinese herbs nephropathy after taking a slimming regimen including Chinese herbs contaminated with Aristolochia fangchi was reported by Belgium groups. These patients experinced a rapid progression to renal failure compared with other interstitial nephropathies. Many patients developed UC (Vanherweghem et al, 1993; Reginster et al, 1997; Cosyns et al, 1998). Aristolochic acid contained in Chinese herbs has been proved to be nephrotoxic and carcinogenic (Thon et al, 1995). Li et al from China reported a 2-center cohort of 1,612 renal transplant recipients, the patients with aristolochic acid nephropathy (AAN) had significantly higher incidence of UC (52.9% vs 0.46% in the control group) (Li et al, 2009). Among these patienst, 88.9% involved the upper urinary tract (37.5% bilateral, 62.5% unilateral). It was more common to see UC cases in the female patients (male to female ratio of 1:3.5). These are very similar to the happenings in Taiwan, i.e., high incedence of UC in the upper urinary tract and female predominence (Hung et al, 2007; Liao et al, 2004; Kang et al, 2004; Kao et al, 2003). Bilateral nephroureterectomy has been a standard procedure for these patients. Synchronous UC in bilateral upper urinary tracts was confirmed in 36.7% of cases (Wu et al, 2004). Among the patients with bilateral upper tract UC, only 25% had bilateral abnormalities in preoperative image studies (Liao et al, 2004). High incidence rate of UUT-UC has been described in some rural areas of the Balkans after year 1950, but it has been decreased significantly in recent 20 years (Markovic et al, 2005). Bilateral involvement (8–10%) and female predominance are the unique characterictics in these patients with BEN which are quite similar to the cases with CHN. Several studies have shown the carcinogenic potential of aristolochic acid contained in Aristolochia fangchi (contamination in some Chinese herbs) and Aristolochia clematis (a plant popularly present in the farm field of the Balkans) (Arlt et al, 2007; Laing et al, 2006; Nortier et al, 2000; Consyns et al, 1999). Debelle et al. proposed to combine BEN and CHN under one name, i.e., aristolochic acid nephropathy (Debelle et al, 2008). Chen et al reported an incresed risk for the professional personels working with Chinese herb medicine to develop chronic renal failure and urinary tract cancer. The age-adjusted relative risks of these professional personels to develop urinary tract cancer were 3.81 for male and 5.86~9.32 for female subjects. This finding supports the hypothesis that urinary tract cancer in Chinese herbalists could be related to the long-term exposure of aristolochic acid -containing herbal medicines (Chen et al, 2009; Yang et al, 2009). Lai et al using the reimbursement database of National Health Insurance from Taiwan to study 4594 patients and 174,701 control subjects (Lai et al, 2010). There was a statistically significant linear dose–response relationship between the cumulative dose of aristolochic acid and the risk of developing urinary tract cancer. Consumption of aristolochic acid–containing Chinese herbal medicine was associated with an increased risk of developing cancer of the urinary tract in a dose-dependent manner and it is independent of arsenic exposure.

2.2.2 Arsenic intoxication

An unusually high incidence of UUT-UC has been described in Taiwan. It occurred in the south-west part of Taiwan where the population was particularly susceptible to the development of UUT-UC which represented 20–25% of all UC cases. This area corresponds to the endemic area of Blackfoot disease (BFD), which is known to be a thromboangiitis of lower limbs leading to gangrene. The majority of cases required amputation of lower limbs. Contamination of drinking water with arsenic has been considered to be the reason for this endemic disease. The cases of UUT-UC in the endemic area of BFD are characterized by female predominance (male to female ratio of 1:2) and more ureteral tumors (twice as common as the renal pelvis tumors) (Tan et al, 2008; Yang et al, 2002; Chiou et al 2001, Chiang et al, 1993). The prevalence of UC in the BFD endemic area improved significantly after the government modernized the water supply system. However, for some reasons, the prevalence of UC in this area is still higher than other parts of Taiwan (Yang et al, 2005; Yang et al, 2002). Arsenic exposure is associated with an increased risk of UC. UC patients had a significantly higher sum of measured urinary arsenic species including inorganic arsenic, monomethylarsonic acid and dimethylarsinic acid (Pu et al, 2002; Chung et al, 2008). Arsenic intoxication also involves the formation of DNA adducts and DNA damage (Kato et al, 1994; Schwerdtle et al, 2003). Association between inorganic arsenic and UC risk focused on the total arsenic ingested from drinking water had been reported (Pu et al, 2002). Subjects of low exposure, were still observed to have higher UC risk in subjects with unfavorable urinary arsenic profile, i.e., pooreer function of arsenic methylation. The primary methylation index (PMI) was defined as the ratio between monomethylarsonic acid and inorganic arsenic. Secondary methylation index (SMI) was defined as the ratio between dimethylarsinic acid and monomethylarsonic acid. Unfavorable PMI and SMI levels indicate an increased risk of developing UC, especially in non-smokers although smoking has been well documented to cause carcionogesis of UC (Zeegers et al, 2000). Undetectable or negligible environmental arsenic still plays an important role (Chung et al, 2008). The arsenic levels allowed in drinking water is not greater than 5µg/L. The WHO established the water quality guidelines for drinking water which included the arsenic levels to be undetectable to less than 10µg/L (WHO 1996/1998). Actually, the average arsenic concentration in Taipei City, the capital of Taiwan, is ranged from undetectable level to 4.0 µg/L. Smoking is associated with an increased risk of UC in a dose dependent manner (Kato et al, 1994). Arsenic contamination in drinking water and smoking are synergestic in the carcinogesis of UC (Chung et al, 2008).

2.2.3 Role of virus in the carcinogenesis of urothelial carcinoma

Polyoma virus (PV), BK virus (BKV), human papillomavirus may play a role in the pathogesis of UC following renal transplantation. There is lack of data to indicate a definitive association between BKV and human cancers (Noel et al, 1994; Husain et al, 2009; Abend et al, 2009; Wang et al, 2009; Roberts et al, 2008; Chen et al, 2010). Presence of polyoma virus in the biopsy specimen may mimick high grade transitional cell carcinoma (Seftel et al, 1996).

2.2.4 Urothelial carcinoma in hemodialysis patients and renal transplant recipients

In Taiwan, UC is the most common type of urological cancer in patients with end stage renal disease (Chang et al, 2007). The cumulative incidence of UC was between 0.77% to 1.7% in hemodialysis patients and 3.1% to 4.1% in renal transplant recipients. The cases of UC in hemodialysis patients and renal transplant recipients have similar characteristics of BEN, CHN and BFD. As compared with the incidence of UC in the general population of Taiwan (10.09/100,000), the standardized incidence ratio of UC in hemodialysis is very high (48.2). Women and middle-aged patients had a higher risk. Physicians who are taking care of hemodialysis patients and renal transplant recipients should be highly alert with presence of hematuria which warrants detailed study of the entire urinary system and image study of the native and transplanted kidneys (Wang et al, 2010; Tai et al, 2009; Liao et al, 2004). Only 19.4% of patients had history of long-term consumption of Chinese herbs and 3.1% had history of using analgesic compounds (Wang et al, 2011). Contamination of drinking water is considered to be another carcinogenic factor.

3. Treatment of Urothelial carcinoma after kidney transplantation

Patients with upper tract lesions are recommended to undergo bilateral nephroureterectomy and bladder cuff resection in one session or in separate sessions (Glassman et al, 2001; Kao et al, 2004; Zhang et al, 2009). Whether postoperative intravesical instillation of chemotherapeutic agents reduces the incidence of bladder recurrence is debating. Wu et al reported that intravesical instillation of epirubicin or mitomycin C appeared to be effective in preventing bladder recurrence and in prolonging time to first bladder recurrence (Wu et al, 2010). Transurethral resection of the bladder tumor is indicated in patients with concomitant or superficial bladder lesions. Intravesical chemotherapy is started after transurethral resection and immunosuppressants are adjusted (Li et al, 2008). Laparoscopic bilateral nephroureterectomy and bladder cuff excision can be performed safely and gives similar oncologic results in experinced hands (Chen et al, 2003; Liao et al, 2004). Laparoscopic bilateral nephroureterectomy can be performed in a single session without repositioning of the patient if a specially designed inflatable cuff is used (Chueh et al, 2002). Retroperitoneal laparoscopic nephroureterectomy with bladder cuff excision can be safely performed by combining cystoscopic resection with open transperitoneal dissection. This might be a safe and feasible alternative for native UUT-UC ipsilateral to a transplanted kidney (Ye et al, 2010). Lymphovascular invasion was reported to be the only significant predictor of cancer specific survival in the univariate and multivariate analyses (Chung et al, 2009). The benefit of routine lymphadenectomy during nephroureterectomy of UC is debatable. The benefit of conversion from calcineurin inhibitors to mammalian targe of rapamycin (mTOR) inhibitors (proliferation signal inhibitors) is another debating issue. Many patients experinced recurrence of UC after bilateral nephroureterctomy and conversion to mTOR inhibitors (Chung et al, 2008; Wang et al 2008; Hu et al, 2009). Systemic chemotherapy can be performed on these patients safely and effectively (Matzkies et al, 2000; Lin et al, 2006).

4. Conclusion

UC is the leading cause of malignancy in renal transplant recipeints in some Asian countries such as China, Iran, Taiwan, Thailand, etc. It is characterized with female predominance, frequent bilateral upper urinary tract lesions. The pathogenesis of UC in renal transplant recipients is still under investigation. Aristolochic acid, arsenic intoxication, smoking and some virus may play important and complicated roles. Transplant physicians should be very alert with hematuria, hydronephrosis of native urinary tract which frequently implicates presence of UC. Bilateral nephroureterectomy in a single session or in separate sessions is recommended

5. References

Abend, JR., Mengxi Jiang, M.& Imperiale, MJ. (2009). BK Virus and Human Cancer: Innocent until Proven Guilty. *Seminar of Cancer Biology*. Vol. 19, No. 4, pp. 252–260.

Alberu, J. (2010). Clinical insights for cancer outcomes in renal transplant patients. *Transplantation Proceedings*. Vol. 42, No.9 Suppl, pp.S36-40.

Arlt, VM., Stiborova, M., vom Brocke, J.,.Simo˜es, ML., Lord, GH., Nortier , JL., Hollstein, M., Phillips, DH.& Schmeiser , HH. (2007). Aristolochic acid mutagenesis: molecular clues to the aetiology of Balkan endemic nephropathy-associated urothelial cancer. *Carcinogenesis*. Vol. 28, No.11, pp.2253-2261.

Ativitavas, T., Jirasiritham, S., Ngorsakun, P., Pipatpannawong, K.& Mavichak, V. (2008). Malignancies in renal transplant patients: 15 years experience in Thailand. *Transplantation Proceedings*. Vol. 40, No.7, pp.2403-2404.

Besarani, D., Cranston, D. (2007) Urological malignancy after renal transplantation. *British Journal of Urology International*. Vol. 100, No.3, pp.502-505.

Chang, CH., Yang, CM.& Yang,AH.(2007). Renal diagnosis of chronic hemodialysis patients with urinary tract transitional cell carcinoma in Taiwan. *Cancer*. Vol. 109, Issue 8, pp. 1487–1492.

Chen, CH.,Huan, SK., Lin, JT.& Chiu, AW. (2003). Laparoscopic bilateral nephroureterectomy and bladder cuff excision for native renal pelvic and ureteral transitional cell carcinoma after renal transplantation. *Journal of Postgraduate Medicine*. Vol. 49,No.2,pp.148-150.

Chen, CH., Wen, MC., Wang, M., Lian, JD., Cheng, CH., Wu, MJ., Yu, TM., Chuang YW., Chang, D.,& Shu, KH. (2010). High incidence of malignancy in polyomavirus-associated nephropathy in renal transplant recipients.

Transplantation Proceedings. Vol. 42,No.3, pp.817-8.

Chen, KS., Lai, MK., Huang, CC., Chu, SH.& Leu, ML. (1995). Urologic cancers in uremic patients. *American Journal of Kidney Diseases*. Vol.25, No.5, pp.694-700.

Chen, PC., Chang, PJ.& Wang, JD. (2009). Chronic Renal Failure and Urinary Tract Cancer in Chinese Herbalists: Implications for the Safety Issues of Herbal Medicine. *Epidemiology*. Vol. 20,Issue 6 , pp.S200.

Chiang, HS., Guo, HR., Hong, CL., Lin, SM.& Lee, GF. (1993). The incidence of bladder cancer in the black foot disease endemic area in Taiwan. *British Journal of Urology*. , pp. 274–278.

Chiou, HY., Chiou, ST., Hsu, YH., Chou, YL., Tseng, CH., Wei, ML.& Chen, CJ. (2001). Incidence of transitional cell carcinoma and arsenic in drinking water: a follow-up study of 8102 residents in an arseniasis-endemic area in northeastern Taiwan. *American Journal of Epidemiology*. Vol. 153, No.5, pp. 411-418.

Chueh, SC., Chen, J., Hsu, WT., Hsieh, MH.& Lai, MK. (2002). Hand assisted laparoscopic bilateral nephroureterectomy in 1 session without repositioning patients is facilitated by alternating inflation cuffs. *Journal of Urology*. Vol.167, No.1, pp.44-47.

Chung, CJ., Huang, CJ., Pu, YS., Su, CT., Huang, YK., Chen, YT.& Hsueh, YM. (2008). Urinary 8-hydroxydeoxyguanosine and urothelial carcinoma risk in low arsenic exposure area. *Toxicology and Applied Pharmacology*. Vol. 226, Issue 1, pp.14–21.

Chung, SD., Lai, MK., Wang, SM., Liao, CH., Yu, HJ. & Chueh, SC. (2008). Urothelial carcinoma in kidney transplant recipients: conversion from calcineurin inhibitor to proliferation signal inhibitor? Comment on: Am J Kidney Dis. 2008 Mar;51(3):471-7. *American Journal of Kidney Disease*. Vol. 52, No.3, pp.630; author reply 631.

Chung, SD., Wang, SM., Lai, MK., Huang, CY., Liao, CH.;,Huang, KH., Pu, YS.; Chueh, SC.& Yu, HJ. (2009).Lymphovascular invasion predicts poor outcome of urothelial carcinoma of renal pelvis after nephroureterectomy. *British Journal of Urology International*. Vol. 103, No.8, pp.1047-1051.

Colin, P., Koenig, P., Ouzzane, A., Berthon, N., Villers, A., Biserte, J.& Rouprêt, M (2009).Environmental factors involved in carcinogenesis of urothelial cell carcinomas of the upper urinary tract. *British Journal of Urology International*. Vol. 104, No.10, pp.1436–1440.

Consyns, JP., Jadoul, M., Squifflet, JP., Wese, FX.& van Ypersels de,.SC. (1999). Urothelial lesions in Chinese-herb nephropathy. *American Journal of Kidney Disease*. Vol. 33, Issue 6, pp.1011–1017.

Cosyns, JP., Goebbels, RM., Liberton, V., Schmeiser, HH., Bieler, CA. & Bernard ,AM. (1998). Chinese herbs nephropathy-associated slimming regimen induces tumours in the forestomach but no interstitial nephropathy in rats. *Archives of Toxicology*. Vol.72, No.11, pp.738-743.

Debelle, FD.; Vanherweghem, JL.; Nortier, JL. (2008). Aristolochic acid nephropathy: a worldwide problem. *Kidney International.* Vol. 74, No.2, pp.158-169.

Einollahi,B., Simforoosh,N., Lessan-Pezeshki, M., Basiri, A., Nafar, M., Pour-Reza Gholi, F., Firouzan, A., Ahmadpour, P., Makhdomi, K., Ghafari, A., Taghizadeh, A., & Tayebi Khosroshahi, H. (2009). Genitourinary tumor following kidney transplantation: a multicenter study. *Transplantation Proceedings.* Vol. 41, No.7, pp.2848-2849.

Gaya, SB., Rees, AJ., Lechler, RI., Williams, G. & Mason, PD. (1995). Malignant disease in patients with long-term renal transplants. *Transplantation.* Vol. 59 No. 12, pp.1705-1709.

Glassman, DT. & Sklar, GN. (2001). Complete genitourinary exenteration for multifocal transitional cell carcinoma in renal transplant recipient. *Journal of Urology.* Vol.166, No.3, pp.986-987.

Hall, MC., Womack,S., Sagalowsky,AI., Carmody,T.; Erickstad,MD.& Roehrborn,CG. (1998). Prognostic factors, recurrence, and survival in transitional cell carcinoma of the upper urinary tract: a 30-year experience in 252 patients. *Urology.* Vol.52, No.4, pp.594-601.

Hu, XP., Ma, L., Wang, Y., Yin, H., Wang, W., Yang, XY.& Zhang, XD. (2009). Rapamycin instead of mycophenolate mofetil or azathioprine in treatment of post-renal transplantation urothelial carcinoma. *Chinese Medical Journal.* Vol. 122, No.1 , pp.35-38.

Hung, YM., Chou, KJ., Hung, SY., Chung, HM.& Chang, JC. (2007). De novo malignancies after kidney transplantation. *Urology.* Vol. 69, No.6, pp.1041-1044.

Husain, E., Prowse, DM., Ktori, E., Shaikh, T., Yaqoob, M., Junaid, I.& Baithun, S.(2009). Human papillomavirus is detected in transitional cell carcinoma arising in renal transplant recipients. *Pathology.* Vol. 41, No.3, pp.245-247.

Husain, E., Khawaja, A., Shaikh, T., Yaqoob, M., Junaid, I.& Baithun, S. (2009). Transitional cell carcinoma of the urinary tract in renal transplant recipients. *Pathology.* Vol. 41, No.4, pp.406-408.

Kang, CH., Yu, TJ., Hsieh, HH., Yang, JW., Shu, K.& Shiue, YL. (2004). Synchronous bilateral primary transitional cell carcinoma of the upper urinary tracts: ten patients with more than five years of follow-up. *Urology.* Vol.63, No.2, pp.380-382.

Kao, YL., Ou, YC., Yang, CR., Ho, HC., Su, CK. & Shu, KH. (2003). Transitional cell carcinoma in renal transplant recipients. *World Journal of Surgery.* Vol.27, No.8, pp.912-916.

Kao, YL., Yang, CR. & Chen, CH. (2004). Urinary exenteration on a renal transplant recipient with multifocal urothelial cancers and prostatic adenocarcinoma. Journal of the Chinese Medical Association. Vol.67, No. 8, pp.422-424.

Kapoor, A.(2008). Malignancy in kidney transplant recipients. Drugs, Vol. 68, No. Suppl 1, pp.11-9.

Kato, K., Hayashi,H., Hasegawa,A., Yamanaka,K.& Okada, S. (1994). DNA damage induced in cultured human alveolar (L-132) cells by exposure to dimethylarsinic acid. *Environmental Health Perspect.* Vol.102, Suppl 3, pp.285–288.

Lai, MN., Wang, SM., Chen,PC., Chen, YY.& Wang, JD. (2010).

Population-Based Case–Control Study of Chinese Herbal Products Containing Aristolochic Acid and Urinary Tract Cancer Risk. *Journal of National Cancer Institute.* Vol.102, No.3, pp.179–186.

Laing, C., Hamour, S., Sheaff, M., Miller, R.& Woolfson, R. (2006). Chinese herbal uropathy and nephropathy? *Lancet.* Vol.368, Issue 9545, pp.1416.

Li, HZ., Xia, M., Han, Y., Xu, XG..& Zhang, YS. (2009.). De novo urothelial carcinoma in kidney transplantation patients with end-stage aristolochic acid nephropathy in China. [Erratum appears in Urol Int. 2010;84(4):484] *Urologia Internationalis.* Vol.83, No.2, pp.200-205.

Li, XB., Xing, NZ., Wang, Y., Hu, XP., Yin, H.& Zhang, XD. (2008). Transitional cell carcinoma in renal transplant recipients: A single center experience. *International Journal of Urology.* Vol. 15, Issue 1, pp. 53–57.

Liao, CH., Chueh, SC., Lai, MK.& Chen J. (2004). Transitional cell carcinoma in renal transplant recipients. Transplantation Proceedings. Vol. 36, No.7, pp.2152-2153.

Lin, CC. , Hsu, CH. & Pu, YS. (2006).Complete response of urothelial carcinoma to chemotherapy in renal allograft recipients: a two-case study. *Anticancer Research.* Vol. 26, No.4B, pp.3191-3195.

Lutz, J., Heemann, U. (2003). Tumours after kidney transplantation. *Current Opinions in Urology.* Vol. 13, No.2, pp.105-109.

Markovic, N., Ignjatovic, I., Cukuranovic, R., Petrovic, B., Kocic, B.& Stefanovic, V. (2005). Decreasing incidence of urothelial cancer in a Balkan endemic nephropathy region in Serbia. A surgery based study from 1969 to 1998. *Pathologie Biologie.* Vol. 53, Issue 1, pp.26-29.

Master, VA., Meng, MV., Grossfeld, GD., Koppie, TM., Hirose, R. & Carroll, PR. (2004). Treatment and outcome of invasive bladder cancer in patients after renal transplantation. *Journal of Urology.* Vol. 171, No. 3, pp.1085-1088.

Matzkies, FK., Tombach, B., Dietrich, M., Kisters, K., Barenbrock, M., Schaefer, RM., Berdel, WE. & Rahn, KH. (2000). MVAC-therapy for advanced urothelial carcinoma in an anuric renal transplant recipient. *Nephrology Dialysis and Transplantation.* Vol. 15, No.1, pp.110-112.

Melchior, S., Franzaring, L., Shardan, A., Schwenke, C., Plumpe, A., Schnell, R., Dreikorn, K. (2011). Urological de novo malignancy after kidney transplantation: a case for the urologist. Journal of Urology. Vol. 185, No. 2, pp.428-432.

Noel, JC., Peny, MO., Mat, O., Antoine, M., Firket, C., Detremmerie, O., Thiry, L., Verhest, A. & Vereerstraeten, P. (1994). Human papillomavirus type 16 associated with multifocal transitional cell carcinomas of the bladder in two transplanted patients. *Transplant International.* Vol. 7, No.5, pp.340-343.

Nortier, JL., Martinez, MCM., Schmeiser, HH., Arlt, VM., Bieler, CA., Petein, M., Depierreux, MF., De Pauw, L., Abramowicz, D., Vereerstraeten, P.& Vanherweghem, JL. (2000). Urothelial carcinoma associated with the use of a Chinese herb (Aristolochia fangchi). *New England Journal of Medicine.* Vol. 342, No. 23, pp.1686-1692.

Penn, I.(2000). Cancers in renal transplant recipients. *Advance in Renal Replacement Therapy.* Vol. 7, No. 2, pp.147-156.

Pu, YS., Hour, TC., Chen, J., Huang, CY., Guan, JY.& Lu, SH. (2002).Arsenic trioxide as a novel anticancer agent against human transitional carcinoma-characterizing its apoptotic pathway. *Anti-Cancer Drugs.* Vol. 13, Issue 3 , pp.293-300.

Rama, I., Grinyo, JM. (2010). Malignancy after renal transplantation: the role of immunosuppression. *Nature Reviews in Nephrology.* Vol. 6, No.9, pp.511-519.

Ravaud, A., Ballanger, P., Ferriere, JM., Wallerand, H., Elkentaoui, H., Robert, G.., Pasticier, G.., Bernhard, JC., Couzi, L.& Merville, P. (2010). Therapeutic management of de novo urological malignancy in renal transplant recipients: the experience of the French Department of Urology and Kidney Transplantation from Bordeaux. *Urology.* Vol. 75, No. 1, pp.126-132.

Reginster, F., Jadoul, M.& van Ypersele de Strihou, C. (1997). Chinese herbs nephropathy presentation, natural history and fate after transplantation. *Nephrology Dialysis Transplantation.* Vol.12, No.1, pp.81-86.

Roberts, ISD., Besarani, D., Mason, P., Turner, G., Friend, PJ.& Newton, R. (2008). Polyoma virus infection and urothelial carcinoma of the bladder following renal transplantation. *British Journal of Cancer.* Vol. 99, No.9, pp.1383–1386.

Schwerdtle, T., Walter, I., Mackiw, I.& Hartwig, A. (2003). Induction of
oxidative DNA damage by arsenite and its trivalent and pentavalent
methylated metabolites in cultured human cells and isolated DNA. *Carcinogenesis.* Volume24, Issue5, pp.967-974.

Seftel, AD., Matthews, LA., Smith, MC. & Willis, J. (1996). Polyomavirus mimicking high grade transitional cell carcinoma. *Journal of Urology.* Vol.156,No. 5, pp. 1764

Swindle, P., Falk, M., Rigby, R., Petrie, J., Hawley, C.& Nicol, D. (1998). Transitional cell carcinoma in renal transplant recipients: the influence of compound analgesics. *British Journal of Urology.* Vol.81, No.2, pp.229-233.

Tai, HC., Lai, MK., Wang, SM., Chueh, SC. & Yu, HJ. (2009). High incidence of urinary tract malignancy among patients with haematuria following kidney transplantation in Taiwan. *Transplant International.* Vol.22, No. , pp.403–407.

Tan, LB., Chen, KT.& Guo, HR. (2008). Clinical and epidemiological features of patients with genitourinary tract tumour in a blackfoot disease endemic area of Taiwan. *British Journal of Urology International.* Vol. 102, No. 1, pp. 48-54.

Thon, WF., Kliem, V., Truss, MC., Anton, P., Kuczyk, M., Stief, CG..& Brunkhorst, R. (1995). Denovo urothelial carcinoma of the upper and lower urinary tract in kidney--transplant patients with end-stage analgesic nephropathy. *World Journal of Urology.* Vol.13, No.4, pp.254-261.

Vanherweghem, JL., Tielemans, C., Abramowicz, D., Depierreux, M., Vanhaelen-Fastre, R., Vanhaelen, M., Dratwa, M., Richard, C., Vandervelde, D., Verbeelen, D., & Jadoul,M. (1993). Rapidly progressive interstitial renal fibrosis in young women: association with slimming regimen including Chinese herbs. *Lancet.* Vol. 341, Issue 8842, pp. 387-391

Wang, HB., Hsieh, HH., Chen, YT., Chiang, CY.& Cheng YT. (2002). The outcome of post-transplant transitional cell carcinoma in 10 renal transplant recipients. *Clinical Transplantation.* Vol.16, No.6, pp.410-413.

Wang, HH., Liu, KL., Chu, SH., Tian, YC, Lai, PC.& Chiang, YJ. (2009). BK virus infection in association with posttransplant urothelial carcinoma. *Transplant Proceedings.* Volume 41, Issue 1, pp. 165-166.

Wang, LJ., Wong, YC.& Huang, CC. (2010). Urothelial carcinoma of the native ureter in a kidney transplant recipient. *Journal of Urology*. Vol.184, No.2, pp.728.

Wang, SM., Tai, HC., Chueh, SC., Chung, SD.& Lai, MK. (2008).Sirolimus does not absolutely abolish the occurrence/recurrence of urothelial carcinoma in renal transplant recipients. *Transplant Proceedings*. Vol. 40, No.7, pp.2395-2396.

Wang, TY., Hu, CJ., Kuo, CW., Chen, Y., Lin, JL., Yang, CW.& Yen, TH. (2011), High incidence and recurrence of transitional cell carcinoma in Taiwanese patients with end-stage renal disease. *Nephrology*. Vol. 16, Issue 2 , pp. 225–231.

WHO 1996/1998 Guidelines for Drinking Water Quality. Second edition (1996) Vol. 2, pp 940–949; and 1998 addendum to Vol. 2, pp 281–283. *World Health Organization*, Geneva.

Wu,MJ., Lian, JD., Yang, CR., Cheng, CH., Chen, CH., Lee, WC., Shu, KH.& Tang, MJ. (2004). High cumulative incidence of urinary tract transitional cell carcinoma after kidney transplantation in Taiwan. *American Journal of Kidney Diseases*. Vol.43, No.6, pp.1091-1097.

Wu, WJ., Ke, HL., Yang, YH., Li, CC., Chou, YH.& Huang, CH. (2010).Should patients with primary upper urinary tract cancer receive prophylactic intravesical chemotherapy after nephroureterectomy? *Journal of Urology*. Volume 183, Issue 1, pp.56-61.

Yang, CY., Chiu, HF., Chang, CC., Ho, SC.& Wu, TN. (2005). Bladder cancer mortality reduction after installation of a tap-water supply system in an arsenious-endemic area in southwestern Taiwan. *Environmental Research*. Vol. 98, No.1, pp.127–132.

Yang, HY., Wang, JD., Lo, TC.& Chen, PC. (2009). Increased Mortality Risk for Cancers of the Kidney and Other Urinary Organs among Chinese Herbalists. *Journal of Epidemiology*. Vol.19, No.1, pp.17-23.

Yang, MH., Chen, KK., Yen, CC., Wang, WS., Chang, YH., Huang, WJ., Fan, FS., Chiou, TJ., Liu, JH.& Chen, PM. (2002). Unusually high incidence of upper urinary tract urothelial carcinoma in Taiwan. *Urology*. Vol. 59, No.5, pp.681-687.

Yang, TC., Shu, KH., Cheng, CH., Wu, MJ.& Lian JD. (1998). Malignancy following renal transplantation. *Chung Hua i Hsueh Tsa Chih - Chinese Medical Journal*. Vol.61, No.5, pp.281-288.

Ye, J., Ma, L., Huang, Y., Hou, X., Xiao, C., Zhao, L., Wang, G., Hong, K. & Lu, J. (2010).Retroperitoneal laparoscopic nephroureterectomy with bladder cuff excision for native upper tract transitional cell carcinoma ipsilateral to a transplanted kidney. *Urology*. Vol. 76,No. 6, pp.1395-1399.

Zeegers, MP., Tan, FE., Dorant, E.& van Den Brandt, PA. (2000). The impact ofcharacteristics of cigarette smoking on urinary tract cancer risk: a metaanalysisof epidemiologic studies. *Cancer*. Vol. 89, Issue 3, pp.630–639.

Zhang, P., Wang, Y., Zhang, XD., Hu, XP., Wang, W., Zhang, Y. & Yin, H. (2009).Clinical character of renal transplant recipients with bilateral native upper urinary transitional cell carcinoma. *Chung-Hua i Hsueh Tsa Chih [Chinese Medical Journal]*. Vol. 89,No. 4, pp.248-250.

Zhou, M., Zhu, Y., Wang, L., Wang, Y., Fu, S.& Min, Z. (2006). Urological malignancy as a complication of renal transplantation: a report of twelve clinical cases. *Clinical Transplants*. pp.395-398.

4

Immune Monitoring of Kidney Recipients: Biomarkers to Appreciate Immunosuppression-Associated Complications

Philippe Saas, Jamal Bamoulid, Béatrice Gaugler and Didier Ducloux
UMR645, INSERM, EFS, Université de Franche-Comté –Service de Néphrologie, CHU, Besançon
France

1. Introduction

The use of nonspecific immunosuppressive drugs has significantly reduced the incidence of acute kidney graft rejection (Sayegh & Carpenter, 2004). This led to a significant improvement in first-year graft survival rates that are "almost close to perfect", as mentioned in a recent review (Lamb et al., 2011). However, the benefits of such immunosuppressive therapies on chronic rejection and overall long-term graft survival are uncertain (Meier-Kriescher et al., 2004a; McDonald et al., 2007). Thus, long term graft survival remains unchanged over decades (Meier-Kriescher et al., 2004a; Meier-Kriescher et al., 2004b). Persistent excessive immunosuppression −related to these immunosuppressive drugs− exposes renal transplant recipients to long-term toxicities including: increased incidence of cancers, severe infectious complications and "metabolic" diseases (for instance, diabetes, and accelerated atherosclerosis leading to cardiovascular diseases).
An excess risk of cancer after renal transplantation has been increasingly recognized over recent decades (Penn et al., 1979; Kasiske et al., 2004; Grulich et al., 2007; Villeneuve et al., 2007; Webster et al., 2007; van Leeuwen et al., 2009), as advances in medicine have extended the life of renal transplant recipients. A meta-analysis including five studies of cancer risks in organ transplant recipients, including 31'977 organ transplant recipients −among which 97% have received a kidney graft− from Denmark, Finland, Sweden, Australia, and Canada shows an increase in the incidence of cancers related to infection with Epstein-Barr virus (EBV), human herpesvirus 8 (HHV8), hepatitis viruses B and C (HBV and HCV), and *Helicobacter pylori* with comparison to the general population (Grulich et al., 2007). However, cancer incidence after transplantation is not restricted to virus-induced cancers, since kidney cancer, myeloma, leukaemia, melanoma as well as bladder and thyroid cancers are more frequent in transplant recipients than the general population (Grulich et al., 2007). Common epithelial cancers (e.g., breast and prostate) occur at the same rate as the general population (Grulich et al., 2007). However, despite a cancer incidence similar with the general population, an interesting study reported a highly aggressive course of tumors and unresponsiveness to "classical" anti-tumoral chemotherapy in renal transplant recipients (Fiebiger et al., 2009). This report confirmed a pioneer work (Barrett et al., 1993) showing the more aggressive course of cancers in renal transplant recipients. Thus, malignancy is now one of the leading causes of patient's

death with functional graft. A recent study analyzing 1'606 renal transplant recipients reports that malignancies accounted for 12 % of death among patients with a functioning renal allograft (Kahwaji et al., 2011). Immunosuppression and its extent directly influence cancer occurrence after transplantation (Dantal et al., 1998; van Leeuwen et al., 2009).

The other main cause of patient's death with functional graft is cardiovascular diseases (Kahwaji et al., 2011) related to accelerated atherosclerosis associated with kidney transplantation (Sarnak et al., 2003; Ojo, 2006). The incidence of cardiovascular diseases is at least 3 to 5 times higher than in the general population (Sarnak et al., 2003). For instance, while left ventricular hypertrophy prevalence in the general population is estimated to 20%, this prevalence increases to 50 to 70% in renal transplant recipients (Sarnak et al., 2003). Depending on the considered reports, cardiovascular disease is reported to be the most common cause of death in patients with functional graft ranging from 24% to 55% (Kasiske et al., 1996; Ojo et al., 2000; Sarnak et al., 2003; Kahwaji et al., 2011). Risk factors for cardiovascular diseases in renal transplant recipients are multiple. They include traditional cardiovascular disease risk factors (e.g., tobacco use, exercise, hypertension, diabetes, or hyperlipidemia), which are highly prevalent, as well as nontraditional risk factors related to a long history of poor kidney function (e.g., hyperhomocysteinemia, chronic inflammation or anemia) (Kasiske et al., 1996; Ducloux et al., 2000; Sarnak et al., 2003; Liefeldt & Budde, 2010; Kahwaji et al., 2011). Moreover, factors related to transplantation itself, including the direct effects of immunosuppression or rejection episodes as well as new-onset diabetes after transplant (NODAT), impact on cardiovascular disease occurrence after kidney transplantation (Kasiske et al., 1996; Sarnak et al., 2003; Ducloux et al., 2005a; Liefeldt & Budde, 2010; Kahwaji et al., 2011).

Thus, it appears that excessive immunosuppression is involved in both increased cancer and cardiovascular disease incidence observed after kidney transplantation. A greater understanding of risk factors leading to excessive immunosuppression may help physicians to determine high-risk recipient profiles and optimize pre- and post-transplantation treatment strategies. In other words, identification of biomarkers predictive of immunosuppression-associated complications may improve late kidney transplantation outcome. In this chapter, we will report efforts of our laboratory to identify immunological factors that can predict the two main complications associated with kidney transplantation, namely cancer and accelerated atherosclerosis that leads to cardiovascular diseases. We focus on: i) $CD4^+$ T cell lymphopenia, a consequence of anti-thymocyte globulin (ATG) administration and ii) recipient innate immune genetic factors appreciated by single nucleotide polymorphism (SNP) analysis. The analysis of these biomarkers was considered only in the settings of transplantation from deceased donors in a Caucasian population. Identification of biomarkers predicting chronic allograft dysfunction is beyond the scope of this review, despite significant advances reported recently in this field (please see a recent commentary in the *Journal of Clinical Investigation;* Schroppel & Heeger, 2010). In contrast to the search for biomarkers predicting chronic allograft dysfunction where immune monitoring was performed in the serum, peripheral blood mononuclear cells (PBMC), urine and the allograft through biopsy (Mannon, 2010), our investigations were focused on non-invasive blood samples (*i.e.,* serum and PBMC).

2. $CD4^+$ T cell lymphopenia as a biomarker for immunosuppression-associated complications

$CD4^+$ T cell lymphopenia in renal transplant recipients results mainly from ATG administration. Despite a limited treatment duration (until 4 days), $CD4^+$ T cell lymphopenia persists for several years in some transplanted patients (Muller et al., 1997; Louis et al., 2007). We previously demonstrated that persistent $CD4^+$ T cell lymphopenia is correlated with enhanced risks of cancers –including skin cancers (Ducloux et al., 1998a), monoclonal gammapathies (Ducloux et al., 1999), lymphomas as well as other non skin cancers such as colon or lung cancers (Ducloux et al., 2002a)–, of opportunistic infections (Ducloux et al., 1998b) and atherosclerotic events (Ducloux et al., 2003) in renal transplant recipients. In contrast, $CD4^+$ T cell lymphopenia seems not to be associated with *de novo* genitourinary malignancies (Guichard et al., 2008). Moreover, we recently associated $CD4^+$ T cell lymphopenia and renal transplant recipient mortality (Ducloux et al., 2010). In this work, the two identified main causes of death in these patients were cancers (36% in the prevalent cohort of 302 consecutive stable renal transplant recipients with a mean follow-up of 92 $\pm$ 7 months) and cardiovascular diseases (39%)(Ducloux et al., 2010). Thus, $CD4^+$ T cell lymphopenia may be considered as an adequate marker for excessive immunosuppression leading to immunosupression-associated complications, at least in patients receiving depletion therapy. However, all transplanted patients treated with ATG did not present a prolonged $CD4^+$ T cell lymphopenia (Ducloux et al., 2003; Ducloux et al., 2010). Thus, the next step was to identify factors responsible for this prolonged severe $CD4^+$ T cell lymphopenia allowing us to distinguish patients that will develop prolonged $CD4^+$ T cell lymphopenia from patients that will not. Some studies (Willoughby et al., 2009; Cai & Terasaki, 2010) reported a benefit of ATG over nondepleting induction therapy mainly on early acute graft rejection occurrence, but also ultimately in preserving allograft function. The benefit of ATG is, however, not similar in each patient (Brennan et al., 2006; Noel et al., 2009). Thus, the choice of a complication risk level could vary according to the supposed benefit of ATG. A high benefit of ATG may lead to accept a higher risk, whereas a slight benefit could lead to prefer a lower risk. Biomarkers, such as $CD4^+$ T cell lymphopenia, may help to select ATG as an appropriate induction therapy. In the next part of this paragraph §2, we will discuss factors that may affect $CD4^+$ T cell reconstitution after ATG-induced T cell depletion as well as factors that may explain the duration, intensity or variability of $CD4^+$ T cell depletion among patients. In addition to ATG, Campath-1H, a humanized anti-CD52 monoclonal antibody called Alemtuzumab, can be used as induction immunosuppression causing T cell depletion (Kaufman et al., 2005; Cianco & Burke, 2008). Whether data obtained with ATG can be transposed to Alemtuzumab remains to be determined. Nevertheless, few clinical studies are available regarding the $CD4^+$ T cell lymphopenia induced by Alemtuzumab administration (Scarsi et al., 2010) not always in the context of kidney transplantation (Cox et al., 2005).

2.1 A role for an altered immune reconstitution on persistent $CD4^+$ T cell lymphopenia after anti-thymocyte globulin administration?

We will describe below factors identified as participating to $CD4^+$ T cell reconstitution (*i.e.*, thymic function, homeostatic proliferation and cytokines involved in this latter process). Most of the works in this field were performed in the setting of hematopoietic cell transplantation. The identification of these factors in the setting of kidney transplantation will enable to use these factors as biomarkers to adapt immunosuppressive regimen and accelerate $CD4^+$ T cell recovery in patients.

2.1.1 The role of the thymic activity on immune reconstitution after T cell depletion

Diseases (e.g., human immunodeficiency virus [HIV] infection), but also treatments (total body irradiation, high dose anti-cancer chemotherapy or depleting antibodies) may be responsible for profound lymphopenia. Studying immune reconstitution after hematopoietic cell transplantation or following anti-HIV therapy has caught the attention of many teams (see below). Understanding factors involved in accelerated –or in contrast delayed– immune reconstitution may limit side effects of these therapies. Based on studies performed in animal models, Mackall and colleagues proposed several years ago that immune reconstitution after T cell depletion arises from two main pathways: thymopoiesis and homeostatic proliferation expansion of residual host lymphocytes or, in the context of hematopoietic cell transplantation, of graft-derived mature T cells (Fig. 1; Mackall et al., 1997). The latter pathway remains the major pathway early after hematopoietic cell transplantation, until donor-derived prothymocytes migrate to the recipient thymus, where they undergo maturation (Moss & Rickinson, 2005). Several evidences in human settings support today the hypothesis sustained by Mackall *et al.* (1997) due to the development of innovative tools allowing discrimination of recent thymic emigrants (RTE, a reflect of thymic activity/output) from other lymphopenia-induced expanded T cells (*i.e.*, naive or memory/activated). A significant improvement to assess thymic function was performed by Douek and colleagues in 1998, when they reported that circulating T cell excision circle (TREC) levels are a direct reflect of thymic function (Douek et al., 1998). These TREC correspond to the episomal DNA circles generated during the rearrangement of the VDJ genes of the TCR α and β chains. TREC are stably retained during cell division, but do not replicate, thus becoming diluted among the daughter cells. In addition to this initial study performed in HIV patients (Douek et al., 1998), circulating TREC level determination was performed in patients after allogeneic hematopoietic cell transplantation. In this setting, pre-transplant TREC levels were found to be a factor predicting T cell reconstitution both in adults and in pediatric patients (Chen et al., 2005; Clave et al., 2005). This assay was also a useful tool to identify RTE early after allogeneic hematopoietic cell transplantation (Douek et al., 2000; Hochberg et al., 2001; Hazenberg et al., 2002; Borghans et al., 2006). Moreover, TREC level determination was also used to assess T cell neogenesis in autologous hematopoietic cell transplantation (Farge et al., 2005). Recently, expression of surface markers –including CD45RA, CD31 or protein tyrosine kinase 7 (PTK7)– on $CD4^+$ T cells has been shown to identify RTE and to attest to an efficient thymopoiesis (Haines et al., 2009; or for a recent review, Kohler & Thiel, 2009). In contrast, homeostatic proliferation expansion is characterized by T cells expressing the CD45RO isoform (Fig.1). Homeostatic proliferation of naive T cells induces the acquisition of a memory/activated phenotype (Fig.1).

A critical issue during T cell recovery is the reconstitution of a most diverse polyclonal T cell repertoire. While thymopoiesis generates "new" T cells with a polyclonal TCR repertoire, homeostatic proliferation expansion results in a very limited TCR repertoire diversity (Fig. 1). Thus, patients exhibiting impaired immune reconstitution due to altered thymic function are less equipped to respond to pathogens or even to control tumors than patients presenting an efficient T cell reconstitution with a fully diverse TCR repertoire (for a review, Williams et al., 2007).

A last concern is that the thymus involutes with age and injury, but keeps its capacity for renewal. This is well illustrated in clinical settings associated with T cell recovery (Dion et al., 2004) where the thymus expands and may become greater than the normal size with intense cellular density, as attested by computerized tomography (Williams et al., 2007). Radiographic measurement of thymus by computer tomographs correlates with circulating TREC levels (Harris et al., 2005). However, thymus renewal capacity declines with age (for a review, Williams et al., 2007). In consequence, circulating TREC levels are inversely correlated with age (Gruver et al., 2007). Over the age of 45-50, thymic activity/output is reduced and naive T cell recovery may take until 5 years after severe iatrogenic lymphopenia (Williams et al., 2007).

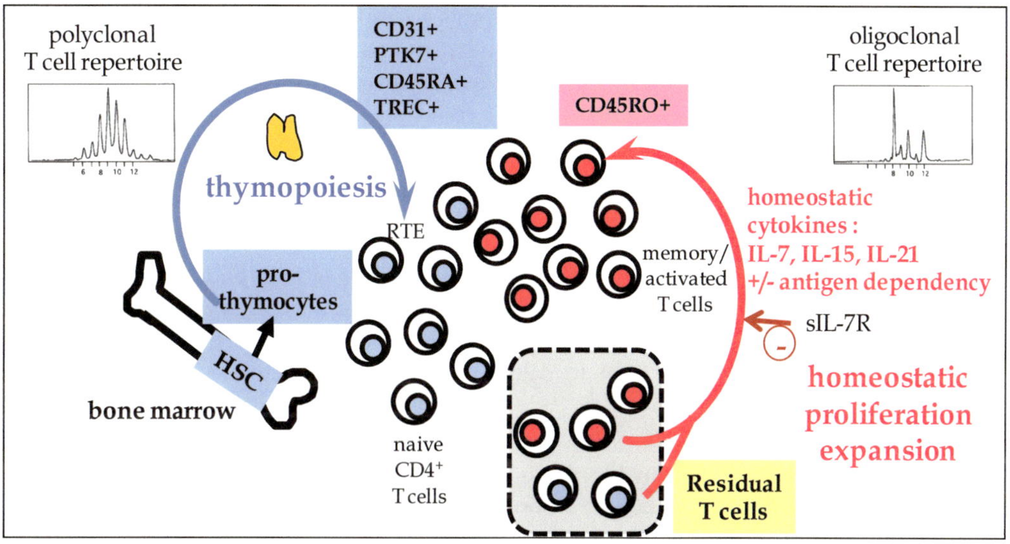

Fig. 1. The main pathways leading to immune reconstitution following CD4+ T cell depletion. The thymic pathway (thymopoiesis) depends on thymic activity. This activity has been shown to decline with age. This pathway generates new T cells, called RTE expressing the following markers: CD31+ CD45RA+ PTK7+ and not CD45RO. These RTE express CD127 (IL-7Rα) and are sensitive to IL-7. Interleukin-7 participates to RTE expansion without inducing CD31 expression loss (Azevedo et al., 2009) or skewing T cell repertoire (Sportes et al., 2008). These RTE contribute to a diverse polyclonal T cell repertoire allowing patients to respond to multiple infectious and/or tumoral antigens. The homeostatic proliferation expansion depends on both residual T cells (*i.e.*, spared by ATG or depleting therapy) and homeostatic cytokine availability. These cytokines are IL-7, IL-15 and IL-21. Interleukin-7 is involved in CD4+ T cell expansion, whereas IL-15 and IL-21 are rather implicated in CD8+ T cell expansion (Boyman et al., 2009). Interleukin-7 activity may be neutralized by a soluble form of IL-7 receptor α (sIL-7R) (Rose et al., 2009). Although IL-7 expands RTE or naive T cells, memory phenotype cells express high levels of CD127, thus allowing them to respond to physiological levels of IL-7 for their survival and homeostatic proliferation. This pathway contributes to a limited T cell repertoire. Abbreviations used: HSC, hematopoietic stem cells; sIL-7R; soluble form of CD127 or IL-7Rα; RTE, recent thymic emigrants.

Few data are available to date concerning the human thymic function and CD4+ T cell recovery after kidney transplantation. Nickel *et al.* (2005) reported stable frequencies of RTE -assessed by CD31, CD45RA CD4 phenotype- 6 months after transplantation. These authors concluded that uremia due to past history of chronic renal dysfunction has no impact on thymic activity (Nickel et al., 2005). However, only 7 patients among 48 received depleting induction therapy (Nickel et al., 2005). This renders difficult to interpret the effects of thymic activity in the context of lymphopenia. In contrast, Scarsi *et al.* (2010) reported a massive reduction of RTE one year post-transplantation after Campath-1H administration. This supports that naive $CD4^+$ T cells −including RTE− may be highly sensitive to ATG (Louis et al., 2007; Gurkan et al., 2010)(see also below, paragraph §2.1.2) and that time is necessary for RTE "replenishment" after T cell depletion. The role of the thymic function at the time of kidney transplantation was not assessed in human. Several years ago, Monaco *et al* reported that thymectomy prior to ATG prolongs T cell lymphopenia in mice (Monaco et al., 1965). We recently identified the thymic activity (as assessed by circulating TREC levels) at the time of kidney transplantation as a major factor predicting $CD4^+$ T cell immune reconstitution after ATG administration (Ducloux et al., 2010). We found a TREC value lower than 2'000 per 150'000 $CD3^+$ cells at the time of transplantation to be the best threshold for the subsequent development of post-ATG $CD4^+$ T cell lymphopenia (Ducloux et al., 2010). Renal transplant recipients with lower TREC levels at time of transplantation exhibited a higher morbidity and mortality risk due to cancers as well as cardiovascular diseases. Determination of circulating TREC levels at the time of transplantation may help to identify patients at high risk of persistent ATG-induced $CD4^+$ T cell lymphopenia and post-transplant cancer occurrence (Ducloux et al., 2010). The strength/efficacy of this new biomarker could be a valuable tool to select the induction treatment (ATG *versus* non depleting anti-CD25 antibodies).

2.1.2 The role of homeostatic proliferation expansion and homeostatic cytokines on immune reconstitution after T cell depletion

The second pathway of immune reconstitution after induction therapy-induced lymphopenia is the homeostatic proliferation of residual T cells. This process, also called lymphopenia-induced proliferation, has been extensively studied in mice (for a review, Boyman et al., 2009). In murine models, this homeostatic proliferation expansion requires homeostatic cytokines (e.g., IL-7) and sometimes cognate antigen-driven interactions (Fig.1; Boyman et al., 2009). Several features with clinical consequences for lymphopenic patients are associated with homeostatic proliferation expansion: a limited TCR repertoire diversity, a shift from naive to memory/activated phenotype in the proliferating cells, a competition for limiting levels of homeostatic cytokines (increasing TCR repertoire skewing, hence decreasing the capacity of the host to respond to antigen challenge), a more delayed T cell recovery (Williams et al., 2007), a possibility to lose transplantation tolerance (Wu et al., 2004) or to favor autoimmunity by expanding autoreactive memory T cells (Monti et al., 2008).

Homeostatic proliferation expansion is the first pathway to be triggered when peripheral T cells decline acutely. This decrease in circulating T cell counts reduces IL-7 consumption, hence leads to enhanced levels of IL-7. This cytokine is then available for residual T cell expansion. High serum levels of IL-7 were found in allografted patients with severe lymphopenia after treatment depletion (Bolotin et al., 1999). However, IL-7 levels decrease rapidly with lymphocyte recovery (Bolotin et al., 1999). Interleukin-7 can be considered as a true regulator of the naive T cell pool size, driving homeostatic proliferation of $CD4^+$ $CD31^+$ RTE with sustained CD31 expression (Azevedo et al., 2009). Memory $CD4^+$ T cells express high levels of CD127 (Boyman et al., 2009), then compete with RTE for IL-7. Dependency on IL-15 or IL-21 for homeostatic proliferation expansion is less marked for $CD4^+$ T cells than $CD8^+$ T cells. Thus, IL-7 levels after lymphopenia are a critical factor to be considered after depletion therapy. Cox *et al* have studied the IL-7 pathway (circulating IL-7 levels and CD127 expression on T cells) in lymphopenic multiple sclerosis patients receiving Campath-

1H treatment. No significant defect was observed (Cox et al., 2005). Data are needed to confirm this observation in the context of kidney transplantation. This is particularly interesting since recombinant human IL-7 has been used in clinical trials (Sportes et al., 2010). Interleukin-7 administration results in an expansion of both naive and memory $CD4^+$ T cells and CD8 T^+ cells with a tendency toward enhanced CD8 T^+ cell expansion. Lymphopenic or normal older patients receiving IL-7 develop an expanded circulating T cell pool with increased T cell repertoire diversity. Moreover, recombinant human IL-7 administration exhibits a favorable toxicity profile, opening the perspective of potential future usage in renal transplant recipients with severe prolonged $CD4^+$ T cell lymphopenia if this IL7 pathway will be found altered. Furthermore, IL-7 treatment of human thymus –*in vitro* or in a xenogeneic model– has been shown to increase thymic activity as attested by elevated TREC levels (Okamoto et al., 2002). Thus, IL-7 treatment may improve thymic activity after kidney transplantation.

2.2 $CD4^+$ T cell subsets, sensitivity to anti-thymocyte globulin administration and immunosuppression-associated complications: the example of accelerated atherosclerosis

Anti-thymocyte globulins are a complex mixture of antibodies with multiple specificities directed against different molecules expressed by T cells, but also non T cells (Bonnefoy-Berard et al., 1991; Rebellato et al., 1994). Several authors believe that ATG exerts its effects through depletion as well as depletion-independent mechanisms. It has been reported that the different $CD4^+$ T cell subsets were not equally sensitive to ATG-induced depletion. Initial works in mice showed that regulatory T cells (Treg) -playing a key role in the control and maintenance of tolerance (Fig.2)– were spared by anti-lymphocyte serum (ALS) (Minamimura et al., 2006), by a mechanism dependent of OX40 signaling pathway present in Treg with a memory phenotype (Kroemer et al., 2007). Moreover, in *in vitro* experiments, ATG has been reported to induce the conversion of Treg from naive $CD25^-$ $CD4^+$ T cells without acquisition of FoxP3 and CTLA-4 expression (Lopez et al., 2006). The source of ATG (from rabbit or horse) may impact Treg conversion with only rabbit-derived ATG allowing Treg conversion (Feng et al., 2008). An increase of Treg after rabbit ATG treatment has been reported *in vivo* in renal transplant recipients (Gurkan et al., 2010). Analysis of CD45RA, CD45RO, CD27 and CD31 marker expression on T cells from both adult and pediatric renal transplant recipients suggests that Treg comes from both RTE and peripheral expansion in adult patients, while they are mainly derived from thymus in children (Gurkan et al., 2010). Furthermore, ATG may also alter T cell migration (LaCorcia et al., 2009) and naive T cells have to home to secondary lymphoid organs in order to maintain a stable population size. A subset of stromal cells present in the secondary lymphoid organs, called fibroblastic reticular cells supports T cell survival (Link et al., 2007). Moreover, secondary lymphoid organs are an important source of IL-7 (Boyman et al., 2009), which participates to naive $CD4^+$ T cell expansion after lymphopenia (see paragraph §2.1.2). Thus, altered T cell homing in the second lymphoid organs after ATG may participate to delayed immune reconstitution.

A thoroughly study in non human primates reported that ATG treatment induced a dose-dependent T cell depletion in the peripheral blood, the spleen and in the lymph nodes. T cell apoptosis in secondary lymphoid organs was identified as the main depletion mechanism (Preville et al., 2001). This supports that lymphocyte depletion is the major mechanism by which ATG preparation exerts its immunosuppressive effect. Another study in mice

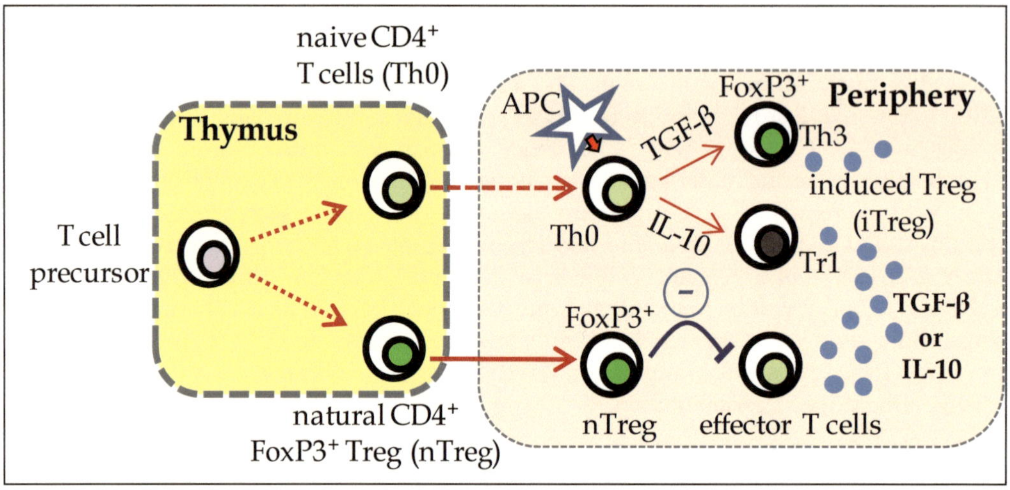

Fig. 2. The two main origins of CD25+ CD4+ regulatory T cells. The role of Treg is to control and maintain immune tolerance (Sakaguchi et al., 2010). These cells may be generated in the thymus and called natural Treg (nTreg). They express FoxP3 and exert their suppressive activity on effector T cells through cell contact, immunosuppressive cytokine secretion, and/or metabolic perturbations as well as by inhibiting antigen presenting cells (APC) (Vignali et al., 2008; Sakaguchi et al., 2010). Regulatory T cells may be also generated from conversion of naive CD25- Th0 CD4+ T cells into induced Treg (iTreg)(see also, Fig.3). This conversion depends on cytokines present during T cell activation by APC. While IL-10 induces FoxP3 neg T regulatory 1 (Tr1) cells that produce IL-10 (Groux et al., 1997; Vieira et al., 2004), a TGF-β-rich microenvironment favors FoxP3+ Th3 that express membrane bound TGF-β and secrete high amount of TGF-β (Chen et al., 2003). Interleukin-10 and TGF-β inhibit effector T cell functions and also neutralize innate immune responses (see Fig.4).

reported that all CD4+ T cell subsets are equally sensitive to mouse ATG, but that naive T cells expand very quickly after homeostatic proliferation with the acquisition of a memory phenotype (Sener et al., 2009). This may explain why initial studies reported that memory phenotype T cells are more resistant to ATG-induced death (see above). The hypothesis of a different susceptibility to ATG-induced death or an imbalance in CD4+ T cell subset reconstitution is tantalizing to explain the relationship between CD4+ T cell lymphopenia and accelerated atherosclerosis after kidney transplantation. Depending on the cytokine microenvironment in which naive CD4+ T cells are primed, different effector CD4+ T helper cell (Th) subsets have been described (Fig.3). Whether ATG or immune recovery following ATG-induced lymphopenia may differently affect CD4+ Th subsets remains to be determined in renal transplant recipients. A study in renal transplant recipients suggested that Th2 subsets were less sensitive than Th1 subsets to ATG treatment (Weimer et al., 2005). However, other Th subsets –such as Th17 (Betteli et al., 2006; Mangan et al., 2006), or the putative Th9 (Dardahlon et al., 2008; Veldhoen et al., 2008) or Th22 (Duhen et al., 2009; Trifari et al., 2009) subsets (Fig.3)– have not been explored. Experimental mouse models of atherosclerosis using atherosclerosis prone apolipoprotein-E deficient or low density lipoprotein (LDL) receptor deficient mice permitted to distinguish pro-atherogenic from anti-atherogenic CD4+ T cell subsets (for recent reviews, Taleb et al., 2010a; Hansson & Hermansson, 2011; Fig.3). One may hypothesize that ATG-induced CD4+ T cell lymphopenia may favor a preferential expansion of pro-atherogenic Th1 cells in detriment of anti-atherogenic Treg (*i.e.*, nTreg and iTreg subsets; Fig. 3). This remains to be determined in the future. Nevertheless, patients with end stage renal disease awaiting kidney transplantation exhibit an inflammatory state including high circulating levels of C reactive protein (CRP) (Ducloux et al., 2002b; Ducloux et al., 2004). Thus, immune reconstitution after depletion therapy occurs in the context of inflammation. One can speculate that pro-inflammatory and pro-atherogenic Th subsets are favored over anti-atherogenic T cells.

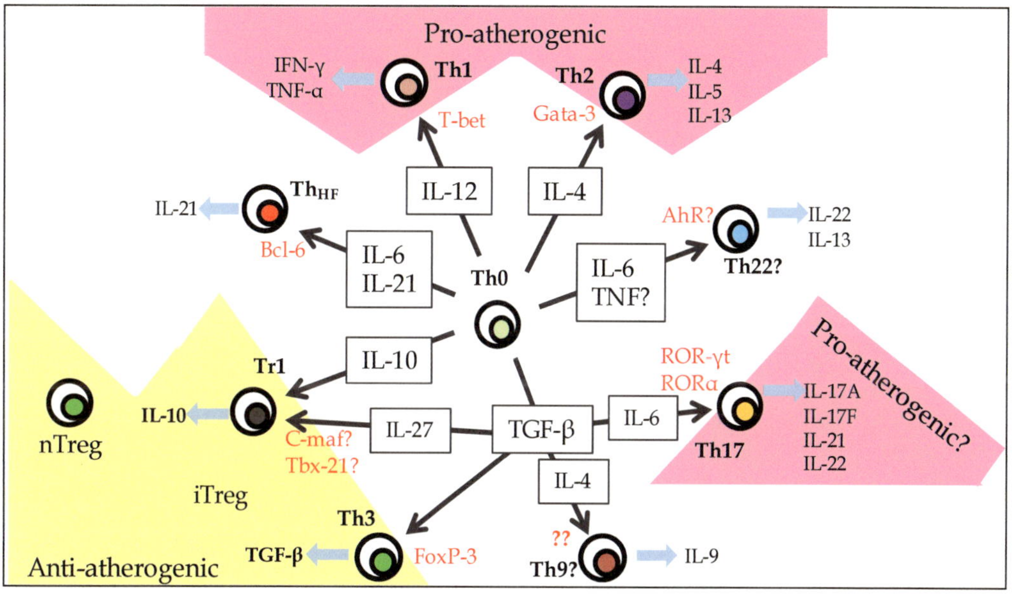

Fig. 3. CD4+ T cell subsets and their role in atherosclerosis. This figure summarizes cytokines involved in Th cell commitment, transcription factors necessary for this process as well as cytokines secreted by the different Th subsets. Transcription factors involved in Th commitment are indicated in red, while secreted cytokines are indicated after the blue arrow. According to cytokine microenvironment, distinct Th subsets can be generated: naive (Th0) T cell priming in the presence of IL-12 induces Th1 cells characterized by TNF-α and IFN-γ secretion and the transcription factor, t-bet. These Th1 cells are pro-atherogenic (in pink) and are found within atherosclerotic plaques (Taleb et al., 2010a). Th0 priming in the presence of IL-4 induces Th2 cells characterized by IL-4, IL-5 and IL-13 secretion and the transcription factor Gata-3. These Th2 cells favor atherosclerotic plaque disruption/instability (Taleb et al., 2010a), a late event in atherosclerosis (Hansson, 2005). Induced Treg (iTreg), already described in Fig.2, protect mice from atherosclerosis and thus are anti-atherogenic (in yellow) (Mallat et al., 2003). Natural Treg –directly produced in the thymus– exert the same anti-atherogenic effect (Ait-Oufella et al., 2006). Th0 priming in the presence of TGF-β and IL-6 leads to Th17 cells characterized by IL-17A, IL-22 and IL-21 secretion and the transcription factors ROR-γt and RORα. These Th17 cells seem to be pro-atherogenic (in pink) (Erbel et al., 2009; Gao et al., 2010; Ait-Oufella et al., 2010; for a recent commentary: Taleb et al., 2010b). The other Th subsets, namely the putative Th9 and Th22 or the helper follicular Th cells (Th_{HF} found in germinal centers and participating to B cell activation) have not been studied in the setting of atherosclerosis. Question mark indicates when data are not confirmed or not available.

As mentioned above, atherosclerosis is a chronic immune-mediated disease implicating both adaptive and innate immunity (Yan & Hansson, 2007; Woollard & Geismann, 2010; Hansson & Hermansson, 2011). In this review, we focused on CD4+ T cells to explain the increased incidence of atherosclerotic events associated with ATG administration. However, accelerated atherosclerosis is not only associated with induction therapy responsible for persistent CD4+ T cell lymphopenia, since cardiovascular diseases are observed in most renal transplant recipients (please see paragraph §1). This is why we also explore innate immune genetic factors to explain accelerated atherosclerosis. Most of the widely used immunosuppressive drugs target T cells and sometimes B cells (Halloran, 2004), while innate cells or factors are not always affected. For instance, calcineurin inhibitors may prevent Treg suppressive functions (Zeiser et al., 2006; Bonnefoy et al., 2008). Thus, regulatory functions are certainly unpaired in renal transplant recipients receiving calcineurin inhibitors. It was shown in mice that Treg dysfunction or blockade increases innate cell activation through Toll-like receptor (TLR) ligands (De Wilde et al., 2008). If this occurs in atherosclerotic plaques, this will favor atherosclerosis progression (Fig.4).

3. Recipient innate immune genetic factors as biomarkers of immunosuppression-associated complications

Inflammation plays a major role in atherosclerosis processes (Hansson, 2005). The atherosclerotic lesions contain large numbers of immune cells, particularly macrophages (Stary et al., 1995) and CD4+ T cells (Zhou et al., 1996). Macrophages are present in atherosclerotic lesions at early stages and play a critical role in lipid accumulation as well as in the plaque rupture (Hansson, 2005). The plaque rupture is responsible in coronary thrombosis (Hansson, 2005). Furthermore, atherosclerosis is associated with systemic immune responses and signs of inflammation. Histopathological and clinical investigations point at inflammatory activation of atherosclerotic plaques as a cause of acute coronary syndromes (Hansson, 2005), and sero-epidemiological studies have suggested links between atherosclerosis and microbial infections (Morre et al., 2000; Neumann et al., 2000). Moreover, several epidemiological studies and therapeutic trials have underlined the importance of inflammation in cardiovascular clinical end-points (Ridker, 2001; Ridker et al., 2009). The relevance of inflammation in atherosclerotic complications in humans is well illustrated by the JUPITER trial showing that achieving CRP levels under 2 mg/L with Rosusvastatin is associated with a 31% decrease in major cardiovascular events (Ridker et al., 2009).
In order to explore how inflammation and cells from the innate immunity may influence the complications associated with kidney transplantation, the analysis of different SNPs was performed in our laboratory. We followed the recommendations provided by *Nature Genetics* (1999) that are: a plausible/expected link between the analyzed protein or its gene promoter and the pathology, a functional characterization of the SNP, and a validation in independent cohorts. Moreover, the size of patient cohort has to be adapted to the frequency of mutated SNP. The following SNPs were analyzed in the settings of kidney transplantation outcome: TLR-4 (Ducloux et al., 2005b) and NOD2/CARD15 (Courivaud et al., 2006), as these two pattern recognition receptors (PRR) are involved in the recognition of pathogens and in the initiation of inflammatory immune responses (Fig.4). Sero-epidemiological studies have suggested a link between atherosclerosis and microbial infections (Morre et al., 2000; Neumann et al., 2000) and the atherosclerotic lesions contain large numbers of immune cells, particularly macrophages and dendritic cells (Woollard &

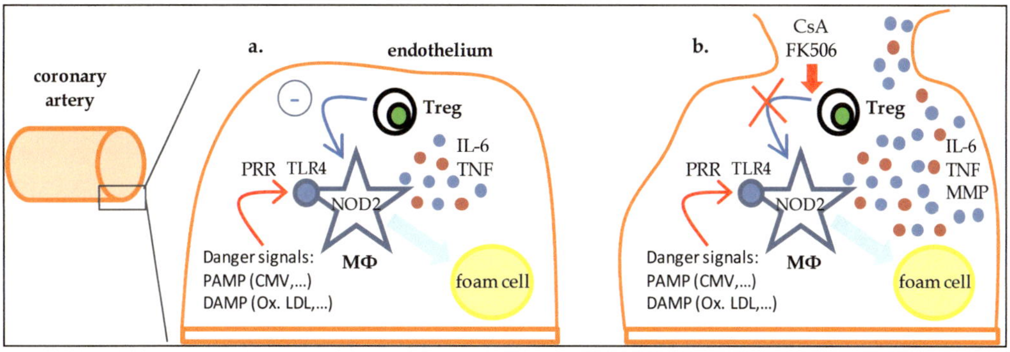

Fig. 4. Accelerated atherosclerosis in renal transplant recipients may result from a hyper-response of innate immune cells to Danger signals and a regulatory T cell deficiency in atherosclerotic lesions. Atherosclerotic lesions are asymmetric focal thickenings of the innermost layer of the artery, the intima. A view of the intima is shown with cells infiltrating this intima and lipid accumulation occurs *via* foam cells. (**a**) Treg controls the pro-inflammatory response and CPA activation. This limits atherosclerosis progression. (**b**) However, in case of Treg deficiency due to, for instance, calcineurin inhibitor (e.g., ciclosporin A, CsA or FK506) administration, pattern recognition receptor (PRR) stimulation by Danger signals induces an increased secretion of inflammatory cytokines, including IL-6 and TNF (De Wilde et al., 2008) as well as other factors involved in atherosclerosis progression such as matrix metalloproteinases (MMP; Hansson, 2005). This leads to atherosclerotic lesion progression and induces the activation and rupture of the plaque (**b**), thrombosis, and ischemia. Which innate immune cells are involved in plaque rupture? Macrophages (MΦ) are present in atherosclerotic lesions at early stages (Stary et al., 1995). They differentiate in foam cells after lipid accumulation, but also increase local inflammatory responses when stimulated by Danger signals. According to Polly Matzinger (1994), these signals may correspond to pathogen-associated molecular patterns (PAMPs, linked to *Cytomegalovirus* [CMV] or *Chlamydia* infections both potentially implicated in atherosclerosis progression (Morre et al., 2000; Neumann et al., 2000) or to damage-associated molecular patterns (DAMPs, related to long history of end stage renal disease favoring hyaluronan accumulation or to increased oxidized LDL [Ox. LDL] production after lipid metabolism perturbations) that stimulate PRR, including TLR2 (Scheibner et al., 2006), TLR4 or NOD2/CARD15. DAMPs lead to sterile inflammatory responses that may favor auto-immune disease occurrence (Rock et al., 2010). For a recent review on Danger signals, please also refer to Kono & Rock (2008).

Geissmann, 2010; Fig.4). Thus, we hypothesized that an enhanced inflammatory response (including inflammatory cytokines, such as IL-6 or TNF-α) in the intima of the artery walls due to a "hyper-responsive" PRR (*i.e.*, TLR4 or NOD2/CARD15) may exert proatherogenic functions (Fig.4). We also studied other SNPs -that did not concern coding regions as for TLR4 and NOD2/CARD12– but rather the promoter gene region. In this setting, this promoter gene region regulates the levels of gene "production". For instance, we analyzed SNP in the *IL-6* or *COX-2* promoter gene (Bamoulid et al., 2006; Courivaud et al., 2009a; Courivaud et al., 2009b; Aubin et al., 2010). We correlated *IL-6* promoter gene SNP at position -174 with NODAT in overweight patients (Bamoulid et al., 2006). We reported, as already published in the general population (Fishman et al., 1998), that renal transplant recipients carrying the G allele (GG or GC genotype carriers) produce higher levels of IL-6 and exhibit higher levels of CRP (Bamoulid et al., 2006). Diabetes is a traditional risk factor of cardiovascular diseases. Thus, NODAT may participate to accelerated atherosclerosis in renal transplant recipients. As previously reported in the general population (Kiechl et al., 2002), 2 TLR4 SNPs were also found associated with atherosclerotic events in renal transplant recipients (Ducloux et al., 2005b). In contrast, no association between NOD2/CARD15 polymorphisms (Courivaud et al., 2006) or *COX-2* promoter gene SNP at position -765 (Courivaud et al., 2009a) and atherosclerotic events after kidney transplantation was observed. Data obtained in the former study (Courivaud et al., 2006) may rely on a minor role of NOD2/CARD15 in the atherosclerotic plaques. NOD2/CARD15 is preferentially located in the intestine (in crypts from the terminal ileum [Kobayashi et al., 2005] and in Paneth cells [Ogura et al., 2003]) and exerts mainly its function in the intestinal tract, as demonstrated in NOD2/CARD15 deficient mice (Kobayashi et al., 2005) and supported by the role of this PRR in gastrointestinal tract-associated pathologies (*i.e.*, Crohn's disease and intestinal graft-versus-host disease) (Hampe et al., 2002; Heliö et al., 2003; Holler et al., 2004). The latter study analyzing *COX-2* promoter gene polymorphism (Courivaud et al., 2009a) is interesting, since an opposite result was obtained according to the analyzed transplant patient cohort. An increased risk of atherosclerotic events was observed in the first cohort, whereas in the second independent cohort the same SNP was associated with a protective effect on atherosclerotic event occurrence. This study (Courivaud et al., 2009a) illustrates perfectly the recommendations made by the editors of *Nature Genetics* concerning "genetic association studies" (1999). The current literature does not provide a clear landscape of SNP associated with complication outcome after kidney transplantation. Several causes may explain the discrepancy between the different studies, such as the cohort size and the functional validation of the SNP in the setting of immunosuppression. In order to increase the cohort size, most of the renal transplant recipients were included but they did not receive the same immunosuppressive regimen or alternatively the year of the graft was very different and thus clinical practices were difficult to compare. To limit these troubles, we are conducting a prospective study involving several renal transplantation centers to recruit a large cohort of patients in a limited time course. However, again, one may mention that clinical follow-up between different centers may be different. Thus, validation studies may be necessary to confirm or infirm SNP studies.

4. Conclusion

Overall, the aim of this review is to report our experience on the identification of biomarkers ($CD4^+$ T cell lymphopenia after ATG, TREC levels at the time of transplantation, and innate immune genetic factors) predicting transplantation-related complications (mainly atherosclerosis and cancer occurrence), and to propose to the use these biomarkers in patient follow up and/or in immunosuppressive strategy design. Furthermore, we propose other "tracks" to improve the clinical relevance of these biomarkers as well as to understand their implications in the occurrence of immunosuppression-associated complications. The efficacy of these identified biomarkers should be tested and validated in prospective clinical trials in order to select the most appropriate immunosuppressive strategy. In the future, one could imagine that these biomarkers may help physicians to manage risks of cancers and cardiovascular diseases in renal transplant recipients. The management of these risks is of great interest as attested by recent reviews (Webster et al., 2008; Wang & Kasiske, 2010).

5. Acknowledgment

We would like to thank Sarah Odrion for excellent editorial assistance and the Centre d'Investigation Clinique intégré en Biothérapies du CHU de Besançon (CBT-506) for its support. Our work in the fields was supported by grants from the Programme Hospitalier de Recherche Clinique 2011 (to D.D), the Fondation de France (Appel d'offre "Maladies cardiovasculaires" 2007, #2007 001859, to P.S.), the DHOS/INSERM/INCa (Appel d'offre Recherche Translationnelle 2008, to D.D. and P.S.), and the APICHU 2010 (SIGAL project to J.B.).

6. References

Ait-Oufella H, Herbin O, Bouaziz JD, Binder CJ, Uyttenhove C, Laurans L, Taleb S, Van Vre E, Esposito B, Vilar J, Sirvent J, Van Snick J, Tedgui A, Tedder TF, Mallat Z. (2010). B cell depletion reduces the development of atherosclerosis in mice. *Journal of Experimental Medicine*, Vol.207, No.8, (August 2010), pp. 1579-87, ISSN 0022-1007.

Ait-Oufella H, Salomon BL, Potteaux S, Robertson AK, Gourdy P, Zoll J, Merval R, Esposito B, Cohen JL, Fisson S, Flavell RA, Hansson GK, Klatzmann D, Tedgui A, Mallat Z. (2006). Natural regulatory T cells control the development of atherosclerosis in mice. *Nature Medicine*, Vol.12, No.2, (February 2006), pp. 178-80, ISSN 1078-8956.

Aubin F, Courivaud C, Bamoulid J, Loupy A, Deschamps M, Ferrand C, Le Corre D, Tiberghien P, Chalopin JM, Legendre C, Thervet E, Humbert P, Saas P, Ducloux D. (2010). Influence of cyclooxygenase-2 (COX-2) gene promoter polymorphism at position -765 on skin cancer after renal transplantation. *Journal of Investigative Dermatology*, Vol.130, No.8, (August 2010), pp. 2134-6, ISSN 0022-202X.

Azevedo RI, Soares MV, Barata JT, Tendeiro R, Serra-Caetano A, Victorino RM, Sousa AE. (2009). IL-7 sustains CD31 expression in human naive CD4+ T cells and preferentially expands the CD31+ subset in a PI3K-dependent manner. *Blood*, Vol.113, No.13, (March 2009), pp. 2999-3007, ISSN 0006-4971.

Bamoulid J, Courivaud C, Deschamps M, Mercier P, Ferrand C, Penfornis A, Tiberghien P, Chalopin JM, Saas P, Ducloux D. IL-6 promoter polymorphism -174 is associated with new-onset diabetes after transplantation. *Journal of the American Society of Nephrology*, Vol.17, No.8, (August 2006), pp. 2333-40, ISSN 1046-6673.

Barrett WL, First MR, Aron BS, Penn I. (1993). Clinical course of malignancies in renal transplant recipients. *Cancer*, Vol.72, No.7, (October 1993), pp. 2186-9, ISSN 1097-0142.

Bettelli E, Carrier Y, Gao W, Korn T, Strom TB, Oukka M, Weiner HL, Kuchroo VK. (2006). Reciprocal developmental pathways for the generation of pathogenic effector TH17 and regulatory T cells. *Nature*, Vol.441, No7090, (May 2006), pp. 235-8, ISSN 0028-0836.

Bolotin E, Annett G, Parkman R, Weinberg K. (1999). Serum levels of IL-7 in bone marrow transplant recipients: relationship to clinical characteristics and lymphocyte count. *Bone Marrow Transplant*, Vol.23, No.8, (April 1999), pp. 783-8, ISSN 0268-3369.

Bonnefoy F, Masson E, Perruche S, Marandin A, Borg C, Radlovic A, Shipman B, Tiberghien P, Saas P, Kleinclauss F. (2008). Sirolimus enhances the effect of apoptotic cell infusion on hematopoietic engraftment and tolerance induction. *Leukemia*, Vol.22, No.7, (July 2008), pp. 1430-4, ISSN 0887-6924.

Bonnefoy-Berard N, Vincent C, Revillard JP. (1991). Antibodies against functional leukocyte surface molecules in polyclonal antilymphocyte and antithymocyte globulins. *Transplantation*, Vol.51, No.3, (March 1991), pp. 669-73, ISSN 0041-1337.

Borghans JA, Bredius RG, Hazenberg MD, Roelofs H, Jol-van der Zijde EC, Heidt J, Otto SA, Kuijpers TW, Fibbe WE, Vossen JM, Miedema F, van Tol MJ. (2006). Early determinants of long-term T-cell reconstitution after hematopoietic stem cell transplantation for severe combined immunodeficiency. *Blood*, Vol.108, No.2, (July 2006), pp. 763-9, ISSN 0006-4971.

Boyman O, Letourneau S, Krieg C, Sprent J. (2009). Homeostatic proliferation and survival of naive and memory T cells. *European Journal of Immunology*, Vol.39, No.8, (August 2009), pp. 2088-94, ISSN 1521-4141.

Brennan DC, Daller JA, Lake KD, Cibrik D, Del Castillo D. (2006). Rabbit antithymocyte globulin versus basiliximab in renal transplantation. *New England Journal of Medicine*, Vol.355, No.19, (November 9, 2006), pp. 1967-77, ISSN 0028-4793.

Cai J, Terasaki PI. (2010). Induction immunosuppression improves long-term graft and patient outcome in organ transplantation: an analysis of United Network for Organ Sharing registry data. *Transplantation*, Vol.90, No.12, (December 27, 2010), pp. 1511-5, ISSN 0041-1337.

Chen W, Jin W, Hardegen N, Lei KJ, Li L, Marinos N, McGrady G, Wahl SM. (2003). Conversion of peripheral CD4+CD25- naive T cells to CD4+CD25+ regulatory T cells by TGF-beta induction of transcription factor Foxp3. *Journal of Experimental Medicine*, Vol.198, No.12, (December 15, 2003), pp. 1875-86, ISSN 0022-1007.

Chen X, Barfield R, Benaim E, Leung W, Knowles J, Lawrence D, Otto M, Shurtleff SA, Neale GA, Behm FG, Turner V, Handgretinger R. (2005). Prediction of T-cell reconstitution by assessment of T-cell receptor excision circle before allogeneic hematopoietic stem cell transplantation in pediatric patients. *Blood*, Vol.15, No.105, (January 15, 2005), pp. 886-93, ISSN 0006-4971.

Ciancio G, Burke GW, 3rd. (2008). Alemtuzumab (Campath-1H) in kidney transplantation. *American Journal of Transplantation*, Vol.8, No.1, (January 2008), pp. 15-20, ISSN 1600-6143.

Clave E, Rocha V, Talvensaari K, Busson M, Douay C, Appert ML, Rabian C, Carmagnat M, Garnier F, Filion A, Socie G, Gluckman E, Charron D, Toubert A. (2005). Prognostic value of pretransplantation host thymic function in HLA-identical sibling hematopoietic stem cell transplantation. *Blood*, Vol.105, No.6, (March 15, 2005), pp. 2608-13, ISSN 0006-4971.

Courivaud C, Bamoulid J, Loupy A, Deschamps M, Ferrand C, Le Corre D, Tiberghien P, Chalopin JM, Legendre C, Thervet E, Saas P, Ducloux D. (2009b). Influence of cyclooxygenase-2 (COX-2) gene promoter polymorphism -765 on graft loss after renal transplantation. *American Journal of Transplantation*, Vol.9, No.12, (December 2009), pp. 2752-7, ISSN 1600-6143.

Courivaud C, Bamoulid J, Tiberghien P, Saas P, Chalopin JM, Ducloux D, Legendre C, Thervet E. (2009a). G-765C COX-2 gene promoter polymorphism and risk of atherosclerosis after kidney transplantation. *Transplantation*, Vol.88, No.6, September 27, 2009), pp. 851-2, ISSN 0041-1337.

Courivaud C, Ferrand C, Deschamps M, Tiberghien P, Chalopin JM, Duperrier A, Saas P, Ducloux D. (2006) No evidence of association between NOD2/CARD15 gene polymorphism and atherosclerotic events after renal transplantation. *Transplantation*, Vol.81, No.8, (April 27, 2006), pp. 1212-5, ISSN 0041-1337.

Cox AL, Thompson SA, Jones JL, Robertson VH, Hale G, Waldmann H, Compston DA, Coles AJ. (2005). Lymphocyte homeostasis following therapeutic lymphocyte depletion in multiple sclerosis. *European Journal of Immunology*, Vol.35, No.11, (November 2005), pp. 3332-42, ISSN 1521-4141.

Dantal J, Hourmant M, Cantarovich D, Giral M, Blancho G, Dreno B, Soulillou JP. (1998). Effect of long-term immunosuppression in kidney-graft recipients on cancer incidence: randomised comparison of two cyclosporin regimens. *Lancet*, Vol.351, No.9103, (February 28, 1998), pp. 623-8, ISSN 0140-6736.

Dardalhon V, Awasthi A, Kwon H, Galileos G, Gao W, Sobel RA, Mitsdoerffer M, Strom TB, Elyaman W, Ho IC, Khoury S, Oukka M, Kuchroo VK. (2008). IL-4 inhibits TGF-beta-induced Foxp3+ T cells and, together with TGF-beta, generates IL-9+ IL-10+ Foxp3(-) effector T cells. *Nature Immunology*, Vol.9, No.12, (December 2008), pp. 1347-55, ISSN 1529-2908.

De Wilde V, Benghiat FS, Novalrivas M, Lebrun JF, Kubjak C, Oldenhove G, Verdebout JM, Goldman M, Le Moine A. (2008). Endotoxin hyperresponsiveness upon CD4+ T cell reconstitution in lymphopenic mice: control by natural regulatory T cells. *European Journal of Immunology*, Vol.38, No.1, (January 2008), pp. 48-53, ISSN 1521-4141.

Dion ML, Poulin JF, Bordi R, Sylvestre M, Corsini R, Kettaf N, Dalloul A, Boulassel MR, Debre P, Routy JP, Grossman Z, Sekaly RP, Cheynier R. (2004). HIV infection rapidly induces and maintains a substantial suppression of thymocyte proliferation. *Immunity*, Vol.21, No.6, (December 2004), pp. 757-68, ISSN 1074-7613.

Douek DC, McFarland RD, Keiser PH, Gage EA, Massey JM, Haynes BF, Polis MA, Haase AT, Feinberg MB, Sullivan JL, Jamieson BD, Zack JA, Picker LJ, Koup RA. (1998). Changes in thymic function with age and during the treatment of HIV infection. *Nature*, Vol.396, No.6712, (December 17, 1998), pp. 690-5, ISSN 0028-0836.

Douek DC, Vescio RA, Betts MR, Brenchley JM, Hill BJ, Zhang L, Berenson JR, Collins RH, Koup RA. (2000). Assessment of thymic output in adults after haematopoietic stem-cell transplantation and prediction of T-cell reconstitution. *Lancet*, Vol355, No. 9218, (May 27, 2000), pp. 1875-81, ISSN 0140-6736.

Ducloux D, Bresson-Vautrin C, Kribs M, Abdelfatah A, Chalopin JM. (2002b). C-reactive protein and cardiovascular disease in peritoneal dialysis patients. *Kidney International*, Vol.62, No. 4, (October 2002), pp. 1417-22, ISSN 0085-2538.

Ducloux D, Carron P, Racadot E, Rebibou JM, Bresson-Vautrin C, Hillier YS, Chalopin JM. (1999). T-cell immune defect and B-cell activation in renal transplant recipients with monoclonal gammopathies. *Transplant International*. Vol.12, No.4, (April 1999), pp. 250-3, ISSN 0934-0874.

Ducloux D, Carron PL, Motte G, Ab A, Rebibou JM, Bresson-Vautrin C, Tiberghien P, Saint-Hillier Y, Chalopin JM. (2002a). Lymphocyte subsets and assessment of cancer risk in renal transplant recipients. *Transplant International*, Vol.15, No.8, (September 2002), pp. 393-6, ISSN 0934-0874.

Ducloux D, Carron PL, Racadot E, Rebibou JM, Bresson-Vautrin C, Saint-Hillier Y, Chalopin JM. (1998b). CD4 lymphocytopenia in long-term renal transplant recipients. *Transplantation Proceedings*, Vol.30, No.6, (September 1998), pp. 2859-60, ISSN 0041-1345.

Ducloux D, Carron PL, Rebibou JM, Aubin F, Fournier V, Bresson-Vautrin C, Blanc D, Humbert P, Chalopin JM. (1998a). CD4 lymphocytopenia as a risk factor for skin cancers in renal transplant recipients. *Transplantation*, Vol.65, No.9, (May 15, 1998), pp. 1270-2, ISSN 0041-1337.

Ducloux D, Challier B, Saas P, Tiberghien P, Chalopin JM. (2003). CD4 cell lymphopenia and atherosclerosis in renal transplant recipients. *Journal of the American Society of Nephrology*, Vol.14, No.3, (March 2003), pp. 767-72, ISSN 1046-6673.

Ducloux D, Courivaud C, Bamoulid J, Vivet B, Chabroux A, Deschamps M, Rebibou JM, Ferrand C, Chalopin JM, Tiberghien P, Saas P. (2010). Prolonged CD4 T cell lymphopenia increases morbidity and mortality after renal transplantation. *Journal of the American Society of Nephrology*, Vol.21, No.5, (May 2010), pp. 868-75, ISSN 1046-6673.

Ducloux D, Deschamps M, Yannaraki M, Ferrand C, Bamoulid J, Saas P, Kazory A, Chalopin JM, Tiberghien P. (2005b). Relevance of Toll-like receptor-4 polymorphisms in renal transplantation. *Kidney International*, Vol.67, No.6, (June 2005), pp. 2454-61, ISSN 0085-2538.

Ducloux D, Kazory A, Chalopin JM. (2004). Predicting coronary heart disease in renal transplant recipients: a prospective study. *Kidney International*, Vol.66, No.1, (July 2004), pp. 441-7, ISSN 0085-2538.

Ducloux D, Kazory A, Chalopin JM. (2005a). Posttransplant diabetes mellitus and atherosclerotic events in renal transplant recipients: a prospective study. *Transplantation*, Vol.79, No.4, (February 27, 2005), pp. 438-43, ISSN 0041-1337.

Ducloux D, Motte G, Challier B, Gibey R, Chalopin JM. (2000). Serum total homocysteine and cardiovascular disease occurrence in chronic, stable renal transplant recipients: a prospective study. *Journal of the American Society of Nephrology*, Vol. 11,No.1, (January 2000), pp. 134-7, ISSN 1046-6673.

Duhen T, Geiger R, Jarrossay D, Lanzavecchia A, Sallusto F. (2009). Production of interleukin 22 but not interleukin 17 by a subset of human skin-homing memory T cells. *Nature Immunology*, Vol.10, No.8, (August 2009), pp. 857-63, ISSN 1529-2908.

Editors. (1999). Freely associating. *Nature Genetics*, Vol.22, No.1, (May 1999), pp. 1-2, ISSN 1061-4036.

Einecke G, Reeve J, Sis B, Mengel M, Hidalgo L, Famulski KS, Matas A, Kasiske B, Kaplan B, Halloran PF. (2010). A molecular classifier for predicting future graft loss in late kidney transplant biopsies. *Journal of Clinical Investigation*, Vol.120,No.6, (Jun 1, 2010), pp. 1862-72, ISSN 0021-9738.

Erbel C, Chen L, Bea F, Wangler S, Celik S, Lasitschka F, Wang Y, Bockler D, Katus HA, Dengler TJ. (2009). Inhibition of IL-17A attenuates atherosclerotic lesion development in apoE-deficient mice. *Journal of Immunology*, Vol.183,No.12, (December 15, 2009), pp. 8167-75, ISSN 0022-1767.

Farge D, Henegar C, Carmagnat M, Daneshpouy M, Marjanovic Z, Rabian C, Ilie D, Douay C, Mounier N, Clave E, Bengoufa D, Cabane J, Marolleau JP, Gluckman E, Charron D, Toubert A. (2005). Analysis of immune reconstitution after autologous bone marrow transplantation in systemic sclerosis. *Arthritis & Rheumatism*, Vol.52, No5, (May 2005), pp. 1555-63, ISSN 0004-3591.

Feng X, Kajigaya S, Solomou EE, Keyvanfar K, Xu X, Raghavachari N, Munson PJ, Herndon TM, Chen J, Young NS. (2008). Rabbit ATG but not horse ATG promotes expansion of functional CD4+CD25highFOXP3+ regulatory T cells in vitro. *Blood*, Vol.111, No7, (Apr 1, 2008), pp. 3675-83, ISSN 0006-4971.

Fiebiger W, Kaserer K, Rodler S, Oberbauer R, Bauer C, Raderer M. (2009). Neuroendocrine carcinomas arising in solid-organ transplant recipients: rare but aggressive malignancies. *Oncology*, Vol. 77,No.5, (May 2009), pp. 314-7, ISSN 0030-2414.

Fishman D, Faulds G, Jeffery R, Mohamed-Ali V, Yudkin JS, Humphries S, Woo P. (1998). The effect of novel polymorphisms in the interleukin-6 (IL-6) gene on IL-6 transcription and plasma IL-6 levels, and an association with systemic-onset juvenile chronic arthritis. *Journal of Clinical Investigation*, Vol.102, No.7, (Oct 1, 1998), pp. 1369-76, ISSN 0021-9738.

Gao Q, Jiang Y, Ma T, Zhu F, Gao F, Zhang P, Guo C, Wang Q, Wang X, Ma C, Zhang Y, Chen W, Zhang L. (2010). A critical function of Th17 proinflammatory cells in the development of atherosclerotic plaque in mice. *Journal of Immunology*, Vol.185, No.10, (Nov 15, 2010), pp. 5820-7, ISSN 0022-1767.

Groux H, O'Garra A, Bigler M, Rouleau M, Antonenko S, de Vries JE, Roncarolo MG. (1997) A CD4+ T-cell subset inhibits antigen-specific T-cell responses and prevents colitis. *Nature*, Vol.389, No.6652, (October 16, 1997), pp.737-42, ISSN 0028-0836.

Grulich AE, van Leeuwen MT, Falster MO, Vajdic CM. (2007). Incidence of cancers in people with HIV/AIDS compared with immunosuppressed transplant recipients: a meta-analysis. *Lancet*, Vol.370, No.9581, (July 7, 2007), pp. 59-67, ISSN 0140-6736.

Gruver AL, Hudson LL, Sempowski GD. (2007). Immunosenescence of ageing. *Journal of Pathology*, Vol.211, No.2, (January 2007), pp.144-56, ISSN 1096-9896.

Guichard G, Rebibou JM, Ducloux D, Simula-Faivre D, Tiberghien P, Chalopin JM, Bittard H, Saas P, Kleinclauss F. (2008). Lymphocyte subsets in renal transplant recipients with de novo genitourinary malignancies. *Urologia Internationalis*, Vol.80, No3, (March 2008), pp. 257-63, ISSN 0042-1138.

Gurkan S, Luan Y, Dhillon N, Allam SR, Montague T, Bromberg JS, Ames S, Lerner S, Ebcioglu Z, Nair V, Dinavahi R, Sehgal V, Heeger P, Schroppel B, Murphy B. (2010). Immune reconstitution following rabbit antithymocyte globulin. *American Journal of Transplantation*, Vol.10, No.9, (September 2010), pp. 2132-41, ISSN 1600-6143.

Haines CJ, Giffon TD, Lu LS, Lu X, Tessier-Lavigne M, Ross DT, Lewis DB. (2009). Human CD4+ T cell recent thymic emigrants are identified by protein tyrosine kinase 7 and have reduced immune function. *Journal of Experimental Medicine*, Vol.206, No.2, (February 16, 2009), pp. 275-85, ISSN 0022-1007.

Halloran PF. (2004). Immunosuppressive drugs for kidney transplantation. *New England Journal of Medicine*, Vol.351, No.26, (December 23, 2004), pp. 2715-29, ISSN 0028-4793.

Hampe J, Grebe J, Nikolaus S, Solberg C, Croucher PJ, Mascheretti S, Jahnsen J, Moum B, Klump B, Krawczak M, Mirza MM, Foelsch UR, Vatn M, Schreiber S. (2002). Association of NOD2 (CARD 15) genotype with clinical course of Crohn's disease: a cohort study. *Lancet*, Vol.359, No.9318, (May 11, 2002), pp. 1661-5, ISSN 0140-6736.

Hansson GK, Hermansson A. (2011). The immune system in atherosclerosis. *Nature Immunology*, Vol.12, No.3, (March 2011), pp. 204-12, ISSN 1529-2908.

Hansson GK. (2005). Inflammation, atherosclerosis, and coronary artery disease. *New England Journal of Medicine,* Vol.352, No.16, (April 21, 2005), pp. 1685-95, ISSN 0028-4793.

Harris JM, Hazenberg MD, Poulin JF, Higuera-Alhino D, Schmidt D, Gotway M, McCune JM. (2005). Multiparameter evaluation of human thymic function: interpretations and caveats. *Clinical Immunology,* Vol.115, No.2, (May 2005), pp.138-46, ISSN 1521-6616.

Hazenberg MD, Otto SA, de Pauw ES, Roelofs H, Fibbe WE, Hamann D, Miedema F. (2002). T-cell receptor excision circle and T-cell dynamics after allogeneic stem cell transplantation are related to clinical events. *Blood,* Vol.99, No.9, (May 1, 2002), pp. 3449-53, ISSN 0006-4971.

Helio T, Halme L, Lappalainen M, Fodstad H, Paavola-Sakki P, Turunen U, Farkkila M, Krusius T, Kontula K. (2003). CARD15/NOD2 gene variants are associated with familially occurring and complicated forms of Crohn's disease. *Gut,* Vol.52, No.4, (April 2003), pp. 558-62, ISSN 0017-5749.

Hochberg EP, Chillemi AC, Wu CJ, Neuberg D, Canning C, Hartman K, Alyea EP, Soiffer RJ, Kalams SA, Ritz J (2001). Quantitation of T-cell neogenesis in vivo after allogeneic bone marrow transplantation in adults. *Blood,* Vol.98, No.4, (August 15, 2001), pp. 1116-21, ISSN 0006-4971.

Holler E, Rogler G, Herfarth H, Brenmoehl J, Wild PJ, Hahn J, Eissner G, Scholmerich J, Andreesen R. (2004). Both donor and recipient NOD2/CARD15 mutations associate with transplant-related mortality and GvHD following allogeneic stem cell transplantation. *Blood,* Vol.104, No.3, (August 1, 2004), pp. 889-94, ISSN 0006-4971.

Kahwaji J, Bunnapradist S, Hsu JW, Idroos ML, Dudek R. (2011). Cause of death with graft function among renal transplant recipients in an integrated healthcare system. *Transplantation,* Vol.91, No2, (January 27, 2011), pp. 225-30, ISSN 0041-1337.

Kasiske BL, Guijarro C, Massy ZA, Wiederkehr MR, Ma JZ. (1996). Cardiovascular disease after renal transplantation. *Journal of the American Society of Nephrology.* Vol.7, No.1, (January, 1996), pp.; 158-65, ISSN 1046-6673.

Kasiske BL, Snyder JJ, Gilbertson DT, Wang C. (2004). Cancer after kidney transplantation in the United States. *American Journal of Transplantation,* Vol.4, No.6, (June 2004), pp. 905-13, ISSN 1600-6143.

Kaufman DB, Leventhal JR, Axelrod D, Gallon LG, Parker MA, Stuart FP. (2005). Alemtuzumab induction and prednisone-free maintenance immunotherapy in kidney transplantation: comparison with basiliximab induction--long-term results. *American Journal of Transplantation,* Vol.5, No.10, (October 2005), pp. 2539-48, ISSN 1600-6143.

Kiechl S, Lorenz E, Reindl M, Wiedermann CJ, Oberhollenzer F, Bonora E, Willeit J, Schwartz DA. (2002). Toll-like receptor 4 polymorphisms and atherogenesis. *New England Journal of Medicine,* Vol.347, No.3, (July 18, 2002), pp. 185-92, ISSN 0028-4793.

Kobayashi KS, Chamaillard M, Ogura Y, Henegariu O, Inohara N, Nunez G, Flavell RA. (2005). Nod2-dependent regulation of innate and adaptive immunity in the intestinal tract. *Science,* Vol.307, No. 5710, (February 4, 2005), pp. 731-4, ISSN 0036-8075.

Kohler S, Thiel A. (2009). Life after the thymus: CD31+ and CD31- human naive CD4+ T-cell subsets. *Blood*, Vol.113, No.4, (January 22, 2009), pp. 769-74, ISSN 0006-4971.

Kono H, Rock KL. (2008). How dying cells alert the immune system to danger. *Nature Reviews in Immunology*, Vol.8, No.4, (April 2008), pp. 279-89, ISSN 1474-1733.

Kroemer A, Xiao X, Vu MD, Gao W, Minamimura K, Chen M, Maki T, Li XC. (2007). OX40 controls functionally different T cell subsets and their resistance to depletion therapy. *Journal of Immunology*, Vol.179, No.8, (October, 15 2007), pp. 5584-91, ISSN 0022-1767.

LaCorcia G, Swistak M, Lawendowski C, Duan S, Weeden T, Nahill S, Williams JM, Dzuris JL. (2009). Polyclonal rabbit antithymocyte globulin exhibits consistent immunosuppressive capabilities beyond cell depletion. *Transplantation*, Vol.87, No.7, (April 15, 2009), pp. 966-74, ISSN 0041-1337.

Lamb KE, Lodhi S, Meier-Kriesche HU. (2011). Long-term renal allograft survival in the United States: a critical reappraisal. *American Journal of Transplantation*, Vol.11, No.3, (March 2011), pp. 450-62, ISSN 1600-6143.

Liefeldt L, Budde K. (2010). Risk factors for cardiovascular disease in renal transplant recipients and strategies to minimize risk. *Transplant International*, Vol.23, No.12, (December 2010), pp. 1191-204, ISSN 0934-0874.

Link A, Vogt TK, Favre S, Britschgi MR, Acha-Orbea H, Hinz B, Cyster JG, Luther SA. (2007). Fibroblastic reticular cells in lymph nodes regulate the homeostasis of naive T cells. *Nature Immunology*, Vol.8, No.11, (November 2007), pp. 1255-65, ISSN 1529-2908.

Lopez M, Clarkson MR, Albin M, Sayegh MH, Najafian N. (2006). A novel mechanism of action for anti-thymocyte globulin: induction of CD4+CD25+Foxp3+ regulatory T cells. *Journal of the American Society of Nephrology*. Vol.17, No.10, (October 2006), pp. 2844-53, ISSN 1046-6673.

Louis S, Audrain M, Cantarovich D, Schaffrath B, Hofmann K, Janssen U, Ballet C, Brouard S, Soulillou JP. (2007). Long-term cell monitoring of kidney recipients after an antilymphocyte globulin induction with and without steroids. *Transplantation*, Vol.83, No.6, (March 27, 2007), pp. 712-21, ISSN 0041-1337.

Mackall CL, Hakim FT, Gress RE. (1997). T-cell regeneration: all repertoires are not created equal. *Immunology Today*. Vol.18, No.5, (May 1997), pp. 245-51, ISSN 0167-5699.

Mallat Z, Gojova A, Brun V, Esposito B, Fournier N, Cottrez F, Tedgui A, Groux H. (2003). Induction of a regulatory T cell type 1 response reduces the development of atherosclerosis in apolipoprotein E-knockout mice. *Circulation*, Vol.108, No.10, (September 9, 2003), pp.1232-7, ISSN 0009-7322.

Mangan PR, Harrington LE, O'Quinn DB, Helms WS, Bullard DC, Elson CO, Hatton RD, Wahl SM, Schoeb TR, Weaver CT. (2006). Transforming growth factor-beta induces development of the T(H)17 lineage. *Nature*, Vol.441, No.7090, (May 11, 2006), pp. 231-4, ISSN 0028-0836.

Mannon RB. (2010). Immune monitoring and biomarkers to predict chronic allograft dysfunction. *Kidney International*, Vol.78, NoSuppl 119, (December 2010), pp. S59-65, ISSN *0085-2538*.

Matzinger P. (1994). Tolerance, danger, and the extended family. *Annual Review of Immunology*, Vol.12, No., pp. 991-1045, ISSN 0732-0582.

McDonald S, Russ G, Campbell S, Chadban S. (2007). Kidney transplant rejection in Australia and New Zealand: relationships between rejection and graft outcome. *American Journal of Transplantation*, Vol.7, No.5, (May 2007), pp. 1201-8, ISSN 1600-6143.

Meier-Kriesche HU, Schold JD, Kaplan B. (2004b). Long-term renal allograft survival: have we made significant progress or is it time to rethink our analytic and therapeutic strategies? *American Journal of Transplantation.*, Vol. 4, No.8, (August 2004), pp. 1289-95, ISSN 1600-6143.

Meier-Kriesche HU, Schold JD, Srinivas TR, Kaplan B. (2004a). Lack of improvement in renal allograft survival despite a marked decrease in acute rejection rates over the most recent era. *American Journal of Transplantation.*, Vol.4, No.3, (March 2004), pp. 378-83, ISSN 1600-6143.

Minamimura K, Gao W, Maki T. (2006). CD4+ regulatory T cells are spared from deletion by antilymphocyte serum, a polyclonal anti-T cell antibody. *Journal of Immunology*,Vol.176, No.7, (Apr 1, 2006), pp. 4125-32, ISSN 0022-1767.

Monaco AP, Wood ML, Russell PS. (1965). Adult Thymectomy: Effect on Recovery from Immunologic Depression in Mice. *Science*, Vol.149, No.3682, (July 23, 1965), pp. 432-5, ISSN 0036-8075.

Monti P, Scirpoli M, Maffi P, Ghidoli N, De Taddeo F, Bertuzzi F, Piemonti L, Falcone M, Secchi A, Bonifacio E. (2008). Islet transplantation in patients with autoimmune diabetes induces homeostatic cytokines that expand autoreactive memory T cells. *Journal of Clinical Investigation*, Vol.118, No.5, (May 2008), pp. 1806-14, ISSN 0021-9738.

Morre SA, Stooker W, Lagrand WK, van den Brule AJ, Niessen HW. (2000). Microorganisms in the aetiology of atherosclerosis. *Journal of Clinical Pathology*, Vol.53, No.9, (September 2000), pp. 647-54, ISSN 0021-9746.

Moss P, Rickinson A. Cellular immunotherapy for viral infection after HSC transplantation. *Nature Reviews Immunology*, Vol.5, No.1, (January 2005), pp. 9-20, ISSN 1474-1733.

Muller TF, Grebe SO, Neumann MC, Heymanns J, Radsak K, Sprenger H, Lange H. (1997). Persistent long-term changes in lymphocyte subsets induced by polyclonal antibodies. *Transplantation*, Vol.64, No.10, (November 27, 1997), pp. 1432-7, ISSN 0041-1337.

Neumann FJ, Kastrati A, Miethke T, Pogatsa-Murray G, Seyfarth M, Schomig A. (2000). Previous cytomegalovirus infection and risk of coronary thrombotic events after stent placement. *Circulation*, Vol.101, No.1, (January 4-11, 2000), pp. 11-3, ISSN 0009-7322.

Nickel P, Kreutzer S, Bold G, Friebe A, Schmolke K, Meisel C, Jurgensen JS, Thiel A, Wernecke KD, Reinke P, Volk HD. (2005). CD31+ naive Th cells are stable during six months following kidney transplantation: implications for post-transplant thymic function. *American Journal of Transplantation*, Vol.5, No.7, (July 2005), pp. 1764-71, ISSN 1600-6143.

Noel C, Abramowicz D, Durand D, Mourad G, Lang P, Kessler M, Charpentier B, Touchard G, Berthoux F, Merville P, Ouali N, Squifflet JP, Bayle F, Wissing KM, Hazzan M. (2009). Daclizumab versus antithymocyte globulin in high-immunological-risk renal transplant recipients. *Journal of the American Society of Nephrology*, Vol.20, No.6, (June 2009), pp. 1385-92, ISSN 1046-6673.

Ogura Y, Lala S, Xin W, Smith E, Dowds TA, Chen FF, Zimmermann E, Tretiakova M, Cho JH, Hart J, Greenson JK, Keshav S, Nunez G. (2003). Expression of NOD2 in Paneth cells: a possible link to Crohn's ileitis. *Gut,* Vol.52,No.11, (November 2003), pp. 1591-7, ISSN 0017-5749.

Ojo AO, Hanson JA, Wolfe RA, Leichtman AB, Agodoa LY, Port FK. (2000). Long-term survival in renal transplant recipients with graft function. *Kidney International,* Vol.57,No.1, (January 2000), pp. 307-13, ISSN 0085-2538.

Ojo AO. (2006). Cardiovascular complications after renal transplantation and their prevention. *Transplantation,* Vol.82, No.5, (September 15, 2006), pp. 603-11, ISSN 0041-1337.

Okamoto Y, Douek DC, McFarland RD, Koup RA. (2002). Effects of exogenous interleukin-7 on human thymus function. *Blood,* Vol.99, No.8, (April 15, 2002), pp. 2851-8, ISSN 0006-4971.

Penn I. (1979). Tumors in allograft recipients. *New England Journal of Medicine,* Vol.301, No.7, (August 16, 1979), pp. 385, ISSN 0028-4793.

Preville X, Flacher M, LeMauff B, Beauchard S, Davelu P, Tiollier J, Revillard JP. (2001). Mechanisms involved in antithymocyte globulin immunosuppressive activity in a nonhuman primate model. *Transplantation,* Vol.71, No.3, (February 15, 2001), pp. 460-8, ISSN 0041-1337.

Rebellato LM, Gross U, Verbanac KM, Thomas JM. (1994). A comprehensive definition of the major antibody specificities in polyclonal rabbit antithymocyte globulin. *Transplantation,* Vol.57, No.5, (March 15, 1994), pp. 685-94, ISSN 0041-1337.

Ridker PM, Danielson E, Fonseca FA, Genest J, Gotto AM, Jr., Kastelein JJ, Koenig W, Libby P, Lorenzatti AJ, Macfadyen JG, Nordestgaard BG, Shepherd J, Willerson JT, Glynn RJ. (2009). Reduction in C-reactive protein and LDL cholesterol and cardiovascular event rates after initiation of rosuvastatin: a prospective study of the JUPITER trial. *Lancet,* Vol.373, No.9670, (April 4, 2009), pp. 1175-82, ISSN 0140-6736.

Ridker PM. (2001). Role of inflammatory biomarkers in prediction of coronary heart disease. *Lancet,* Vol.358, No.9286, (September 22, 2001), pp. 946-8, ISSN 0140-6736.

Rock KL, Latz E, Ontiveros F, Kono H. (2010). The sterile inflammatory response. *Annual Review of Immunology.* Vol.28, No., (March 2010), pp. 321-42, ISSN 0732-0582.

Rose T, Lambotte O, Pallier C, Delfraissy JF, Colle JH. (2009). Identification and biochemical characterization of human plasma soluble IL-7R: lower concentrations in HIV-1-infected patients. *Journal of Immunology.* Vol.182, No.12, (June 15 2009), pp. 7389-97, ISSN 0022-1767.

Sakaguchi S, Miyara M, Costantino CM, Hafler DA. (2010). FOXP3+ regulatory T cells in the human immune system. *Nature Reviews Immunology,* Vol.10, No.7, (July 2010), pp. 490-500, ISSN 1474-1733.

Sarnak MJ, Levey AS, Schoolwerth AC, Coresh J, Culleton B, Hamm LL, McCullough PA, Kasiske BL, Kelepouris E, Klag MJ, Parfrey P, Pfeffer M, Raij L, Spinosa DJ, Wilson PW. (2003). Kidney disease as a risk factor for development of cardiovascular disease: a statement from the American Heart Association Councils on Kidney in Cardiovascular Disease, High Blood Pressure Research, Clinical Cardiology, and Epidemiology and Prevention. *Circulation,* Vol.108, No.17, (October 28, 2003), pp. 2154-69, ISSN 0009-7322.

Sayegh MH, Carpenter CB. (2004). Transplantation 50 years later--progress, challenges, and promises. *New England Journal of Medicine,* Vol.351, No.26, (December 23, 2004), pp. 2761-6, ISSN 0028-4793.

Scarsi M, Bossini N, Malacarne F, Valerio F, Sandrini S, Airo P. (2010). The number of circulating recent thymic emigrants is severely reduced 1 year after a single dose of alemtuzumab in renal transplant recipients. *Transplant International,* Vol.23, No.8, (August 2010), pp. 786-95, ISSN 0934-0874.

Scheibner KA, Lutz MA, Boodoo S, Fenton MJ, Powell JD, Horton MR. (2006). Hyaluronan fragments act as an endogenous danger signal by engaging TLR2. *Journal of Immunology,* Vol.177, No.2, (July 15, 2006), pp. 1272-81, ISSN 0022-1767.

Schroppel B, Heeger PS. (2010). Gazing into a crystal ball to predict kidney transplant outcome. *Journal of Clinical Investigation,* Vol.120, No.6, (June 2010), pp. 1803-6, ISSN 0021-9738.

Sener A, Tang AL, Farber DL. (2009). Memory T-cell predominance following T-cell depletional therapy derives from homeostatic expansion of naive T cells. *American Journal of Transplantion,* Vol.9, No.11, (November 2009), pp. 2615-23, ISSN 1600-6143.

Sportes C, Babb RR, Krumlauf MC, Hakim FT, Steinberg SM, Chow CK, Brown MR, Fleisher TA, Noel P, Maric I, Stetler-Stevenson M, Engel J, Buffet R, Morre M, Amato RJ, Pecora A, Mackall CL, Gress RE. (2010). Phase I study of recombinant human interleukin-7 administration in subjects with refractory malignancy. *Clinical Cancer Research,* Vol.16, No.2, (January 15, 2010), pp. 727-35, ISSN 1078-0432.

Sportes C, Hakim FT, Memon SA, Zhang H, Chua KS, Brown MR, Fleisher TA, Krumlauf MC, Babb RR, Chow CK, Fry TJ, Engels J, Buffet R, Morre M, Amato RJ, Venzon DJ, Korngold R, Pecora A, Gress RE, Mackall CL. (2008). Administration of rhIL-7 in humans increases in vivo TCR repertoire diversity by preferential expansion of naive T cell subsets. *Journal of Experimental Medicine,* Vol.205, No.7, (July 7, 2008), pp. 1701-14, ISSN 0022-1007.

Stary HC, Chandler AB, Dinsmore RE, Fuster V, Glagov S, Insull W, Jr., Rosenfeld ME, Schwartz CJ, Wagner WD, Wissler RW. (1995) A definition of advanced types of atherosclerotic lesions and a histological classification of atherosclerosis. A report from the Committee on Vascular Lesions of the Council on Arteriosclerosis, American Heart Association. *Circulation,* Vol.92, No.5, (September 1, 1995), pp. 1355-74, ISSN 0009-7322.

Taleb S, Tedgui A, Mallat Z. (2010a). Adaptive T cell immune responses and atherogenesis. *Current Opinion in Pharmacology,* Vol.10,No.2, (April 2010), pp. 197-202, ISSN 1471-4892.

Taleb S, Tedgui A, Mallat Z. (2010b). Interleukin-17: friend or foe in atherosclerosis? *Current Opinion in Lipidology,* Vol.21, No.5, (October 2010), pp. 404-8, ISSN 0957-9672.

Trifari S, Kaplan CD, Tran EH, Crellin NK, Spits H. (2009). Identification of a human helper T cell population that has abundant production of interleukin 22 and is distinct from T(H)-17, T(H)1 and T(H)2 cells. *Nature Immunology,* Vol.10, No.8, (August 2009), pp. 864-71, ISSN 1529-2908.

van Leeuwen MT, Grulich AE, Webster AC, McCredie MR, Stewart JH, McDonald SP, Amin J, Kaldor JM, Chapman JR, Vajdic CM. (2009). Immunosuppression and other risk factors for early and late non-Hodgkin lymphoma after kidney transplantation. *Blood*, Vol.114, No.3, (July 2009), pp. 630-7, ISSN 0006-4971.

Veldhoen M, Uyttenhove C, van Snick J, Helmby H, Westendorf A, Buer J, Martin B, Wilhelm C, Stockinger B. (2008). Transforming growth factor-beta 'reprograms' the differentiation of T helper 2 cells and promotes an interleukin 9-producing subset. *Nature Immunology*, Vol.9, No.12, (December 2008), pp. 1341-6, ISSN 1529-2908.

Vieira PL, Christensen JR, Minaee S, O'Neill EJ, Barrat FJ, Boonstra A, Barthlott T, Stockinger B, Wraith DC, O'Garra A.(2004). IL-10-secreting regulatory T cells do not express Foxp3 but have comparable regulatory function to naturally occurring CD4+CD25+ regulatory T cells. *Journal of Immunol*, Vol.172, No.10, (May 15, 2004), pp. 5986-93, ISSN 1521-4141.

Vignali DA, Collison LW, Workman CJ. (2008). How regulatory T cells work. *Nature Reviews Immunology*, Vol.8, No.7, (July 2008), pp. 523-32, ISSN 1474-1733.

Villeneuve PJ, Schaubel DE, Fenton SS, Shepherd FA, Jiang Y, Mao Y. (2007). Cancer incidence among Canadian kidney transplant recipients. *American Journal of Transplantation*, Vol. 7, No.4, (April 2007), pp. 941-8, ISSN 1600-6143.

Wang JH, Kasiske BL. Screening and management of pretransplant cardiovascular disease. *Current Opinion in Nephrology and Hypertension*, Vol.19, No.6, (November 2010), pp. 586-91, ISSN 1062-4821.

Webster AC, Craig JC, Simpson JM, Jones MP, Chapman JR. (2007).Identifying high risk groups and quantifying absolute risk of cancer after kidney transplantation: a cohort study of 15,183 recipients. *American Journal of Transplantation*, Vol.7, No. 9, (September 2007), pp. 2140-51, ISSN 1600-6143.

Webster AC, Wong G, Craig JC, Chapman JR. (2008). Managing cancer risk and decision making after kidney transplantation. *American Journal of Transplantation*, Vol.8, No.11, (November 2008), pp. 2185-91, ISSN 1600-6143.

Weimer R, Staak A, Susal C, Streller S, Yildiz S, Pelzl S, Renner F, Dietrich H, Daniel V, Rainer L, Kamali-Ernst S, Ernst W, Padberg W, Opelz G. (2005). ATG induction therapy: long-term effects on Th1 but not on Th2 responses. *Transplant International*, Vol.18, No.2, (February 2005), pp. 226-36, ISSN 0934-0874.

Williams KM, Hakim FT, Gress RE. (2007). T cell immune reconstitution following lymphodepletion. *Seminars in Immunology*, Vol.19, No.5, (October 2007), pp. 318-30, ISSN 1044-5323.

Willoughby LM, Schnitzler MA, Brennan DC, Pinsky BW, Dzebisashvili N, Buchanan PM, Neri L, Rocca-Rey LA, Abbott KC, Lentine KL. (2009) Early outcomes of thymoglobulin and basiliximab induction in kidney transplantation: application of statistical approaches to reduce bias in observational comparisons. *Transplantation*, Vol.87, No.10, (May 27 2009), pp 1520-9, ISSN 0041-1337.

Woollard KJ, Geissmann F. (2010). Monocytes in atherosclerosis: subsets and functions. *Nature Reviews Cardiology*, Vol.7, No.2 (February 2010), pp. 77-86, ISSN 1759-5002.

Wu Z, Bensinger SJ, Zhang J, Chen C, Yuan X, Huang X, Markmann JF, Kassaee A, Rosengard BR, Hancock WW, Sayegh MH, Turka LA. (2004). Homeostatic proliferation is a barrier to transplantation tolerance. *Nature Medicine*, Vol.10, No.1, (January 2004), pp. 87-92, ISSN 1078-8956.

Yan ZQ, Hansson GK. (2007). Innate immunity, macrophage activation, and atherosclerosis. *Immunological Review*, Vol.219, No., (October 2007), pp. 187-203, ISSN 1600-065X.

Zeiser R, Nguyen VH, Beilhack A, Buess M, Schulz S, Baker J, Contag CH, Negrin RS. (2006). Inhibition of CD4+CD25+ regulatory T-cell function by calcineurin-dependent interleukin-2 production. *Blood*, Vol.108, No.1, (July 1, 2006), pp. 390-9, ISSN 0006-4971.

Zhou X, Stemme S, Hansson GK. (2001). Evidence for a local immune response in atherosclerosis. CD4+ T cells infiltrate lesions of apolipoprotein-E-deficient mice. *American Journal of Pathology*, Vol.149, No.2, (August 1996), pp. 359-66, ISSN 0887-8005.

5

Urinary Fructose-1,6-Bisphosphatase (FBP-1,6) and N-Acetyl-β-Hexosaminidase (HEX) in Monitoring Kidney Transplantation - Literature Review

Alina Kępka[1], Sławomir Dariusz Szajda[2], Napoleon Waszkiewicz[2], Sylwia Chojnowska[3], Paweł Pludowski[1], Jerzy Robert Ładny[2] and Krzysztof Zwierz[3]

[1]The Children's Memorial Health Institute, Warsaw
[2]Medical University, Białystok
[3]Medical Institute, College of Computer Science and Business Administration, Łomża
Poland

1. Introduction

Kidney grafts begin normal function immediately after transplantation, after several, or after dozen or so days delay. **A**cute **K**idney **I**nsufficience (AKI), **N**ephrotic **S**yndrome (NS) and **C**hronic **A**llograft **N**ephropathy (CAN), sometimes defined as "**I**nterstitial **F**ibrosis / **T**ubular **A**trophy (IF/TA) without any specific etiology" (Reuter et al., 2010), are the main types of complications connected with kidney transplantation.

In the diagnosis of the function of transplanted renal allografts, activities of enzymes excreted into urine by particular fragments of nephron are used. Increase of enzymuria precedes some clinical symptoms and is a more sensitive diagnostic marker than tubular proteinuria. Increase of enzymuria may also be useful for determination the time since renal tubules damage took place. Fructose-1,6 – bisphosphatase (FBP-1,6)- the principal enzyme of gluconeogenesis and N-acetyl-β-hexosaminidase (HEX)- the most active of the lysosomal exoglycosidases, taking part in the degradation of glycoconjugates (glycoproteins, glycolipids, proteoglycans), are markers used for monitoring kidney allograft function both in early and late post transplant periods, because of localization in the proximal contorted and straight tubules of nephron.

2. Urinary fructose-1,6-bisphosphatase (FBP-1,6) key enzyme of gluconogenesis

2.1 Renal glucose production

Kidneys require a continuous supply of glucose as a metabolic fuel. In the absence of dietary intake of carbohydrates, glycogen stores (mostly liver's) are able to supply glucose for only ten to eighteen hours. Fortunately liver and kidneys are able to produce glucose via the gluconeogenesis pathway (Champe et al., 2008) [Fig. 1.].

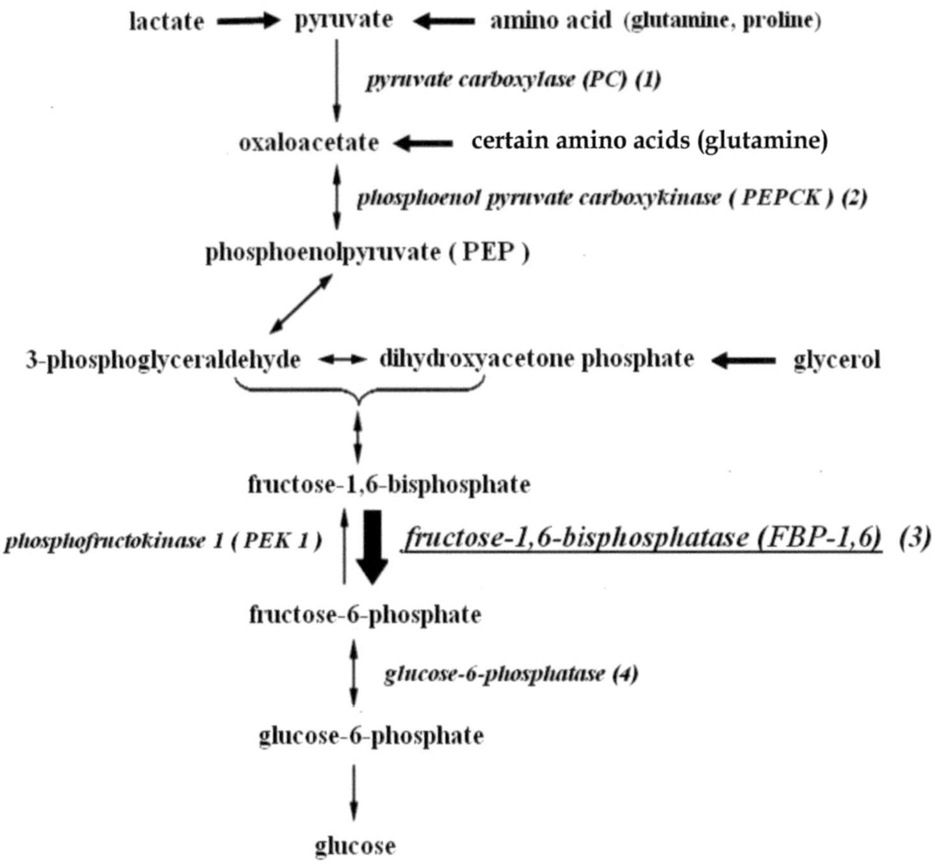

Fig. 1. Renal gluconeogenesis. The key enzymes of gluconeogenesis: (1) **P**yruvate **C**arboxylase (PC), (2) **P**hospho**E**nol **P**yruvate **C**arboxy**K**inase (PEPCK), (3) **F**ructose-**1,6**-**B**is**P**hosphatase (FBP-1,6), (4) glucose-6-phosphatase. The main renal gluconeogenic substrates are: glutamine, lactate, glycerol.

Renal glucose production accounts for between 5% to 25% of the total glucose formed by gluconeogenesis, in the body (Conjard et al., 2001; Meyer et al., 2003). The proximal renal tubules are capable of synthesizing glucose from a variety of precursors, including lactate, pyruvate, glutamine (the main substrate of renal gluconeogenesis), glutamate, and glycerol. The three segments of the renal proximal tubules PCT1, PCT2 and PST [Fig. 2.] can synthesize glucose at different rates from lactate. PCT2 and PST segments synthesize more glucose from lactate than the PCT1 segment (Yáñez et al., 2003; Yáñez et al., 2005). The PCT1 segment is specialized in the reabsorption of lactate in kidney (Yáñez et al., 2005). The segments PCT1, PCT2 and PST synthesize glucose from glutamine with about the same capacity (Conjard et al., 2001), which indicates that glutamine is the main gluconeogenic substrate for the kidney (Stumvoll et al., 1997). Also fructose, propionate and proline are potential candidates for renal glucose precursors (Conjard et al., 2001; Meyer et al., 2003; Stumvoll et al., 1997). Fructose-1,6-bisphosphatase (FBP-1,6. EC 3.1.3.11) [Fig. 1.] is a key regulatory enzyme for renal gluconeogenesis.

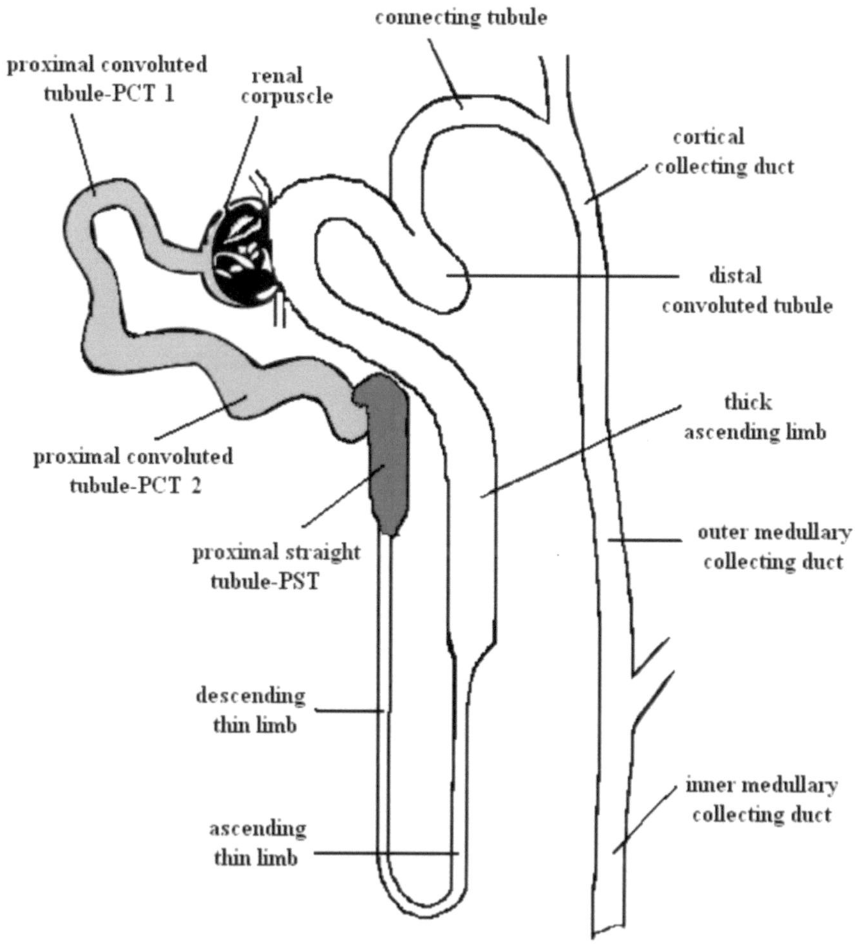

Fig. 2. Localization of FBP-1,6 and HEX in the nephron. FBP -1,6 is confined to the **P**roximal **C**onvoluted **T**ubule -PCT1, PCT2 and **P**roximal **S**traight **T**ubule -PST. Lysosomal N-acetyl-β-D-hexosaminidase (HEX) is distributed along the nephron with highest activity in the proximal convoluted tubule PCT1 and PCT2.

2.2 Structure and action of kidney FBP-1,6

FBP-1,6 catalyzes the irreversible conversion of fructose-1,6-bisphosphate (Fru-1,6-P_2) to fructose-6-phosphate and inorganic phosphate in the reaction:

$$\text{Fructose 1,6-bisphosphate} + H_20 = \text{Fructose-6-phosphate} + \text{phosphate}$$

The mammalian kidney FBP-1,6 is a tetramer composed of four identical subunits with molecular weight ranging from 36 kDa to 41 kDa per subunit (e.g. each subunit of the pig kidney enzyme consists of 337 amino acids), organized as a dimer of dimers [Fig. 3.].

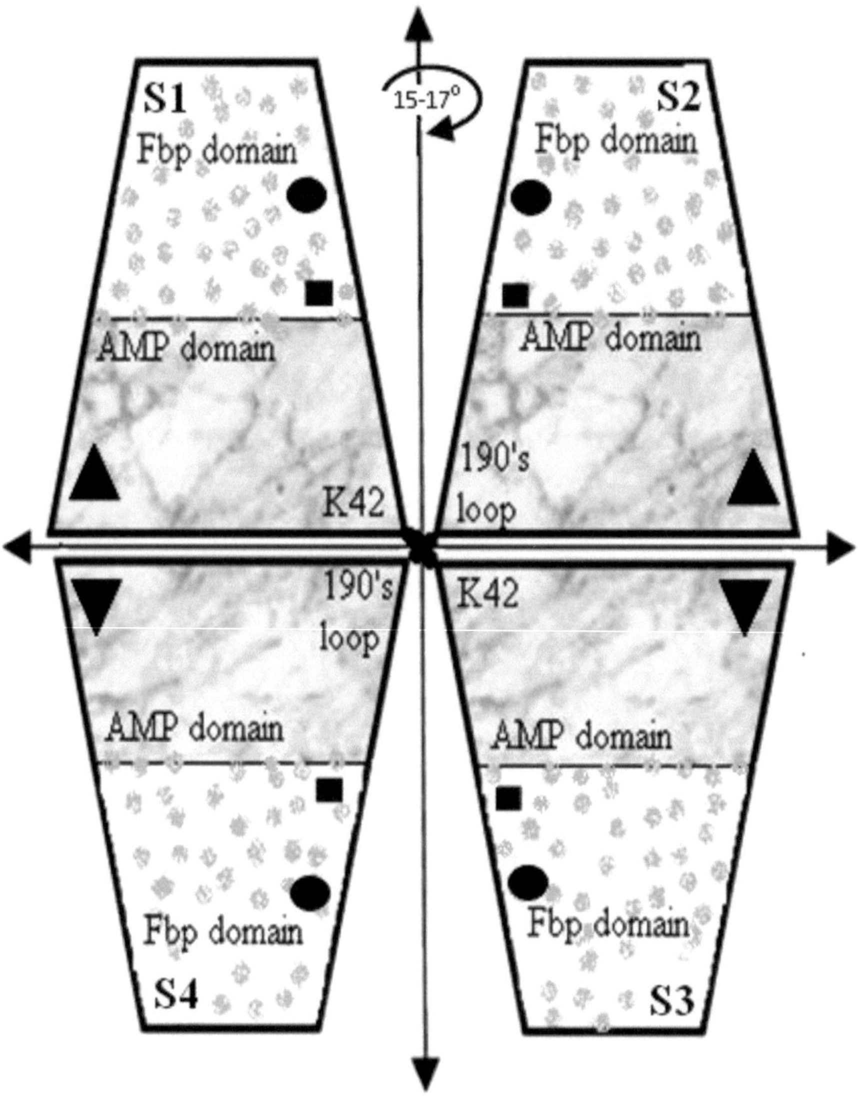

Fig. 3. The quaternary structure of fructose-1,6-bisphosphatase (R-state). The four subunits of FBP-1,6 are designated S1,S2,S3,S4 and are labeled clockwise. The S1 and S2 subunits correspond to the upper dimer, and the S3, S4 subunits correspond to the lower dimer. Each subunit is composed of two folding domains. The AMP domain has the AMP binding site (▲), while the Fru-1,6-P_2 (Fbp) domain contains the active site (•). The divalent metal sites (■) are located between the AMP and Fbp domains. Residues of the 190's loop make critical contacts with Lys-42 (K42). The R→T transition of FBP-1,6 involves a 15°-17° clockwise rotation of the S1:S2 dimer in respect to the S3:S4 dimer.

The tetramer of FBP-1,6 requires divalent cations: magnesium, manganese, zinc or cobalt for its catalytic activity (Dżugaj, 2006; Sáez et al., 1996; Yáñez et al., 2003). In each of four (S1, S2, S3 and S4) subunits, X-ray crystallographic studies have identified that the AMP and FBP domains [Fig. 3.]. Fru-1,6-P_2 (substrate) binding site (•) is located in each of four FBP domains. The AMP-binding sites (▲) are located at AMP domains approximately 30Å from the active site. One divalent metal-binding site (■) is located at each of the FBP domain between the Fru-1,6 P_2 and AMP binding domains of each subunit [Fig. 3.]. Pig kidney FBP-1,6 exists in at least two quaternary conformations called **R** (relaxed)-active, and **T** (tense)-inactive state, depending on the relative concentrations of the FBP-1,6 effectors. The allosteric transition R→ T of kidney FBP-1,6 involves a 15^0-17^0 clock-wise rotation around the vertical axis of the S1:S2 (upper) dimer, with respect to the S3:S4 (lower) dimer (Kelly et al., 1996; Lu et al., 1996; Zhang et al., 1994) [Fig. 3.]. Localization the 190's loops and Lys-42 near the horizontal and vertical molecular symmetry axes is critical for the R→T transition. AMP (reflecting shortage of energy) inhibits the enzyme, shifting FBP-1,6 from the R to the T conformation [Fig. 3.]. In the absence of AMP the FBP-1,6 exists in the active R state. Fructose-1,6-bisphosphate, fructose-6-phosphate and ATP (reflecting excess of energy), as well as metal cations, stabilize the R (active) state (Kelly-Loughane & Kantrowitz, 2001; McIninch & Kantrowitz, 2001). Mammalian kidney FBP-1,6 is activated by high glucagon/insulin ratio, which elevate cAMP level and increase activity of protein kinase A. Increased activity of protein kinase A favors the phosphorylation of bifunctional complex 6-phosphofructo-2-kinase/fructose-2,6-bisphosphatase. Phosphorylated phosphofructokinse-2 is inactive, which decreases the level of fructose 2,6-P_2 (inhibitor of FBP-1,6) (Champe et al., 2008). FBP-1,6 has two synergistic natural inhibitors: mentioned earlier adenosine-5'-monophosphate (AMP), and fru-2,6-P_2, a product of the bifunctional phosphofructokinase-2/ fructose bisphosphatase-2 (Hines et al., 2007; Sáez et al., 1996; Wu et al., 2006). Excess of FBP-1,6 substrate i.e Fru-1,6-P_2, acts as an inhibitor on FBP-1,6. Are novel inhibitors of fructose-1,6-bisphosphatase such as achyrofuran, anilinoquinazoline (also an inhibitor of tyrosine kinase) and 3-(2-carboxyethyl)-4,6-dichloro-1H-indole-2-carboxylic acid (MDL-29951)- also an antagonist of the glycine site of the NMDA receptor (Wright et al., 2001; Wright et al., 2003).

2.3 Ultrastructural localization of the FBP-1,6 in kidney

FBP-1,6 immunoreactivity was detected in kidney cortex cells, but not in the medulla. In the cortex all epithelial cells the PCT1, PCT2, and PST segments, forming the proximal convoluted tubules were FBP-1,6 positive (Yáñez et al., 2003). Aldolase B, but not aldolase A, colocalizes and forms a complex with FBP-1,6 (Yáñez et al., 2005).

Expression FBP-1,6 activity in cytoplasm and apical cells membranes PCT1, PCT2 and PST segments of the proximal tubules was demonstrated (Yáñez et al., 2003) [Fig. 2.]. Expression of FBP-1,6 was also observed in the basolateral membrane region of the PCT1 segment of the proximal tubule and colocalized with the **M**ono**C**arboxilate **T**ransporter 1 (MCT1) (Yáñez et al., 2003; Yáñez et al., 2005). MCT1 contributes to the transport of monocarboxylic acids in many tissues, which suggest that the PCT1 segment is specialized in the reabsorpion of lactate in kidney. The actual level of lactate transporter expression in the PCT1 segment might be the reason for the difference in the rates of glucose neosynthesis from lactate in the human renal proximal tubules (Yáñez et al., 2003).

The subcellular location of kidney FBP-1,6 is similar to liver FBP-1,6. The histochemical analysis revealed that the anti-FBP-1,6 antibody detected two single bands with a molecular weight of 36kDa and 40 kDa, in kidney and liver, respectively (Yáñez et al., 2003). The immunofluorescence and confocal analysis revealed that FBP-1,6 was present in the cytosol and inside the nucleus of hepatocytes and proximal cells of the nephron (Sáez et al., 1996). Nuclear FBP-1,6 function is similar to the function of the cytosolic form. FBP-1,6 can be translocated inside the nuclei of proximal tubule cells (Yáñez et al., 2003; Yáñez et al., 2005). The peroxidase reaction in light microscopy, yielded a strong signal FBP-1,6 in the proximal straight and convoluted tubules located at the cortex, but not in cells of the kidney medulla. The FBP-1,6 reaction is concentrated in the apical membrane region and is also observed in the basolateral membrane region (Yáñez et al., 2005). No immunoreactivity was observed in glomeruli, ascending and descending loops of Henle, collecting tubules, distal tubules and in cell of the kidney medulla (Sáez et al., 1996; Yáñez et al., 2003).

Determination of the fructose-1,6-bisphosphatase activities in the fractions of kidney and liver (assayed spectrophotometrically at 30^{0}C, by following the rate of NADH formation) revealed that FBP-1,6 activity is present in both tissues in the initial homogenate, the cytoplasmic extract and the high speed supernatant. No activity of FBP-1,6 was observed in the nuclear fraction, light or the heavy mitochondrial and microsomal fraction (Sáez et al., 1996).

2.4 Genetics and localization of the FBP-1,6 isozymes in human tissues

Human FBP-1,6 is coded in 2 distinct genes, *FBP1* and *FBP2* (Matsuura et al., 2002). *FBP1* consist of seven exons and spans over 31 kilobases at chromosome 9q22.2-q22.3 and expresses a 362-amino acid (el-Maghrabi et al., 1995). Messenger RNA (mRNA) from liver, kidney and monocytes is identical (Kikawa et al., 1994). *FBP2* which was isolated from muscle, codes 339 amino acids, and shares 77% amino acid sequences identity with *FBP1* (Tillmann & Eschrich, 1998).

FBP-1,6 is expressed in variety of organs such as: liver, kidney, muscle, brain, lung, small intestine, retina (Cloix et al., 1997; Mamczur et al., 2010; Nomura et al., 1994; Velásquez et al., 2010; Yáñez et al., 2003; Yáñez et al., 2005). Existence of four isozymes: muscle, liver, brain and intestine in tissues of vertebrates has been postulated (Dżugaj, 2006). In mammals two isoforms of FBP-1,6 exist, which are encoded by separate genes. In humans L-FBP-1,6 which is expressed mainly in liver and kidney, and M-FBP-1,6 is expressed mainly in muscle. Both isforms (L-FBP-1,6 and M-FBP-1,6) were found in several organs such as lung and brain (Bigl et al., 2008).

3. FBP-1,6 in kidney transplantation

After damage of the epithelial cell membranes, FBP-1,6 is released into urine. Therefore urinary FBP-1,6 activity was recommended for diagnoses of complications in the early post-transplantation period. Urinary FBP-1,6 was assayed in the second morning midstream urine portion in patients after transplantation. Cold ischemia time was 20.6±8.4h (range 3-32h), with a median of 22 h. Urinary FBP-1,6 excretion was significantly lower in grafts stored for a shorter time than 22 hours (0.69±0.42 U/g creatinine) as compared to FBP-1,6 urinary excretion in grafts stored > 22 hours (1.13±0.56 $p=0.035$ U/g creatinine). Multiple regression analysis demonstrated that the cold ischemia time was the only pre-transplant factor, which significantly correlated with early post-transplant urinary FBP-1,6 excretion (multiple $R=0.65$, $F=14.6$, $p<0.001$). After transplantation the patients were given cyclosporine A (CsA), but CsA levels did not correlate with urinary FBP-1,6 activities during the first four postoperative days. The duration of the cold ischemia time is significantly correlated with the degree of urinary excretion of FBP-1,6 during the first four postoperative days (Kotanko et al., 1997).

Sharp increase in the activities of lactate dehydrogenase (LDH), glucose-6-phosphatase (G6Pase), malic enzyme (ME) and fructose-1,6-bisphosphatase (FBP-1,6) was observed in homogenates of renal cortex and medulla, after 5 min of warm ischemia induced by occlusion of rat renal left artery. Warm ischemia lasting 15-60 min resulted in a progressive decrease in the activity of the above enzymes. Reperfusion of rat kidneys for 60 min after prolonged warm ischemia caused complete recovery of the activity of the above enzymes (Khundmiri et al., 2004).

Five to ten day after uncomplicated renal transplantation enzymuria reaches a constant value, which is much higher than the average in healthy humans (Jung et al., 1992). Activity of urinary FBP-1,6 reached a lower level on the 4th day after transplantation, and remained on a stable low rate. During the four first days after transplantation the activity of urinary FBP-1,6 amounted to 0.9±0.5 U/g (0.1±0.06 U/mmol urinary creatinine); range 0.2-2.1 U/g (0.02-0.24 U/mmol)] (Kotanko et al., 1997). However in complicated transplantations urinary excretion of FBP-1,6 significantly increases, contrary to urinary creatinine concentration, which change slowly (Jung et al., 1992).

During experimental transplantation renal grafts taken from non-heart beating donors, fructose- 1,6-bisphosphate was used, for protection graft microcirculation against ischemic damage. Microdialysis probes in the renal cortex of pig kidney were used to monitor pyruvate concentration during hypotermic machine perfusion with a perfusate containing 29.4 mM exogenous fructose-1,6-diphosphate (FDP). During glycolysis fructose-1,6-diphosphate (FDP) is generated from glucose and is transformated into pyruvate. In the absence of oxygen, pyruvate is transformated into lactate rather than acetyl-CoA and is accumulated in the cell. The decrease of pH inhibits glucose conversion to fructose-1,6-diphosphate. Significant increases in pyruvate production ($p<0.05$) were observed after 12h of perfusion in the interstitial fluid of FDP-treated kidneys, as compared to control kidneys. After 24 h of graft perfusion the concentration of pyruvate was 149.1±58.4 μM in the FDP group and 55.6±17.9μM in the control group. The addition of FDP to the fluid during ischemic kidney perfusion, resulted in enhanced pyruvate production in the extracellular space. FDP has rheologic and antioxidant effects in addition to its ability to promote glycolysis and improve red blood cell deformability (Baicu et al., 2004).

FDP prevents the decline of renal cortical Na-K-ATPase activity induced by ischemia end gentamicin toxicity. Lu and Lin (Lu & Lin, 1989) have shown that fructose-1,6-diphosphate (FDP) has the ability to restrain the oxygen-radical related reperfusion injury. They observed reduction in renal Na-K-ATPase activity by 18.6% after 30 min of renal pedicle clamping and 60 min of reflow as well as a 32.5% reduction in renal Na-K-ATPase activity after 90 min of injection 100mg/kg gentamicin. Application of 4g/kg fructose-1,6-diphosphate (FDP) and 60 min infusion after reflow in the ischemic group, and 90 min infusion after injection of the drug in gentamicine-treated group, increased renal Na-K-ATPase activity in the FDP-treated group in comparison to the control kidney (Lu & Lin, 1989).

Expression of urinary FBP-1,6 protein is utilized to evaluate the degree of chronic post transplant nephropathy. Increased expression key renal enzymes of the citrate circle i.e. NAD^+-dependent **I**socitrate **D**e**H**ydrogenase (IDH) and **I**ron-**R**esponsive **E**lement-**B**inding **P**rotein-**1**/aconitase (IREBP1), as well as mitochondrial CK, creatine kinase B-type, ornithine aminotransferase and FBP-1,6 were observed in IF/TA. FBP-1,6 protein was expressed at a significantly lower level in aTX(allogenic graft) than in sTX (syngenic graft) (Reuter et al., 2010). The above data is supported by analysis of gene expression profiles of renal transplants, which revealed reduced FBP-1,6 mRNA level in graft with IF/TA (Scherer et al., 2003).

Determination of urinary FBP-1,6 activity was not only used for evaluation of transplanted kidneys, but also to estimate the degree of damage to renal tubules of diabetic patients (Eid et al., 2006), in idiopatic nephrotic syndrome (Kępka et al., 2008) acute pyelonephritis (Zoch-Zwierz et al., 2004), heavy metal (e.g.$HgCl_2$) or, maleic acid intoxication (Kotanko et al., 1984), after trichloroethylene (TCE) administration (Khan et al., 2009). The urinary FBP-1,6 activity significantly increases after nephrotoxic drugs (ifosfamide, cisplatinum) (Pfaller et al., 1994) prednisolone, and azathioprine (Kotanko et al., 1986), cyclosporine, sirolimus and tacrolimus (Klawitter et al.,2010).

4. HEX - most active exoglycosidase in catabolism of glycoconjugates

All renal glycoconjugates (glycoproteins and glycolipids, present in renal cell membranes, and participating in inter cellular communication and interactions, as well as glycosaminoglycans of the renal cell surfaces, and extra cellular matrix), contain oligosaccharide chains (Gabius, 2009).Glycoconjugates are subject to constant synthesis and degradation. The protein cores of the glycoconjugates are synthesized in the cytoplasm, but glycosylation occurs in endoplasmatic reticulum and Golgi Apparatus (Zwierz et al., 1999). Lysosomes are the principal sites of intracellular digestion of sugar chains of glycoconjugates (Cuervo, 2004). Exoglycosidases which successively release individual sugars from non reducing ends of oligosaccharide chains are localized in lysosomes (Strecker et al., 1988; Winchester, 2005) [Fig. 4].

N-acetyl-β-hexosaminidase (HEX) (EC 3.2.1.52) is the most active of lysosomal exoglycosidases (Popko et al., 2008), taking part in the catabolism of oligosaccharide chains of all types of glycoconjugates (Zwierz et al., 1999). The fact that HEX has the highest activity of amongst exoglycosidases may be explained by the fact that aminohexoses (N-acetyl-glucosamine and N-acetyl-galactosamine) are components of all types of glycoconjugates: glycoproteins, glycolipids and glycosaminoglycans of proteoglycans (Chojnowska et al., 2011). HEX releases monomers of N-acetyl-glucosamine and N-acetyl-galactosamine from the non reducing ends of oligosaccharide chains of glycoconjugates (Zwierz et al., 1999). Isoenzymes of HEX are composed of two polypeptide chains (α and β) which are products of gene duplication (Pennybacker et al., 1996). Of the heat labile isoenzymes S (αα) and A (α,β), heat stable isoenzyme B (ββ) (Pérez & Tutor, 1998) and P (ββ) (Arciuch et al., 1999), HEX A and HEX B are the most common. In the majority of tissues HEX A (MW 96-110 kDa) and HEX B (MW 100-110 kDa) have similar contribution to the total HEX activity, because in normal conditions HEX S has only trace activity (Zwierz et al., 1999), and HEX P appears only in several situations e.g. pregnancy (Arciuch et al., 1999).

Kidneys are a rich source of HEX (Borzym-Kluczyk et al., 2005). HEX activity in the nephron is highest in proximal convoluted tubules. In proximal convoluted tubules HEX activity is three times higher than in renal corpuscles (Jung et al., 1992). HEX A and HEX B with the distinct dominance of HEX A are present in renal medulla and renal cortex (Tassi et al., 2000). In the urine of healthy humans the activity of HEX is low, mainly due to HEX A derived from naturally exfoliated proximal convoluted tubule cells. Urinary excretion of HEX depends on age, sex, race and blood pressure (Agirbasli et al., 1996). Although HEX is present in variety of tissues and body fluids, urinary HEX activity is the most significant (Ostrowska et al., 1993).

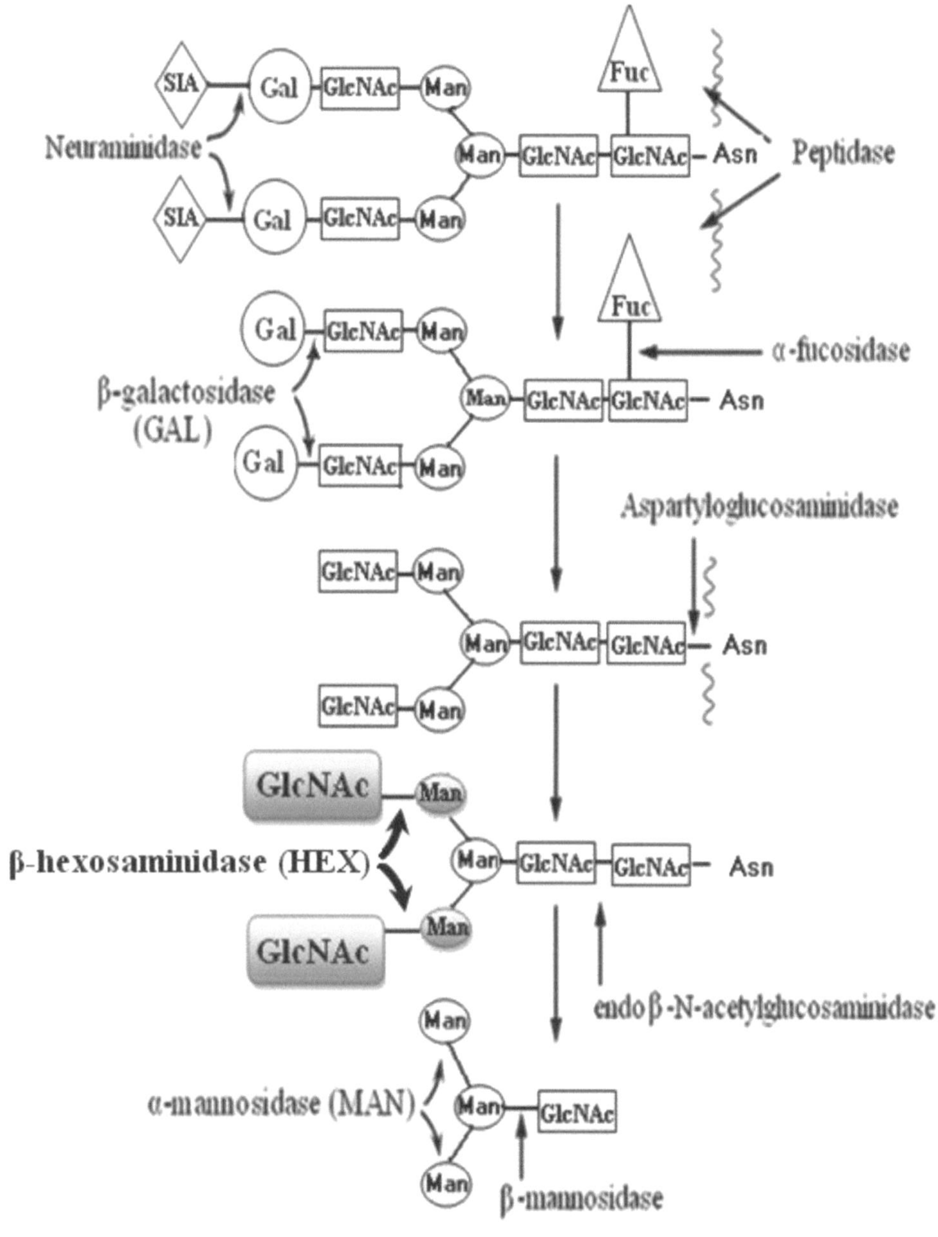

Fig. 4. Catabolism of the sugar chains of N-linked glycoproteins.
Asn- asparagine,Gal-galactose, GlcNAc-N-acetylglucosamine,Fuc-fucose, Man- mannose, SIA – Sialic acid (N-acetylneuraminic acid).

Urinary HEX activity is independent of diuria, diurial variations, low pH, or presence of the morphotic elements of blood (Costigan et al., 1996). Urinary HEX activity increases from several to dozens of times after damage to the epithelium of proximal convoluted tubules cells (Rustom et al., 1998). As cells of renal proximal convoluted tubules are very sensitive to hypoxia, all pathological states occurring with hypoxia, lead to dysfunction of the epithelium of renal proximal convoluted tubules, and leakage of HEX into urine (Chujo et al., 2008). The kidneys are critical targets for toxicity induced by heavy metals e.g. cadmium (Jung et al., 1993), and HEX activity in urine is recommended as a simple, stable, and cheap, screening indicator for early detection of renal dysfunction caused by cadmium (Jung et al., 1993).

5. HEX in renal transplantation

HEX was used for evaluation of the condition of human kidney grafts before transplantation, condition of transplanted kidneys, and estimation of toxicity of drugs used during renal transplantation.

In evaluating the contribution of the Na^+/H^+ antiporter of kidney donors and recipients to post reperfusion injury and recovery after transplantation, HEX urinary excretion rate was treated as independent predictor. Positive association of donor antiport activity with total HEX excreted within the first three days after transplantation reflecting acute post perfusion injury, confirmed antiport active contribution to renal susceptibility to the ischemic insult. Urinary HEX excretion was treated as one of the independent predictors of short-term graft outcome, and the length of the recipient's stay at hospital (Matteucci et al., 1999). Excretion into urine of trimethylamine-N-oxide (TMAO) - derived from renal medullary osmolytes, and metabolites of glycolysis (lactate) or Krebs cycle (acetate, citrate) (reflecting energy supply to the cells) was used for the evaluation of the influence of retrieval conditions (cold storage and reperfusion) on renal medulla injury in an isolated perfused pig kidney model. Determination of the above substances by proton NMR spectroscopy as early markers of ischemia reperfusion injury during cold storage and reperfusion, is a proof that increase in TMAO and metabolites of glycolysis or Krebs cycle are relevant markers of graft damage during cold storage and reperfusion. In the model above HEX was not efficient in assessing tubular damage during cold storage and reperfusion, which may be explained by the fact that increase in TMAO and disregulation of glycolysis and Krebs cycle precede any increase in excretion of HEX connected with damage of cell, and leakage of lysosomal enzymes taking part in the degradation of damaged tissues (Hauet et al., 2000). Working on the same model it was stated that TMAO (trimethylamine-N-oxide), DMA (dimethylamine) and acetate are more efficient parameters for assessing the impact of preservation solutions on renal medulla injury than HEX (Hauet et al., 2000).

HEX activity is an established biomarker for assessing the condition of machine perfused kidneys for transplantation, and for predicting kidney transplant outcome. Out of six biomarkers evaluated (**L**actate **D**e**H**ydrogenase-LDH, **AS**partate **A**mino**T**ransferase-ASAT, **G**lutathione **-S-T**ransferase-GST, HEX, **H**eart type **F**atty **A**cid **B**inding **P**rotein-H-FABP), ROC analysis certifies that only three of them (GST-AUC 0.67, HEX-AUC 0.64, H-FABP-AUC 0.64) measured in machine perfusion perfusate at the end of machine perfusion, are independently associated with the risk of delayed graft failure (Moers et al., 2010). Therefore it was concluded that GST, HEX and H-FABP are independent predictors for delayed graft failure, but not the graft survival. Increased activity of GST, HEX and H-

FABP in the machine perfusate could be an additional factor to consider in adjusting postoperative recipient management, but not in the decision to transplant or discard kidneys donated after brain death (Moers et al., 2010). Urinary excretion of the HEX activity (determined by fluorometric method) was used for the evaluation of the influence of long-term blood pressure and renal function in kidney donors, and of renal tubular function after transplantation. Excretion of HEX was positively correlated with the excretion of total protein, albumin and β_2 - microglobulin ($p= 0.000$, $p<0.007$, and $p= 0.002$, respectively) (Talseth et al., 1986). Renal allograft function during the first 24 h after transplantation was compared with the function of remaining second kidney of the living donor in the first hour after transplantation. A 4-fold (significantly) higher level of HEX excretion in the recipients compared with the donors, falling to 2–fold (significantly) higher level after 6 hours, and only tendening to increase after 24 h after transplantation, was observed (Bugge et al., 1999). HEX is a specific indicator of ischemia/reperfusion injury of proximal tubules and attenuation of this injury by atrial natriuretic peptide (Chujo et al., 2008). During rejection in 92% of renal allografts, a significant increase in total HEX activity, and decrease in urinary activity of HEX A, with simultaneous increase in activity of HEX B, and intermediary forms of HEX, was observed (Whiting et al., 1983). Urines from transplant patients showed HEX isoenzyme patterns similar to the normal urine, but in episodes of rejection, dependent on the degree on severity of rejection, total HEX activity increased. Increase in total HEX activity was caused by intermediate forms which increased more than 10-fold, however with a simultaneous decrease in activity of HEX A and HEX B (Kind, 1982).

Two mathematical models: model A based on excretion of one, and the model B based on excretion of four enzymes were used for evaluation of the applicability of urinary excretion of **F**ructose-1,6-**B**is**P**hosphatase (FBP-1,6), **G**lutathione **S**-**T**ransferase (GST), HEX and **P**yruvate **K**inase (PK), in renal allograft of patients after transplantation, who were given cyclosporin A (CyA group) or azathioprine and prednisolone (CON-group). In excretion of one enzyme (model A) the best results were obtained in the CON-group, using GST or FBP-1,6 urinary activities. Urinary HEX and PK were less efficient than GST and FBP-1,6. In the CyA group, FBP-1,6 or GST recognized 7 out of 9 graft rejections; PK diagnosed 5, but HEX only 4 rejections. In the CON-group, using model B, four of the above urinary activities were sufficient to detect all 12 graft rejections. FBP-1,6 was the best individual marker enzyme, followed by HEX. The combinations HEX/PK/GST and HEX/GST sufficed to detect all 12 rejections in the CON group, but only one in the CyA group (Kotanko et al., 1986).

Daily monitoring of urinary HEX excretion is a helpful adjunct method in diagnosis of renal damage caused by rejection and ischemia (Sandman et al., 1973), as determination of urinary HEX excretion is a reliable, rapid, sensitive and simple method. Excretion of urinary HEX may be a sign of impending rejection of kidney transplant, and daily measurement of HEX output may be useful in the early diagnosis of rejection (Koivula et al., 1978).

It is stressed that urinary HEX activities measured and reported every day are essential, if an early warning of kidney rejection is to be detected. However, during evaluation of increases in urinary HEX activity, causes of increase not connected with rejection (gentamycine toxicity, urinary tract infection, septicemia, pancreatitis, cardiac failure and thrombosis renal artery or vein) should also be considered (Corbett et al., 1978).

Increases in serum (Loko et al., 1991), and urinary total HEX activity in renal transplant patients (Keyser et al., 1976), caused by HEX intermediate forms, which resemble the increase caused by oral contraceptive steroids, pregnancy, diabetes mellitus and liver diseases were reported. Chronic renal failure resulted in a decrease of serum HEX activity. In control serums and serum with elevated HEX activity HEX A was the dominant activity. Activity of HEX B was low or not detected. An intermediate serum HEX peak was present as a minor peak in the control sera, but intermediate forms accounted for about 40% of serum HEX activity in the renal transplant group. Urinary HEX provided a sensitive indicator of active renal disease (Thompson et al., 1977). Increased urinary HEX preceded the increase of serum creatinine, and was therefore the earliest detectable indication of rejection. Determinations the urinary HEX available to the clinician on the same day are possible without preservation of urine, and they are not subject to bacterial contaminations. There is agreement that the determination of HEX in urine will provide a slightly earlier results than with other methods, however HEX urinary activities may have a serious limitation in cases of bacterial or toxic complications (Keyser et al., 1976; Thompson et al., 1977).

During evaluation of HEX and **A**lanine **A**mino**P**eptidase (AAP) activities, **C**orrected to baseline **F**ractional **E**xcretion (CFE), and in differential diagnosis of **C**yclo**s**porine **A**cute **N**ephrotoxicity (CsAN) or in **A**cute **R**ejection (AR) crisis, after renal transplantation, CFE values above normal for both HEX and AAP, were more frequently found in episodes of acute rejection, than in cyclosporine acute nephrotoxicity episodes (76vs 0%; $p<0.001$). Consequently a rise in CFE levels for both HEX and AAP is strongly suggestive of acute rejection crisis (Bornstein et al., 1996). Using a spectrophotometric method for HEX, and separation of urinary inhibitors on Sephadex G-25, the CFE normal value for HEX was 4.26 ± 3.23, and the abnormal was 10.76 + 2SD. Out of 21 AR episodes, 16 had abnormal CFE values for both HEX and AAP, 4 for HEX alone and 1 for AAP alone. Abnormal CFE values for both HEX and AAP were more frequently found in AR episodes than in CsAN episodes (76 vs 0%; $p<0.001$). The sensitivity, specificity, positive predictive value and diagnostic efficiency in regard to AR and CsAN is 0.84; 0.66; 0.7; 0.73 for HEX alone, and 0.63; 0.95; 0.93; 0.80, for HEX and AAP, respectively. On the basis of above results it was concluded that determination of both enzymes presents a rapid, reliable, cheap, noninvasive and easily available method to help assessing the postoperative period of patients undergoing renal transplantation (Bornstein et al., 1996). Evaluating HEX and AAP as indicators of graft function in renal transplant recipients taking cimetidine, urinary HEX and AAP, excretions were found to be normal throughout the period of treatment with cimetidine, which indicated that observed continuously high concentrations of creatinine in serum were not due to impairment of graft function (Krishna et al., 1986). Therefore urinary activities of HEX and AAP may be valuable as complementary renal-function tests in transplant recipients receiving cimetidine, in addition to being useful as early markers of rejection (Krishna et al., 1986).

Urinary HEX activity is a valuable indicator of drug nephrotoxicity. Very high and overlapping urinary excretion of HEX in about 35% of renal transplant patients treated with cyclosporin and prednisolne, or prednisolone with azathioprine, was reported (Tataranni et al., 1992). However, in the group of patients affected by autoimmune steroid-unsensitive uveitis treated with cyclosporin at progressively decreasing doses, urinary HEX activity decreased in parallel to decreasing cyclosporin doses. HEX release to the tissue culture medium was used as a specific marker of renal tubular cell injury for in vitro evaluation the nephrotoxicity of two immunosuppressive drugs: FK506 and cyclosporin A (Moutabarrik et al., 1992). HEX release to the medium from tubular cells incubated with 0.1 and 1 μM FK506, as well as 1 μM cyclosporin A for 10, 24, and 48 hr, was not different from that of the control. In contrast to the above statement, 50 μM of FK506, and CsA induced a significant release of HEX to the medium from tubular cells treated for 10, 24, and 48hr ($p<0.01$) with these drugs, whereas 10 μM CsA significantly increases HEX release only after 48hr incubation. At the same concentrations, CsA seemed to induce a greater HEX release than FK506 ($p<0.01$) (Moutabarrik et al., 1992). Gentamicin nephrotoxicity accompanied by increased urinary excretion of HEX and β-galactosidase, appeared consistently within three days after the start of treatment, and fell towards pre-treatment levels a week after stopping the treatment (Wellwood et al., 1978). Other antimicrobial agents (ampicillin, ampicillin+cloxacilin, cephalexin, sulphonamides, nalidixic acid, nitrofurantoin, tetracycline) did not change urinary HEX excretion. It is worth of noting that increase in urinary HEX excretion after gentamicine treatment, preceded increase in serum creatinine and urinary proteins. Causes of impairment in renal function in patients with renal allografts are often difficult to determine, therefore rejection of the graft must always be taken into consideration. Graft nephrectomy in two patients and hemodialysis in another two were reported, after gentamycin treatment, and it is concluded that increase in urinary HEX should not be interpreted as an indicator of rejection of renal allograft when the patient is receiving gentamycin (Wellwood et al., 1978). During determination of HEX excretion 24 hr before and 24 hr after intravenous application of ioxaglate (contrast medium) in renal transplant patients, none of the patients receiving ioxaglate, experienced altered urinary HEX excretion, but only a tendency to increase, even in patients treated with cyclosporine, and patients with GFR <60ml/min. (Deray et al., 1995). The only objection to that results is the short time of determination of HEX urinary excretion after application of ioxaglate, as another researchers (Wellwood et al., 1978) observed increase in urinary HEX excretion three days after administration of gentamycine. However, it was found on the rat model, that ioxaglate induced a smaller increase in urinary HEX excretion than diatrizoate sodium meglumine (Deray et al., 1990). It was reported that **P**en**T**o**X**ifylline (PTX) seemed to be temporarily effective in reducing proteinuria and stabilizing renal graft function in more than half of patients at the end of 6 month follow-up in **C**hronic **A**llograft **N**ephropathy(CAN) (Shu et al., 2007). However in CAN, PTX increased urinary HEX excretion in the 3rd month of follow-up, but stabilized in the 6th month, although urinary HEX excretion was still significantly higher than before PTX treatment. Some researchers (Shu et al., 2007) believe that the failure to reduce urinary HEX by PTX implies that renal tubular damage is not modified by PTX, which decrease both proteinuria and urinary HEX excretion in Type 2 diabetic patients (Navarro et al., 2003).

6. Stabilization of FBP-1,6 and HEX activities in human urine

Excretion of enzymes into urine depends on circadian rhythm. The highest urinary excretion rates of arylsulphatase A, α-glucosidase, β-galactosidase and β-glucuronidase, during 24 hour collection, were found betwen 6^{00} – 9^{00} AM, and the lowest between 1^{00} -9^{00} PM. Therefore, collection of urine for 3-hours between 6^{00}- 9^{00} AM was recommended for determination urinary enzymes (Werner et al., 1970). Other authors (Jung et al., 1992) recommend 2-hour collection of urine, i.e. between 6^{00}-8^{00}AM. *Kotanko P.* and *Pfaller W.* (Kotanko et al., 1997; Pfaller et al., 1994) recommend collection of urine from second morning midstream, as an appropriate specimen for analysis of urinary enzymes. The first portion of urine voided after night, should be definitely avoided, as storage of enzymes in urine during the night, may cause enzyme denaturation (Maruhn, 1983; Werner et al., 1970). Actually, urinary enzymes are commonly determined in urine of the second morning midstream collection, and calculated on gram or mole of excreted creatinine in this urine (Kotanko et al., 1997). Daily urinary creatinine excretion is stable and depends essentially on the muscle mass of the examined person.

During preparation of urine for analysis, epithelia and blood cells (Jung et al., 1992) should be removed by centrifugation in 3000-4500 rev/min by 5-10 min. Low molecular enzyme inhibitors e.g urea, should be removed by gel filtration on Sephadex G-25 or dialysis (Jung et al., 1992; Maruhn, 1979). Fresh urine stored in room temperature for several hours retain activity of the majority of enzymes. Freezing of fresh urine may decrease the activity of some enzymes. It was reported that freezing of urine after dialysis or gel filtration on Sephadex G-25 did not decrease the activity of the majority of urinary enzymes (Jung et al., 1992; Maruhn, 1979; Maruhn, 1983).

FBP-1,6 activity is comparatively stable in fresh urine stored at + 4°C. Therefore for preservation and determination of FBP-1,6, we (Kępka et al., 2009) recommend adjusting the pH of urine to pH 5.5-7.5, as FBP-1,6 activity decreased by 48% and 95%, respectively, in urine stored at pH 4.5, and 8.5. We (Kępka et al., 2009) do not recommend storage of unprotected urine, as the activity of FBP-1,6 stored for 6 days at a temperature of +4°C at pH 4.5 to 8.5, decreased significantly when compared to its initial activity. The pH 5.5-7.5 was optimal for determination and preservation the activity of FBP-1,6 in urine at a temperature of +4°C for 6 days with addition of protective substances. Positive effect of 2-mercaptoethanol (a two-fold increase in FBP-1,6 activity, with 2-mercaptoethanol added) was observed in the homogenate of the renal cortex (Burch et al., 1978). In our experience, the 2-mercaptoethanol (to protect –SH groups) added to urine may be used for successful protection of FBP-1,6 activity in urine stored for 7 days at +4°C (Kępka et al., 2009). Also adding 2-mercaptoethanol, and sodium azide (to prevent bacterial growth) into urine, had a statistically significant positive effect on FBP-1,6 activity during 7 days storage at +4°C. Our results suggest that 2-mercaptoethanol may be used for successful protection of FBP-1,6 activity in urine stored for 7 days at +4°C. We obtained the best protection of FBP-1,6 activity in urine stored for 7 days with 2-mercaptoethanol and sodium azide.

Addition of EDTA into urine had a statistically significant positive effect on FBP-1,6 stability during 4 days of storage at +4°C, but after storage longer than 5 days, significant decrease in FBP-1,6 activity was observed (Kępka et al., 2009). Our results are in agreement with the reports of Pfaller et al. (Pfaller et al., 1994) who, after storing urine for not longer than 5 days at a temperature of +4°C with the addition of EDTA, did not observed a significant decrease in FBP-1,6 activity.

There is the possibility of determining FBP-1,6 in urine stored with EDTA for 4 days at +4°C, because of an insignificant decrease in FBP-1,6 activity (by 4.6%).

HEX and majority of urinary enzymes were stable at pH 5.5-7.5 (Jung et al., 1983). The mean of total HEX activity in urine of normal males and females was 6.8 units (unit= μ mol of methylumbelliferone released from the substrate per hour per litre of urine) /mmol of creatinine, with CV within- batch of 3% and between-batch of 8%. Storage of urine samples at 4°C or at -20°C had little effect on the total HEX activity. Repeated analysis after urine storage for 2 weeks at 4°C showed a decrease which was newer greater than 5% of the total activity. During continuous flow analysis of urinary HEX isoenzymes separated on DEAE cellulose column in normal urine, a large HEX A and

smaller HEX B components were always present, usually in the ratio approximately 4:1. Slight traces of intermediate components, I_1 and I_2 were present in some normal urines, but contributed less than 2% of total activity. The reproducibility of isoenzyme profiles have CV 7.2%, and inclusion of 5% methiolate altered isoenzyme profile by less than 1%. Effect of dialysis on the activity of urinary HEX was minimal with CV of 5.6% (Kind, 1982). HEX is inactivated at urine pH higher than pH 8.0 (Islekel et al., 2007; Jung et al., 1982; Jung et al., 1983), but HEX- B isozyme is comparatively stable in alkaline urine (Islekel et al., 2007).
Urinary HEX activity is stable in fresh urine at room temperature for up to 3 hours, in temp. 4°C ≤ 50 days, and at -20°C for one year. HEX activity in crude urine conserved with 30% glycerol or ethylene glycol, was maintained for over 1 year in -20°C; in gel filtrate or dialyzate for 3 months in 4°C or -20°C (Jung et al., 1992). It was shown that using albumin solution for urine dilution is essential for stability of HEX in diluted urine (Sandman et al., 1973).

7. Conclusion

The literature review revealed that urinary FBP-1,6 and HEX are good markers for monitoring kidney to be transplanted, degree of the ischemic damage of kidney from the moment of resection to transplantation, as well as condition of the patient and transplanted kidney after transplantation. There were reports of cases where enzymuria precedes proteinuria and clinical symptoms of rejection. Determination of urinary FBP-1,6 is more complicated than HEX, because it requires more expensive reagents and strict conditions of urine handling and storage. FBP-1,6 and HEX present a rapid, reliable, cheap (particularly HEX), noninvasive and easily available methods to help assessing the postoperative period of patients undergoing renal transplantation. However, during evaluation of increase in urinary FBP-1,6 and HEX activities, causes of increase not connected with rejection, should also be considered.

8. Acknowledgment

We are grateful do Dr Tony Merry from Manchester University for critical reading of the manuscript.

9. References

Agirbasli, M.; Radhakrishnamurthy, B.; Jiang, X.; Bao, W. & Berenson, GS. (1996). Urinary N-acetyl-beta-D-glucosaminidase changes in relation to age, sex, race, and diastolic and systolic blood pressure in a young adult biracial population. The Bogalusa Heart Study. *Am J Hypertens*, 9, 2, 157-161.

Arciuch, LP.; Bielecki, D.; Borzym, M.; Południewski, G.; Arciszewki, K.; Różański, A. & Zwierz ,K. (1999). Isoenzymes of N-acetyl-beta-hexosaminidase in complicated pregnancy. *Acta Biochim Pol*, 46, 4, 977-983.

Baicu, SC.; Simmons, PM.; Campbell, LH.; Taylor, MJ. & Brockbank, KG. (2004). Interstitial fluid analysis for assessment of organ function. *Clin Transplant*, 18, Suppl.12, 16-21.

Bigl, M.; Jandrig, B.; Horn, LC. & Eschrich, K. (2008). Aberrant methylation of human L- and M-fructose 1,6-bisphosphatase genes in cancer. *Biochem Biophys Res Commun,* 377, 2, 720-724.

Bornstein, B.; Arenas, J.; Morales, JM.; Praga, M.; Rodicio, JL.; Martinez, A. & Valdivieso, L. (1996). Cyclosporine nephrotoxicity and rejection crisis: diagnosis by urinary enzyme excretion. *Nephron,* 72, 3, 402-406.

Borzym- Kluczyk, M.; Darewicz, B.; Knaś, M.; Szajda, S.; Sulik, M.; Olszewska, E. & Zwierz, K. (2005). The activity of N-acetyl-beta-glucosaminidase and its isoenzymes in the renal tissue, serum and urine of patients with renal cancer. *Contemp Oncol,* 9, 7, 287-290.

Bugge, JF.; Hartmann, A.; Osnes, S.; Bentdal, O. & Stenstrøm, J. (1999). Immediate and early renal function after living donor transplantation. *Nephrol Dial Transplant,* 14, 2, 389-393.

Burch, HB.; Narins, RG.; Chu, C.; Fagioli, S.; Choi, S.; McCarthy, W. & Lowry, OH. (1978). Distribution along the rat nephron of three enzymes of gluconeogenesis in acidosis and starvation. *Am J Physiol,* 235, 3, F246–253.

Champe, PC.; Harvey, RA. & Ferrier, DR. (2008). Biochemistry (4th edition), *Wolter Kluwer, Lippincott Williams &Wilkins, Philadelphia. Baltimore. New York. London. Buenos Aires. Hong Kong. Sydney. Tokyo.* 117-124.

Chojnowska, S.; Kępka, A.; Szajda, SD.; Waszkiewicz, N.; Bierć, M. & Zwierz, K. (2011). Exoglycosidase markers of diseases. *Biochem Soc Trans,* 9, 39 ,1, 406-409.

Chujo, K.; Ueki, M.; Asaga, T. & Taie, S. (2008). Atrial natriuretic peptide attenuates ischemia/reperfusion-induced renal injury by reducing neutrophil activation in rats. *Tohoku J Exp Med,* 215, 3, 257-266.

Cloix, JF.; Beaulieu, E. & Hevor, T. (1997). Varius fructose-1,6-bisphosphatase m RNAs in mouse brain, liver, kidney and heart. *Neuroreport,* 8, 3, 617-622

Conjard, A.; Martin, M.; Guitton, J.; Baverel, G. & Ferrier, B. (2001). Gluconeogenesis from glutamine and lactate in the isolated human renal proximal tubule: longitudinal heterogeneity and lack of response to adrenaline. *Biochem J,* 360, 371-377.

Corbett, CR.; Thompson, AE. & Pric,e RG. (1978). Urinary enzymes and renal transplantation: the early warning controversy. *Clin Chem,* 24, 4, 724-725.

Costigan, MG.; Rustom, R.; Bone, JM.; Shenkin, A.; Costigan, MG.; Rustom, R.; Bone, JM. & Shenkin, A. (1996). Origin and significance of urinary N-acetyl-beta-D-glucosaminidase (NAG) in renal patients with proteinuria. *Clin Chim Acta,* 29, 255, 2, 133-144.

Cuervo AM. (2004). Autophagy: in sickness and in health. *Trends Cell Biol,* 14, 2, 70-77.

Deray, G.; Mouquet, C.; Ourhama, S.; Bellin, MF.; Jacquiaud, C.; Luciani, J.; Bitker, MO. & Jacobs, C. (1995). Effects on renal haemodynamics and tubular function of the contrast medium Ioxaglate in renal transplant patients. *Clin Radiol,* 50, 7, :476-478.

Deray, G.; Dubois, M.; Martinez, F.; Baumelou, B.; Beaufils, H.; Bourbouze, R.; Baumelou, A. & Jacobs, C. (1990). Renal effects of radiocontrast agents in rats: a new model of acute renal failure. *Am J Nephrol,* 10, 6, 507-513.

Dżugaj, A. (2006). Localization and regulation of muscle fructose-1,6-bisphosphatase, the key enzyme of glyconeogenesis. *Adv Enzyme Regul*, 48, 1, 57-71.

Eid, A.; Boding, S.; Ferrier, B.; Delage, H.; Boghossian, M.; Martin, M.; Baverel, G. & Conjard, A. (2006). Intrinsic gluconeogenesis is enhanced in renal proximal tubules of Zucker diabetic fatty rats. *J Am Soc Nephrol*, 17, 2, 398-405.

el-Maghrabi, MR.; Lange, AJ.; Jiang, W.; Yamagata, K.; Stoffel, M.; Takeda, J.; Fernald, AA.; Le Beau, MM.; Bell, GI. & Baker, L. (1995). Human fructose-1,6-bisphosphatase gene (FBP1): exon-intron organization, localization to chromosome bands 9q22.2-q22.3, and mutation screening in subject with fructose-1,6-bisphosphatase deficiency. *Genomics*, 27, 520-525.

Gabius, HJ. (2009). The sugar code, fundamentals of glycosciences. *Willey-VCH Verlag GmbH&Co. KGaA: Weiheim, FRG.*

Hauet, T.; Baumert, H.; Gibelin, H.; Hameury, F.; Goujon, JM.; Carretier, M. & Eugene, M. (2000). Noninvasive monitoring of citrate, acetate, lactate, and renal medullary osmolyte excretion in urine as biomarkers of exposure to ischemic reperfusion injury. *Cryobiology*, 41, 4, 280-291.

Hines, JK.; Chen, X.; Nix, JC.; Fromm, HJ. & Honzatko, RB. (2007). Structures of mammalian and bacterial fructose-1,6-bisphosphatase reveal the basis for synergism in AMP/fructose 2,6-bisphosphate inhibition. *J Biol Chem*, 282, 49, 36121-36131.

Islekel,H; Soylu,A; Altun, Z; Yis, U; Turkmen, M.& Kavukcu, S.(2007). Serum and urine cystatin C levels in children with post-pyelonephritic renal scarring: a pilot study. *Int Urol Nephrol*, 39, 4, 1241-1250.

Jung, K.; Pergande, M.; Schreiber, G. & Schröder, K. (1983). Stability of enzyme in urine at 37 degrees C. *Clin Chim Acta*, 131, 3, 185-191.

Jung, K.; Mattenheimer, H. & Burchardt, U. (1992). Urinary enzymes in clinical and experimental medicine. *Berlin, Springer-Verlag*, 8-202.

Jung, K.; Pergande, M.; Schröder, K. & Schreiber, G. (1993). Influence of pH on activity of enzymes in urine at 37^{0}C. *Clin Chem*, 28, 8, 1814.

Jung, K.; Pergande, M.; Graubaum, HJ.; Fels, LM.; Endl, U. & Stolte, H. (1993). Urinary proteins and enzymes as early indicators of renal dysfunction in chronic exposure to cadmium. *Clin Chem*, 39, 5, 757-765.

Kelley, N.; Giroux, EL.; Lu, G. & Kantrowitz, ER. (1996). Glutamic acid residue 98 is critical for catalysis in pig kidney fructose-1,6-bisphosphatase. *Biochem Biophys Res Commun*, 219, 848-852.

Kelly-Loughane, N. & Kantrowitz, ER. (2001). AMP inhibition of pig kidney fructose-1,6-bisphosphatase. *Biochim Biophys Acta*, 1548, 66-71.

Keyser, JW.; Watkins, GL. & Salaman, JR. (1976). N-acetylglucosaminidase and gamma-glutamyltransferase in urine of patients with renal transplants: not an early indicator of rejection. *Clin Chem*, 22, 6, 925-926.

Kępka, A.; Szajda, SD.; Stypułkowska, A.; Waszkiewicz, N.; Jankowska, A.; Chojnowska, S. & Zwierz, K. (2008). Urinary fructose-1,6-bisphosphatase activity as a marker of the damage to the renal proximal tubules in children with idiopathic nephrotic syndrome. *Clin Chem Lab Med*, 46, 6, 831-835.

Kępka, A.; Szajda, SD.; Waszkiewicz, N.; Zalewska, A.; Płudowski, P.; Zwierz-Gugała, D.; Zalewska-Szajda, B.; Borzym-Kluczyk, M.; Kryśkiewicz, E. & Zwierz, K. (2009). Stabilizing the urinary activity of fructose-1,6- bisphosphatase with EDTA and mercaptoethanol. *Clin Biochem*, 42, 1487-1489.

Khan, S.; Priyamvada, S.; Khan, SA.; Khan, W.; Farooq, N.; Khan, F. & Yusufi, AN. (2009). Effect of trichloroethylene (TCE) toxicity on the enzymes of carbohydrate metabolism, brush border membrane and oxidative stress in kidney and other rat tissues. *Food Chem Toxicol*, 47, 7, 1562-1568.

Khundmiri, SJ.; Asghar, M.; Khan, F.; Salim, S. & Yusufi, AN. (2004). Effect of ischemia and reperfusion on enzymes of carbohydrate metabolism in rat kidney. *J Nephrol*, 17, 3, 377-383.

Kikawa, Y.; Inuzuka, M.; Takano, T.; Shigematsu, Y.; Nakai, A.; Yamamoto, Y.; Jin, BY.; Koga, J.; Taketo, A. & Sudo, M. (1994). cDNA sequences encoding human fructose-1,6-bisphosphatase from monocytes, liver and kidney: application of monocytes to molecular analysis of human fructose-1,6-bisphosphatase deficiency. *Biochem Biophys Res Commun*, 199, 687-693.

Kind, PR. (1982). N-Acetyl-beta-D-glucosaminidase in urine of patients with renal disease, and after renal transplants and surgery. *Clin Chim Acta*, 26, 119, 1-2), 89-97.

Klawitter, J.; Klawitter, J.; Kushner, E.; Jonscher, K.; Bendrick-Peart, J.; Leibfritz, D.; Christians, U. & Schmitz, V. (2010). Association of immunosuppressant-induced protein changes in the rat kidney with changes in urine metabolite patterns:a proteo-metabonomic study. *J Proteome Res*, 9, 2, 865-875.

Koivula, T.; Pitkänen, E.; Turto, H. & Tötterman, T. (1978). The excretion of urinary N-acetyl-beta-glucosaminidase and beta-glucuronidase as a sign of impending rejection of kidney transplants. *Ann Clin Res*, 10, 5, 288-290.

Kotanko, P.; Gstraunthaler, G. & Pfaller, W. (1984). Urinary enzymes in the non-invasive diagnosis of kidney epithelial lesions in acute kidney failure. *Wien Kin Wochenschr*, 96, 16, 625-629.

Kotanko, P.; Keiler, R.; Knabl, L.; Aulitzky, W.; Margreiter, R.; Gstraunthaler, G. & Pfaller, W. (1986). Urinary enzyme analysis in renal allograft transplantation. *Clin Chim Acta*, 160, 2, 137-144.

Kotanko, P.; Margreiter, R. & Pfaller, W. (1997). Graft ischemia correlates with urinary excretion of the proximal marker enzyme fructose-1,6-bisphosphatase in human kidney transplantation. *Nephron*, 77, 1, 62-67.

Krishna, KS.; Kirubakaran, MG. & Kanagasabapathy, AS. (1986). Urinary enzymes as indices of graft function in renal transplant recipients taking cimetidine. *Clin Chem*, 32, 1 Pt 1, 201.

Loko, F.; Robic, D.; Bondiou, MT. & Bourbouze, R. (1991). Concentrations of N-acetyl-beta-D-glucosaminidase and its intermediate isoenzymes in serum of patients with renal transplants. *Clin Chem*, 37, 4, :583-584.

Lu, FM. & Lin SY. (1989). Effect of FDP and Danshen on renal cortical Na-K-ATPase activity in rats after treatment with renal ischemia and gentamycin. *Chin Med J*, 102, 7, 516-523.

Lu, G.; Stec, B.; Giroux, EL. & Kantrowitz, ER. (1996). Evidence for an active T-state pig kidney fructose-1,6-bisphosphatase:interface residue Lys-42 is important for allosteric inhibition and AMP cooperativity. *Protein Science*, 5, 2333-2342.

Maruhn, D. (1979). Preparation of urine for enzyme determination by gel filtration. In: Diagnostic significance of enzymes and proteins in urine. *Dubach UC Schmidt U Hrsg, Bern-Studgard-Wien: H. Huber. 22-29.*

Maruhn, D. (1983). Methodological aspects of urinary enzymology. *Z Gesamte Inn Med*, 38, 557-564.

Matsuura, T.; Chinen, Y.; Arashiro, R.; Katsuren, K.; Tamura, T.; Hyakuna, N. & Ohta, T. (2002). Two newly identified genomic mutations in a Japanese female patients with fructose-1,6-bisphosphatase (FBPase) deficiency. *Mol Genet Metab*, 76, 207-210.

Mamczur, P.; Mazurek, J. & Rakus, D. (2010). Ubiquitous presence of gluconeogenic regulatory enzyme, fructose-1,6-bisphosphatase, within layers of rat retina. *Cell Tissue Res*, 341, 213-221.

Matteucci, E.; Carmellini, M.; Mosca, F. & Giampietro, O. (1999). The contribution of Na+/H+ exchange to postreperfusion injury and recovery of transplanted kidney. *Biomed Pharmacother*, 53, 9, 438-444.

McIninch, JK. & Kantrowitz, ER. (2001). Use of silicate sol-gels to trap the R and T quaternary conformational states of pig kidney fructose-1,6-bisphosphatase. *Biochim Biophys Acta*, 1547, 2, 320-328.

Meyer, C.; Stumvoll, M.; Welle, S.; Woerle, HJ.; Haymond, M. & Gerich, J. (2003). Relative importance of liver, kidney and substrates in epinephrine-induced increased gluconeogenesis in humans. *Am J Physiol Endocrinol Metab*, 285, 4, E819-826.

Moers, C.; Varnav, OC.; van Heurn, E.; Jochmans, I.; Kirste, GR.; Rahmel, A.; Leuvenink, HG.; Squifflet, JP.; Paul, A.; Pirenne, J.; van Oeveren, W.; Rakhorst, G. & Ploeg, RJ. (2010). The value of machine perfusion perfusate biomarkers for predicting kidney transplant outcome. *Transplantation*, 15, 90, 9, 966-973.

Moutabarrik, A.; Ishibashi, M.; Fukunaga, M.; Kameoka, H.; Kawaguchi, N.; Takano, Y.; Kokadom, Y.; Sonoda, T.; Onishi, S. & Takahara, S. (1992). FK506-induced kidney tubular cell injury. *Transplantation*, 54, 6, 1041-1047.

Navarro, JF.; Mora, C.; Muros, M.; Maca, M. & Garca, J. (2003). Effects of pentoxifylline administration on urinary N-acetyl-beta-glucosaminidase excretion in type 2 diabetic patients: a short-term, prospective, randomized study. *Am J Kidney Dis*, 42, 2, 264-270.

Nomura, M.; Takihara, Y.; Yasunaga, T. & Shimada, K. (1994). One of the retinoic acid-inducible cDNA clones in mouse embryonal carcinoma F9 cell encodes a novel isoenzyme of fructose-1,6-bisphosphatase. *FEBS Lett*, 348, 201-205.

Ostrowska, L.; Zwierz, K.; Koniusz, Z. & Gindzieński, A. (1993). Function, properties and clinical significance of N-acetyl-beta-D-hexosaminidase. *Post Hig Med Dosw*, 47, 1, 67-79.

Pennybacker, M.; Liessem, B.; Moczall, H.; Tifft, CJ.; Sandhoff, K. & Proia, RL. (1996). Identification of domains in human beta-hexosaminidase that determine substrate specificity. *J Biol Chem*, 19, 271, 29, 17377-17382.

Pérez, LF. & Tutor, JC. (1998). Assay of beta-N-acetylhexosaminidase isoenzymes in different biological specimens by means of determination of their activation energies. *Clin Chem*, 44, 2, 226-231.

Pfaller, W.; Thorwartl, U.; Nevinny-Stickel, M.; Krall, M.; Schober, M.; Joannidis, M. & Hobisch, A. (1994). Clinical value of fructose-1,6-diphosphatase in monitoring renal tubular injury. *Kidney Internat*, 46, Suppl 47, S68–75.

Popko, J.; Marciniak, J.; Ilendo, E.; Knas, M.; Guszczyn, T.; Stasiak-Barmuta, A.; Moniuszko, T.; Zwierz, K. & Wysocka, J. (2008). Profile of exoglycosidases in synovial cell cultures derived from human synovial membrane. *Cell Biochem Biophys*, 51, 2-3, 89-95.

Reuter, S.; Reiermann, S.; Wörner, R.; Schröter, R.; Edemir, B.; Buck, F.; Henning, S.; Peter-Katalinic, J.; Vollenbröker, B.; Amann, K.; Pavenstädt, H.; Schlatter, E. & Gabriëls, G. (2010). IF/TA-related metabolic changes-proteome analsis of rat renal allografs. *Nephrol Dial Transplant*, 25, 8, 2492-24501.

Rustom, R.; Costigan, M.; Shenkin, A. & Bone, JM. (1998). Proteinuria and renal tubular damage: urinary N-acetyl-beta-D-glucosaminidase and isoenzymes in dissimilar renal disease. *Am J Nephrol*, 18, 3, 179-185.

Sandman, R.; Margules, RM. & Kountz, SL. (1973). Urinary lysosomal glycosidases after renal allotransplantation: correlation of enzyme excretion with allograft rejection and ischemia. *Clin Chim Acta*, 30, 45, 4, 349-359.

Sáez, DE.; Figueroa, CD.; Concha, II. & Slebe, JC. (1996). Localization of the fructose-1.6-bisphosphatase at the nuclear periphery. *J Cell Biochem*, 15, 63(4), 453-462.

Scherer, A.; Krause, A.; Walker, JR.; Sutton, SE.; Serón, D.; Raulf, F. & Cooke, MP. (2003). Optimized protocol for linear RNA amplification and application to gene expression profiling of human renal biopsies. *Biotechniques*, 34, 3, 546-550, 552-554, 556.

Shu, KH.; Wu, MJ.; Chen, CH.; Cheng, CH.; Lian, JD. & Lu, YS. (2007). Effect of pentoxifylline on graft function of renal transplant recipients complicated with chronic allograft nephropathy. *Clin Nephrol*, 67, 3, 157-163.

Strecker, G.; Michalski, JC. & Montreuil, J. (1988). Lysosomal catabolic pathway of N-glycosylprotein glycans. *Biochimie*, 70, 11, 1505-1510.

Stumvoll, M.; Meyer, C.; Mitrakou, A.; Nadkarni, V. & Gerich, JE. (1997). Renal glucose production and utilization: new aspects in humans. *Diabetologia*, 40, 749-757.

Talseth, T.; Fauchald, P.; Skrede, S.; Djøseland, O.; Berg, KJ.; Stenstrøm, J.; Heilo, A.; Brodwall, EK. & Flatmark, A. (1986). Long-term blood pressure and renal function in kidney donors. *Kidney Int*, 29, 5, 1072-1076.

Tassi, C.; Abbritti, G.; Mancuso, F.; Morucci, P.; Feligioni, L. & Muzi, G. (2000). Activity and isoenzyme profile of N-acetyl-beta-D-glucosaminidase in urine from workers exposed to cadmium. *Clin Chim Acta*, 29, 1-2, 55-64.

Tataranni, G.; Zavagli, G.; Farinelli, R.; Malacarne, F.; Fiocchi, O.; Nunzi, L.; Scaramuzzo, P. & Scorrano, R. (1992). Usefulness of the assessment of urinary enzymes and microproteins in monitoring ciclosporin nephrotoxicity. *Nephron*, 60, 3, 314-318.

Thompson, AE.; Tucker, SM. & Price, RG. (1977). Assay of N-acetyl-beta-D-glucosaminidase in urine of patients with renal transplants as an indicator of rejection. *Clin Chem*, 23, 2 PT. 1, 301-302.

Tillmann, H. & Eschrich, K. (1998). Isolation and characterization of an allelic cDNA for human muscle fructose-1,6-bisphosphatase. *Gene*, 212, 295-304

Velásquez, ZD.; Pérez, M.; Morán, MA.; Yanez, AJ.; Avila, J.; Slebe, JC. & Gómez-Ramos, P. (2010). Ultrastructural localization of fructose-1,6-bisphosphatase in mouse brain. *Microsc Res Tech*, © 2010 Wiley-Liss, Inc. DOI: 10.1002/jemt.20911.

Wellwood, JM.; Davies, D.; Leighton, M. & Thompson, AE. (1978). Urinary N-acetyl-beta-D-glucosaminidase assay in renal transplant recipients. *Transplantation*, 26, 6, 396-400.

Werner, M.; Heilbron, DC.; Maruhn, D. & Atoba, M. (1970). Patterns of urinary enzyme excretion in healtly subject. *Clin Chim Acta*, 29, 437-449.

Whiting, PH.; Petersen, J.; Power, DA.; Stewart, RD.; Catto, GR. & Edward, N. (1983). Diagnostic value of urinary N-acetyl-beta-D-glucosaminidase, its isoenzymes and the fractional excretion of sodium following renal transplantation. *Clin Chim Acta*, 15, 130, 3, 369-376.

Winchester, B. (2005). Lysosomal metabolism of glycoproteins. *Glycobiology*, 15, 6, 1R-15R.

Wright, SW.; Hageman, DL.; McClure, LD.; Carlo, AA.; Treadway, JL.; Mathiowetz, AM.; Withka, JM. & Bauer, PH. (2001). Allosteric inhibition of fructose-1,6-bisphosphatase by anilinoquinazolines. *Bioorg Med Chem Lett*, 11, 17-21.

Wright, SW.; Carlo, AA.; Danley, DE.; Hageman, DL.; Karam, GA.; Mansour, MN.; McClure, LD.; Pandit, J.; Schulte, GK.; Treadway, JL.; Wang, IK. & Bauer, PH. (2003). 3-(2-carboxy-ethyl)-4,6-dichloro-1*H*-indole-2-carboxylic acid: an allosteric inhibitor of fructose-1,6-bisphosphatase at the AMP site. *Bioorg Med Chem Lett*, 13, 2055-2058.

Wu, C.; Khan, SA.; Peng, LJ. & Lange, AJ. (2006). Roles for fructose-2,6-bisphosphate in the control of fuel metabolism: beyond its allosteric effects on glycolytic and gluconeogenic enzymes. *Adv Enzyme Regul*, 46, 72-88.

Yáñez, AJ.; Bertinat, R.; Concha, II. & Slebe, JC. (2003). Nuclear localization of liver FBPase in kidney and liver. *FEBS Lett*, 550, 35-40.

Yánez, AJ.; Nualart, F.; Droppelmann, C.; Bertinat, R.; Brito, M.; Concha, II. & Slebe, JC. (2003). Broad expression of fructose-1,6-bisphosphatase and phosphoenolopyruvate carboxykinase provide evidence for gluconeogenesis in human tissues other than liver and kidney. *J Cell Physiol*, 197, 2, 189-197.

Yañez, AJ.; Ludwig, HC.; Bertinat, R.; Spichiger, C.; Gatica, R.; Berlien, G.; Leon, O.; Brito, M.; Concha, II. & Slebe, JC. (2005). Different involvement for aldolase isoenzymes in kidney glucose metabolism: aldolase B but not aldolase A colocalizes and forms a complex with FBPase. *J Cell Physiol*, 202, 743-753.

Zhang, Y.; Liang, JY.; Huang, S. & Lipscomb, WN. (1994). Toward a mechanism for the allosteric transition of pig kidney fructose-1,6-bisphosphatase. *J Mol Biol*, 244, 5, 609-624.

Zoch-Zwierz, W.; Kępka, A.; Tomaszewska, B.; Wasilewska, A.; Wierciński, R.; Smółko, M.; Winiecka, W. & Porowski, T. (2004). Assesement of fructose-1,6-bisphosphatase in urine of children with acute pyelonephritis. *Pol Merk Lek*, XVI, 91, 56-59.

Zwierz, K.; Zalewska, A. & Zoch-Zwierz, W. (1999). Isoenzymes of N-acetyl-beta-hexosaminidase. *Acta Biochim Pol*, 46, 3, 739-751.

6

Evaluation of CTLA-4, CD28 and CD86 Genes Polymorphisms in Acute Renal Allograft Rejection among Tunisian Patients

Henda Krichen et al.*
Research laboratory of transplantation Immunopathology (LR03SP01), Tunis El Manar university, Charles Nicolle hospital, Tunisia

1. Introduction

Kidney transplantation is the preferred therapy for most patients with end-stage renal disease (Sui et al., 2008; Turgeon et al., 2009). Transplantation improves both quality of life and survival (Chavez et al., 2008). Unfortunately, the rate of renal allograft rejection remains important. With the aim of reducing the level of transplantation failure, several researches were achieved to elucidate the immunological mechanisms involved in this process. Thus, it was well established that allograft rejection is an immune response strongly depending on T cells proliferation. In fact, T lymphocytes play a crucial role in the initiation and the regulation of the adaptive immune response to foreign or native antigen (Vincenti, 2008). Herein, we focused on the costimulatory molecules: CTLA-4 and CD28: two receptors of T lymphocytes, and CD86: their common ligand on the antigen presenting cells (APC).

2. Costimulatory molecules pathway of t lymphocytes activation

The activation of naïve T cells requires two distinct signals. The first one is mediated by the association of the T cell receptor (TCR) with the Major Histocompatibility Complex (MCH) molecules, known in humans as the Human Leukocyte Antigen (HLA) (Thomas, 2007) and expressed on the antigen presenting cells (APCs). This interaction mediates the specificity of a T cell response by the recognition of specific epitopes of the presented antigen. The second signal is provided by the interaction between CD28 on the T cell surface and CD86 (B7-1) or CD80 (B7-2) on the APCs (Alegre et al., 2001; Handa et al., 2005). This co-stimulatory signal leads to clonal-T lymphocytes expansion and differentiation and to cytokines expression

* Imen Sfar[1], Taieb Ben Abdallah[1], Rafika Bardi[1], Ezzeddine Abderrahim[2], Saloua Jendoubi-Ayed[1], Mouna Makhlouf[1], Houda Aouadi[1], Hammadi Ayadi[2], Khaled Ayed[1] and Yousr Gorgi[1]
[1]*Research laboratory of transplantation Immunopathology (LR03SP01), Tunis El Manar university, Charles Nicolle hospital,*
[2]*Center of Biotechnology of Sfax.*
[3]*National Health Institute,*
[4]*Department of Nephrology, Charles Nicolle hospital, Tunisia*

(Melichar et al., 2000; Seliger et al., 2008). In fact, the ligation of CD28 and CD3 (a T cell co-receptor) promotes the production of interleukins IL-4 and IL-5 and seems to be unique in its ability to induce very high levels of IL-2 production by prolonging the nuclear residency of nuclear factor of activated T cells (NFAT). These interleukins enhance T-helper-cell differentiation. CD28 engagement also confers critical survival signals to T cells which provides resistance to apoptosis and induces long-term expansion of T-cells (Beier et al., 2007; Wang et al., 2004) (Figure 1).

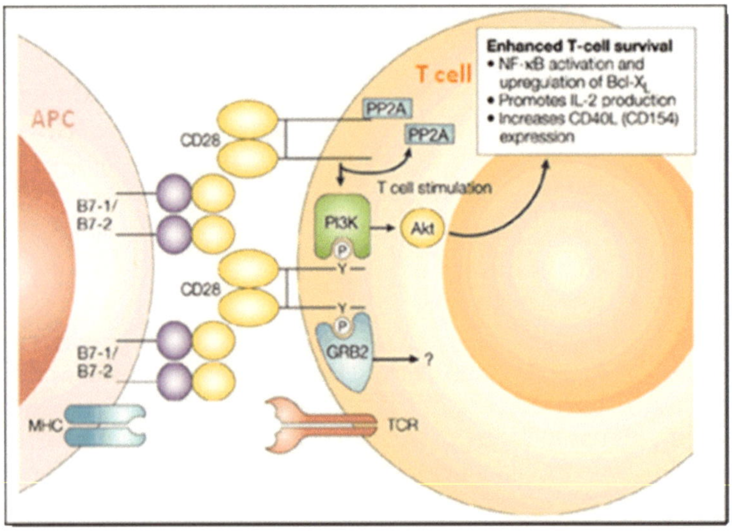

Fig. 1. Engagement of CD28 (Sharp, 2002). Signaling through CD28 promotes cytokine (IL-2) mRNA production and entry into the cell cycle, T-cell survival (at least in part by induction of Bcl-X_L), T-helper-cell differentiation and immunoglobulin isotype switching. (NF-kB, nuclear factor kappa b; PI3K, phosphatidylinositol 3-kinase; PP2A, protein phophatase 2A)

Following T cell activation, the expression on the T lymphocytes surface of the Cytotoxic T Lymphocyte Antigen-4 (CTLA-4), the counter receptor of the CD28, is rapidly up-regulated. CTLA-4 is the higher affinity receptor for both CD80 and CD86. The binding of CTLA-4 to these ligands down-regulates T lymphocytes proliferation (Beier, 2007; Collins, 2002; Wang, 2004). In fact, the engagement of CTLA-4 delivers negative signals, which inhibit IL-2 mRNA production, cytokines synthesis, cell cycle progression and then terminate T cell responses (Sharp, 2002) (Figure 2).

Several mechanisms by which CTLA-4 down-regulates T cells activation have been proposed. Thus, CTLA-4 might successfully compete with CD28 for CD80/86 and thereby inhibit the costimulatory effect of CD28. CTLA-4 could prevent constitutive expression of downstream signaling pathways by interacting with the protein tyrosine kinases (PTKs) Lck, Fyn and ZAP-70 through SHP1 phosphatase; now these PTKs play a key role in the TCR signaling. CTLA-4 might also directly interact with the TCR-CD3 complex at the immunological synapse to disrupt T-cell activation by binding and blocking the immunoreceptor tyrosine-based activation motif (ITAM) which serves as substrate to the PTKs, and, when its tyrosine residue is phosphorylated, induces the activation of ZAP-70 (Brand, 2005; Chuang et al., 1999) (Figure 3).

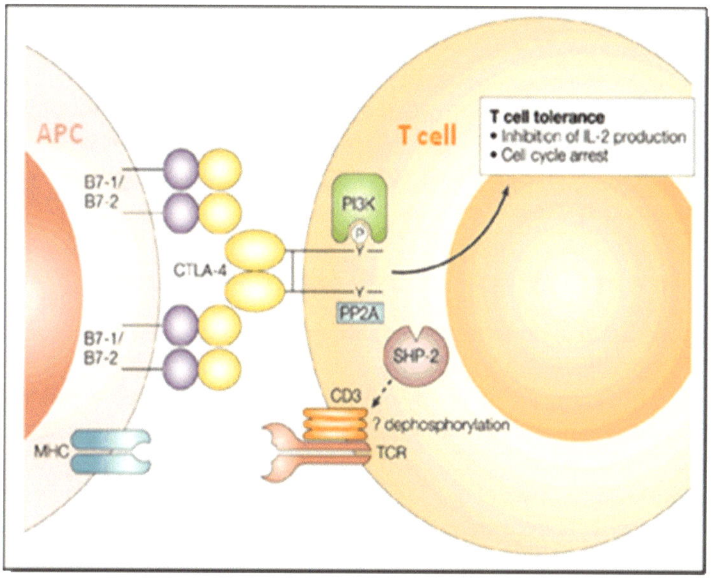

Fig. 2. Engagement of CTLA-4 (Sharp, 2002). Each CTLA-4 dimer can bind two independent B7-1/B7-2 homodimers. The crystal structure of B7-1/B7-2–CTLA-4 indicates that a linear zipper-like structure might form between B7-1/B7-2 and CTLA-4 homodimers.

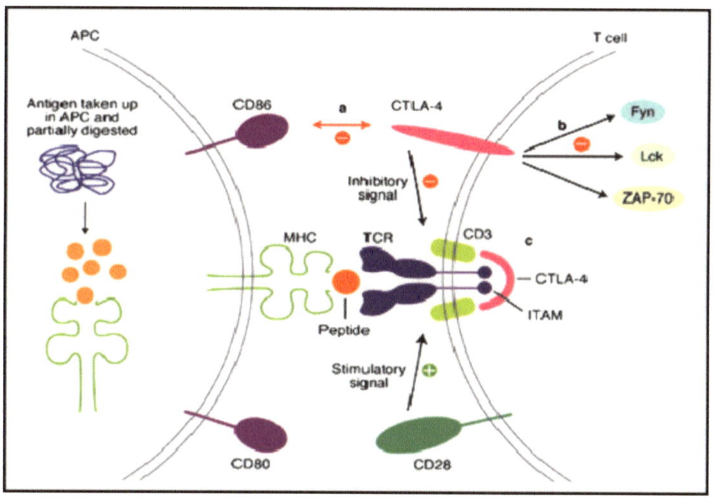

Fig. 3. Proposed mechanisms by which CTLA-4 inhibits T-cell activation (Brand, 2005)

Such down-regulation of T lymphocytes proliferation may induce immune tolerance, which is fundamental for allograft acceptance. Thus, the outcome of an immune response involves a balance between CD28-mediated T cell activation and CTLA-4-mediated inhibition.
Previous studies also focused on the costimulatory pathway of T lymphocytes activation. For instance, Minguela et al. analyzed the expression of costimulatory molecules in liver transplant and demonstrated that up-regulation of CD28/CTLA-4/CD86 molecules is associated with acute rejection of liver allograft (Minguela et al., 2000). Furthermore, it has

been demonstrated that the blockade of CD28-CD86 binding prolongs graft survival and induces specific tolerance (Akalin et al., 1996; Lenschow et al., 1995; Sayegh, 1998). Therefore, the genes of the costimulatory molecules were candidate for a large spectrum of autoimmune diseases such as rheumatoid arthritis (Matsuchita et al., 2000), asthma (Cotydon et al., 2007), systemic lupus erythematosus (Wong et al., 2005) or multiple sclerosis (Van Veen et al., 2003). Thus, numerous polymorphic markers have been reported to cause abnormal expression or dysfunction of the proteins.

3. Polymorphisms in the CTLA-4, CD28, and CD86 genes

The CTLA-4 and the CD28 genes are homologous and closely linked in the 2q33 chromosomal region. CD28 is constitutively expressed on almost all resting human CD4+ T-cells and 50–80% of all CD8+ T-cells. In contrast, CTLA-4 is only expressed after T-cell activation. It is usually located intra-cellularly and moves rapidly to the cell surface at the site of T-cell/APC interaction (Bier, 2007). CD80 and CD86 are encoded by homologous genes located in the 3q21 chromosomal region (Dalla-Costa et al., 2010). The expression kinetics of CD80 and CD86 also differ: CD86 is constitutively expressed at low levels and rapidly up-regulated, whereas CD80 is inducibly expressed later than CD86 on APCs (Greenwald et al., 2002).

Among the most characterized polymorphisms in CTLA-4 costimulatory molecule, an A/G transition at position (+49) of the exon 1 (rs231775) causes a Threonine/Alanine substitution in the leader peptide and could affect the inhibitory function of CTLA-4. The (+49) A allele had been identified as protective, whereas the G allele was associated with greater susceptibility to autoimmune diseases (Liu et al., 2010). A single nucleotide polymorphism (SNP) at position (-318) C/T in the promoter region (rs5742909) influences promoter activity and the expressions of both CTLA-4 mRNA in un-stimulated cells and cell-surface CTLA-4 on activated cells (Kusztal et al., 2010). The (+6230) A/G polymorphism (or CT60) in the 3′untraslated region (UTR) of the CTLA-4 gene (rs3087243) has been shown to be associated with the mRNA level of soluble CTLA-4. This later SNP was associated with the levels of membrane and cytoplasmic CTLA-4 in CD4 T lymphocytes from multiple sclerosis patients and with the variation of serum soluble CTLA-4 level in Graves' disease patients (Kusztal et al., 2010). Also in the 3′UTR of CTLA-4 gene, a microsatellite (AT)n has been identified at position 642. The variation in the number of the dinucleotide (AT) repeat is associated with the stability of mRNA transcripts (Liu, 2010). It has been established that a low number of (AT) repeats is responsible for favorable mRNA stability, which results in lower T cell proliferation (Kusztal et al., 2010).

For the CD28 gene, a T/C SNP at position (+17) of the intron 3 (rs3116496) or IVS3 (+17) is identified. The functional role of this SNP is not yet clearly established, but it is known that this polymorphic site is within a region where regulatory elements could bind (Marín et al., 2005).

In the CD86 gene, a (+1057) G/A polymorphism in the exon 8 (rs1129055) results in an Alanine/Threonine substitution at codon 304 located in the CD86 cytoplasmic tail which contains putative phosphorylation sites for protein kinase C (PKC). This substitution could modify the phosphorylation level in this region and influence the APC-signal transmission pathway by CD86 (Pawlak et al., 2010).

Since the regulation of T lymphocytes activation is crucial during the allograft rejection process, we focused on the relationship between CTLA-4, CD28 and CD86 gene polymorphisms and renal transplant outcomes. Herein, we examined the genotypic distribution of the (+49) A/G, (-318) C/T, (+6230) G/A and (AT)n microsatellite of CTLA-4, (+17) T/C of CD28 and (+1057) G/A of CD86 gene in a cohort of Tunisian kidney allograft recipients.

4. Subjects and methods

4.1 Patients

We retrospectively investigated 127 renal transplant recipients who underwent transplantation between 1986 and 2008. Based on the important impact of HLA disparity between donor and recipient on transplantation outcomes, patients were classified into two groups according to the HLA-haplotype similarity between donor and recipient:

- Group I: included 23 HLA-identical haplotype allograft recipients
- Group II: included 104 recipients showing one or more mismatches in the HLA haplotype.

The acute rejection diagnosis was made by clinical, histological, and biochemical standard assessment (Banff criteria). As maintenance immunosuppression, all patients received prednisolone, tacrolimus and/or mycophenolate mofetil. Patients of Group II received rabbit anti-thymocyte globulin (ATG) as induction therapy. ATG was also administrated after an acute rejection episode in 13 patients of Group I and 8 of Group II.

Prior to transplantation, the sera of 124 patients, 23 from Group I and 101 from Group II, were tested for anti-HLA antibodies by the microlymphocytotoxicity assay. The main characteristics of our patients are summarized in Table 1.

Features	*Patients (n=127)*	*Group I (n=23)*	*Group II (n=104)*
Age (years)	32.08±10.92	31.74± 6.70	32.36±11.51
Sex ratio (Males/ Females)	1.71	2.22	1.60
Donor type (%)			
RLD	79.53	100	75
DD	16.53	0	20.19
ULD	3.94	0	4.81
Fallow-up time (months)	85 ± 63.59	129±73.83	75±57.06
Initial nephropathy (%)			
Glomerulonephritis	40.94	56.52	37.35
Unspecified Chronic nephropathy	28.35	4.35	33.65
Tubulointerstitial nephropathy	18.11	13.04	16.35
Vascular nephropathy	7.09	8.07	6.73
Rapidly evolutionary nephropathy	3.15	-	2.89
Gravidic nephropathy	0.79	-	0.96
Hereditary nephropathy	0.79	-	0.96
Hemolytic and uremic syndrome	0.79	-	0.96
Acute rejection (%)	31 (24.41)	5 (21.74)	26 (25)
Anti-HLA antibodies presence in pre-transplantation	19/124	4/23	15/101

Table 1. Epidemiological features of the kidney allograft recipient
RLD: related living donor; DD: deceased donor; ULD: unrelated living donor.

4.2 Controls

As a control group, we examined 83 ethnically and geographically matched healthy subjects recruited from the blood donors of the same area than patients. The study was approved by the local ethics committee

4.3 Molecular biology methods

4.3.1 DNA extraction

Genomic DNA was isolated from EDTA-anticoagulated peripheral blood samples of unrelated healthy blood donors and renal recipients, and extracted by a standard salting-out procedure.

4.3.2 Polymorphisms genotyping

4.3.2.1 CTLA-4 (+49) A/G and CTLA-4 (+6230) A/G

Typing of the CTLA-4 exon 1 A/G transition at position 49 and 3'UTR (+6230) A/G polymorphism was achieved by the polymerase chain reaction-restriction fragment length polymorphism (PCR-RFLP) method using a PCR System 2700 Thermal Cycler (Applied Biosystems, Gene Amp®). The PCR protocol and the primers used are listed in Table 2.
PCR was carried out in a final volume of 20 µl containing 100ng of genomic DNA, 1.5 mM $MgCl_2$, 0.2 mM dNTP, 10 pmol of each primer and 0.5U of Taq DNA polymerase (Promega, USA). The restriction enzymes used were *Kpn I* for (+49) A/G and *Nco I* for (+6230) A/G.

4.3.2.2 CTLA-4 (-318) C/T and CD28 (+17)T/C

To determine genotypes of the CTLA-4 (-318) C/T in the gene promoter of CTLA-4 and of the CD28 (+17) T/C polymorphism a PCR-SSP (sequence specific primer) was used in a 25µl final volume mixed solution, containing 100 ng genomic DNA, 1.5 mM $MgCl_2$, 0.2 mM dNTP, 10 pmol of each the various allele-specific forward and reverse primers, and 0.5U of Taq DNA polymerase (Promega, USA). The PCR protocol and the primers used are listed in Table 2.

4.3.2.3 CTLA-4 (AT)n

The genotyping of (AT) repeat in the UTR of the CTLA-4 gene was performed by length-fragments analysis method using an automated sequencer (Perkin-Elmer ABI Prims 310 Genetic Analyzer) and Peak Scanner software. A lane size standard (ROX-500) and the Formamide Hi-Di were added to all samples according to each manufacturer's instructions. A PCR was previously realized in a final volume of 20 µl containing 50 ng of genomic DNA, 1.5 mM $MgCl_2$, 0.2 mM dNTP, 10 pmol of each primer and 0.5U of Taq DNA polymerase (Promega, USA) with the protocol and the couple of primers summarized in Table 2.

4.3.2.4 CD86 (+1057) G/A

For the amplification of a DNA fragment containing the (+1057) G/A polymorphism on the exon 8 of the CD86 gene, a PCR was performed using a PCR System 2700 Thermal Cycler (Applied Biosystems, Gene Amp®) in a final volume of 20µl containing 50ng of genomic DNA, 1.5 mM $MgCl_2$, 0.2 mM dNTP, 10 pmol of each primer and 0.5U of Taq DNA polymerase (Promega, USA) with the protocol and the couple of primers summarized in Table 2. The amplified fragments were then sequenced in forward direction using the Ex 8/3 primer in an ABI PRISM Dye Terminator Cycle Ready Reaction kit (Applied Biosystems) under recommended conditions. Sequenced samples were purified using Centri-Sep columns (Dye EXTm 2.0 Spin Kit, Qiagen) according to manufacturer's instructions, loaded in a PE ABI Prisms 310 Genetic Analyzer (Perkin Elmer) and analyzed using ABI Prisms Navigator Software. The two alleles G and A at position (+1057) were observed as different fluorescence peaks in that position.

4.3.3 Statistical analysis

Allelic and genotypic frequencies were evaluated by direct counting. Statistical comparisons were performed, between patients and controls, by χ^2 test calculated on 2x2 contingency tables using the Statcalc program (Epi Info version 20010; Centers for Disease Control and Prevention, Atlanta, GA, USA). Fisher's exact test was used when an expected cell value was less than 5. p value < 0.05 was considered to be statistically significant. Odd ratio(OR), with 95% confidence intervals (95%CI), was calculated using the same software.
Haplotype frequencies and Hardy-Weinberg equilibrium p values were estimated by the Thesias 3.1 program (DA Tregouet, INSERM U525, Paris, France).

Polymorphisms	*Primers*	*Temperature, time and cycles for PCR*
CTLA-4 (+49) A/G	**Forward:** 5'CAAGGCTCAGCTGAACCTGGGT3' **Reverse:** 5'TACCTTTAACTTCTGGCTTTG3'	Initial denaturation for 4 min at 94°C, 35 cycles of 30 sec at 94°C, 30 sec at 67°C and 1 min at 72°C and final elongation 5 min at 72°C.
CTLA-4 (-318) C/T	**Specific primers:** F10: 5' ACTTAGTTATCCAGATCCAC 3' F11: 5' ACTTAGTTATCCAGATCCAT 3' **Common primer:** R10: 5' AGGCTCTTGAATAGAAAGC 3'	Initial denaturation for 2 min at 94°C, 35 cycles of 30 sec at 94°C, 30 sec at 55°C and 45 sec at 72°C and final elongation 2 min at 72°C.
CTLA-4 (+6230) A/G	**Forward** CT60 Sens: 5' CACCACTATTTGGGATATACC 3' **Reverse** CT60 Antis: 5' AGCTCTATATTTCAGGAAGGC 3'	Initial denaturation for 5 min at 94°C, 30 cycles of 40 sec at 94°C, 30 sec at 61°C and 50 sec at 72°C and final elongation 7 min at 72°C.
CTLA-4 (AT)n	**Forward** (AT)n R: 5'TGGTGTATTAGTGTCCTG 3' **Reverse** (AT)n F: 5' Fam GATGCTAAAGGTTGTATT 3'	Initial denaturation for 2 min at 94°C, 3 cycles of 30 sec at 94°C, 30 sec at 54°C and 30 sec at 72°C and final elongation 7min at 72°C.
CD28 (+17) T/C	**Specific primers:** CD28 T: 5' CTGGGTAAGAGAAGCGCAAT 3' CD28 C: 5' CTGGGTAAGAGAAGCGCAAC 3' **Common primer:** CD28 Com: 5' CTCAATGCCTTCTGGAAATC 3'	Initial denaturation for 2 min at 94°C, 35 cycles of 30 sec at 94°C, 30 sec at 60°C and 30 sec at 72°C and final elongation 5 min at 72°C.
CD86 (+1057) G/A	**Forward** Ex 8/3 5'CTCCTCATTGCTGTTCCAATGGCAACC 3' **Reverse** Ex 8/4 5'CATGAGCCATTAAGCTGGGCTTGGCCC 3'.	Initial denaturation for 4 min at 94°C, 35 cycles of 30 sec at 94°C, 30 sec at 67°C and 1 min at 72°C and final elongation 5min at 72°C.

Table 2. Sequences of primers and PCR conditions

5. Results

5.1 Patient characteristics

No significant differences were found between groups of patients in gender, age, ethnicity or primary disease (Table 1).

Thirty-one patients (24.41%) developed at least one acute rejection episode within the first six months after transplantation. The rate of acute rejection was lower in Group I (21.74%) than in Group II (25%) or in the global group of patients (24.41%) (Table 1).

Before transplantation, 19/124 recipients were sensitized (anti-HLA positive): 4/23 in Group I, two of them developed an acute rejection episode and 5/101 in Group II, including 7 with an acute rejection episode. Among the 105 anti-HLA negative recipients, 19 were in Group I (3 of them undergone an acute rejection) and 86 were in Group II (18 with acute rejection).

The incidence of acute rejection was statistically associated with the presence of anti-HLA antibodies before transplantation in the 124 patients (p=0.01) and in Group II (p=0.04) (Table3).

	Patients (n=124)		*Group I (n=23)*		*Group II (n=101)*	
	AR (+) n= 30	**AR (-) n= 94**	**AR(+) n=5**	**AR (-) n= 18**	**AR(+) n= 25**	**AR (-) n= 76**
AHA(+)	9	10	2	2	7	8
AHA (-)	21	84	3	16	18	68
p	0.01[a]		0.19		0.04[b]	

AHA: anti-HLA antibodies; AR(+): acute rejection; AR(-): non acute rejection

[a]: $p = 0.01$; OR=3.60; 1.12<OR<11.20; 95% CI

[b]: $p = 0.04$; OR=3.31; 0.88<OR<11.91; 95% CI

Table 3. Association between acute rejection and the presence of anti-HLA antibodies in pre-transplantation

5.2 Distribution of genotypes and alleles frequencies in patients and controls

The genotyping of the microsatellite (AT)n in the UTR of the CTLA-4 gene showed 22 distinct alleles of size ranging from 88 to 146 bp. The shortest allele of 88 bp was the most frequent in controls and patients.

For all polymorphisms, no differences were found in the frequencies of genotypes and alleles between the global cohort of patients and controls (Table 4).

5.3 Polymorphisms and acute rejection

Comparing the genotypes distribution between acute rejection and non acute rejection patients, we noticed that the (+49) G/G and (+6230) A/A genotypes of the CTLA-4 gene and the (+1057) G/G genotype on the CD86 gene were more frequent in case of acute rejection (Table 5).

The frequencies of the alleles: (+49) G, (+6230) A and (AT) 120bp of the CTLA-4 gene and of (+1057) G allele of the CD86 gene were higher in acute rejection patients than in non-acute rejection ones (Figure 3).

Polymorphisms	*Patients (n=127)*	*Controls (n=83)*	*p (HWE)*
CTLA-4 (+49)A/G			
Genotypes			
A/A	18.90	7.23	
A/G	42.52	37.35	
G/G	38.58	55.42	
Alleles			
A	0.402	0.260	0.194
G	0.598	0.740	
CTLA-4 (-318) C/T			
Genotypes			
C/C	88.98	90.36	
C/T	10.24	8.43	
T/T	0.78	1.20	
Alleles			
C	0.941	0.946	0.373
T	0.059	0.054	
CTLA-4 (+6230) A/G			
Genotypes		2	
G/G	34.65	5.03	
A/G	48.03	48.19	
A/A	17.32	26.50	
Alleles			
G	0.587	0.493	0.913
A	0.413	0.506	
CTLA-4 (AT)n			
Genotype			
88 bp/88 bp	17.32	29.07	
Allele 88 bp	0.417	0.518	
CD28 (+17) T/C			
Genotypes			
T/T	48.03	55.42	
T/C	33.07	38.55	
C/C	18.90	6.02	
Alleles			
T	0.646	0.747	0.001
C	0.354	0.253	
CD86 (+1057) G/A			
Genotypes	52.76	60.24	
G/G	38.58	36.14	
G/A	8.66	3.62	
A/A			
Alleles			
G	0.720	0.783	0.635
A	0.280	0.217	

p (HWE): Hardy-Weinberg equilibrium *p* value

Table 4. Genotypes and alleles frequencies in patients and controls (%)

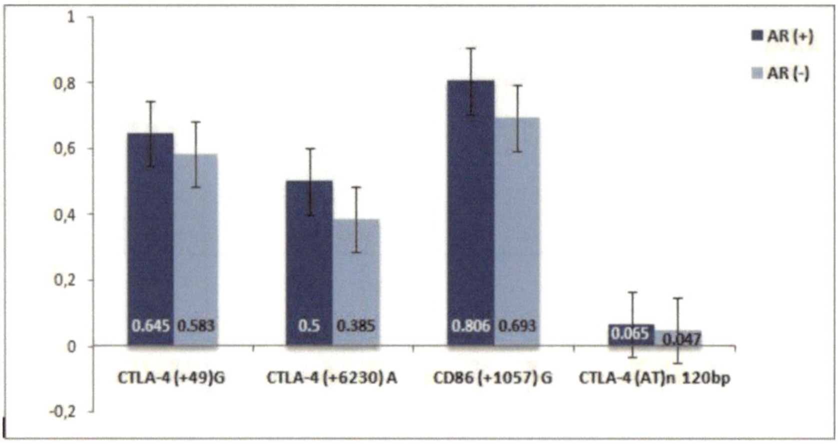

AR(+): acute rejection; AR(-): non acute rejection

Fig. 3. Allele frequencies in acute rejection and in non-acute rejection patients

On the other hand, no differences were found in the distribution of alleles or genotypes frequencies of (-318) C/T polymorphism of the CTLA-4 gene or (+17) T/C of the CD28 gene. In addition, in negative anti-HLA recipients (105 patients), the 120 bp allele of (AT)n microsatellite in CTLA-4 gene was more frequent in acute rejection patients (0.071) than in non-acute rejection ones (0.055).
Moreover, in the negative anti-HLA recipients of the Group I (19 patients), the alleles (+49) G and (+6230) A of CTLA-4 were also more frequent in acute rejection patients than in non-acute rejection ones (0.833 *vs* 0.625 and 0.5 *vs* 0.281 respectively).

Polymorphisms	*Patients (n = 127)*		*Group I (n = 23)*		*Group II (n =104)*	
	AR(+) n=31 n(%)	*AR(-) n=96 n(%)*	*AR(+) n=5 n(%)*	*AR(-) n=18 n(%)*	*AR(+) n=26 n(%)*	*AR(-) n=78 n(%)*
CTLA-4 (+49) A/G						
Genotypes						
G/G	14 (46.16)	35 (36.46)	4 (80)	6 (33.33)	10 (38.46)	29 (37.18)
G/A	12 (38.71)	42 (43.75)	1 (20)	11 (61.11)	11 (42.31)	31 (39.74)
A/A	5 (16.13)	19 (19.79)	0	1 (5.56)	5 (19.23)	18 (23.08)
Alleles						
G	0.645	0.583	0.900	0.689	0.596	0.570
A	0.355	0.417	0.100	0.361	0.404	0.430
CTLA-4 (-318) C/T						
Genotypes						
C/C	27 (87.1)	86 (89.58)	4 (80)	16 (88.89)	23 (88.46)	70 (89.74)
C/T	4 (12.9)	9 (3.38)	1 (20)	1 (5.56)	3 (11.54)	8 (10.26)
T/T	0	1 (1.04)	0	1 (5.56)	0	0
Alleles						
C	0.935	0.943	0.900	0.917	0.942	0.949
T	0.065	0.057	0.100	0.083	0.058	0.051

CTLA-4 (+6230) G/A						
Genotypes						
G/G	8 (25.81)	36 (37.50)	0	8 (44.44)	8 (30.77)	28 (35.90)
G/A	15 (48.38)	46 (47.92)	4 (80)	10 (55.56)	11 (42.31)	36 (46.15)
A/A	8 (25.81)	14 (14.58)	1 (20)	0	7 (29.92)	14 (17.95)
Alleles						
G	0.500	0.615	0.400	0.722	0.519	0.590
A	0.500	0.385	0.600	0.278	0.481	0.410
CTLA-4 (AT)n						
Genotypes						
88bp/88bp	7 (22.58)	15 (15.62)	1 (20)	1 (5.56)	6 (23.08)	14 (17.95)
120bp/120bp	0	1 (1.04)	0	0	0	1 (1.18)
120bp/other	7 (22.58)	21 (21.88)	1 (20)	5 (27.78)	5 (19.23)	6 (7.69)
Allele 120 bp	0.065	0.047	0	0.138	0.115	0.155
CD28 (+17) T/C						
Genotypes						
T/T	14 (46.16)	47 (48.96)	1 (20)	9 (50)	13 (50)	38 (48.27)
T/C	12 (38.71)	30 (31.25)	3 (60)	2 (11.11)	9 (34.62)	28 (35.90)
C/C	5 (16.13)	19 (19.79)	1 (20)	7 (38.89)	4 (15.38)	12 (15.38)
Alleles						
T	0.645	0.646	0.500	0.556	0.673	0.667
C	0.355	O.354	0.500	0.444	0.327	0.333
CD86 (+1057) A/G						
Genotypes						
G/G	20 (64.52)	47 (48.96)	3 (60)	8 (44.44)	17 (65.38)	39 (50)
G/A	10 (32.26)	39 (40.62)	1 (20)	7 (38.89)	9 (34.62)	32 (41.03)
A/A	1 (3.22)	10 (10.42)	1 (20)	3 (16.17)	0	7 (8.97)
Alleles						
G	0.806	0.693	0.700	0.639	0.827	0.705
A	0.914	0.307	0.300	0.361	0.173	0.295

Table 5. Genotypes frequencies in renal transplant recipients: comparison between acute rejection (AR+) and non acute rejection (AR-)

Haplotype	*Patients*		*Group I / anti-HLA(-)*	
	RA(+) n=31	*RA(-) n=96*	*RA(+) n=3*	*RA(-) n=16*
AGA	0.041	0.084	0.167	0.177
AGG	0.235	0.266	-	0.198
AAA	0.023	0.027	-	-
AAG	0.055	0.040	-	-
GGA	0.098	0.129	0.042	0.063
GGG	0.125	0.136	0.291	0.280
GAG	0.390	0.251	0.209	0.177
GAA	0.031	0.068	0.291	0.103

Table 6. Haplotype frequencies of the SNPs (+49) A/G and (+6230) G/A of CTLA-4 and (+1057) A/G of CD86 in acute rejection and non acute rejection patients

We also estimated the haplotype frequencies considering the three SNPs: (+49) A/G and (+6230) G/A of CTLA-4 and of CD86 in acute rejection and non acute rejection recipients (Table6). Our results showed that the association CTLA-4(+49)G/CTLA-4(+6230)A/ CD86(+1057)G was more frequent in patients who undergone an acute rejection comparing with those who do not in the total cohort: 0.390 *versus* 0.251, and especially in the anti-HLA negative patients of the Group I: 0.209 *versus* 0.177.

6. Discussion

The interactions of CTLA-4 and CD28 with their ligands CD80 and CD86 represent an important co-stimulatory signal that regulates T-cell activation. The genes encoding these molecules may be candidates for the susceptibility to acute renal allograft rejection. In our study, we sought to investigate the most characterized polymorphisms in the CTLA-4, the CD28 and the CD86 genes among 83 healthy subjects and 127 renal transplants.

Based upon the important impact of HLA disparity between donor and recipient on transplantation outcomes, we subdivided the patients into two groups. Indeed, the rate of acute rejection in our cohort was lower in the recipients showing similar HLA haplotype with their donors.

It is also established that pre-formed anti-HLA antibodies in allograft recipients can induce sever vascular disease of organ transplant, particularly an antibody-mediated rejection (humoral rejection), which has become a major clinical challenge since the rejection caused by antibodies resists treatment by conventional drug regimens. In renal transplant, hyper acute rejection is the most often caused by anti-HLA antibodies produced by the graft recipient (Chang et al., 2009; Poli, 2009). Moreover, donor-specific anti-HLA antibodies developed after transplantation transduce signals that are both pro-inflammatory than pro-proliferative suggesting mechanistic roles in acute and chronic antibody-mediated rejection (Li et al., 2009). Thus, antibody response to donor HLA class I and class II antigens represents a significant risk factor for kidney transplant failure. That's why, prior to transplantation, recipient sera are tested for HLA antibodies and a determination of donor mismatch acceptability increases transplant success. Sensitization occurs through exposure to HLA antigens via blood transfusions, previous grafts, or pregnancies (Karahan et al., 2009). In our study, sensitized patients were statistically more susceptible to develop acute rejection than non-sensitized ones. This result corroborates those of previous studies which reported that patients with pre-transplantation high levels of panel-reactive antibody show an increased risk of graft failure (Chang et al., 2009; Karahan et al., 2009).

A recent analysis in end-stage renal disease patients among Turkish population proposed also that de novo synthesis of these antibodies after transplantation could be detrimental for the graft. However, we did not detect a significant difference in acute rejection incidence between patients which developed anti-HLA antibodies in post transplantation and those which do not. In fact, the influence of anti-HLA antibodies on the development of rejection episodes depends probably on patient-specific clinical factors differing among patients (Karahan et al., 2009).

The distribution of genotype and allele frequencies in our study highlighted a trend toward an increase of CTLA-4 (+49) G, (+6230) A, 120 bp (AT)n and in CD86 (+1057) G alleles frequencies among patients with acute allograft loss compared to non-acute rejection ones, suggesting that these alleles may enhance the incidence of acute rejection. In order to validate this supposition, we sought to eliminate the other risk factors: the presence of anti-

HLA antibodies and the HLA disparity between donor and recipient. Thus, we compared allele frequencies in non-sensitized patients of the Group I, and we also noticed the rise of these same alleles with the occurrence of acute rejection. However, the wide confidence intervals (CIs) in this analysis reflect the relatively small numbers in some of the subgroups, with a consequent loss of statistical power. A larger patient cohort would therefore be required for us to reduce the width of the CIs and confirm these observations.

Our findings can join those of Kim et al. who reported the implication of the (+49) G allele of CTLA-4 in late acute rejection kidney allograft (Kim et al., 2010), and also those of Marìn et al. who revealed an association of the (+1057) G allele of CD86 and acute rejection in liver allograft (Marìn et al., 2005). In contrast to us, Muro et al. study shows that the potential correlated allele of CTLA-4 gene to liver acute rejection is the (+6230) G (Muro et al, 2008). Slavcheva et al. rather revealed a lack of association between CTLA-4 (+49) A/G polymorphism and renal or liver acute rejection, and a possible implication of alleles 92 and 94 bp of the (AT)n microsatellite (Slacheva et al., 2001).

Our study did not reveal any differences between patients with an acute rejection episode and those free of acute rejection in genotypic or allelic frequencies of the (-318) C/T gene promoter of the CTLA-4 or the (+17) T/C in the intron 3 of the CDE28 gene. Whereas, a recent study reported that the (-318) T allele induces a more important activity of the promoter region, a higher level of CTLA-4 molecular expression, and a more efficient inhibitory effect on T lymphocyte activation than the (-318) C allele (Slacheva et al., 2001). Besides, this SNP has been associated to several autoimmune disorders such as chronic obstructive pulmonary disease (Liu et al., 2010) or sporadic breast cancer (Fan et al., 2004). The exact role of the (+17) T/C polymorphism the CD28 gene is not really clear. It has been rarely correlated directly to autoimmunity dysfunction. Recently, a Polish study on cervical squamous cell carcinoma (CSCC) reported a potential association with the CD28 (+17) T/C polymorphism, but the authors specified that this association is restricted only to the well-differentiated CSCC (Pawlak et al. 2010).

The analysis of the haplotype frequencies distribution in our recipients revealed that the combination of CTLA-4(+49) G/CTLA-4 (+6230) A/CD86 (+1057) G was more frequent in case of acute rejection considering the whole cohort or the anti-HLA (-) patients of the Group I. These results led us to suppose that the simultaneous presence of the alleles CTLA-4 (+49) G, (+6230) A, (AT) 120bp and CD86 (+1057) G could constitute susceptibility haplotype to acute rejection in renal allograft. In fact, alleles at different loci may interact, increasing or decreasing susceptibility to a disease [22]. Thus, we know that the SNPs (AT)n and (+6230) A/G are involved in both the level and the stability of mRNA of the CTLA-4 molecule. Therefore, we suggest that the association CTLA-4 (+49) G-(+6230) A-(AT) 120bp may be linked to reduced expression of CTLA-4 on the T-cell surface, which could lead to reduce CTLA-4 production and subsequently impair inhibitory function and contribute to enhance T lymphocytes proliferation. The phosphorylation site introduced in the cytoplasmic tail of the CD86 molecule caused by the (+1057) A/G SNP affects APC signal transduction. So it is likely to presume that (+1057) G allele leads to a higher capability of T cells activation. Consequently, patients bearing concurrently the CTLA-4 (+49) G, (+6230) A, (AT) 120bp and CD86 (+1057) G alleles could develop elevated level of immune response and then a higher risk of allograft rejection. However, these results should be interpreted with caution due to the low number of patients in some subgroups. This hypothesis can confirm a recent research realized in the same context which investigated the influence of

CTLA-4 gene polymorphism on long-term kidney allograft function. No significant correlation of a particular SNP with the risk of acute rejection was found. However, the combination (+49)AA/(AT)LL haplotype (where L=low AT repeat number) was associated to better allograft function than the GG/HH haplotype (where H=high ,i.e. >82-bp repeats) (Kusztal et al., 2010).

7. Conclusion

In summary, our analysis of the costimulatory molecules genes revealed a genetic profile which may be implied in the enhancement of acute rejection incidence in Tunisian kidney recipients. We suggest that the alleles (+49) G, (+6230) A and (AT) 120bp of CTLA-4 gene and (+1057) G of CD86 gene may have a predisposition effect on acute rejection acting independently of the other risk factors: the presence of anti-HLA antibodies and the HLA disparity between donor and recipient. The (-318) C/T SNP in the promoter of CTLA-4 gene and the (+17) T/C in the CD28 gene seem to not be involved in the susceptibility to renal allograft rejection. More studies are needed in order to clarify if determination of the costimulatory molecules genotypes could be a useful prognostic factor witch interfere in allograft failure.

8. Acknowledgment

Our gratitude is extended to H. Hadj Kacem and to the team of "Unité Cible pour le Diagnostic et de Thérapie" from the CBS (Center of Biotechnology of Sfax, Tunisia) for their contribution in the optimization of the genotyping and the analysis method used in this work.
This study was supported by a grant for Tunisian Kidney Transplantation Research Fund.

9. References

Akalin E., Chandraker A., Russell M.E. et al. (1996). CD28-B7 T cell costimulatory blockade by CTLA4-Ig in the rat renal allograft model: inhibition of cell-mediated and humoral immune responses in vivo. *Transplantation*, Vol. 62, No. 12, pp. 1942-1945.

Alegre M., Fallarino F., Zhou P. et al. (2001). Transplantation and the CD28/CTLA-4/B7 pathway. *Transplantation Proceedings*, Vol. 33, No. 1-2, pp. 209-211.

Beier K.C., Kallinich T. & Hamelmann E. (2007). Master switches of T-cell activation and differentiation. *European Respiratory Journal*, Vol. 29, pp. 804–812.

Brand O., Gaugh S. & Heward J. (2005). HLA, CTLA-4 and PTPN22: the shared genetic master-key to autoimmunity?. *Expert Reviews in Molecular Medicine*. Vol. 17, N. 23, pp. 1-15.

Chang A.T. & Platt J.L. (2009). The role of antibodies in transplantation. *Transplantation Reviews*, Vol. 23, pp. 191–198.

Chavez H., Beaudreuil S., Abbed K. et al. (2007). Absence of CD4 CD25 regulatory T cell expansion in renal transplanted patients treated in vivo with Belatacept mediated CD28-CD80/CD86 blockade. *Transplant Immunology*, Vol. 17, pp. 243-248.

Chuang E., Lee K.M. & Robbins M.D. (1999). Regulation of CTLA-4 by Scr kinases. *Journal of Immunology*, Vol. 162, pp. 1270-1277.

Collins A.V., Brodie D.W., Gilbert R.J.C. et al. (2002). The interaction proprieties of costimulatory molecules revisited. *Immunity*. Vol. 17, pp. 201-210.

Corydon T.J., Haagerup A., Jensen T.G. et al. (2007). A functional CD86 polymorphism associated with asthma and related allergic disorders. *Journal of Medical Genetics*, Vol. 44, pp. 509-515.

Dalla-Costa R., Pincerati M.R., Holsbach Beltrame M. et al. (2010). Polymorphisms in the 2q33 and 3q21 chromosome regions including T-cell coreceptor and ligand genes may influence susceptibility to pemphigus foliaceus. *Human Immunology*, Vol. 71, pp. 809–817.

Fan L.Y., Tu X.Q., Chen Q.B. et al. (2004). CTLA-4 gene polymorphisms confer susceptibility to primary biliary cirrhosis and autoimmune hepatitis in Chinese population. *World Journal of Gastroenterology*, Vol. 10, pp. 3056-3059.

Greenwald G.R., Latchman Y.E., Sharpe A.H. et al. (2002). Negative co-receptors on l ymphocytes. Current Opinion in Immunology, Vol. 14, pp. 391–396.

Handa T., Nagai S., Ito I. et al. (2005). Polymorphism of B7 (CD80 and CD86) genes do not affect disease susceptibility to Sarcoidosis. *Respiration*. Vol. 72, pp. 243-248.

Karahan G.E., Seyhun Y., Oguz F. et al. (2009). Anti-HLA Antibody profile of Turkish patients with end-stage renal disease. Transplantion Procceedings, Vol. 41, pp. 3651–3654.

Kim H.J., Jeon K.H., Lee S.H. et al. (2010). Polymorphisms of the CTLA4 gene and kidney transplant rejection in Korean patients. *Transplant Immunology*, Vol. 24, pp. 40–44.

Kusztal M., Kościelska-Kasprzak K., Drulis-Fajdasz D. et al. (2010). The influence of CTLA-4 gene polymorphism on long-term kidney allograft function in Caucasian recipients. *Transplant Immunology*, Vol. 23, pp. 121–124.

Lenschow D.J., Zeng Y., Hathcock K.S. et al. (1995). Inhibition of transplant rejection following treatment with anti-B-2 and anti-B-1 antibodies. *Transplantation*, Vol. 60, No. 10, pp. 1171-1178.

Li F., Atz M.E. & Reed E.F. (2009) Human leukocyte antigen antibodies in chronic transplant vasculopathy—mechanisms and pathways. *Current Opinion in Immunology*, Vol. 21, pp. 557–562.

Liu Y ., Liang W.B., Gao L.B. et al. (2010). CTLA4 and CD86 gene polymorphisms and susceptibility to chronic obstructive pulmonary disease. *Human Immunology*, Vol. 71, pp. 1141–1146.

Marín L.A., Moya-Quiles M.R., Miras M. et al. (2005). Evaluation of CD86 gene polymorphism at (+1057) position in liver transplant. *Transplant Immunology*, Vol. 15, pp. 69-74.

Matsushita M., Tsuchiya N., Oka T. et al. (2000). New polymorphisms of human CD80 and CD86: lack of association with Rheumatoid arthritis and systemic lupus erythematosus. *Genes and Immunity*. Vol. 1, pp. 428-434.

Melichar B., Nash N.A., Lenzi R. et al. (2000). Expression of costimulatory molecules CD80 and CD86 and their receptors CD28, CTLA-4 on malignant ascites CD3+ tumor-infiltrating lymphocytes (TIL) from patients with ovarian and other types of peritoneal carcinomatosis. *Clinical and Experimental Immunology*, Vol. 119, pp. 19-27.

Minguela A., Marín L., Torío A. et al. (2000). CD28/CTLA-4 and CD80/CD86 costimulatory molecules are mainly involved in acceptance or rejection of human liver transplant. *Human Immunology*, Vol. 61, pp. 658-669.

Muro M., Rojas R., Botella C. et al. (2008). CT60 A/G marker of the 3'UTR region of the CTLA-4 gene and liver transplant. *Transplant Immunology*, Vol. 18, pp. 246-249.

Pawlak, E., Karabon L., Wlodarska-Polinska I. et al. (2010). Influence of CTLA-4/CD28/ICOS gene polymorphisms on the susceptibility to cervical squamous cell carcinoma and stage of differentiation in the Polish population. *Human Immunology*, Vol. 71, pp. 195-200.

Poli F., Cardillo M., Scalamogna M. et al. (2009). Clinical relevance of human leukocyte antigen antibodies in kidney transplantation from deceased donors: The North Italy Transplant program approach. *Human Immunology*, Vol. 70, pp. 631–635.

Sayegh M.H. &Turka L.A. (1998). The role of T-cell costimulatory activation pathways in transplant rejection. *New English Journal of Medicine*. Vol. 338, No. 25, pp. 1813-1820.

Seliger B., Marincola F.M., Ferrone S. et al. (2008). The complex role of B7 molecules in Tumor immunology. *Trends in Molecular Medicine*. Vol. 14, No. 12, pp. 550-559.

Sharpe A.H. & Freeman G.J., The B7–CD28 superfamily. (2002). *Nature Reviews Immunology*, Vol. 2, pp. 116-126

Slavcheva E., Albanis E., Jiao Q. et al. (2001). Cytotoxic T-Lymphocyte Antigen 4 gene polymorphism and susceptibility to acute allograft rejection. *Transplantation*, Vol. 72, No. 5, pp. 935-940.

Sui W., Dai Y., Huang Y.S. et al. (2008). Microarray analysis of MicroRNA expression in acute rejection after renal transplantation. Transplant Immunology, Vol. 19, pp. 81–85.

Suwalska K., Pawlak E., Karabona L. et al. (2008). Association studies of *CTLA-4, CD28,* and *ICOS* gene polymorphisms with B-cell chronic lymphocytic leukemia in the Polish population. Human Immunology, Vol. 69, pp. 193–201.

Thomas I.J., Petrish de Marquesini L.G., Ravanan R. et al. (2007). CD86 has sustained costimulatory effect on CD8 T cells. *Journal of Immunology*, Vol. 179, pp. 5936-5946.

Turgeon N.A., Krik A.D., Iwakosi N.N. et al. (2009). Differential effects of donor-specific alloantibody. Transplantation Reviews, Vol. 23, pp. 25-33.

Van Veen T., Crusius J.B.A., Van Winsen L. et al. (2003). CTLA-4 and CD28 gene polymorphisms in susceptibility, clinical course and progression of multiple sclerosis. *Journal of Neuroimmunology*, Vol. 140, pp.188–193.

Vinceti F. (2008). Costimulation blockade in autoimmunity and transplantation. *Journal of Allergy and Clinical Immunology*, Vol. 121, pp. 299-306.

Wang S. & Chen L. (2004). Co-signaling molecules of the B7-CD28 family in positive and negative regulation of T lymphocyte responses. *Microbes and Infection*. Vol. 6, pp. 759–766.

Wong C.K., Lit L.C.W., Tam L.S. et al. (2005). Aberrant production of soluble costimulatory molecules CTLA-4, CD28, CD80 and CD86 in patients with systemic lupus erythematosus. Rheumatology, Vol. 44, pp. 989-994

7

Urinary Proteomics and Renal Transplantation

Elisenda Banon-Maneus, Luis F Quintana and Josep M Campistol
LENIT (Laboratori Experimental de Nefrologia i Trasplantament)
Hospital Clínic de Barcelona, Catalunya
Spain

1. Introduction

Nearly 60 years after the first successful organ transplantation in humans, it has been an exponential increase in our understanding of the immunological processes involved in organ transplantation. This knowledge has resulted in the identification of immunogenic drug targets and improvement on the management of patient's surveillance. The past 5 decades have also seen an explosive evolution in the fields of molecular biology, chemistry and informatics that have enabled increased data throughput, permitting the study of complete sets of molecules with increasing speed and accuracy using the omics techniques such as, genomics (DNA), transcriptomics (RNA), proteomics (proteins) and metabolomics (metabolites) (Bañón-Maneus et al 2007)

Despite overall improvements in immunosuppression regimens, chronic allograft dysfunction (CAD) continues to have a negative impact on graft and patient survival, even with the use of appropriate doses of immunosuppressive drugs to prevent acute rejection. Successful management requires an early detection along with adequate treatment. (Hariharan et al 2000 and Meier-Kriesche et al 2004)

Available diagnostic methods include clinical presentation, biochemical parameters and biopsies. Currently, the only non-invasive biomarkers for follow up the kidney graft are serum creatinine, glomerular filtration rate (GFR) and proteinuria but neither is particularly sensitive or specific and may not reflect early changes. At present, biopsy allograft is regarded as the gold standard for the diagnosis of CAD allowing its early detection; however, this is a costly procedure which is associated with clinical complications (Ojo et al 2000 and Nankivell et al 2003). The patient's management would be facilitated if there were appropriate biomarkers enabling the diagnosis or prognosis of different states throughout the post transplant course. At that point the proteomics have emerged as a really useful technology for biomarker discovery.

2. Urine as a source of biomarkers

The Biomarkers Definitions Working Group, defined Biomarker as a molecule that it is a characteristic, objectively measured and evaluated as an indicator of normal biological processes, pathogenic processes or pharmacological responses (Biomarkers Definitions Working Group, 2001). The ideal biological sample for detecting biomarkers is the so-called "proximal fluid", the bio fluid in closest contact with the site of disease (Decramer et al 2008). Then, in the context of kidney transplantation the closest biological sample, besides the biopsy, is the urine which represent a fairly simple, non-invasive and inexpensive method for obtaining suitable samples for biomarker analyses, and presents a huge advantage as it can be performed regularly and frequently if necessary.

The human kidney (Fig. 1) is composed of 1 million nephrons, which can be divided in two functional parts: the glomerulous, which filters the plasma yielding the "primitive" urine, and the renal tubule, which reabsorbs most of the primitive urine. However, more than 99% of this primitive urine is reabsorbed. The remainder (the urine) exits the kidney via the urethra into the bladder (Fig. 1) (Decramer et al 2008). Therefore urine may contain

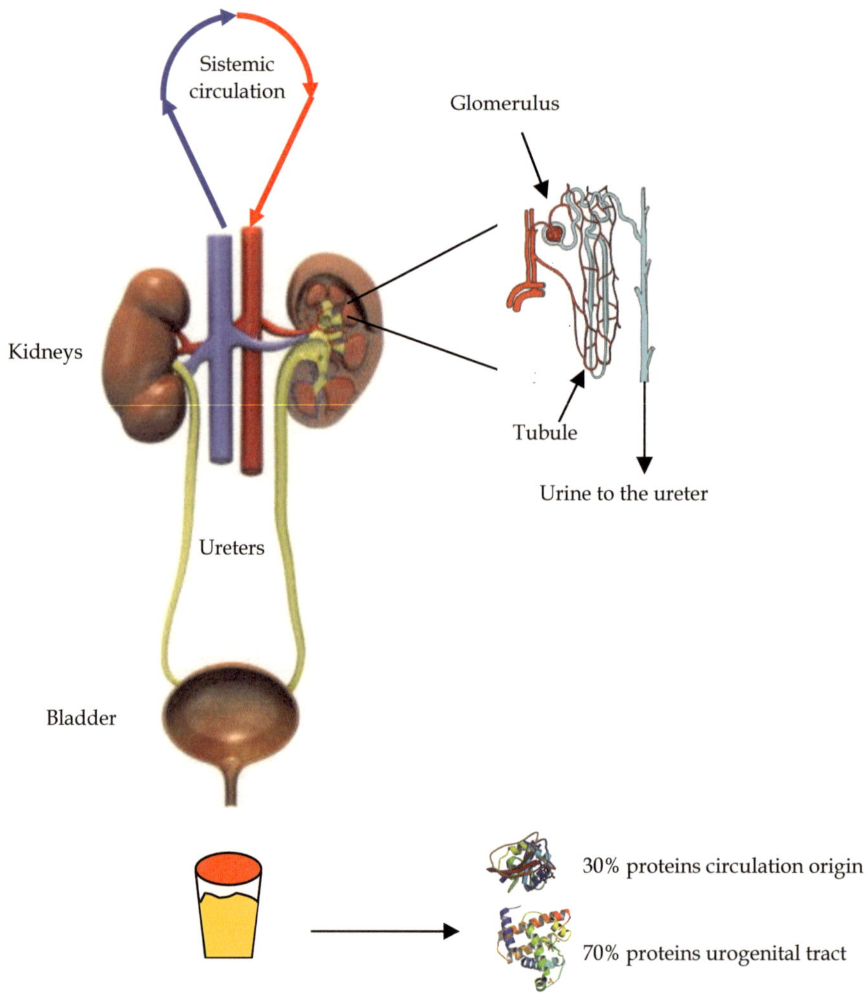

Fig. 1. Urinary proteins origin. Human kidney it is constituted by nephrons. The plasma filtration occurs into the glomerulus and the reabsorption into the tubule. The urine generated exits the kidney via urethra into the bladder. (Adapted Decramer et al 2008) (images from www. turbosquid.com and www.ratical.org)

information not only from the kidney and the urinary tract but also from more distant organs via plasma obtained by glomerular filtration. In healthy individuals, 70% of the urinary proteome originates from the kidney and the urinary tract, whereas the remaining 30% represents proteins filtered by the glomerulus (Thongboonkerd and Malasit 2005).
For these reasons urine is defined as "fluid biopsy" of the kidney and urogenital tract, and many of the changes in kidney and urogenital tract can be detected in the urinary proteome. Furthermore, as blood filtering, urine contains protein components that are similar to those found in the blood. Thus, pathological changes occurring in other organs can be detected in blood plasma and, therefore, can be detected in the urinary proteome. NHGRI (National Human Genome Research Institute) has said that the study of proteomics of fluids is one of the most promising tools for the development of noninvasive tools for early detection of human diseases. Human urine is a fluid that contains immediately accessible useful biomarkers, it is easy to obtain, non invasive, could be stored for long time and other advantages described into Table 1. But the urine has some disadvantages too.

ADVANTAGES	DISADVANTAGES
- can be obtained in large quantities using non-invasive procedures - easy assessment of reproducibility or improvement in sample preparation protocols - urinary peptides and lower molecular mass proteins are generally soluble. (Solubilization of these low molecular weight proteins and peptides is a process with a major influence on the proteomics analysis) - > 30 KDa compounds can be analyzed in a mass spectrometer without additional manipulation - urinary protein is relatively stable probably due to the fact that urine "stagnates" for hours in the bladder - can be stored for several years at -80 °C without significant alteration of its proteome - not only the changes in the kidney and genitourinary tract are reflected by changes in the urinary proteome but also changes at more distant sites	- it widely varies in protein and peptide concentrations mostly because of differences in the daily intake of fluid - standardization based on creatinine or peptides generally present in urine - definition of disease-specific biomarkers in urine, is complicated by significant changes in the proteome during the day - changes are likely caused by variations in the diet, metabolic or catabolic processes, circadian rhythms, and exercise as well as circulatory levels of various hormones

Table 1. Advantages and disadvantages of urine as source of biomarkers (Decramer et al 2008, Fliser et al 2005, Kolch et al 2005, Omenn et al 2005, Schaub et al 2004, Schiffer et al 2006, and Theodorescu et al 2006)

Clinical proteomics is growing significantly in recent years due to the prospect of identifying new targets for treatment and therapeutic intervention and biomarkers for diagnosis, prognosis, and therapeutic efficacy using technologies that allow us to compare proteomic profiles between different conditions pathophysiology. The measurement of protein in the urine has been used for many years for the diagnosis and monitoring of many kidney diseases.

3. Omics strategies and single molecule approaches

The major differences between omics strategies and single molecule approaches lies in throughput (hundreds of thousands versus one or a few), but also in experimental design. Classic single molecule bio medical research is based on hypothesis testing, building new experiments based on prior observations and theory, such that classic scientific research tends towards a reductionist approach in understanding disease and disease processes, owing to the limitations of most technologies and the complex nature of pathological systems. After a first omics hypothesis generating approach, classic single molecule experiments should ensue, in order to delve further into the mechanisms of the newly generated hypotheses. (Naesens and Sarwal, 2010)

The development of genomics and transcriptomics notwithstanding, gene polymorphisms and transcript levels correlate incompletely with the expression level of the functionally active proteins, which more accurately reflect actual cellular events. This poor correlation between genotype, gene expression and the localization or activity of the proteins is caused by the complex regulation of the transcription and the post translational modifications that change the properties of proteins. Proteins therefore provide a better picture of events that occur inside an organism and provide ideal biomarkers for disease conditions. (Abbott 1999, Quintana et al 2010 and Righetti and Boschetti 2007)

4. Proteomics technology

Proteomics methods are also increasingly being used in the field of organ transplantation. Because urine is the ideal non invasive specimen for renal diseases, the number of proteomic studies of urine has surged, and urine proteomics are a promising tool for the non invasive diagnosis of acute rejection and chronic allograft histological damage.

New tools and new applications of chemical technologies have revolutionized proteomics and peptidomics last years. Proteomics tools include gel electrophoresis (like one dimensional gel electrophoresis (1D); two dimensional gel electrophoresis (2D)) and gel free methods using mass spectrometry (like matrix-assisted laser ionization (MALDI); liquid chromatography mass spectrometry (LC-MS); surface-enhanced laser ionizationwith time of flight mass spectrometry (SELDI-TOF-MS)) (Naesens and Sarwal, 2010).

Proteome analysis of urine requires fractionation to reduce complexity of the sample. Fractionation can be obtained by different techniques. These fractions are subsequently analyzed by a mass spectrometer (MS) where the relative abundance of the different proteins and peptides is determined. Bioinformatics treatment of the protein data in combination with the fractionation parameters yields protein profiles representing the partial protein content of samples (Fig. 2)

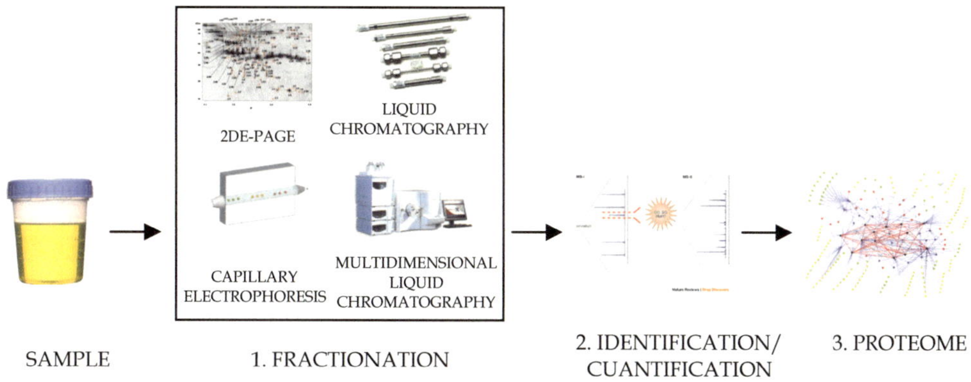

Fig. 2. Proteome analysis of urine requires fractionation to reduce complexity of the sample. Fractionation can be obtained by different chromatographic techniques or 2DE-PAGE. 2 These fractions are subsequently analyzed by a mass spectrometer (MS) 3 Bioinformatics treatment of the obtained data give us the sample proteome.

4.1 Urine sample: Collection, storage and preparation

Sample collection, storage and preparation it is a crucial issue, and many of the techniques described later requires different preparation methods. (Lee et al 2008)

Collection

The volume, protein concentration and composition of urine show considerable variation among the day. There is no ideal time of day to collect urine specimens for proteomics, but it is preferable to obtain samples at the same time of the day to minimize variations. The first morning void could be contaminated by cells from the lower urinary tract and bacteria harbored in the urinary tract. 24 hour samples have the problem of protein degradation. The second void of the morning could be one of the best samples that could be used, because it is easy to obtain when patients come to hospital and could be quickly processed. (O'Riordan et al 2006)

Some intra-patient variability in the urine proteome has been previously observed, but other investigations have identified only minor variations in samples collected for up to a year. Individual fluctuations seem to be minimally affected by diet and exercise. The relative influence of exogenous and endogenous factors needs further exploration, but should be considered when planning protocols and in interpretation of data (Akkina et al 2009).

Storage

The addition of protease inhibitors, filtration, centrifugation before and after freezing to reduce contamination by proteins leaking cellular debris and bacteria it is necessary. It is necessary to do some test to confirm the absence of red blood cells and leukocytes to avoid possible contamination of the samples.

Repeated freezing and thawing is known to fragment certain proteins, such as IgG and α-1-antitrypsin, and should be avoided. Urine stored at 37 °C can exhibit specific protease activity. An advantage of urinary proteomics is that the analytical reproducibility of the urine proteomic profile is unaffected by long term freezing, remaining stable for several years, even when stored at -20ºC (O'Riordan et al 2006).

Preparation

The presence of several excessively abundant urinary proteins, among them albumin and uromodulin (uromodulin is most abundant in normal urine, whereas albumin predominates in urine from diseased kidneys), can interfere with analyses. Depletion of these abundant proteins can increase the relative concentration and odds of detecting lower abundance proteins, but with the depletion we can lose some not abundant proteins (Hewitt et al 2004).
Isolating or concentrating urinary proteins may be essential in low concentration specimens, particularly for gel-based studies. Numerous methods have been compared including precipitation with organic solvents, centrifugal filtration, lyophilization and ultrafiltration but with varying results. Precipitation with Trichloroacetic Acid gave good qualitative yield. Reverse phase extraction has also been shown to be effective in specimen concentration as well as for desalting urinary peptides and segregating lower-molecular weight proteins (Bañón-Maneus et al 2007 and 2011).

4.2 Separation of proteins

Mono-and two-dimensional electrophoresis (2D-PAGE)

Two-dimensional electrophoresis was first described by O'Farrell over 30 years ago. The technology used for separation of proteins is polyacrylamide gel electrophoresis. For many proteomic applications, electrophoresis in one dimension is the method of choice. The proteins are separated according to their mass and how the proteins are solubilized in sodium dodecyl sulfate (SDS) there are generally no problems of solubilization. It is a simple, reproducible and allows the separation of proteins of 10-300 kDa. The 2D-PAGE two-dimensional electrophoresis allows separate thousands of proteins in a single experiment, and is currently the most efficient method for separating very complex protein mixtures. It is based on a separation of proteins according to the isoelectric point, followed by separation of proteins according to their molecular mass (Fig. 3). The first dimension separation is performed by isoelectric focusing, during which proteins are separated in a pH gradient until reaching a position where its net charge is zero, its isoelectric point (Fig. 4A). In a second dimension, proteins are separated by molecular weight in polyacrylamide gels (Fig. 4B). The high resolution of the technique is that the two separations are based on independent parameters. The key innovation for the 2D-PAGE was the development of gels with immobilized pH gradient (IPG). For detection of proteins has traditionally been using the radioactive labeling or staining with Coomassie blue or silver, for greater sensitivity. It also has developed a silver staining method compatible with surface protein digestion and mass spectrometry (Fig. 3) (Bañon-Maneus et al 2010, Oh et al 2004 and Thongboonkerd 2002). A recent development of 2D-PAGE technology is DIGE (Difference in Gel Electrophoresis), explained later.
The 2D-PAGE also has limitations: It is a very demanding technique, is time consuming, and difficult to automate, is limited by the number and type of proteins to solve; the very large or hydrophobic proteins do not enter the gel during the first dimension while proteins very acidic or very basic not well resolved, and in the presence of abundant proteins are difficult to detect low abundance proteins. Some of these problems can be resolved by fractionation,

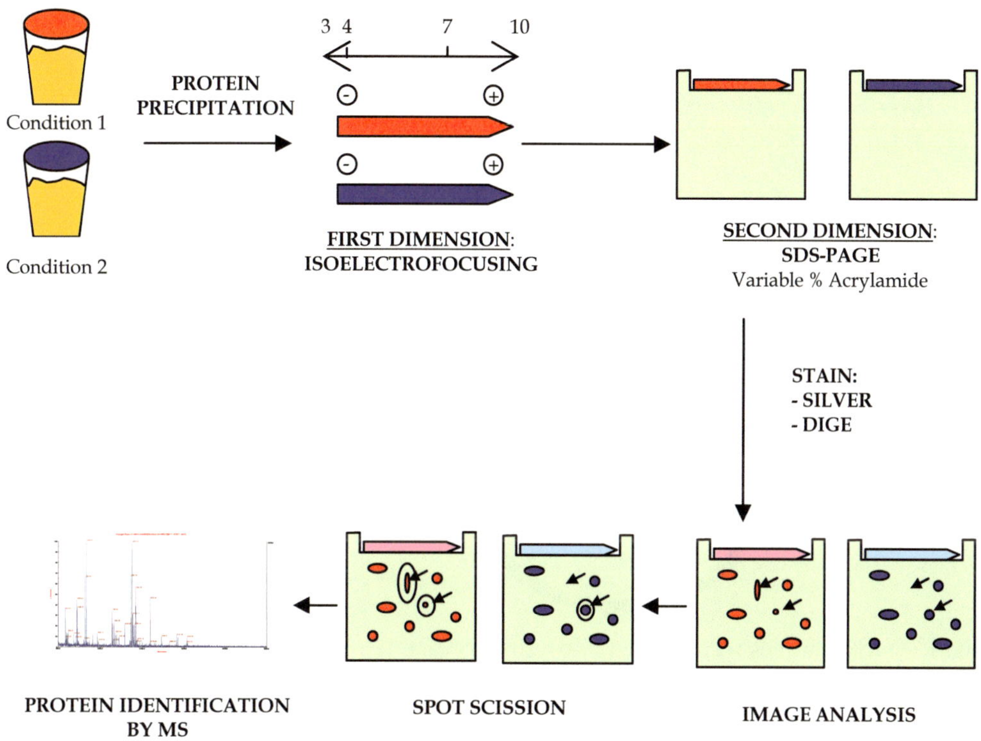

Fig. 3. 2D-PAGE workflow. After the protein extraction of the samples proteins were firs separated by the isoelectric point and after that by molecular weight. After the 2DE-PAGE staining the images were analyzed by finding of differential spots, that after the scission were identified by distinct Mass spectrometry approaches.

the use of certain solubilization conditions and the use of IPGs with different pH ranges. (Table 2) (Yoshida et al 2005)

Liquid chromatography

LC is a physical method of separation based on the distribution of the various components of a mixture into two immiscible phases one stationary and the other mobile. The mobile phase involves a liquid that flows through a column containing the steady phase. Classic LC is carried out in a column which is generally made of glass and filled with the steady phase. The steady phase may be a solid with different chemical properties which give rise to different types of chromatography - ion exchange chromatography, reverse-phase chromatography, and others. The mobile phase may be a pure solvent or mixture of solvents. After placing the sample on the upper part, the mobile phase flows through the column as a result of gravity. To improve the efficiency of separations, the size of steady phase particles was gradually diminished down to microns, and this called for high pressures to ensure mobile phase flow. (Table 2) (Cutillas et al 2003 and Mann et al 2002)

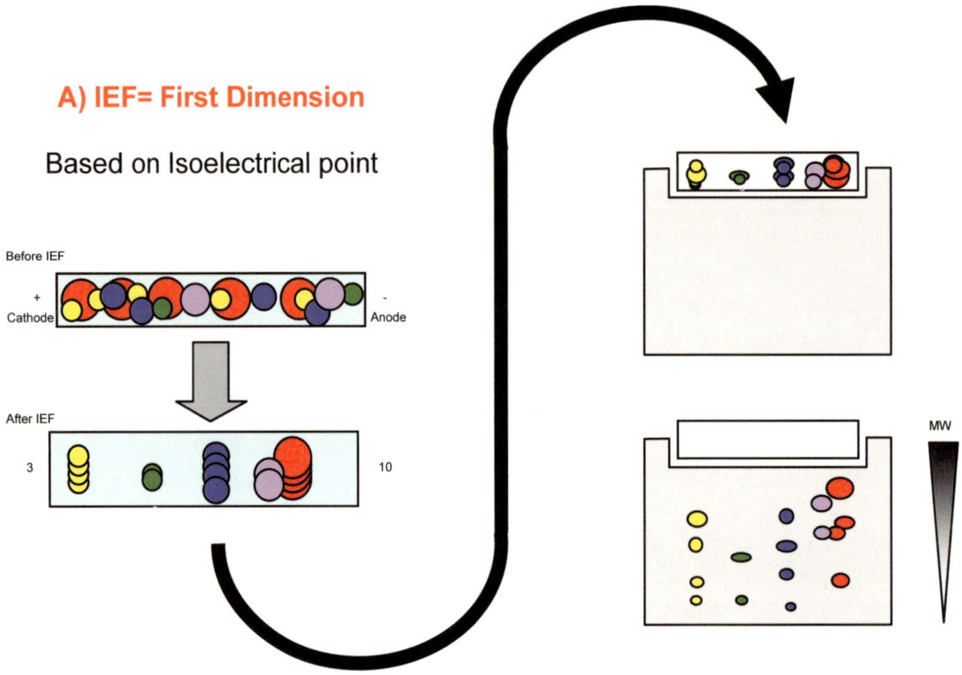

Fig. 4. A) IEF Samples were loaded into a dry polyacrylamide gel strips with an immobilized pH gradient for the separation by isoelectric point B) Second dimension, strips were loaded on the top of polyacrylamide gel and proteins were separated by molecular weight

Technology	ADVANTAGES	DISADVANTAGES
2DE-MS	For large molecules, sequencing of biomarkers easy to perform from spots	Restricted to selected IP, difficult to automate, time consuming, small molecules not detected (<10 kDa)
SELDI-TOF	High throughput, easy-to-use, automation, low sample volume	Restricted to selected proteins, low resolution MS, lack of comparability.
LC-MS	Automation, multidimensional, high sensitivity, used for detection of large molecules (>20 kDa) after tryptic digest, sequence determination of biomarkers provided by MS/MS	Reassembly of tryptic peptides into their precursor molecule can be problematic, time consuming, relatively sensitive toward interfering compounds, medium throughput
CE-MS	Automation, high sensitivity, fast, low sample volume, multidimensional	Generally not suited for larger molecules (>20 kDa)

2DE-MS, Two-dimensional gel-electrophoresis followed by mass spectrometry; LC-MS, liquid chromatography coupled to mass spectrometry, SELDI-TOF, surface-enhanced laser desorption/ionization coupled to mass spectrometry; CE-MS, capillary electrophoresis coupled to mass spectrometry

Table 2. Advantages and disadvantages of proteomic techniques for use in urinary biomarker discovery

High Performance Liquid Chromatography

High-performance liquid chromatography (HPLC) involves dissolving the protein mixture in buffer and pumping it through a series of columns. The columns are composed of materials with various physical, chemical and immunological properties, which bind different proteins with varying degrees of affinity depending on the complementary protein properties. The proteins can then be eluted from the columns. The properties on which separation can be based are numerous; the elements most frequently applied to urine are size exclusion (based on size), reverse phase (based on hydrophobicity), strong and weak cation binding, and affinity binding (i.e. an immunoglobulin adsorbing to protein of interest). (Bañón-Maneus et al 2007)

Capillary electrophoresis

In a silica capillary, proteins or peptides are separated as a function of charge at a desired pH by an electric field in which the capillary is housed. Like HPLC, this method can be applied to intact proteins, as well as digests. Although a powerful separation technique, capillary electrophoresis (CE) does not yield reliable quantitative information. (Table 2) (Schiffer et al 2006)

Mass spectrometry (MS): Identification and characterization of proteins

Proteins can be identified by various means, among which include the sequencing of the N-terminal specific antibody detection, amino acid composition, co-migration with known proteins and over-expression and depletion of genes. All these methods are generally slow, laborious or expensive and therefore not suitable for use as large-scale strategies. However, the MS, because of its rapidity and high sensitivity, has become the preferred method for identifying large-scale protein and the first step to study the proteome of different organisms. It also allows the characterization of post-translational modifications that have physiological relevance, such as glycosylation and phosphorylation. To analyze proteins by mass spectrometry these must be converted into peptides through proteolysis, usually with trypsin (Mauri et al 2009). This so robust technique involves (Fig. 5):

- Conversion of peptides into gas phase ions using soft ionization techniques such as ionization-assisted laser desorption matrix (MALDI) from a sample in solid form, or by electrospray ionization (ESI) of a sample solution.
- Separation of ions according to m/z (mass / charge) in a mass analyzer (e.g. type analyzer TOF (Time Of Flight), quadrupole, ion trap, etc.). Optional Fragmentation of selected peptide ions through goal decomposition stable (or PSD technique: post source decay) or by collision-induced dissociation (CID) conducted in a tandem mass spectrometer combining two different analyzers.
- Measurement of the masses in a detector obtaining a mass spectrum that reflects the abundance of ions versus their value m / z

For protein identification it has been developed two strategies:

- Identification by peptide fingerprint (PMF: peptide mass fingerprinting) or peptide mapping using MALDI-TOF spectrometer type.
- Identification of peptides obtained by fragmentation of whole or partial sequence of amino acids (sequence tag) using a tandem mass spectrometer.

Peptide mass fingerprinting

Peptide mapping is a technique used routinely to identify proteins quickly, usually from SDS-PAGE gels or 2D-PAGE and that is normally performed in a mass spectrometer type

MALDITOF. In this approach the protein is digested with an enzyme, usually trypsin. The sample is incorporated into a metal plate with a matrix and crystals formed upon evaporation. Subsequently, the sample is irradiated with laser to ionize the molecules. The ions are accelerated by an electric field towards a detector, the value m / z of each ion is determined by the flight time from the source reaching the detector.

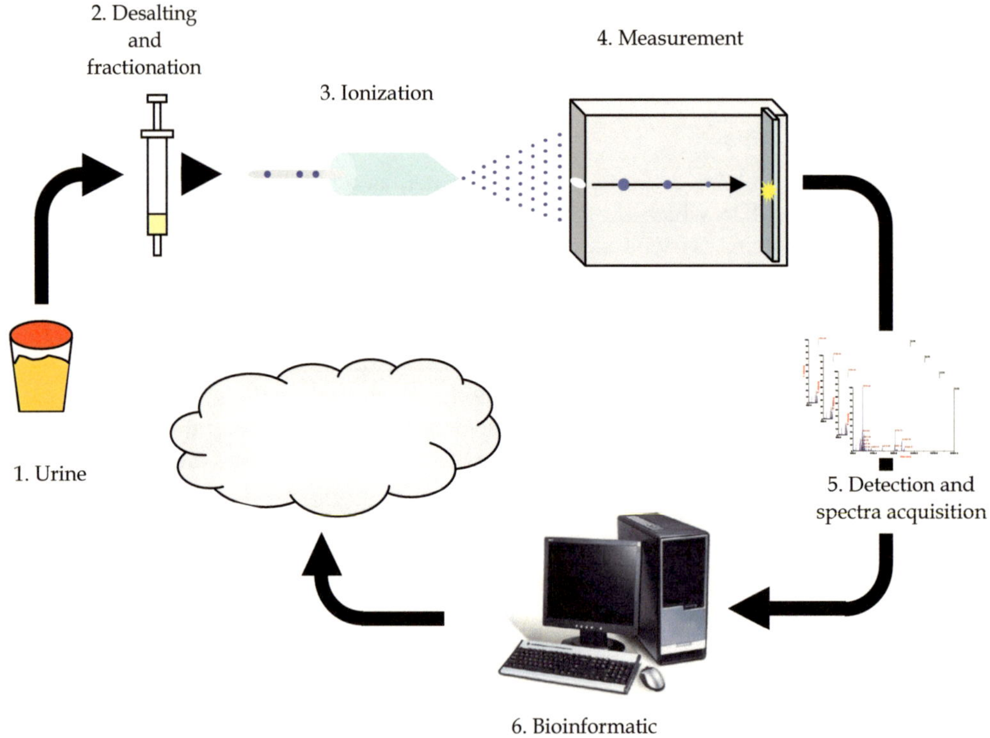

Fig 6. Urine samples were concentrated and separated from organic salts by solid phase. Each sample was applied and dried on an uncoated MALDI target plate using the sandwich technique.

The peptide fingerprint (PMF) of a particular protein is a set of peptides generated by digestion of a specific protease. These experimental peptide masses are compared with theoretical peptide masses of proteins present in databases by developing various algorithms available on the network. For the correct identification of the protein mass requires a large number of peptides matching the theoretical masses of peptides, covering part of the protein sequence database. The limitations of mass spectrometry are that the ionization of peptides is selective and not quantitative. In an equimolar set of peptides derived from digestion of a protein, some peptides may not be detected and the rest of them can be a large variation in signal intensity. If the amount of protein in the gel is small, the number of peptides observed can be small and therefore the protein can not be identified with certainty. The MALDI-TOF MS is of little use to analyze protein mixtures. Very clear protein spots from 2D gels can contain several proteins (Bañón-Maneus et al 2007 and Gazzana and Borlak 2007)

Peptide sequence

It is a strategy to identify proteins not annotated in databases or for the ambiguous identification by MALDI-TOF. The tandem mass spectrometer MS / MS can also determine the amino acid sequence. Ion is selected by a mass spectrometer and fragmented first collision with a gas and the fragments are analyzed in a second spectrometer. Peptide sequence can be done with MALDI ionization source type or ESI. (Gazzana and Borlak 2007)

Surface-enhanced laser desorption/ionization (SELDI)

SELDI-MS incorporates chromatographic and MS principles in a single platform. An activated surface on a 'chip' binds proteins on the basis of their chemical and physical properties; unbound proteins are washed off. A subset of the proteome is thus selected and the chip plugs directly into the mass spectrometer for analysis. This is a high-throughput screening technique that facilitates relative abundance profiling of individual proteins from different samples. Although the approach can be extremely useful for screening peptide/protein samples for recognition of biomarker ions, it does not enable the protein origin of these ions to be reliably discerned. Other disadvantages are use of relatively low-resolution MS, the fact that only a subset of the proteome can be studied on any particular surface, and that the performance varies between different machines (as does performance of a single machine over time). (O´Riordan et al 2006)

4.3 Expression level quantitative techniques

The main application of proteomics is the study of protein expression profile. There are two strategies that enhance the study of differential protein expression between different samples, the gel based and the free gel technologies.

Gel based quantitative proteomics: DIGE

Also recently described an approach based on the labeling of proteins with different fluorophores and the separation of samples by 2D-PAGE in the same gel. This methodology, called DIGE (Differential Gel Electrophoresis), minimizes the variability of the gels decreased analysis time and allows quantification of very specific expression profile. Briefly, two samples are differentially labeled with two different fluorescence CyDyes (p.e, Cy3 and Cy5), mixed, and then resolved simultaneously within the same 2DE gel. The introduction of a pooled internal standard labeled with a third dye (p.e. Cy2) improves the accuracy of protein quantification between samples from different gels allowing detection of small changes in protein levels. Differentially expressed proteins could be identified using protein fingerprinting MS methods as modern matrix-assisted laser desorption/ionization-time of-flight MS (MALDI-TOF-MS) instrumentation. (Alban et al 2003, Shaw et al 2003, Unlu et al 1997 and Wu 2006)

Gel Free quantitative proteomics: ICAT, iTRAQ, SILAC

The ICAT (isotope-coded affinity tags), which can determine the relative amount of protein between two samples. The two protein samples are labeled with the ICAT reagent light or heavy (as hydrogen or deuterium leads). This reagent binds to cystein and contains biotin to facilitate purification. Subsequently, the two samples are mixed and digested with trypsin. The peptides marked with ICAT reagent are separated in an affinity column and analyzed by MS. The relative intensity of the peptides identical in each sample (differ in a mass of 8 Da) are abundant protein from which they came. The fragmentation of the peptide by MS / MS led to the identification of the protein (Sobhani 2010).

An improved approach analogous to ICAT has been developed called iTRAQ (Applied Biosystems). The technique is based upon chemically tagging the N-terminus of peptides generated from protein digests that have been isolated from cells, tissues, biological fluids in two different states (Chen et al 2010). The two labeled samples are then combined, fractionated by nanoLC and analyzed by tandem mass spectrometry. Database searching of peptides data fragmentation provides the identification of the labeled peptides and hence the corresponding proteins. Fragmentation of the tag attached to the peptides generates a low molecular mass reporter ion that is unique to the tag used to label each of the digests. Measurement of the intensity of these reporter ions, enables relative quantification of the peptides in each digest and hence the proteins from where they originate. There are four tags available enabling four different conditions to be multiplexed together in one experiment. (Gigy et al 1999)

Stable isotope labeling with amino acids in cell culture (SILAC) is a simple and straightforward approach for in vivo incorporation of a label into proteins for mass spectrometry (MS)-based quantitative proteomics. SILAC relies on metabolic incorporation of a given 'light' or 'heavy' form of the amino acid into the proteins. The method relies on the incorporation of amino acids with substituted stable isotopic nuclei (e.g. deuterium, 13C, 15N). Thus in an experiment, two cell populations are grown in culture media that are identical except that one of them contains a 'light' and the other a 'heavy' form of a particular amino acid (e.g. 12C and 13C labeled L-lysine, respectively). When the labeled analog of an amino acid is supplied to cells in culture instead of the natural amino acid, it is incorporated into all newly synthesized proteins. After a number of cell divisions, each instance of this particular amino acid will be replaced by its isotope labeled analog. Since there is hardly any chemical difference between the labeled amino acid and the natural amino acid isotopes, the cells behave exactly like the control cell population grown in the presence of normal amino acid. It is efficient and reproducible as the incorporation of the isotope label is 100%. This technology it is not yet available for human urine proteomics but it could be used in experimental models by the administration of pellet food with the isotope enhanced. (Quan et al 2011)

Protein Arrays

Protein arrays are rapidly being developed for the characterization of activities and for detecting protein-protein interactions on a large scale. Like DNA arrays, protein arrays will be essential for basic research and more applied research to drug discovery and development of diagnostic methods. In a pioneering work done by the group of Snyder, we developed a chip with 6,000 yeast proteins to identify new proteins that interact with calmodulin or phospholipids. The proteins were obtained by cloning the corresponding ORFs and each protein was expressed fused to GST (glutathione S-transferase) and a histidine tag. This important work showed that it is possible to prepare microarrays with thousands of proteins and used to study interactions. However, although significant progress has been made for the preparation of the arrays, we still need to face several technological challenges to allow allowing the use of this tool to many researchers. (Zhu et al, 2000)

5. Protein biomarkers for kidney transplantation

Currently follow up of renal transplant recipients is done by the physicians checking serum creatinine and glomerular filtration rate (GFR), but neither is particularly sensitive or specific and may not reflect early alterations (Paul 2009 and Nankivell 2003). At present, biopsy allograft is regarded as the gold standard for the diagnosis of kidney diseases allowing its early detection; however, this is a costly procedure that is associated with clinical complications (Beckingham et al 1994).

5.1 Acute renal allograft rejection

One of the major problems in renal transplantation is acute renal allograft rejection. Acute rejection is one of the key factors that determine long term graft function and survival in renal transplant patients. This fatal complication is inevitable if the diagnosis is delayed.

Mainly for groups reported urinary proteomic approach for acute rejection. Interestingly, each group found a different pattern of protein biomarkers that were associated with allograft rejection. These differences are not surprising, as each study had differences in disease definition, sample collection and handling, protocol for protein and data analysis. (Rush and Nickerson 2011)

Clarke et al reported the comparison between 17 urines from rejecting patients to urines from 15 stable (not biopsied) controls. Proteomic analysis of the urine was done using SELDI15 and ProteinChip Arrays with immobilized metal affinity (IMAC-3) and hydrophobic (H4) surface. The best candidate biomarkers were four proteins of molecular around 7 kd and one of 13.4 kd. A separate analysis using the CART algorithm in the Ciphergen Biomarker Pattern Software using two different proteins of 3.4 kd and 10 kd, respectively, correctly classified 91% of the 34 urine specimens in the training set, producing a sensitivity of 83% and a specificity of 100%. (Clarke et al 2003*)*

O'Riordan *et al* reported on the urine proteome in 23 renal transplant patients with biopsy-proven acute rejection, 22 recipients with stable graft function (characterized by serum creatinine) and 20 healthy volunteers (27). The urine was preadsorbed on four different chip surfaces, and was analyzed by SELDI-TOF. Protein masses that were useful in the construction of the classification algorithms were of approximately 2.0, 2.8, 4.8, 5.8 7.0, 19.0 and 25.6 kd. Patients that had experienced acute rejection could be distinguished from stable patients with a sensitivity of 90.5% to 91.3% and a specificity of 77.2% to 83.3%, depending on the classifier used. (O'Riordan et al 2004)

The main drawback with this two studies is that control samples (stable renal transplant recipients) where characterized by a serum creatinine and no biopsies were done at the time of urine collection.

Wittke et al reported the analysis done by CE-MS from 19 patients with subclinical or clinical rejection, 10 patients with urinary tract infection but without rejection, and 29 patients without acute rejection or urinary tract infection (28). These patients were from a centre that performs protocol biopsies, and the urine samples were obtained at the time of protocol biopsy. An additional cohort of 66 healthy controls was studied. The authors were able to discriminate the rejecting patients from those without rejection in 16 of 19 patients using combinations of 16 polypeptides. (Wittke et al 2005)

Finally, Schaub et al sought to determine whether such candidate proteins can be detected in urine using mass spectrometry. Four patient groups were defined on the basis of allograft function, clinical course, and biopsy result. Four groups where analyzed: acute clinical

rejection, stable transplant, acute tubular necrosis, and recurrent (or de novo) glomerulopathy. Urines were collected the day of the allograft biopsy. As a normal control group, urines from healthy individuals were analyzed, as well as 5 urines from non-transplanted patients with lower urinary tract infection. Three prominent peak clusters were found in 94% of the patients with acute rejection episodes, but only in 18% of patients without clinical and histologic evidence for rejection and in any of normal controls. In addition, the presence or absence of these peak clusters correlated with the clinicopathologic course in most patients. Acute tubular necrosis, glomerulopathies, lower urinary tract infection, and cytomegalovirus viremia were not confounding variables. (Schaub et al 2004)
In conclusion, proteomic technology together with stringent definition of patient groups can detect urine proteins associated with acute renal allograft rejection. Identification of these proteins may prove useful as non-invasive diagnostic markers for rejection and the development of novel therapeutic agents.

5.2 BKV renal allograft nephropathy

BKV renal allograft nephropathy (BKVAN have an important role in development of renal allograft dysfunction (Fishman 2002). About 6-10% of these patients develop BKVAN, and the reported graft loss rate in this group has been as high as 50% (6,7). BKVAN can resemble acute allograft rejection (AR) and differentiation between them can be challenging both at histological and molecular levels (Fishman 2002). The discrimination is important because the treatment is diametrically opposite for the two conditions. In general, immunosuppression needs to be reduced in patients with BKVAN, whereas it is increased in AR. Currently, these two clinical conditions cannot be differentiated in a reliable way on the basis of clinical and laboratory findings and a definitive diagnosis of BKVAN requires allograft biopsy. Even the histological differentiation of BKVAN from AR can be difficult unless viral inclusions are seen on allograft biopsy (Fishman 2002).
Jahnukainen et al used Surface-enhanced laser desorption/ionization (SELDI) time of flight mass spectrometry to compare the urinary of patients with BKVAN, AR and stable graft function. They were able to detect several peaks that were differentially expressed in the BKVAN group compared with both the AR and stable function groups. Peaks that corresponded to m/z values of 5.872, 11.311, 11.929, 12.727, and 13.349 kD were significantly higher in patients with BKVAN. As Mannon *et al* showed significant similarity of transcriptional expression of molecules associated with inflammation and fibrosis between BKVAN and AR (Mannon et al 2005). This probably is due to the similarity of the inflammatory response and leakage of inflammation related small molecular weight proteins into urine in both conditions. The limitations of this study are that all of their analyses were based on a limited sample size, and their results on the sensitivity and the specificity of the various algorithms should be interpreted with caution. A true assessment of sensitivity and specificity of the SELDI technique and the various models tested in this report cannot be determined until an independent validation set that is derived from another set of patients is assessed. Proteomic marker(s) profiles, together with plasma and urine BKV PCR and clinical information, may help in making differentiation of BKVAN from AR in a non-invasive manner. Histological verification of BKVAN probably will continue to be required for the foreseeable future, but it is likely that proteomic biomarkers could be used in deciding when a biopsy is necessary. Further studies on a larger number of patients are needed to validate these findings and to detect the identity of the significantly different peaks to develop robust, non-invasive methods for BKVAN diagnostics. (Fishman 2002).

5.3 Chronic allograft rejection

The survival half-life for kidneys from deceased donors is approximately 11 yr, and the pathogenesis of chronic allograft rejection (CAD) is multifactorial (Mauiyyedi et al, 2001). Analyses of graft histology reflected in the revised Banff criteria indicate CAD can be subcategorized, in part, on the basis of evidence of local inflammation and the presence or absence of interstitial fibrosis and tubular atrophy (IF/TA) (Solez et al, 2008). Although specific inciting factors are difficult to define in each situation, distinct histopathologic entities often correlate with likely causes. For example, calcineurin inhibitor toxicity frequently manifests as IF/TA without inflammation; ongoing cellular alloimmunity presents histologically with tubulitis with or without IF/TA; C4d staining suggests transplant glomerulopathy with or without IF/TA; and detectable, donor-specific serum antibodies underlie antibody-mediated allograft injury (Solez et al, 2008).

Because only a subset of patients develop CAD and at present physicians do not have the ability to reverse chronic fibrotic kidney damage, it is essential that the transplant community develop reliable and noninvasive approaches to predict which patients are most likely to develop graft failure so that appropriate interventions can be instituted before graft failure becomes clinically apparent (Mauiyyedi et al, 2001).

Urine proteomic profiling of CAD has been investigated in a few studies to date. Using SELDI as screening methodology and liquid chromatography coupled to mass spectrometry (LCMS) to obtain protein ID information, O'Riordan et al studied the urinary proteome of 75 renal transplant recipients and 20 healthy volunteers. Patients could be classified into subgroups with normal histology and Banff CAN grades 2-3 with 86% sensitivity and 92% specificity. Several urinary proteins associated with advanced CAN were identified including a1-microglobulin, b2-microglobulin, prealbumin, and endorepellin, the antiangiogenic C-terminal fragment of perlecan. Increased urinary endorepellin was confirmed by ELISA and increased tissue expression of the endorepellin/perlecan ratio by immunofluoresence analysis of renal biopsies (O'Riordan 2008).

Our group is also investigating the utility of proteomic analysis of urinary samples as a non-invasive method to detect and evaluate CAD. We did the two main proteomic approaches, gel based and gel free approach. Proteomics based on two-dimensional electrophoresis (2-DE) has been optimized with the development of Difference Gel Electrophoresis (DIGE). A proteome map of stable renal patients as a reference protein database, to validate the utility of 2D-DIGE technology in finding new candidates as CAD urinary biomarkers were established. Morning spot urine of kidney transplant patients with a biopsy two years after transplantation with CI/CT score 0-I-II/III (n=8/group) was collected. 2D silver stained and mass spectrometry (MS) analyses were used to establish the proteome map and 2D-DIGE and MS were used to identify proteins exhibiting differential abundance. In this work not only the urinary proteome of renal stable patients was established but we were able to identify 11 proteins with elevated levels on advanced CAD: β-2 microglobulin, MASP-2, α-1-β-glycoprotein, leucine-rich α-2-glycoprotein 1, α-1-antitrypsin, Gelsolin precursor, AIF-like mitchondrion-associated inducer of death, heparan sulfate proteoglycan, anti-TNF-α antibody light-chain, immunoglobulin lambda light chain and dimethylarginine-dimethylaminohydrolase 2 and wnt-1. Eight of these proteins, α-1-antitrypsin, angiotensinogen, β-2-microglobulin, dimethyl-arginine dimethylaminohydrolase-2, immunoglobulin lambda light chain, transferrin, trypsin precursor, and Zn-β-2-glycoprotein, have been described in other renal injuries thus reducing their validity as biomarkers of, but we identified wnt-1, a protein from wnt/β-catenin pathway that has been described as a pathway really involved in fibrosis in other organs such as lung (Bañón-Maneus et al 2010).

Proteomic analysis using solid phase extraction as protein purification method and Protein profiling by MALDI-TOF was also performed. This is a relatively simple proteomic approach that allows rapid differential diagnosis of patients and information transfer between the laboratory and the clinical context. Fifty individuals: 32 patients with chronic allograft dysfunction (14 with pure interstitial fibrosis and tubular atrophy, and 18 with chronic active antibody-mediated rejection) and 18 controls (8 stable recipients and 10 healthy controls) were studied. Unsupervised hierarchical clustering showed good segregation of samples in groups corresponding mainly to the four biomedical conditions. Moreover, the composition of the proteome of the pure interstitial fibrosis and tubular atrophy group differed from that of the chronic active antibody-mediated rejection group, and an independent validation set confirmed the results from the training set (Quintana et al 2009). With the gel free approach we detected (by LC-M/MS) and quantified (by LCMS) 6000 polypeptide ions in undigested urine specimens across 39 CAD patients and 32 control individuals. Although unsupervised hierarchical clustering differentiated between the groups when including all the identified peptides, specific peptides derived from uromodulin and kininogen were found to be significantly more abundant in control than in CAD patients and correctly identified the two groups. These peptides are therefore potential biomarkers that might be used for the diagnosis of CAD. In addition, ions at m/z 645.59 and m/z 642.61 were able to differentiate between patients with different forms of CAD with specificities and sensitivities of 90% in a training set and, significantly, of 70% in an independent validation set of samples. Interestingly low expression of uromodulin at m/z 638.03 coupled with high expression of m/z 642.61 diagnosed CAD in virtually all cases (Quintana et al 2009).

This suggests that urinary proteome analysis can be used for the non-invasive monitoring of renal transplant patients, although it awaits validation in larger cohorts.

6. Conclusion

In summary, the application of proteomics in the field of renal and organ transplantation opens important options diagnostic and prognostic purposes. At present, urinary proteomics allows us a more early and accurate diagnosis of acute rejection by the experimental determination of peptides in the urine. The differential detection of peptides at diverse stages of the NCT in acute rejection allows us a better way to understand rejection and tolerance. The combined information derived from genomics and proteomics will lead us to consistently reduce the risk factors for graft failure (acute rejection, ischemia-reperfusion, immunosuppression, NCT), with increased life of the organs and improved patient's quality of life, because proteomics is one of the fields that can help to establish a connection between genomic sequences and biological behavior, constituting an important tool in functional analysis of genes of unknown function. The main advantage of a urine proteomic study as a source of markers for the detection of renal disease in the transplant is that urine is a fluid readily available and non-invasive. There are multiple proteomic techniques although it is noteworthy that, even though the results that each technique offers are very consistent, none is sufficient by itself to obtain and complete proteome and is advisable to combine several of the techniques described. Therefore, the primary application of proteomics is the search for markers that could be the basis for the realization of a microarray of proteins with diagnostic potential.

7. References

Abbott A (1999) A post-genomic challenge: learning to read patterns of protein synthesis. *Nature*. Dec 16;402(6763):715-20.

Akkina SK, Zhang Y, Nelsestuen GL, Oetting WS, Ibrahlm HN. (2009) Temporal stability of the urinary proteome after kidney transplant: more sensitive than protein composition? *J Proteome Res*. Jan;8(1):94-103.

Alban A, David SO, Bjorkesten L, Andersson C, Sloge E, Lewis S, Currie I. (2003) A novel experimental design for comparative two-dimensional gel analysis: Two-dimensional difference gel electrophoresis incorporating a pooled internal standard. *Proteomics* ; Jan;3(1):36-44

Bañon-Maneus E, Diekmann E ; Campistol JM (2007) Utilitat de la proteómica urinària en el trasplantament renal. *Butlletí Trasplantament*. Num. 35 Març

Banon-Maneus E, Diekmann F, Carrascal M, Quintana L.F, Moya-Rull D, Bescós M., Ramírez-Bajo M.J, Rovira J, Gutierrez-Dalmau A, Solé-González A, Abián J, Campistol JM. (2010) 2DE Dige urinary proteomic profile in the search of non immune chronic allograft dysfunction biomarkers. *Transplantation*. Mar 15;89(5):548-58.

Bañon-Maneus E, Quintana LF and Campistol JM (2011) Methods in proteomic análisis, In *Biblioteca de Trasplantes Siglo XXI Volume 8. GENOMICS AND PROTEOMICS IN SOLID ORGAN TRANSPLANT*, pp. (73) Drug Farma S.L., ISBN: 978-84-96724-69-3, Madrid

Beckingham, I. J., Nicholson, M. L., and Bell, P. R. (1994) Analysis of factors associated complications following renal transplant needle core biopsy. *Br. J. Urol.* 73, 13–15

Biomarkers Definitions Working Group. (2001) Biomarkers and surrogate endpoints: preferred definitions and conceptual framework. *Clin Pharmacol Ther*. Mar;69(3):89-95.

Chen YT, Chen CL, Chen HW, Chung T, Wu CC, Chen CD, Hsu CW, Chen MC, Tsui KH, Chang PL, Chang YS, Yu JS. (2010) Discovery of novel bladder cancer biomarkers by comparative urine proteomics using iTRAQ technology *J Proteome Res*. Nov 5;9(11):5803-15.

Clarke W, Silverman BC, Zhang Z, Chan DW, Klein AS, Molmenti EP. (2003) Characterization of renal allograft rejection by urinary proteomic analysis. *Ann Surg*; 237: 660-5.

Cutillas PR, Norden AG, Cramer R, Burlingame AL, Unwin RJ (2003). Detection and analysis of urinary peptides by on-line liquid chromatography and mass spectrometry: application to patients with renal Fanconi syndrome. *Clin Sci(Lond)*. May;104(5):483-90

Dadhania D, Muthukumar T, Ding R, Li B, Hartono C, Serur D, Seshan SV, Sharma VK, Kapur S, Suthanthiran M. (2003) Molecular signatures of urinary cells distinguish acute rejection of renal allografts from urinary tract infection. *Transplantation*; 75: 1752–1754

Decramer S, Gonzalez de Peredo A, Breuil B, Mischak H, Monsarrat B, Bascands JL, Schanstra JP (2008). Urine in clinical proteomics. *Mol Cell Proteomics*. Oct;7(10):1850-62.

Fishman JA. (2002) BK virus nephropathy–polyomavirus adding insult to injury *N Engl J Med*; 347: 527–530.

Fliser, D., Wittke, S., Mischak, H. (2005) Capillary electrophoresis coupled to mass spectrometry for clinical diagnostic purposes. *Electrophoresis* 26, 2708–2716

Gazzana G, Borlak J. (2007) Improved method for proteome mapping of the liver by 2-DE MALDI-TOF MS. *J Proteome Res*; 6: 3143.

Gigy SP, Rist B, Gerber SA, Turecek F, Gelb MH, Aebersold R. (1999). Quantitative analysis of complex protein mixtures using isotope-coded affinity tags. *Nature Biotechnology* 17, 994-999.

Hariharan S, Johnson CP, Bresnahan BA, Taranto SE, McIntosh MJ, Stablein D (2000). Improved graft survival after renal transplantation in the United States, 1988 to 1996. *N Engl J Med*; 342: 605.

Hewitt SM, Dear J, Star RA. (2004) Discovery of protein biomarkers for renal diseases. *J Am Soc Nephrol*. Jul;15(7):1677-89.

Kolch, W., Neususs, C., Pelzing, M., and Mischak, H. (2005) Capillary electrophoresis-mass spectrometry as a powerful tool in clinical diagnosis and biomarker discovery. *Mass Spectrom. Rev.* 24, 959–977

Lee RS, Monigatti F, Briscoe AC, Waldon Z, Freeman MR, Steen H. (2008) Optimizing sample handling for urinary proteomics. *J Proteome Res*. Sep;7(9):4022-30.

Mann M, Ong SE, Grønborg M, Steen H, Jensen ON, Pandey A. (2002) Analysis of protein phosphorylation using mass spectrometry: deciphering the phosphoproteome. *Trends Biotechnol* 20: 261–268

Mannon RB, Hoffmann SC, Kampen RL, Cheng OC, Kleiner DE, Ryschkewitsch C, Curfman B, Major E, Hale DA, Kirk AD. (2005) Molecular evaluation of BK polyomavirus nephropathy. *Am J Transplant*. Dec;5(12):2883-93.

Mauri P, Scigelova M. (2009) Multidimensional protein identification technology for clinical proteomic analysis. *Clin Chem Lab Med.*;47(6):636-46.

Meier-Kriesche HU, Schold JD, Kaplan B. (2004) Long-term renal allograft survival: Have we made significant progress or is it time to rethink our analytic and therapeutic strategies? *Am J Transplant*; 4: 1289.

Naesens M, Sarwal MM. (2010) Molecular diagnostics in transplantation. *Nat Rev Nephrol*. Oct;6(10):614-28.

Nankivell, B. J., Borrows, R. J., Fung, C. L., O'Connell, P. J., Allen, R. D., and Chapman, J. R., Jr. (2003) The natural history of chronic allograft nephropathy. *N. Engl. J. Med.* 349, 2326–2333

Oh J, Pyo JH, Jo EH, Hwang SI, Kang SC, Jung JH, Park EK, Kim SY, Choi JY, Lim J. (2004) Establishment of a near-standard twodimensional human urine proteomic map. *Proteomics*; 4: 3485.

Ojo AO, Hanson JA, Wolfe RA, Leichtman AB, Agodoa LY, Port FK (2000) Long-term survival in renal transplant recipients with graft function. *Kidney Int* 57 : 307– 313,

Omenn GS., States DJ, Adamski M, Blackwell TW, Menon R, Hermjakob H, Apweiler R, Haab BB, Simpson, R. J., Eddes, J. S., Kapp, E. A., Moritz, R. L., Chan, D. W., Rai, A. J., Admon, A., Aebersold, R., Eng, J., Hancock, W. S., Hefta, S. A., Meyer, H., Paik, Y. K., Yoo, J. S., Ping, P., Pounds, J., Adkins, J., Qian, X., Wang, R., Wasinger, V., Wu, C. Y., Zhao, X., Zeng, R., Archakov, A., Tsugita, A., Beer, I., Pandey, A., Pisano, M., Andrews, P., Tammen, H., Speicher, D. W., and Hanash, S. M. (2005) Overview of the HUPO Plasma Proteome Project: results from the pilot phase with 35 collaborating laboratories and multiple analytical groups, generating a core dataset of 3020 proteins and a publicly-available database. *Proteomics* 5, 3226–3245

O'Riordan E, Orlova TN, Mei J J, Butt K, Chander PM, Rahman S, Mya M, Hu R, Momin J, Eng EW, Hampel DJ, Hartman B, Kretzler M, Delaney V, Goligorsky MS. (2004) Bioinformatic analysis of the urine proteome of acute allograft rejection. *J Am Soc Nephrol;* 15: 3240-8.

O'Riordan E, Gross SS, Goligorsky MS. (2006) Technology Insight: renal proteomics-at the crossroads between promise and problems. *Nat Clin Pract Nephrol.* Aug;2(8):445-58.

O'Riordan E, Orlova TN, Mendelev N, et al Urinary proteomic analysis of chronic allograft nephropathy. *Proteomics Clin Appl* 2008; 2: 1025.

Paul, L. C. (1999) Chronic allograft nephropathy: an update. *Kidney Int.* 56, 783–793

Quan H, Peng X, Liu S, Bo F, Yang L, Huang Z, Li H, Chen X, Di W. (2011) Differentially expressed protein profile of renal tubule cell stimulated by elevated uric acid using SILAC coupled to LC-MS *Cell Physiol Biochem.*;27(1):91-8.

Quintana LF, Solé-Gonzalez A, Kalko SG, Bañon-Maneus E, Solé M, Diekmann F, Gutierrez-Dalmau A, Abian J, Campistol JM. (2009) Urine proteomics to detect biomarkers for chronic allograft dysfunction. *J Am Soc Nephrol.* Feb;20(2):428-35.

Quintana LF, Campistol JM, Alcolea MP, Bañon-Maneus E, Solé-Gonzalez A, Cutillas PR. (2009) Application of label-free quantitative peptidomics for the identification of urinary biomarkers of kidney chronic allograft dysfunction. *Mol Cell Proteomics.* Jul;8(7):1658-73.

Quintana LF, Bañon-Maneus E, Solé-Gonzalez A, Campistol JM. (2009) Urine proteomics biomarkers in renal transplantation: an overview. *Transplantation.*;(88): S45-S49

Righetti PG, Boschetti E. (2007) Sherlock Holmes and the proteome-a detective story. *FEBS J.* Feb;274(4):897-905.

Rush D. Nickerson P (2011) Urine proteomics in acute renal transplant rejection, In *Biblioteca de Trasplantes Siglo XXI Volume 8. GENOMICS AND PROTEOMICS IN SOLID ORGAN TRANSPLANT*, pp. (73) Drug Farma S.L., ISBN: 978-84-96724-69-3, Madrid

Schaub, S., Wilkins, J., Weiler, T., Sangster, K., Rush, D., and Nickerson, P. (2004) Urine protein profiling with surface-enhanced laser-desorption/ionization time-of-flight mass spectrometry. *Kidney Int.* 65, 323–332

Schaub S, Rush D, Wilkins J, Gibson IW, Weiler T, Sangster K, Nicolle L, Karpinski M, Jeffery J, Nickerson P. (2004) Proteomic-based detection of urine proteins associated with acute renal allograft rejection *J Am Soc Nephrol.* Jan;15(1):219-27.

Shaw J, Rowlinson R, Nickson J, Stone T, Sweet A, Williams K, Tonge R. (2003) Evaluation of saturation labelling two-dimensional difference gel electrophoresis fluorescent dyes. *Proteomics;* Jul;3(7):1181-95.

Schiffer, E., Mischak, H., and Novak, J. (2006) High resolution proteome/peptidome analysis of body fluids by capillary electrophoresis coupled with MS. *Proteomics* 6, 5615–5627

Sobhani K. (2010) Urine proteomic analysis: use of two-dimensional gel electrophoresis, isotope coded affinity tags, and capillary electrophoresis *Methods Mol Biol.*;641:325-46.

Solez K, Colvin RB, Racusen LC, Haas M, Sis B, Mengel M, Halloran PF, Baldwin W, Banfi G, Collins AB, Cosio F, David DS, Drachenberg C, Einecke G, Fogo AB, Gibson IW, Glotz D, Iskandar SS, Kraus E, Lerut E, Mannon RB, Mihatsch M, Nankivell BJ,

Nickeleit V, Papadimitriou JC, Randhawa P, Regele H, Renaudin K, Roberts I, Seron D, Smith RN, Valente M (2008) Banff 07 classification of renal allograft pathology: Updates and future directions. *Am J Transplant* 8 : 753- 760,

Theodorescu, D., Wittke, S., Ross, M. M., Walden, M., Conaway, M., Just, I., Mischak, H., and Frierson, H. F. (2006) Discovery and validation of new protein biomarkers for urothelial cancer: a prospective analysis. *Lancet Oncol.* 7, 230–240

Thongboonkerd V, McLeish KR, Arthur JM, Klein JB. (2002) Proteomic analysis of normal human urinary proteins isolated by acetone precipitation or ultracentrifugation. *Kidney Int*; 62: 1461.

Thongboonkerd, V., Malasit, P. (2005) Renal and urinary proteomics: current applications and challenges. *Proteomics* 5, 1033–1042

Unlü M, Morgan ME, Minden JS. (1997) Difference gel electrophoresis: A single gel method for detecting changes in protein extracts. *Electrophoresis*; 18: 2071.

Wittke S, Haubitz M, Walden M, Rohde F, Schwarz A, Mengel M, Mischak H, Haller H, Gwinner W. (2005) Detection of acute tubulointerstitial rejection by proteomic analysis of urinary samples in renal transplant recipients. *Am J Transplant*; 5: 2479-88.

Wu TL. (2006) Two-dimensional difference gel electrophoresis. *Methods Mol Biol*; 328: 71.

Yoshida Y, Miyazaki K, Kamiie J, Sato M, Okuizumi S, Kenmochi A, Kamijo K, Nabetani T, Tsugita A, Xu B, Zhang Y, Yaoita E, Osawa T, Yamamoto T. (2005) Two-dimensional electrophoretic profiling of normal human kidney glomerulus proteome and construction of an extensible markup language (XML)-based database. *Proteomics*; 5: 1083.

Zhu H, Bilgin M, Bangham R, Hall D, Casamayor A, Bertone P, Lan N, Jansen R, Bidlingmaier S, Houfek T, Mitchell T, Miller P, Dean RA, Gerstein M, Snyder M. (2001). Global analysis of protein activities using proteome arrays. *Science* 293, 2101-2105

8

Pharmacogenetics and Renal Transplantation

Chi Yuen Cheung
Department of Medicine, Queen Elizabeth Hospital
Hong Kong

1. Introduction

Different patients receiving the same dose of a drug can exhibit a wide range of blood concentrations. This is a main concern regarding the immunosuppressive drugs because of their narrow therapeutic indices. Subtherapeutic blood concentrations are associated with an increased risk of acute rejection while overdosing may increase the risk of over-immunosuppression, with subsequent increased risk of infection and malignancies. Moreover, there are also numerous drug-specific adverse effects. At present, therapeutic drug monitoring (TDM) is used to address the issue of inter-individual variation in pharmacokinetics of immunosuppressive agents. However, TDM cannot influence drug exposure during the first 2-3 days after transplantation. Thus many patients experience a significant delay in achieving target blood concentrations, significantly increasing the risk of acute graft rejection (Clase et al., 2002; Undre et al., 1999). The narrow therapeutic index of these agents prevents use of a strategy based on a higher initial dose for all patients. As a result, there is a clear need for a strategy to allow individualized immunosuppressive drug dosing in the immediate post-transplant period.

After administration, the drug is absorbed and distributed to its site of action, where it interacts with targets such as receptors and enzymes, undergoes metabolism, and is then excreted. Each of these processes might involve clinically significant genetic variations. In the general population, it is estimated that genetics accounts for 20% to 95% of the variability in drug disposition and effects (Kalow et al., 1998). Other non-genetic factors, such as hepatic or renal function, drug interactions, and nature of diseases will also influence the effects of medication. With the introduction of tools for genomic analysis, the DNA variants responsible for the differences in drug-metabolizing capacities were discovered. Subsequently, individuals can be characterized as efficient or poor metabolizers for a particular drug based on their gene polymorphisms encoding protein variants that metabolize the drug. The genetic polymorphisms in drug-metabolizing enzymes together with drug transporters and drug receptors led to the hypothesis that genetic factors may be implicated in the inter-individual variability of the pharmacokinetic or pharmacodynamic characteristics of immunosuppressive drugs, major side effects, and immunologic risks.

By definition, pharmacogenetics is the study of genetic variation that gives rise to differing responses to drugs, whereas pharmacogenomics is the application of genomic technologies to drug discovery (Goldstein et al., 2003; Phillips & Van Bebber, 2005; Stoughton & Friend, 2005). Nowadays, the two terms are often used interchangeably. The promising role of pharmacogenetics and pharmacogenomics illustrates the concept of personalized medicine, in which the characterization of the patients' genotype may help to identify the right drug and dose for each patient. The wider use of pharmacogenetic testing is also currently viewed as an important tool to improve drug safety and efficacy (Hesselink et al., 2005a; Shastry, 2005).

2. Pharmacokinetics and pharmacogenetics

The relationship between genetic variation and drug response was first observed in the 1950s for drugs metabolized by N-acetyltransferase. Based on the blood concentrations of drugs metabolized by this enzyme, patients were classified into "fast and slow acetylators". However, the molecular genetic basis for such inherited traits began to be elucidated only in the late 1980s, with the initial cloning and characterization of polymorphic human genes encoding for drug metabolizing enzymes.

Whether pharmacogenetics can be applied successfully in daily clinical practice depends on our understanding of the enzymes which metabolize the drugs. When a drug is administered, it is first absorbed in the intestine, and different proteins in the intestinal wall can determine the amount that finally passes into the blood. The calcineurin inhibitors (CNIs), the mammalian target of rapamycin (mTOR) inhibitors and corticosteroids are all metabolized by the oxidative enzymes in the cytochrome (CYP) 3A family (Dai et al., 2004, 2006; Kamdem et al., 2005) and are substrates for the P-glycoprotein (P-gp) (Miller et al., 1997; Saeki et al., 1993). They work together to form an active barrier to drug absorption, limiting the oral bioavailability of the CNIs and mTOR inhibitors (Zhang & Benet, 2001). Some drugs require binding proteins before their delivery to the targets, such as CNIs that bind to immunophilins as part of their mechanism of action. As a result, only a proportion of an administered drug can reach the target. In order to define the association between the genotypes and the pharmacokinetics of a drug, a group of individuals are given the same dose of a drug, and the blood concentrations will then be measured at different intervals (Dunn et al., 2001; Schiff et al., 2007). These individuals are genotyped for polymorphisms at certain candidate genes, and the association between the genotypes and the pharmacokinetics is subsequently statistically analyzed. The ultimate goal is to find out the gene variants that can help in predicting the pharmacokinetics of a drug, and identifying patients who need a higher dose to reach the desired blood concentration (Evans & McLeod, 2003; McLeod & Evans, 2001). The combined analysis of gene variants encoding the different proteins that mediate the drug action may help to determine the final dose necessary to obtain a pharmacological effect (Kruger et al., 2008). This complicated picture shows that a successful pharmacogenetics approach would require the genotyping of several genes in each patient.

3. P-glycoprotein

Many drugs, including some immunosuppressive agents, are pumped out of the endothelial cells by P-gp, encoded by adenosine triphosphate-binding cassette subfamily B member 1 (ABCB1) gene (formerly called multidrug resistance-1 [MDR1] gene) (Benet et al., 1999; Lown et al., 1997). One of the main functions of P-gp is to ensure the energy-dependent cellular efflux of substrates. The P-gp expression in the intestinal wall and in the proximal tubular cells of the kidneys suggests that it may have a role in the absorption and excretion of xenobiotics. In the gut, alteration in its expression, function, or both raises the absorption of its substrates (Ambudkar et al., 1999). Individuals with a genotype with high intrinsic P-gp activity have a lower proportion of the drug that reaches the blood stream compared with a genotype with less P-gp activity (Choudhuri & Klaassen, 2006). Various single nucleotide polymorphisms (SNPs) have been identified within the *ABCB1* gene over the recent few years (Kim, 2002). An SNP, located in exon 26 (exon 26 3435C>T), was associated with variations in the intestinal expression and function of P-gp. However, this SNP is a silent polymorphism that does not result in any amino acid changes. It was suggested that it may be in linkage disequilibrium with other functional polymorphisms within the *ABCB1* gene. A co-segregation of exon 26 3435T with the T allele of the non-synonymous exon 21 SNP (exon 21 2677G>T), resulting in an A893S amino acid change, and also with the T allele of the synonymous exon 12 SNP (exon 12 1236C>T) was reported. This disequilibrium led to haplotype analysis of the ABCB1 gene and identification of the links between the genomic variations represented by each haplotype on ABCB1 function. This approach takes into account the combination of SNPs present in an allele (Kim, 2002) and might be more predictive of changes in response to drugs than SNP-based approaches.

4. CYP3A

CYP3A proteins can be classified into families and subfamilies on the basis of amino acid sequence similarities. Members of the CYP3A subfamily are implicated in the metabolism of structurally diverse endobiotics, drugs, and protoxic or procarcinogenic molecules. Substantial inter-individual differences in CYP3A expression contribute greatly to variations in the oral bioavailability and systemic clearance of CYP3A substrates (Nebert & Russell, 2002). Human CYP3A activities reflect the heterogeneous expression of at least three CYP3A members, CYP3A4, CYP3A5, and CYP3A7, which are adjacent to each other on chromosome band 7q21. CYP3A7 is normally only expressed in fetal liver. CYP3A4 and CYP3A5 have been identified as the major enzymes responsible for the disposition of drugs (Sattler et al., 1992). In enterocytes, CYP3A4 and CYP3A5 are involved in intestinal metabolism, preventing systemic uptake of immunosuppressive agents; while in the liver, they provide a further layer contributing to first-pass metabolism, thus affecting the drug clearance. For example, CYP3A5 variants alter the dose requirement of tacrolimus (Tac). Since CYP3A5 is involved in Tac deactivation, patients with a genotype that encodes for lower enzyme activity would have an increase drug exposure. Thus a lower dose will be required to be within the target blood concentration. The normal (wild-type) sequences of CYP3A4 and CYP3A5 are designated as CYP3A4*1 and CYP3A5*1. The most frequent CYP3A4 SNP linked to different enzymatic activities is -392 A>G in the gene promoter. The -392 G allele (also called CYP3A4*1B) increased CYP3A4 expression in vitro (Rebbeck et al., 1998; Westlind et al., 1999). This SNP is common in individuals of African descent (30%–70%) but rare among whites (1%–10%) (Makeeva et al., 2008; Quaranta et al., 2006). On the other hand, the most important SNP of the CYP3A5 gene leading to the alteration of gene expression and enzymatic activity is the SNP 6986 A>G in intron 3. Analysis revealed that only individuals with at least one CYP3A5*1 allele (A at position 6986) produce high levels of full-length CYP3A5 mRNA and express CYP3A5, which then accounts for at least 50% of the total CYP3A content. Those with the CYP3A5*3 allele (G at position 6986) display sequence variability in intron 3 that creates a cryptic splice site and encodes an aberrantly spliced mRNA with a premature stop codon, leading to the absence of protein expression (Kuehl et al., 2001).

5. Tacrolimus

Among the factors which have been investigated for the possible influence on CNIs pharmacokinetics, polymorphisms in genes coding for CYP3A (3A4 and 3A5) and P-gp received much attention. The impact of CYP3A4, CYP3A5, and MDR1 SNPs on Tac pharmacokinetics has been analyzed extensively in recent years. CYP3A5 expressers, who are carriers of at least one CYP3A5*1 allele, would have higher Tac clearance and lower dose-normalized C_0 at different times after renal transplantation compared with CYP3A5*3 homozygotes (Haufroid et al., 2004; Haufroid et al., 2006; Hesselink et al., 2003; Macphee et al., 2005; Mourad et al., 2006; Roy et al., 2006; Tada et al., 2005; Thervet et al., 2003; Tsuchiya et al., 2004; Zhang et al., 2005; Zhao et al., 2005). A study of 118 kidney recipients examined the relationship between CYP3A5*1/*3 and Tac dose-normalized concentrations at 1 week, 1 month, and 3 months post-transplantation. At 1 week, the mean dose-normalized blood concentration was significantly lower in CYP3A5*1 carriers (33 ng/mL per mg/kg/day) compared with CYP3A5*3 homozygotes (102 ng/mL per mg/kg/day). This difference remained significant at 1 month and 3 months post-transplant (Zhang et al., 2005). A temporal change in Tac oral bioavailability has been reported by Kuypers et al. The dose-normalized exposure to Tac increased progressively over a 5-year period in individuals predicted to be CYP3A5 non-expressers but not in CYP3A5 expressers (Kuypers et al., 2007). The frequency of these alleles depends on the population studies: the CYP3A5*1 allele is present in 15 % of the Caucasian, 45% of the African-American (Kuehl et al., 2001), and 25% of the Chinese population (Balram et al., 2003). Since many genetic differences exist between races, it is also important to examine whether the described polymorphisms are related to differences in pharmacokinetic and dosing of Tac in different population. In a study of 103 stable Chinese renal transplant recipients (Cheung et al., 2006), a strong significant genetic effect between CYP3A5*3 polymorphism and both the dose-normalized $AUC_{0\text{-}12}$ and the daily Tac dose has been demonstrated. In fact, the CYP3A5*3 polymorphism may explain 35.3% of the variation in the daily Tac dose observed in the renal transplant recipients. In another study involving Caucasian population (Op den Buijsch et al., 2007), significantly higher dose-normalized C_0, dose-normalized $AUC_{0\text{-}12}$ and dose-normalized peak concentrations (C_{max}) is demonstrated in carriers of the CYP3A5*3 allele in both early and late post renal transplant recipient groups than in patients homozygous for CYP3A5*1. In their centre, a complete Tac pharmacokinetic profile was usually requested early for patients who failed to achieve the target Tac concentration shortly after transplantation. Since the CYP3A5*1 allele was over-represented in this early phase group in their study, the authors concluded that renal transplant recipients carrying this allele have more difficulties in achieving and maintaining Tac concentrations compared to homozygous carriers of the CYP3A5*3 variant. This might be of importance for the Chinese population in which the CYP3A5*1 allele has a much higher prevalence than in the Caucasian population.

CYP3A5 is closely linked to the CYP3AP1 pseudogene, and the CYP3AP1*1 allele (-44 G) was in strong linkage disequilibrium with the low-expression CYP3A5*3 allele. In fact, the CYP3AP1 genotype resembles the CYP3A5 genotype (Kuehl et al., 2001). A significant association was found between the CYP3AP1 polymorphism and three parameters, namely, drug concentrations during the first week post-transplant, time to reach the target blood concentrations, and the risk of early allograft rejection (MacPhee et al., 2002, 2004).

On the other hand, the impact of the CYP3A4 and ABCB1 polymorphisms in Tac pharmacokinetics is not clear. Most studies failed to show any association between

CYP3A4 gene polymorphisms and Tac pharmacokinetics although at least one group has reported lower C_0 concentrations at 3 and 12 months post-transplantation in carriers of the CYP3A4*1B allele than in the CYP3A4*1 homozygotes (Hesselink et al., 2003). Similarly, there has been conflicting pubished data about the influence of the polymorphisms of the ABCB1 system on the pharmacokinetics of Tac. A number of studies have reported that there seems to be no association between the ABCB1 polymorphisms and Tac dose-normalized C_0 (Haufroid et al., 2004; Hebert et al., 2003; Hesselink et al., 2003; Mai et al., 2004; Zhang et al., 2005) or the dose-normalized AUC (Tada et al., 2005; Tsuchiya et al., 2004). However, some studies found a correlation between individual ABCB1 polymorphisms and a higher Tac dose (MacPhee et al., 2002; Zheng et al., 2003; Zheng et al., 2004). Carriers of the 2677T or the 3435T MDR1 alleles showed higher dose-normalized Tac C_0 concentrations compared with 2677 G-homozygous (GG) and 3435 C-homozygous (CC) patients (Akbas et al., 2006; Anglicheau et al., 2003; Li et al., 2006). Because of differences in design and study populations it might be that a polymorphism, that has a minor influence on the Tac blood concentrations, demonstrates contrasting results among these studies. Moreover, there are several SNPs that may occur together, resulting in different haplotypes. The correlation of these haplotypes with the pharmacokinetics of Tac has not yet been described extensively. In one study, a correlation between the ABCB1 1236C-2677G-3435C haplotype and a higher Tac dose was found (Anglicheau et al., 2003). However, in another study of 63 Caucasian renal transplant recipients with a complete 9-point 12-hour AUC of Tac, 3 SNPs in the ABCB1 system were genotyped. Neither the individual ABCB1 polymorphisms nor the ABCB1 haplotypes were associated with any pharmacokinetic parameter (Op den Buijsch et al., 2007). On the other hand, in a study of Chinese renal transplant recipients (Cheung et al., 2006), individuals carrying the 2677TT or 3435TT genotype has a significantly lower dose-normalized AUC_{0-12}, but no correlation was found between ABCB1 system haplotype and dose-normalized AUC_{0-12}. In multiple regression analysis the 2677TT and 3435TT genotype was not shown to be significant if the CYP3A polymorphism was included. Therefore, the published correlation of SNPs of the ABCB1 system with dose-normalized AUC of Tac might be related to genetic linkage of the ABCB1 system with other polymorphisms, such as the CYP3A system. Individuals with the mutant genotype appear to be over-represented in the CYP3A5 expresser population and under-represented in the CYP3A5 non-expresser population. Thus the interaction between P-gp and CYP3A5 further complicates the analysis of interaction between ABCB1 genotype and Tac pharmacokinetics.

Despite the fact that expression of CYP3A5 results in higher Tac dose requirements and significant delay in achieving target blood concentrations early after transplantation, most of the previous studies failed to identify the association of the genetic polymorphisms with increased incidence of acute rejection (Hesselink et al., 2008; Macphee et al., 2004). However, in a recent prospective study of 62 patients who underwent 10-day scheduled renal graft biopsy, significantly higher overall incidences of early T-cell-mediated rejection of at least Banff grade 1 in severity were detected in CYP3A5 expressers. The severity was also associated with the CYP3A5 genotypes. Moreover, the estimated glomerular filtration rate in CYP3A5 expressers was lower than that of the non-expressers until one month after transplantation (Min et al., 2010). However, further large-scale long-term outcome studies are necessary to confirm the clinical relevance of the findings.

6. Cyclosporine

Healthy volunteers who are CYP3A5*1 carriers had a lower cyclosporine (CsA) AUC when compared with individuals with homozygous for CYP3A5*3 (Min et al., 2004). Moreover, renal transplant recipients who carry CYP3A5*1 were also found to exhibit lower dose-normalized CsA C_0 (Haufroid, et al., 2004). However, this association has not been confirmed by most authors (Anglicheau et al., 2004; Hesselink et al., 2003, 2004; Kreutz et al., 2004). This is strange because the clear influence of CYP3A5 genotype on Tac absorption could not be shown similarly in CsA (as both are CNIs). A possible explanation is that the molar dose of CsA administered is approximately 30-fold higher than that for Tac and it blocks a saturable barrier to drug absorption more effectively than for Tac (Higgins et al., 1999). The association between CYP3A4 SNPs and CsA pharmacokinetics is also controversial. The CYP3A4*1B allele has been linked to significantly higher CsA clearance compared with wild-type homozygotes (Hesselink et al., 2004; Min & Ellingrod, 2003). However, this association was not confirmed in other studies (Rivory et al., 2000; von Ahsen et al., 2001). In whites, the 3A4*1B occurs at a low frequency (Coto & Tavira, 2009), and recruitment of the minimum number of carriers to reach statistical significance is difficult.

The association between ABCB1 SNPs and CsA pharmacokinetics is also controversial. In a study involving 106 renal transplant recipients, carriers of the ABCB1 1236 wild-type allele had a lower dose-normalized C_{max} and lower increased AUC when compared with the 1236 T allele homozygotes (Anglicheau et al., 2004). In another study with 69 renal transplant recipients, a significantly lower AUC and C_2 in carriers of the ABCB1 3435 T allele was shown at day 3 post-transplant but the difference did not remain significant at 1 month (Foote et al., 2007). However, most of the large studies did not find an association between any of the ABCB1 polymorphisms and CsA pharmacokinetics (Haufroid et al., 2004; Kuzuya et al., 2003; Mai et al., 2003). On the other hand, the influence of ABCB1 genotype on pharmacodynamics seems more compelling. The incidence of CsA nephrotoxicity was significantly higher when the donor had the ABCB1 3435TT genotype (Hauser et al., 2005). This is consistent with the hypothesis that local levels of P-gp expression in renal tubular epithelial cells can explain the susceptibility to CNI nephrotoxicity. It has been shown that lower levels of P-gp expression were found in renal biopsies in patients with CNI nephrotoxicity (Joy et al., 2005). CsA nephrotoxicity is also exacerbated by concomitant use of sirolimus, which can be explained by the inhibitory effect of sirolimus on P-gp-mediated efflux and subsequent increased cellular concentration of CsA (Anglicheau et al., 2006). Moreover, another study also found that ABCB1 polymorphisms in donors influence long-term graft outcome. The donor ABCB1 haplotype 1236T/2677T/3435T was significantly associated with increase graft loss, acute rejection episodes and greater decrease in renal function (Woillard et al., 2010).

In addition to CYP and ABCB1 genes, other gene variants can also affect CNIs pharmacokinetics and clinical outcomes. In a study of subpopulation of patients participating in the CAESAR study, 4 gene polymorphisms including ABCB1 G2677T/A, IMPDH2 T3757C, IL-10 C-592A and TNF-alpha G-308A demonstrated a statistically significant association with biopsy-proven acute rejection at 12 months post-transplant (Grinyo et al., 2008). CsA action is mediated by its binding to the cyclophilins (Cyp). In a study involving 290 kidney-transplanted patients, the effect of two CypA polymorphisms on CsA pharmacokinetics and clinical outcomes was analyzed (Moscoso-Solorzano et al.,

2008). In vitro studies showed that a promoter SNP (-11 G/C) affected gene expression but was not related to differences in C_0 and C_2 dose-normalized levels. However, an association between the high expression allele and nephrotoxicity was found but these results need further confirmation.

7. Azathioprine

Most of the pharmacogenetic traits first identified were discovered by phenotypic analysis detecting a bi- or trimodality of an enzymatic activity (Weinshilboum, 2003). Azathioprine, metabolized in part by S-methylation catalyzed by the enzyme thiopurine methyltransferase (TPMT), is an example. Large inter-individual differences were reported in TPMT activity, which was found to be inherited in an autosomal codominant fashion (Weinshilboum et al., 1999). When individuals with low or undetectable TPMT activity received standard doses of azathioprine, they had high concentrations of the active metabolites 6-thioguanine nucleotides and drug-induced myelosuppression. On the other hand, azathioprine efficacy will be reduced in patients with very high levels of TPMT activity which can be attributed to its rapid metabolization (Chocair et al., 1992; Soria-Royer et al., 1993). TPMT activity correlates with both short- and long-term results after renal transplantation (Thervet et al., 2001). Subsequently, these variations in TPMT activity were shown to be attributed to genetic polymorphisms within the TPMT gene. At present, 20 variant alleles (TPMT*2 - *18) have been identified, which are associated with decreased activity when compared with the TPMT*1 wild type allele. TPMT*3A, the most common variant allele responsible for low TPMT activity in whites, encodes a protein with two single nucleotide polymorphisms (SNP), G460A in exon 7 and A719G in exon 10, leading to modifications in the amino acid sequence. The phenotypic test for TPMT activity determination in red blood cells and, subsequently, DNA-based tests, were among the first pharmacogenetic tests to be used in clinical practice.

8. Mycophenolic acid

Mycophenolic acid (MPA) is the active derivative of the prodrug mycophenolate mofetil but MPA itself is also available as enteric coated sodium salt tablet. MPA is metabolized by uridine-glucuronyl-transferase (UGT), primarily UGT1A8 and 1A9, to the inactive metabolite 7-O-glucuronide (MPAG). MPAG is primarily excreted by kidneys, although a proportion is secreted in bile by the drug efflux pump multidrug resistance associated protein 2 (MRP2), now also called ABCC2. Deconjugation by intestinal bacterial flora results in a second peak of absorption at 6 to 8 hours due to enterohepatic recirculation. This second peak accounts for 30-50% of the total AUC. As a result, co-administration with medication that inhibit ABCC2, such as CsA, can result in a significantly reduced MPA exposure (Hesselink et al., 2005b). Several SNPs have been found in the ABCC2 gene (Ito et al., 2001). It has been found that ABCC2 C-24T and C-3972T polymorphisms can protect the renal transplant recipients from a decrease in MPA exposure associated with mild liver dysfunction. Moreover, C-24T SNP was associated with significantly high dose-normalized MPA trough levels at steady state (Naesens et al., 2006).
Polymorphisms have also been identified in both UGT1A9 and 1A8 genes. In vitro studies have shown that polymorphisms in the UGT1A9 gene result in significant alteration of the UGT enzymatic activity. Two polymorphisms in the promoter region of the UGT1A9 gene,

namely C-275T>A and C-2152C>T, result in higher MPA glucuronidation rates (Girard et al., 2004). It has been demonstrated that in renal transplant recipients, carriers of either or both polymorphisms had lower MPA AUC and C_0 (Johnson et al, 2008; Kuypers et al., 2005; van Schaik et al., 2009). On the other hand, UGT1A8*3 (P277C>Y) polymorphism results in an approximately 30-fold reduction in MPAG formation (Bernard et al., 2006).
MPA inhibits inosine monophosphate dehydrogenase (IMPDH), a key enzyme in the pathway for purine synthesis.. The two isoforms of IMPDH, IMPHD1 and IMPDH2, have similar enzymatic activity. Individuals with low levels of lymphocyte IMPDH activity are more likely to experience toxicity with MPA and those with high levels are more likely to have rejection (Glander et al., 2004). There were different variants of the IMPDH2 gene and the 263L>F variant resulted in a reduction in enzyme activity to 10% of the wild-type (Wang et al., 2007). Several mutants of IMPDH had decreased affinity for MPA (Farazi et al., 1997). However, there are no clinical associations for this SNP. On the other hand, 2 SNPs in the IMPDH1 gene, namely +125G>A and -106G>A, were found to be associated with increase risk of rejection after kidney transplantation but the underlying mechanism remains uncertain (Wang et al., 2008). Despite of availability of different candidate genes, there are still insufficient data to support the use of pharmacogenetic strategy for mycophenolate.

9. Mammalian target of rapamycin inhibitors

There is only limited data concerning the pharmacogenetics of mTOR inhibitors. Usually it takes longer time for sirolimus to achieve desired therapeutic range because of its long half-life (approximately 60 hours). Thus use of pharmacogenetic strategy seems to be an ideal option for sirolimus dosage adjustment. However, the data in literature is controversial. While there were studies showing reduced oral bioavailability of sirolimus in CYP3A5 expressors (Anglicheau et al., 2005; Le Meur et al., 2006), similar association was not found in other studies (Mourad et al., 2005; Renders et al., 2007). Moreover, none of the studies could show the influence of ABCB1 genotype on sirolimus exposure (Anglicheau et al., 2005; Mourad et al., 2005; Renders et al., 2007). As a result, pharmacogenetics is still not suitable for sirolimus dosing.

10. Conclusion and future perspective

Currently TDM is the gold standard for monitoring and titration of immunosuppressive drugs in order to ensure adequate immunosuppression but avoid side effects. However, many patients experience significant delay in achieving therapeutic blood concentrations, resulting in a higher risk of acute rejection. As a result, selection of the best drug with an accurate dose is important. Pharmacogenetics have generated considerable enthusiasm in transplantation medicine in recent years and it is widely believed that "personalized medicine" is the ultimate goal of use of immunosuppressive drugs. Although many genetic factors have been shown to influence pharmacokinetics for the immunosuppressive drugs, only CYP3A5 genotyping may help to guide individual tacrolimus dosing in clinical practice. Moreover, the focus of pharmacogenetic studies has recently shifted from pharmacokinetics to transplantation outcomes, such as renal allograft dysfunction. Although there is substantial evidence that intrarenally expressed ABCB1 is implicated in the pathogenesis of CNI nephrotoxicity, there is no direct evidence in human that the association between ABCB1 genotype and CNI nephrotoxicity is indeed caused by higher intrarenal concentration of CNIs (Hesselink et al., 2010). Further prospective and intervention studies involving genetic profile and transplant outcome are required for recommendation of widespread use of pharmacogenetic testing in routine clinical practice.

11. References

Akbas, S.H.; Bilgen, T.; Keser, I.; Tuncer, M.; Yucetin, L.; Tosun, O.; Gultekin, M. & Luleci, G. (2006). The effect of MDR1 (ABCB1) polymorphism on the pharmacokinetic of tacrolimus in Turkish renal transplant recipients. *Transplant Proc,* Vol.38, No.5, pp.1290-1292

Ambudkar, S.V.; Dey, S.; Hrycyna, C.A.; Ramachandra, M.; Pastan, I.& Gottesman, M.M. (1999). Biochemical, cellular, and pharmacological aspects of the multidrug transporter. *Annu Rev Pharmacol Toxicol,* Vol.39, pp.361-398

Anglicheau, D.; Verstuyft, C.; Laurent-Puig, P. ; Becquemont , L. ; Schlageter, M.H.; Cassinat, B. ; Beaune, P. ; Legendre, C. ;& Thervet, E. (2003). Association of the multidrug resistance-1 gene single-nucleotide polymorphisms with the tacrolimus dose requirements in renal transplant recipients. *J Am Soc Nephrol,* Vol.14, No.7, pp.1889-1896

Anglicheau, D. ; Thervet, E. ; Etienne, I. ; Hurault De Ligny, B. ; Le Meur, Y. ; Touchard, G. ; Buchler, M. ; Laurent-Puig, P. ; Tregouet, D. ; Beaune, P. ; Daly, A. ; Legendre, C. & Marquet, P. (2004). CYP3A5 and MDR1 genetic polymorphisms and cyclosporine pharmacokinetics after renal transplantation. *Clin Pharmacol Ther,* Vol.75, No.5, pp.422-433

Anglicheau, D.; le Corre, D.; Lechaton, S. ; Laurent-Puig, P. ; Kreis, H. ; Beaune, P. ; Legendre, C. & Thervet, E. (2005). Consequences of genetic polymorphisms for sirolimus requirements after renal transplant in patients on primary sirolimus therapy. *Am J Transplant,* Vol.5, No.3, pp.595-603

Anglicheau, D.; Pallet, N.; Rabant, M.; Marquet, P. ; Cassinat, B. ; Meria, P. ; Beaune, P. ; Legendre, C. & Thervet, E. (2006). Role of P-glycoprotein in cyclosporine cytotoxicity in the cyclosporine-sirolimus interaction. *Kidney Int,* Vol.70, No.6, pp.1019-1025

Balram, C.; Zhou, Q.; Cheung, Y.B. & Lee, E.J. (2003). CYP3A5*3 and *6 single nucleotide polymorphisms in three distinct Asian populations. *Eur J Clin Pharmacol,* Vol.59, No.2, pp.123-126

Benet, L.Z.; Izumi, T.; Zhang,Y.; Silverman, J.A. & Wacher, V.J. (1999). Intestinal MDR transport proteins and P-450 enzymes as barriers to oral drug delivery. *J Control Release,* Vol.62, No.1-2, pp.25-31

Bernard, O.; Tojcic, J.; Journault, K.; Perusse, L. & Guillemette, C. (2006). Influence of nonsynonymous polymorphisms of UGT1A8 and UGT2B7 metabolizing enzymes on the formation of phenolic and acyl glucuronides of mycophenolic acid. *Drug Metab Dispos,* Vol.34, No.9, pp.1539-1545

Cheung, C.Y.; Op den Buijsch, R.A.; Wong K.M.; Chan, H.W.; Chau, K.F.; Li, C.S.; Leung, K.T.; Kwan, T.H.; de Vries. J.E.; Wijnen, P.A.; van Dieijen-Visser, M.P. & Bekers, O. (2006). Influence of different allelic variants of the cytochrome 3A and adenosine triphosphate-binding cassette B1 gene on the tacrolimus pharmacokinetic profile of Chinese renal transplant recipients. *Pharmacogenomics,* Vol.7, No.4, pp.563-574

Chocair, P.R.; Duley, J.A.; Simmonds, H.A. & Cameron, J.S. (1992). The importance of thiopurine methyltransferase activity for the use of azathioprine in transplant recipients. *Transplantation,* Vol.53, No.5, pp.1051-1056

Choudhuri, S.& Klaassen, C.D. (2006). Structure, function, expression, genomic organization, and single nucleotide polymorphisms of human ABCB1 (MDR1), ABCC (MRP), and ABCG2 (BCRP) efflux transporters. *Int J Toxicol,* Vol.25, No.4, pp.231-259

Clase, C.M.; Mahalati, K. ; Kiberd, B.A. ;Lawen, J.G. ; West, K.A.; Fraser, A.D. & Belitsky P. (2002). Adequate early cyclosporin exposure is critical to prevent renal allograft rejection: patients monitored by absorption profiling. *Am J Transplant,* Vol.2, No.8, pp.789-795

Coto, E. & Tavira, B. (2009). Pharmacogenetics of calcineurin inhibitors in renal transplantation. *Transplantation,* Vol.88, No.3S, pp.S62-S67

Dai, Y.; Iwanaga, K.; Lin, Y.S.; Hebert, M.F.; Davis, C.L.; Huang, W.; Kharasch, E.D. & Thummel, K.E. (2004). In vitro metabolism of cyclosporine A by human kidney CYP3A5. *Biochem Pharmacol,* Vol.68, No.9, pp.1889-1902

Dai, Y.; Hebert, M.F.; Isoherranen, N.; Davis, C.L.; Marsh, C.; Shen, D.D. & Thummel, K.E. (2006). Effect of CYP3A5 polymorphism on tacrolimus metabolic clearance in vitro. *Drug Metab Dispos,* Vol.34, No.5, pp.836-847

Dunn, C.J.; Wagstaff, A.J.; Perry, C.M.; Plosker, G.L. & Goa, K.L. (2001). Cyclosporin: An updated review of the pharmacokinetic properties, clinical efficacy and tolerability of a microemulsion-based formulation (Neoral)1 in organ transplantation. *Drugs,* Vol.61, No.13, pp.1957-2016

Evans, W.E. & McLeod, H.L. (2003). Pharmacogenomics—Drug disposition, drug targets, and side effects. *N Engl J Med,* Vol.348, No.6, pp.538-549

Farazi, T.; Leichman, J.; Harris, T.; Cahoon, M. & Hedstrom, L. (1997). Isolation and characterization of mycophenolic acid-resistant mutants of inosine-5'-monophosphate dehydrogenase. *J Biol Chem,* Vol.272, No.2, pp.961-965

Foote, C.J.; Greer, W.; Kiberd, B.; Fraser, A.; Lawen, J.; Nashan, B. & Belitsky, P. (2007). Polymorphisms of multidrug resistance gene (MDR1) and cyclosporine absorption in de novo renal transplant patients. *Transplantation,* Vol.83, No.10, pp.1380-1384

Girard, H.; Court, M.H.; Bernard, O.; Fortier, L.C.; Villeneuve, L.; Hao, Q.; Greenblatt, D.J.; von Moltke, L.L.; Perussed, L. & Guillemette, C. (2004). Identification of common polymorphisms in the promoter of the UGT1A9 gene: evidence that UGT1A9 protein and activity levels are strongly genetically controlled in the liver. *Pharmacogenetics,* Vol.14, No.8, pp.501-515

Glander, P; Hambach, P.; Braun, K.P.; Fritsche, L.; Giessing, M.; Mai, I.; Einecke, G.; Waiser, J.; Neumayer, H.H. & Budde, K. (2004). Pre-transplant inosine monophosphate dehydrogenase activity is associated with clinical outcome after renal transplantation. *Am j Transplant,* Vol.4, No.12, pp.2045-2051

Goldstein, D.B.; Tate, S.K. & Sisodiya, S.M. (2003). Pharmacogenetics goes genomic. *Nat Rev Genet,* Vol.4, No.12, pp. 937-947

Grinyo, J.; Vanrenterghem, Y.; Nashan, B.; Vincenti, F.; Ekberg, H.; Lindpaintner, K.; Rashford, M.; Nasmyth-Miller, C.; Voulgari, A.; Spleiss, O.; Truman, M. & Essioux, L. (2008). Association of four DNA polymorphisms with acute rejection after kidney transplantation. *Transplantation,* Vol. 21, No.9, pp.879-891

Haufroid, V.; Mourad, M.; Van Kerckhove, V.; Wawrzyniak, J.; De Meyer, M.; Eddour, D.C.; Malaise, J.; Lison, D.; Squifflet, J.P. & Wallemacq, P. (2004). The effect of CYP3A5 and MDR1 (ABCB1) polymorphisms on cyclosporine and tacrolimus dose requirements and trough blood levels in stable renal transplant patients. *Pharmacogenetics*, Vol.14, No.3, pp.147-154

Haufroid, V.; Wallemacq, P.; VanKerckhove, V.; Elens, L.; De Meyer, M.; Eddour, D.C.; Malaise, J. ; Lison, D. & Mourad, M. (2006). CYP3A5 and ABCB1 polymorphisms and tacrolimus pharmacokinetics in renal transplant candidates: Guidelines from an experimental study. *Am J Transplant*, Vol.6, No.11, pp.2706-2713

Hauser, I.A. ; Schaeffeler, E.; Gauer, S. ; Scheuermann, E.H. ; Wegner, B. ; Gossmann, J. ; Ackermann, H. ; Seidl, C. ; Hocher, B. ; Zanger, U.M.; Geiger, H.; Eichelbaum, M. & Schwab, M. (2005). ABCB1 genotype of the donor but not of the recipient is a major risk factor for cyclosporine-related nephrotoxicity after renal transplantation. *J Am Soc Nephrol*, Vol.16, No.5, pp.1501-1511

Hebert, M.F.; Dowling, A.L.; Gierwatowski, C.; Lin, Y.S.; Edwards, K.L.; Davis, C.L.; Marsh, C.L.; Schuetz, E.G. & Thummel, K.E. (2003). Association between ABCB1 (multidrug resistance transporter) genotype and post-liver transplantation renal dysfunction in patients receiving calcineurin inhibitors. *Pharmacogenetics*, Vol.13, No.11, pp.661-674

Hesselink, D.A.; van Schaik, R.H.; van der Heiden, I.P.; van der Werf, M.; Gregoor, P.J.; Lindemans, J.; Weimar, W. & van Gelder, T. (2003). Genetic polymorphisms of the CYP3A4, CYP3A5, and MDR-1 genes and pharmacokinetics of the calcineurin inhibitors cyclosporine and tacrolimus. *Clin Pharmacol Ther*, Vol.74, No.3, pp.245-254

Hesselink, D.A.; van Gelder, T.; van Schaik, R.H.; Balk, A.H.; van der Heiden, I.P.; van Dam, T.; van der Werf, M.; Weimar, W. & Mathot, R.A. (2004). Population pharmacokinetics of cyclosporine in kidney and heart transplant recipients and the influence of ethnicity and genetic polymorphisms in the MDR-1, CYP3A4, and CYP3A5 genes. *Clin Pharmacol Ther*, Vol.76, No.6, pp.545-556

Hesselink, D.A.; van Gelder, T. & van Schaik, R.H. (2005a). The pharmacogenetics of calcineurin inhibitors: One step closer toward individualized immunosuppression? *Pharmacogenomics*, Vol. 6, No.4, pp.323-337

Hesselink, D.A.; van Hest, R.M.; Mathot, R.A.; Bonthuis, F.; Weimar, W.; de Bruin, R.W. & van Gelder, T. (2005b). Cyclosporine interacts with mycophenolic acid by inhibiting the multidrug resistance-associated protein 2. *Am J Transplant*, Vol.5, No.5, pp.987-994

Hesselink, D.A.; van Schaik, R.H.; van Agteren, M.; de Fijter, J.W.; Hartmann, A.; Zeier, M.; Budde, K.; Kuypers, D.R.; Pisarski, P.; Le Meur, Y.; Mamelok, R.D. & van Gelder, T. (2008). CYP3A5 genotype is not associated with a higher risk of acute rejection in tacrolimus-treated renal transplant recipients. *Pharmacogenet Genomics*, Vol.18, No.4, pp.339-348

Hesselink, D.A.; Bouamar, R. & van Gelder, T. (2010). The pharmacogenetics of calcineurin inhibitor-related nephrotoxicity. *Ther Drug Monit*, Vol.32, No.4, pp.387-393

Higgins, R.M.; Morlidge, C.; Magee, P.; McDiarmaid-Gordon, A.; Lam, F.T. & Kashi, H. (1999). Conversion between cyclosporin and tacrolimus --30-fold dose prediction. *Nephrol Dial Transplant*, Vol.14, No.6, pp1609

Ito, S.; Ieiri, I.; Tanabe, M.; Suzuki, A.; Higuchi, S. & Otsubo, K. (2001). Polymorphism of the ABC transporter genes, MDR1, MRP1 and MRP2/cMOAT, in healthy Japanese subjects. *Pharmacogenetics,* Vol.11, No.2, pp.175-184

Johnson, L.A.; Oetting, W.S.; Basu, S.; Prausa, S.; Matas, A. & Jacobson, P.A. (2008). Pharmacogenetic effect of the UGT polymorphisms on mycophenolate is modified by calcineurin inhibitors. *Eur J Clin Pharmacol,* Vol.64, No.11, pp.1047-1056

Joy, M.S.; Nickeleit, V.; Hogan, S.L., Thompson, B.D. & Finn, W.F. (2005). Calcineurin inhibitor-induced nephrotoxicity and renal expression of P-glycoprotein. (2005). *Pharmacotherapy,* Vol.25, No.6, pp779-789

Kamdem, L.K.; Streit, F.; Zanger, U.M.; Brockmoller, J.; Oellerich, M.; Armstrong, V.W. & Wojnowski, L. (2005). Contribution of CYP3A5 to the in vitro hepatic clearance of tacrolimus. *Clin Chem,* Vol.51, No.8, pp.1374-1381

Kalow, W.; Tang, B.K. & Endrenyi, L. (1998). Hypothesis: Comparisons of inter- and intra-individual variations can substitute for twin studies in drug research. *Pharmacogenetics,* Vol.8, No.4, pp.283–289

Kim, R.B. (2002). MDR1 single nucleotide polymorphisms: Multiplicity of haplotypes and functional consequences. *Pharmacogenetics,* Vol.12, No.6, pp.425-427

Kreutz, R.; Zurcher, H.; Kain, S.; Martus, P.; Offermann, G. & Beige, J. (2004). The effect of variable CYP3A5 expression on cyclosporine dosing, blood pressure and long-term graft survival in renal transplant patients. *Pharmacogenetics,* Vol.14, No.10, pp.665-671

Krüger, B.; Schröppel, B. & Murphy, B.T. (2008). Genetic polymorphisms and the fate of the transplanted organ. *Transplant Rev (Orlando)* Vol.22, No.2, pp.131-140

Kuehl, P.; Zhang, J.; Lin. Y.; Lamba, J.; Assem, M.; Schuetz, J.; Watkins, P.B.; Daly, A.; Wrighton, S.A.; Hall, S.D.; Maurel, P.; Relling, M.; Brimer, C.; Yasuda, K.; Venkataramanan, R.; Strom, S.; Thummel, K.; Boguski, M.S. & Schuetz, E. (2001). Sequence diversity in CYP3A promoters and characterization of the genetic basis of polymorphic CYP3A5 expression. *Nat Genet,* Vol.27, No.4, pp.383-391

Kuypers, D.R.; Naesens, M.; Vermeire, S. & Vanrenterghem, Y. (2005). The impact of uridine diphosphate-glucuronosyltransferase 1A9 (UGT1A9) gene promoter region single-nucleotide polymorphisms T-275A and C-2152T on early mycophenolic acid dose-interval exposure in de novo renal allograft recipients. *Clin Pharmacol Ther,* Vol.78, No.4, pp.351-361

Kuypers, D.R.; de Jonge, H.; Naesens, M.; Lerut, E.; Verbeke, K. & Vanrenterghem, Y. (2007). CYP3A5 and CYP3A4 but not MDR1 single-nucleotide polymorphisms determine long-term tacrolimus disposition and drug-related nephrotoxicity in renal recipients. *Clin Pharmacol Ther,* Vol.82, No.6, pp.711-725

Kuzuya, T. ; Kobayashi, T.; Moriyama, N.; Nagasaka, T.; Yokoyama, .; Uchida, K.; Nakao, A. & Nabeshima, T. (2003). Amlodipine, but not MDR1 polymorphisms, alters the pharmacokinetics of cyclosporine A in Japanese kidney transplant recipients. *Transplantation,* Vol.76, No.5, pp.865-868

Le Meur, Y.; Djebli, N.; Szelag, J.C. ; Hoizey, G. ; Toupanoe, O.; Rerolle, J.P. & Marquet, P. (2006). CYP3A5*3 influences sirolimus oral clearance in de novo and stable renal transplant recipients. *Clin Pharmacol Ther,* Vol.80, No.1, pp.51-60

Li, D. ; Gui, R. ; Li, J. ; Huang, Z. & Nie, X. (2006). Tacrolimus dosing in Chinese renal transplant patients is related to MDR1 gene C3435T polymorphisms. *Transplant Proc,* Vol.38, No.9, pp.2850-2852

Lown, K.S.; Mayo, R.R.; Leichtman, A.B.; Hsiao, H.L.; Turgeon, D.K.; Schmiedlin-Ren, P.; Brown, M.B.; Guo, W.; Rossi, S.J.; Benet, L.Z. & Watkins, P.B. (1997). Role of intestinal P-glycoprotein (mdr1) in interpatient variation in the oral bioavailability of cyclosporine. *Clin Pharmacol Ther,* Vol.62, No.3, pp.248-260

MacPhee, I.A.; Fredericks, S.; Tai, T.; Syrris, P.; Carter, N.D.; Johnston, A.; Goldberg, L. & Holt, D.W. (2002). Tacrolimus pharmacogenetics: Polymorphisms associated with expression of cytochrome p4503A5 and P-glycoprotein correlate with dose requirement. *Transplantation,* Vol.74, No.11, pp. 1486–1489.

MacPhee, I.A.; Fredericks, S.; Tai, T.; Syrris, P.; Carter, N.D.; Johnston, A.; Goldberg, L. & Holt, D.W. (2004). The influence of pharmacogenetics on the time to achieve target tacrolimus concentrations after kidney transplantation. *Am J Transplant,* Vol.4, No.6, pp.914-919

MacPhee, I.A.; Fredericks, S.; Mohamed, M.; Moreton, M.; Carter, N.D.; Johnston, A.; Goldberg, L. & Holt, D.W. (2005). Tacrolimus pharmacogenetics: The CYP3A5*1 allele predicts low dose-normalized tacrolimus blood concentrations in whites and South Asians. *Transplantation,* Vol.79, No.4, pp.499-502

Mai, I. ; Stormer, E. ; Goldammer, M. ; Johne, A. ; Kruger, H. ; Budde, K. & Roots, I. (2003). MDR1 haplotypes do not affect the steady-state pharmacokinetics of cyclosporine in renal transplant patients. *J Clin Pharmacol,* Vol.43, No.10, pp.1101-1107

Mai, I.; Perloff, E.S.; Bauer, S.; Goldammer, M.; Johne, A.; Filler, G.; Budde, K. & Roots, I. (2004). MDR1 haplotypes derived from exons 21 and 26 do not affect the steady-state pharmacokinetics of tacrolimus in renal transplant patients. *Br J Clin Pharmacol,* Vol.58, No.5, pp.548-553

Makeeva, O.; Stepanov, V.; Puzyrev, V.; Goldstein D.B. & Grossman, I. (2008). Global pharmacogenetics: Genetic substructure of Eurasian populations and its effect on variants of drug-metabolizing enzymes. *Pharmacogenomics,* Vol.9, No.7, pp.847-868

McLeod, H.L. & Evans, W.E. (2001). Pharmacogenomics: Unlocking the human genome for better drug therapy. *Annu Rev Pharmacol Toxicol,* Vol.41, pp.101-121

Miller, D.S.; Fricker, G. & Drewe, J. (1997). P-glycoprotein-mediated transport of a fluorescent rapamycin derivative in renal proximal tubule. *J Pharmacol Exp Ther,* Vol.282, No.1, pp.440-444

Min, D.I. & Ellingrod, V.L. (2003). Association of the CYP3A4*1B 5 flanking region polymorphism with cyclosporine pharmacokinetics in healthy subjects. *Ther Drug Monit,* Vol.25, No.3 pp. 305-309

Min, D.I.; Ellingrod, V.L.; Marsh, S.& McLeod, H. (2004). CYP3A5 polymorphism and the ethnic differences in cyclosporine pharmacokinetics in healthy subjects 1. *Ther Drug Monit,* Vol.26, No.5, pp.524-528

Min, S.I.; Kim, S.Y.; Ahn, S.H.; Min, S.K.; Kim, S.H., Kim, Y.S.; Moon, K.C.; Oh, J.M.; Kim, S.J. & Ha, J. (2010). CYP3A5*1 allele: impacts on early acute rejection and graft function in tacrolimus-based renal transplant recipients. *Transplantation,* Vol.90, No.12, pp.1394-1400

Moscoso-Solorzano, G.T.; Ortega, F.; Rodríguez, I.; Garcia-Castro, M.; Gomez, E.; Diaz-Corte, C.; Baltar, J.M.; Alvarez, V.; Ortiz, A. & Coto, E. (2008). A search for cyclophilin-A gene variants in cyclosporine A-treated renal transplanted patients. *Clin Transplant*, Vol.22, No.6, pp.722-729

Mourad, M. ; Mourad, G. ; Wallemacq, P. ; Garrigue, V. ; Van Bellingen, C. ; Van Kerkhove, V. ; De Meyer, M.; Malaise, J.; Chaib Eddour, D.; Lison, D. ; Squifflet, J.P. & Haufroid, V. (2005). Sirolimus and tacrolimus trough concentrations and dose requirements after kidney transplantation in relation to CYP3A5 and MDR1 polymorphisms and steroids. *Transplantation*, Vol.80, No.7, pp.977-984

Mourad, M. ; Wallemacq, P. ; De Meyer, M. ; Brandt, D. ; Van Kerkhove, V. ; Malaise, J.; Chaib Eddour, D.; Lison, D. & Haufroid, V. (2006). The influence of genetic polymorphisms of cytochrome P450 3A5 and ABCB1 on starting dose- and weight-standardized tacrolimus trough concentrations after kidney transplantation in relation to renal function. *Clin Chem Lab Med*, Vol.44, No.10, pp.1192-1198

Naesens, M.; Kuypers, D.R.; Verbeke, K. & Vanrenterghem, Y. (2006). Multidrug resistance protein 2 genetic polymorphisms influence mycophenolic acid exposure in renal allograft recipients. *Transplantation*, Vol.82, No.8, pp.1074-1084

Nebert, D.W.; & Russell, D.W. (2002). Clinical importance of the cytochromes P450. *Lancet*, Vol.360, No.9340, pp.1155-1162

Op den Buijsch, R.A.; Christiaans, M.H.; Stolk, L.M., de Vries, J.E.; Cheung, C.Y.; Undre, N.A.; van Hooff, J.P.; van Dieijen-Visser, M.P.& Bekers, O. (2007). Tacrolimus pharmacokinetics and pharmacogenetics: influence of adenosine triphosphate-binding cassette B1 (ABCB1) and cytochrome (CYP) 3A polymorphisms. *Fundam Clin Pharmacol*, Vol.21, No.4, pp.427-435

Phillips, K.A. & Van Bebber, S.L. (2005). Measuring the value of pharmacogenomics. *Nat Rev Drug Discov*, Vol.4, No.6, pp.500-509

Quaranta, S.; Chevalier, D.; Allorge, D.; Lo-Guidice, J.M.; Migot-Nabias, F.; Kenani, A.; Imbenotte, M.; Broly, F.; Lacarelle, B. & Lhermitte, M. (2006). Ethnic differences in the distribution of CYP3A5 gene polymorphisms. *Xenobiotica*, Vol.36, No.12, pp.1191-1200

Rebbeck, T.R.; Jaffe, J.M.; Walker, A.H.; Wein, A.J. & Malkowicz, S.B. (1998). Modification of clinical presentation of prostate tumors by a novel genetic variant in CYP3A4. *J Natl Cancer Inst*, Vol.90, No.16, pp.1225-1229

Renders, L.; Frisman, M.; Ufer, M.; Mosyagin, I.; Haenisch, S.; Ott, U.; Caliebe, A.; Dechant, M.; Braun, F.; Kunzendorf, U. & Cascorbi, I. (2007). CYP3A5 genotype markedly influences the pharmacokinetics of tacrolimus and sirolimus in kidney transplant recipients. *Clin Pharmacol Ther*, Vol.81, No.2, pp. 228-234

Rivory, L.P.; Qin, H.; Clarke, S.J.; Eris, J.; Duggin, G.; Ray, E.; Trent, R.J. & Bishop, J.F. (2000). Frequency of cytochrome P450 3A4 variant genotype in transplant population and lack of association with cyclosporin clearance. *Eur J Clin Pharmacol*, Vol.56, No.5, pp.395-398

Roy, J.N. ; Barama, A. ; Poirier, C. ; Vinet, B. & Roger, M. (2006). Cyp3A4, Cyp3A5, and MDR-1genetic influences on tacrolimus pharmacokinetics in renal transplant recipients. *Pharmacogenet Genomics*, Vol.16, No.9, pp.659-65

Saeki, T.; Ueda, K.; Tanagawara, Y.; Hori, R. & Komano, T. (1993). Human P-glycoprotein transports cyclosporine A and FK506. *J Biol Chem*, Vol. 268, No.9, pp.6077-6080

Sattler, M.; Guengerich, F.P.; Yun, C.H.; Christians, U. & Sewing, K.F. (1992). Cytochrome P-450 3A enzymes are responsible for biotransformation of FK506 and rapamycin in man and rat. *Drug Metab Dispos*, Vol.20, No.5, pp.753-761

Schiff, J.; Cole, E. & Cantarovich, M. (2007). Therapeutic monitoring of calcineurin inhibitors for the nephrologist. *Clin J Am Soc Nephrol*, Vol.2, No.2, pp.374-384

Shastry, B.S. (2005). Genetic diversity and new therapeutic concepts. *J Hum Genet*, Vol. 50, No. 7, pp. 321-328

Soria-Royer, C.; Legendre, C.; Mircheva, J. ; Premel, S. ; Beaune, P. & Kreis, H. (1993). Thiopurine-methyl-transferase activity to assess azathioprine myelotoxicity in renal transplant recipients. *Lancet*, Vol.341, No.8860, pp.1593–1594

Stoughton, R.B. & Friend, S.H. (2005). How molecular profiling could revolutionize drug discovery. *Nat Rev Drug Discov*, Vol.4, No.4, pp.345-350

Tada, H.; Tsuchiya, N.; Satoh, S.; Kagaya, H.; Li, Z.; Sato, K.; Miura, M.; Suzuki, T.; Kato, T. & Habuchi, T. (2005). Impact of CYP3A5 and MDR1(ABCB1) C3435T polymorphisms on the pharmacokinetics of tacrolimus in renal transplant recipients. *Transplant Proc*, Vol.37, No.4, pp.1730-1732

Tsuchiya, N.; Satoh, S.; Tada, H.; Li, Z.; Ohyama, C.; Sato, K.; Suzuki, T.; Habuchi, T. & Kato, T. (2004). Influence of CYP3A5 and MDR1 (ABCB1) polymorphisms on the pharmacokinetics of tacrolimus in renal transplant recipients. *Transplantation*, Vol.78, No. 8, pp.1182-1187

Thervet, E.; Anglicheau, D.; Toledano, N.; Houllier, A.M. ; Noel, L.H. ; Kreis, H. ; Beaune, P. & Legendre, C. (2001). Long-term results of TMPT activity monitoring in azathioprine-treated renal allograft recipients. *J Am Soc Nephrol*, Vol.12, No.1, pp.170-176

Thervet, E.; Anglicheau, D.; King, B.; Schlageter, M.H.; Cassinat, B.; Beaune, P.; Legendre, C. & Daly, A.K. (2003). Impact of cytochrome p450 3A5 genetic polymorphism on tacrolimus doses and concentration-to-dose ratio in renal transplant recipients. *Transplantation*, Vol.76, No.8, pp.1233-1235

Undre, N.A.; van Hooff, J.; Christiaans, M.; Vanrenterghem, Y.; Donck, J.; Heeman, U.; Kohnle, M.; Zanker, B.; Land, W.; Morales, J.M.; Andres, A.; Schafer, A. & Stevenson, P. (1999). Low systemic exposure to tacrolimus correlates with acute rejection. *Transplant Proc*, Vol.31, No.1-2, pp.296-298

Van Schaik, R.H.; van Agteren, M.; de Fijter, J.W.; Hartmann, A.; Schmidt, J.; Budde, K.; Kuypers, D.; Le Meur, Y.; van der Werf, M.; Mamelok, R. & van Gelder, T. (2009). UGT1A9 -275T>A/-2152C>T polymorphisms correlate with low MPA exposure and acute rejection in MMF/tacrolimus-treated kidney transplant patients. *Clin Pharmcol Ther*, Vol.86, No.3, pp.319-327

von Ahsen, N.; Richter, M.; Grupp, C.; Ringe, B.; Oellerich, M. & Armstrong, V.W. (2001). No influence of the MDR-1 C3435T polymorphism or a CYP3A4 promoter polymorphism (CYP3A4-V allele) on dose-adjusted cyclosporin A trough concentrations or rejection incidence in stable renal transplant recipients. *Clin Chem*, Vol.47, No.6, pp.1048-1052

Wang, J.; Zeevi, A.; Webber, s.; Girnita, D.M.; Addonizio, L.; Selby, R.; Hutchinson, I.V. & Burckart G.J. (2007). A novel variant L263F in human inosine 5′-monophosphate dehydrogenase 2 is associated with diminished enzyme activity. *Pharmacogenet Genomics*, Vol.17, No.4, pp.283-290

Wang, J.; Yang, J.W.; Zeevi, A.; Webber, S.A.; Girnita, D.M.; Selby, R.; Fu, J.; Shah, T.; Pravica, V.; Hutchinson, I.V. & Burckart, G.J. (2008). IMPDH gene polymorphisms and association with acute rejection in renal transplant recipients. *Clin Pharmacol Ther,* Vol.83, No.5, pp.711-717

Weinshilboum, R.M.; Otterness, D.M. & Szumlanski, C.L. (1999). Methylation pharmacogenetics: Catechol O-methyltransferase, thiopurine methyltransferase, and histamine N-methyltransferase. *Annu Rev Pharmacol Toxicol,* Vol.39, pp.19–52.

Weinshilboum, R. (2003). Inheritance and drug response. *N Engl J Med,* Vol.348, No.6, pp.529–537

Westlind, A.; Löfberg, L.; Tindberg, N. Andersson, T.B. & Ingelman-Sundberg, M. (1999). Interindividual differences in hepatic expression of CYP3A4: Relationship to genetic polymorphism in the 5'-upstream regulatory region. *Biochem Biophys Res Commun,* Vol.259, No.1, pp.201-205

Woillard, J.B.; Rerolle, J.P.; Picard, N.; Rousseau, A.; Guillaudeau, A,; Munteanu, E.; Essig, M.; Drouet, M.; Le Meur, Y. & Marquet, P. (2010). Donor P-gp polymorphisms strongly influence renal function and graft loss in a cohort of renal transplant recipients on cyclosporine therapy in a long-term follow-up. *Clin Pharmacol Ther,* Vol.88, No.1, pp.95-100

Zhang, X.; Liu, Z.H.; Zheng, J.M.; Chen, Z.H.; Tang, Z.; Chen, J.S. & Li, L.S. (2005). Influence of CYP3A5 and MDR1 polymorphisms on tacrolimus concentration in the early stage after renal transplantation. *Clin Transplant,* Vol.19, No.5, pp.638-643

Zhang, Y. & Benet, L.Z. (2001). The gut as a barrier to drug absorption. Combined role of cytochrome P4503A and P-glycoprotein. *Clin Pharmacokinet,* Vol.40, No.3, pp.159-168

Zhao, Y.; Song, M.; Guan, D.;Bi, S.; Meng, J.; Li, Q. & Wang, W. (2005). Genetic polymorphisms of CYP3A5 genes and concentration the cyclosporine and tacrolimus. *Transplant Proc,* Vol.37, No.1, pp.178-181

Zheng, H.; Webber, S.; Zeevi, A.; Schuetz, E.; Zhang, J.; Bowman, P.; Boyle, G.; Law, Y.; Miller, S.; Lamba, J. & Burckart, G.J. (2003). Tacrolimus dosing in pediatric heart transplant patients is related to CYP3A5 and MDR1 gene polymorphisms. *Am J Transplant,* Vol.3, No.4, pp.477–483

Zheng, H.; Zeevi, A.; Schuetz, E.; Lamba, J.; McCurry, K.; Griffith, B.P.; Webber, S.; Ristich, J.; Dauber, J.; Iacono, A.; Grgurich, W.; Zaldonis, D.; McDade, K.; Zhang, J. & Burckart, G.J. (2004). Tacrolimus dosing in adult lung transplant patients is related to cytochrome P4503A5 gene polymorphism. *J Clin Pharmacol,* Vol.44, No.2, pp.135-140

9

Tolerance in Kidney Transplantation

Faouzi Braza, Maud Racape, Jean-Paul Soulillou and Sophie Brouard
University of Nantes, Inserm U643
France

1. Introduction

Advances in immunosuppressive treatments led us to better control acute rejection and improve graft survival in organ transplantation. However, immunosuppressive drugs, due to their toxicity, are also responsible for many side effects as opportunistic infections, renal failure, cardiovascular disease and malignancy (Stegall et al, 1997; Soulillou et al, 2001; Ojo et al, 2003; Fishman et al, 2007). Then, establishing long-term graft acceptance without the continuous utilisation of immunosuppression, also called "tolerance" is a highly desirable therapeutic goal.

Many strategies have been developed to achieve this goal in transplantation but whereas achievable in rodent models (Tomita et al,. 1994), it remains very difficult in human because of many differences between their immune system. The definition of true tolerance has been proposed by Billingham et al in 1953, as a well-functioning graft lacking histological lesions of rejection, in the absence of immunosuppression in an immunocompetent host accepting a second graft of the same donor, while able to reject a third-party graft. In clinic some cases of spontaneous tolerance, who stopped their immunosuppressive treatments and display a good graft function, were reported in the last decades in 20 % of liver transplanted recipients (Leruta et al., 2006) but also in kidney transplantation (Roussey-Kesler et al., 2006) suggesting that tolerance exist in human. Because several keys elements of transplant tolerance in rodents cannot be demonstrated in humans, this state has been referred to as "operational tolerance". Thanks to these patients, the scientific community aims to identify prognostic and diagnostic biomarkers that could help physicians to detect tolerance (Brouard et al, 2007; Newell et al, 2010; Sagoo et al) to safely reduce immunosuppression in transplanted recipients.

2. Long-term graft acceptance exploiting the central tolerance

Billingham et al. first demonstrated in 1953 the feasibility of "actively acquired tolerance" in contrast with "actively acquired immunity" in their neonatal mouse model (Billingham et al., 1953). They demonstrated that injection of foreign antigens to mice at a foetal stage induced tolerance to a skin graft of the same donor at the adult stage. They thus reported on a phenomenon of "acquired tolerance" defined as a well-functioning graft lacking histological lesions of rejection, in the absence of immunosuppression, in an immunocompetent host accepting a second graft of the same donor, while able to reject a third-party graft. Moreover, they deduced from these experiments that immune system formation and lymphocyte education to self-antigens were taking place early during embryonic development. Mechanisms of central tolerance are based on positive and negative selection of T lymphocytes in the thymus permitting the discrimination of self and nonself (Von Boehmer et al., 1990; Nossal., 1994). Consequently, two main strategies were developed in experimental and clinical transplantation to exploit the natural process of self-reactive T lymphocyte depletion in the thymus: intrathymic injection of alloantigens (Ildstad et al, 1985; Ildstad et al, 1986; Posselt et al, 1990) and mixed chimerism (Kurtz et al., 2004) to induce central tolerance to foreign antigens, allowing the acceptance of the graft.

2.1 Tolerance induction by intrathymic injection of alloantigens

One strategy for the induction of tolerance is the introduction of foreign alloantigens into the adult thymus to re-educate T cells of the host to recognize such antigens as self and tolerate them. There was a huge interest in this approach after the demonstration by Posselt et al that intrathymic injection of allogeneic islets induced donor-specific transplant tolerance in rat (Posselt et al., 1990). Many reports have since confirmed this observation. In experimental kidney transplantation, Remuzzi et al generated tolerance in Lewis rats by injecting in the thymus isolated glomeruli from Brown-Norway rat kidneys. They observed a donor specific unresponsiveness that permitted the renal allograft to survive indefinitely without immunosuppression (Remuzzi et al., 1991). Later, Nick D. Jones and colleagues demonstrated that the delivery of alloantigens to the thymus could lead to the induction of tolerance in vivo in adult mice (Jones et al., 1998). Indeed they showed that intrathymic injections of H-2k^{b+} splenocytes combined with peripheral T cell depletion trigger the long-term graft survival of H-2k^{b+} cardiac allograft in transgenic mice expressing a specific TCR against H-2k^{b+} (Jones et al., 1998). In their mouse model, tolerance was performed by clonal deletion of alloreactive T cells.

Similarly, Oluwole and colleagues showed that intrathymic injections of a combination of seven major histocompatibility peptides from RT1.Au rat to ACI rat induced tolerance to cardiac and islet allografts from RT1.Au donor. In a second report they identified five immunodominant peptides inducing tolerance in ACI rats and studied the cytokine profile in grafts, thymus and lymphoid tissues of each tolerant and rejecting rat by ELISA and RT-PCR (Oluwole et al., 1993). They demonstrated that injection of a single immunodominant tolerant peptide induced an antigen specific down-regulation of Th1 responses, in both graft and lymphoid tissues, and an augmentation of Th2 cytokines (IL-4 and IL-10) in the graft. In contrast they observed a strengthless Th1 response in rejected graft correlating with the events in lymphoid tissues (Oluwole et al., 1993). These different reports showed that direct intrathymic injection of donor cells generates specific unresponsiveness and clonal deletion of host T cells. The first attempt to extend this approach in human has been performed in cardiac allografts (Remuzzi et al., 1995). This study showed that the injection of donor cells in thymus before transplantation was safe but did not allow a continuous provision of donor alloantigen and was insufficient to induce long term graft survival.

2.2 Tolerance induction by mixed chimerism in rodents

Other studies demonstrated that bone marrow infusions of the donor associated with total body or thymic irradiation to deplete peripheral T cells could provide a source of stem cells able to establish mixed chimerism (recipient and donor) and induce tolerance in transplantation (Kurtz et al., 2004). The engraftment of allogenic bone marrow in the recipient allows having a permanent source of donor antigens and produces cells involved in the T lymphocyte selection, such as thymic progenitors which repopulate the peripheral T cell repertory, and dendritic cells which allow negative selection in the thymus. All new mature T lymphocytes of host and donor, recognizing donor and host antigens, are eliminated during the step of central tolerance. Finally, the donor is considered as «self» by the new developing immune system. As long as donor and host bone marrow coexist, the thymus will not generate mature T cells with reactivity against the donor or the host (Kurtz et al., 2004). This intrathymic deletion of donor-reactive thymocytes was shown to be the dominant mechanism for the maintenance of tolerance in mixed chimerism transplantation (Kurtz et al., 2004). First animal studies with antisera or monoclonal antibodies against lymphocytes showed that engraftment of donor bone marrow could enhance long-term survival of transplanted tissues without the need of a complete and potentially lethal ablation of host's immune system induced by irradiation (S.P.Cobbold et al., 1986). Later, Yedida Sharabi and David H. Sachs were the first to induce tolerance by mixed chimerism using a nonlethal conditioning regimen in mice skin allograft model (Sharabi et al., 1989). They showed that mixed hematopoietic chimerism can induce robust donor-specific tolerance, even across full MHC mismatched. This method involved a nommyeloablative conditioning regimen in which mice were pretreated with an anti-CD4 and an anti-CD8 to deplete peripheral T cells, following total body and thymic irradiations and an injection of donor bone marrow cells. In their experiment, all mice displayed a stable chimerism and long-term graft survival without graft versus host diseases. Most of their tolerant mice also displayed a cell-mediated lympholysis and a mixed lymphocyte reaction tolerance (Sharabi et al., 1989). Megan Sykes's team clearly identified in 1994 the mechanism of B10.A skin allograft tolerance in B10.A ==> B10 chimeric mice after specific conditioning regimen followed by B10.A bone marrow cell injection (Figure 1). For that, they followed the clonal

B10 mice	B10. A mice
H-2b; Kb Ab E- Db I-E- TCR Vβ-11 +	H2-a; Kk Ak E+ Dk Dd Ld TCR Vβ-11 - I-E+ (no antigen recognized by TCR Vβ-11)

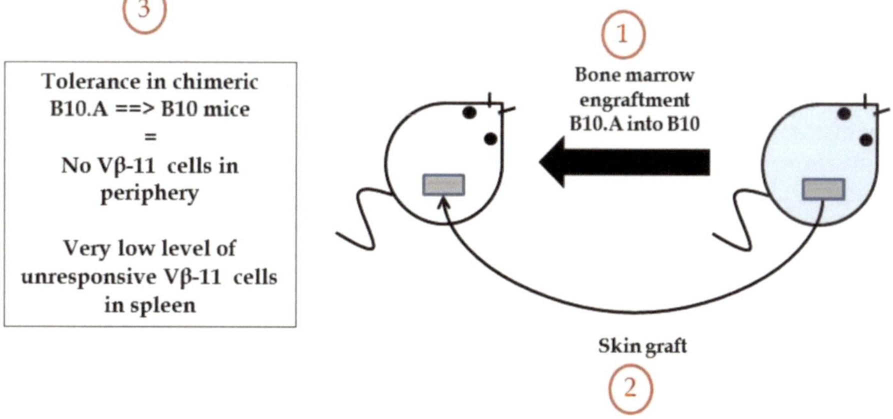

deletion of VB11+T cells in their tolerant mice, these cells being normally deleted in I-E+ B10.A mice, but not in B10 mice. In their work, they demonstrated that most of VB11+ T cells of tolerant chimeras B10.A ==> B10 were deleted. They didn't detect VB11+ cells in periphery but very low level in spleen of tolerant mice. These cells were anergic following TCR stimulation in vitro (Tomita et al,. 1994).
No evidence of peripheral mechanisms could be found in these models (Khan et al,. 1996). Indeed, depletion of donor chimeric cells with donor class I MHC-specific monoclonal antibody broke tolerance in these mice, and was associated with the appearance in blood of T cells with receptors recognizing donor antigens (Khan et al,. 1996). But if the thymus was removed just before depletion, specific tolerance to the donor persisted in the absence of donor chimerism, and donor-reactive T cells did not appear in the periphery. Thus, the major factor for tolerance in this model is to give a constant source of donor antigen presenting cells to permit intrathymic deletion of new thymocytes, which continued to be generated (Khan et al,. 1996). Similar approaches were performed in monkeys with success. But in this model, tolerance was associated with the loss of mixed chimerism suggesting the implication of peripheral mechanisms to maintain tolerance in non-human primates (Kawai et al., 1995).

2.3 Tolerance induction by mixed chimerism in human kidney transplantation

The proof of concept that the tolerance of an organ can be obtained when the transplanted organ is followed by engrafting of bone marrow of the same donor was shown in humans in a few cases. Indeed two patients, who received a HLA-matched bone marrow transplantation, were able to accept few years later a kidney graft from the same donor without immunosuppressive drugs (Sayegh et al., 1991). Some teams developed a clinically relevant non-myeloablative preparative regimen permitting an induction of tolerance in human kidney transplantation. They performed this approach in both HLA-matched (Scandling et al., 2008) and HLA-mismatched situation (Kawai et al., 2008).
For the HLA-matched study six patients were enrolled in the protocol but only results of one patient were published. This patient has undergone a post-transplantation conditioning regimen of total lymphoid irradiation and injection of rabbit anti-thymocyte immunoglobulins allowing the engraftment of donor's kidney and bone marrow. In these patients, they observed a stable mixed chimerism and a well-functioning graft despite the withdrawal of all immunosuppressors. Also, few experiments were accomplished in order to study the immune system of these operationally tolerant recipients. They tested immune responses and showed a good immune reconstitution after the conditioning regimen without opportunistic infections, normal in vitro T-cells responses against virus, bacteria and third-party allogenic cells. In contrast, there was a global unresponsiveness of host T cells against donor dendritic cells. This study demonstrated that it was possible to achieve persistent chimerism and tolerance to the graft without graft versus host disease (Scandling et al., 2008).
The study by Kawai et al. has reported a stable renal allograft-function after complete removal of all immunosuppressors (Kawai et al., 2008). Five patients with end-stage renal disease have undergone combined bone marrow and kidney transplantation from HLA mismatched donors after specific conditioning regimen including a strong immunosuppressive treatment and a thymic irradiation before transplantation (figure 2). Because of the death of one patient during the study, the conditioning regimen protocol was modified. Then, physicians performed a progressive diminution of immunosuppressive

drugs during the first months until complete withdrawal. The clinical follow-up of the patients was achieved by controlling creatinine and proteinuria levels and making biopsy surveillance (immunofluorescence microscopy including C4d deposition). Thus, all patients displayed stable creatinine level and graft function despite the presence of antidonor HLA II antibodies and C4d deposits in three of the four recipients. Authors were unable to detect mixed chimerism after 14 days. The authors noticed a specific unresponsiveness of host T cells against donor antigens in vitro (Kawai et al., 2008). Tolerated grafts exhibited a high level of Foxp3 expression and no expression of granzyme B suggesting a role of regulatory T cells (Tregs) in the maintenance of tolerance as previously described in monkey (Kawai et al., 1995). This study suggests some evidences for a cooperation of central and peripheral tolerance mechanisms in operational tolerance. Indeed, mixed chimerism permits to suppress alloreactive T cells whereas intragraft regulatory T cells maintain a global unresponsiveness of allogenic surviving T cells permitting the long term survival of the graft. In spite of encouraging results, a few patients waiting for an allograft can receive an HLA-identical allograft, used in most of these protocols and giving the best results. Moreover, this protocol is uneasy to apply in clinic because of the possibility for the patient to develop a graft versus host disease, associated with the bone marrow engraftment. Finally, the conditioning regimen must be mastered and safe for patients. There are too much non acceptable conditions just to induce tolerance.

Conditionning regiment undergone by each patient to induce mixed chimerism and tolerance (Kawai et al., 2008)

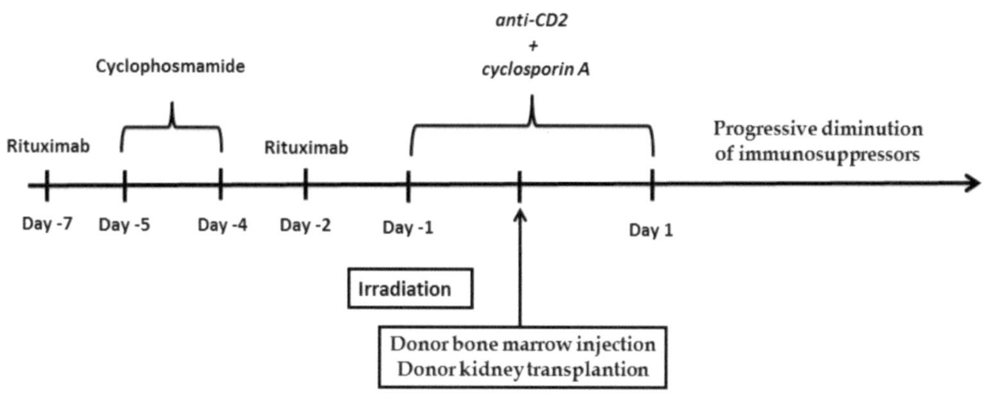

3. Kidney transplantation tolerance induction by manipulating peripheral mechanisms

Clinicians use immunosuppressive drugs to suppress immune reactions against the graft (Philip et al., 2004). Basically, these drugs can be classified in three groups: anti-inflammatory of the corticosteroid family as prednisone; cytotoxic treatment as cyclophosphamide; and fungus or bacteria derived molecule as Cyclosporin A, Tacrolimus and Sirolimus inhibiting T cell signaling. All these drugs have a large spectrum of action and suppress deleterious functions as well as protective functions of our immune system

(Galon et al., 2002). Thus, although immunosuppressive drugs demonstrated good impact in graft survival, they are responsible for large dangerous side effects.
The development of monoclonal antibodies gave the possibility to target particular processes of the immune response (Kohler et al., 1975). These antibodies were used in clinical transplantation to deplete reactive T lymphocytes (Strober et al., 1984) to improve long term survival of the graft, but also to induce tolerance notably through costimulatory blockade and induction of regulatory immune mechanisms (Kirk et al., 1997). Another approach for tolerance induction is to rebalance the pool of regulatory cells in transplanted patients in order to restore the cellular homeostasis. During the last decades, many regulatory populations were identified in animals and also in humans. They represent a strong potential clinical tool for the establishment of tolerance in human transplantation. Thus, many studies try to develop different protocols able to generate specific allogenic regulatory cells in order to promote donor-specific tolerance.

3.1 The use of monoclonal antibodies: T cell depletion and blockade of costimulatory signals

T cell activation requires three signals to enhance a strong immune response. The two first signals depend on the interaction of T cells with antigen presenting cells. Interaction between MHC-peptide and TCR provides the specificity of the response. The second signal, called the "costimulatory signal", is given by molecules on antigen presenting cells that interact with particular costimulatory receptors on T cells. In the absence of costimulation, T cells that recognize antigen either fail to respond and die or enter a state of unresponsiveness known as anergy (Schwartz et al., 1990). Thus, costimulation is a key determinant of T cell response. The third signal is provided by cytokines and her respective receptors. There are different kinds of cytokines that can enhance proliferation, survival, but also orientate the immune response. Anti-thymocyte globulin preparations were first used to deplete alloreactive peripheral T cells, in combination with total lymphoid irradiation (Stroberet al., 1984, Strober et al 1989). However, it was suggested that the T cell depletion induced by ATG was not sufficient to induce tolerance (ref). OKT3, a monoclonal murine antibody directed against CD3 molecule of the TCR (Cosimi et al., 1981) was then used to block activation of T cell in vitro and induce depletion of T cells in vivo. Although several studies demonstrated the efficacy of OKT3 in the prevention and treatment of acute rejection (Vincenti et al., 1998; Webster et al., 2006) its clinical use was limited by many serious side effects. Administration of the drug is often followed by a cytokine storm with high fever, arterial hypertension and pulmonary oedema as result of capillary leak. Secondly, some patients can develop antibodies against the xenogeneic epitope that are responsible for decreased efficacy. Lastly, a higher incidence of infectious complications and malignancies has been reported, suggesting a too strong immunosuppression (Ortho Multicenter Transplant Study Group et al., 1985).
To limit the over-immunosuppression generated by OKT3, another monoclonal antibody was developed that was targeting the interleukin 2 receptor, a molecule specifically involved in proliferation and activation of T lymphocytes. Such treatments spare T lymphocytes not involved in the recognition of donor antigen, decreasing the over-immunosuppression. Monoclonal antibodies that are specific for rodents IL-2R can abrogate proliferation of activated T cells in vitro, prevent and reverse acute heart rejection in mice (Kirkman et al., 1985) and delay kidney rejection in monkeys (Shapiro et al., 1987). In human kidney transplantation, the efficacy of a rat monoclonal antibody (33B1.3) was studied and

confirmed in a randomized clinical trial in combination with immunosuppressors (Soulillou et al., 1987). The 33B1.3 blocks the α and β chain association preventing the interaction between IL-2 and its receptor. The efficacy of this treatment to prevent acute rejection is similar to rabbit antithymocyte globulin treatment with fewer side effects (Soulillou et al., 1990). Nowadays it's clearly demonstrated that treatments with anti-IL2R associated with cyclosporin A and steroids ameliorate the survival of the graft and decrease opportunistic infections, but nevertheless with a little more acute rejection (Brennan et al., 2006) and a decrease of Tregs in periphery (Bluestone et al., 2008).

Alentuzumab (Campath-1H), a humanized rat monoclonal antibody, binds CD52, a glycoprotein expressed by T and B lymphocytes, monocytes and granulocytes (Xia et al., 1993). Injection of Alentuzumab leads to massive depletion of peripheral lymphocytes. It has been used for the treatment of lymphoma (Hale et al., 2002) but also in kidney transplantation. Indeed, in combination with low dose of cyclosporin A, this treatment could induce tolerance (Calne et al., 1998). Moreover, it has been showed that Alentuzumab treatment followed by low dose of tacrolimus permit to decrease acute rejection and opportunistic infections but also increase the number of Tregs (Ciancio et al., 2008). But recent data demonstrated that the use of high dose of Alentuzumab to treat acute rejection must be made with caution because of the high risk of early infection-associated death (Clatworthy et al., 2009).

Belatacept (LEA29Y), a selective costimulation blocker, binds surface costimulatory ligands (CD80 and CD86) of antigen-presenting cells. Then there is a blockade of second signal inducing death and anergy of effector T cells (Schwartzet al., 1990; Sayegh et al., 1998). Belatacept is derived from Abatacept, a human fusion protein combining the extracellular domain of cytotoxic T-lymphocyte–associated antigen 4 with the constant region fragment of human IgG1 (CTLA4Ig). Treatment with Belatacept permit to have effective immunosuppression, superior renal function and reduced incidence of chronic allograft nephropathy than in patients treated with cyclosporin A (Vincenti et al., 2005). Treatments with Belatacept have no adverse effects on Tregs and even improve their infiltration in the graft (Bluestone et al., 2008). A recent study has tested the immunoregulatory effect of selective CD28 blockade on kidney and heart allograft in primates (ref). It has been showed that CD28 blockade reduced alloreactivity and increased the pool of peripheral T regulatory cells. In addition, authors observed a strong infiltration of Tregs in graft. Thus, this treatment permits to manipulating and rebalance the regulatory mechanisms in transplanted primates (Poirier et al., 2010). Selective CD28 blockade has significant advantages relative to CD80/86 blockade by Belatacept (Vincenti et al., 2005). Indeed with Belatacept, all B7 molecules are targeted, preventing activator and inhibitory signals by CD28 and CTLA-4 respectively. With CD28 antagonist we block just effector T cells and not Tregs that constitutively express CTLA-4 for their immunosuppressive activity (Wing et al., 2008)

Blockade of CD40 pathway in non-human primates also allows the long term graft survival. The first study in monkey demonstrated the good effect with an anti-CD40 injection in kidney transplantation (Kirk et al., 1999). But the first generation of this antibody induced serious side effects as thromboembolic complications (Kawai et al., 2000). Recently a new human monoclonal anti-CD40 antibody (4D11) was developed and studied in kidney graft model in cynomolgus monkeys. 4D11 was described as a potential effective immunosuppressive drug inducing a diminution of graft lesions and alloantibody production (Imai 2007). Thus, it was shown that the blockade of both CD40 and ICOS pathways in a rat heart transplantation model ameliorates the graft survival (Guillonneau et

al 2005). Also, injection of anti-ICOS in transgenic CD40Ig rat preferentially inhibits chronic rejection, decreases leucocyte infiltration in the graft and cytotoxic activity of T cells.
A lot of differences, in the immune system, exist between human and animal, notably the strong presence of human memory cells which play a central role in chronic rejection. They present different characteristics which prevent their manipulation in vivo. Indeed, it was shown that memory cells are resistant to depletion (Gallon et al., 2006), costimulatory blockade (Yang et al., 2007) and apoptosis (Wu et al., 2004) and can be activated by low antigenic signal and without costimulation (Cho et al., 2000). A lot of studies thus try to specifically target human memory T cells by neutralizing the tumor necrosis factor which is an important factor for the generation of memory T cells (Croft, 2003; Yuan et al., 2003) or by blocking adhesion molecules, then inhibiting the infiltration of such T cells in the graft (Ellis and Krueger., 2001; Dedrick et al., 2002; Vicenti et al., 2007).

3.2 Tolerogenic cellular therapy

Recently, new protocols to induce tolerance were developed in experimental transplantation. It is a "tolerogenic cellular therapy" approach mainly developed in rodents (Bluestone et al., 2005; Morelli et al., 2007) (figure 5). In fact, in the last decades a lot of regulatory immune populations were isolated and identified as potential suppressors of allogenic responses. Thus, Tregs (Sakaguchiet al., 1995; Qin et al., 1998; Hori et al., 2003) tolerogenic dendritic cells, myeloid-derived suppressor cells, NKT cells (Seino et al., 2001) and B cells (Fuchs ansMatzinger., 1991) were described to induce and transfer tolerance in experimental transplantation. Thus, CD4+ T cells with regulatory function have been shown to play a critical role in the maintenance of transplantation tolerance (Qin et al., 1998). The CD25+ fraction of CD4+ T cells mediates tolerance on adoptive transfer into a naive host (Hara et al., 2001; Graca et al., 2002). These cells were shown to be potent suppressors of activated T cells in vitro (Thornton et al., 1998) and to be crucial for the control of the effector function of alloreactive CD4+ and CD8+T cells in transplantation models in vivo (Maurik et al., 2002). The precise mechanisms by which these Treg cells exert their suppressive function remain to be defined, but we know that surface molecules such as CTLA-4 (Read et al., 2000), the glucocorticoid-induced tumor necrosis factor receptor (GITR) (Shimizu et al., 2002), and cytokines such as TGF-β and IL-10 (Hara et al., 2001) play roles for the maintenance of tolerance. Several studies have demonstrated that the regulation mediated by Treg cells is dependent on a continuous supply of alloantigens (Scully et al., 1998; Sanchez-Fueyo et al., 2001) suggesting that these cells have specificity for alloantigens. In transplantation, alloreactive CD4+ T cells with indirect allospecificity are thought to play a key role in chronic rejection, and the control of these pathogenic effector cells by donor-specific Treg cells could, therefore, result in transplantation tolerance (Wise et al., 1998; Graca et al., 2002). However, the possibility of using Treg cells as immunotherapy for the induction of antigen-specific tolerance is limited by cell number. Indeed, the entire pool of Treg cells accounts for only 5% to 10% of CD4+T cells in the peripheral blood of healthy persons. Consequently, a lot of teams focused their efforts on the possibility to expand *ex-vivo* human allogenic Tregs. In mice, ex-vivo stimulation of Tregs by anti-CD3 and anti-CD28 promotes strong proliferation of these cells (Nadig et al., 2010; Issa et al., 2010). In humans other studies described the possibility to induce specific allogenic Tregs by using tolerogenic dendritic cells (Bacchetta et al., 2010) or CD40-activated B cells (Zheng et al., 2010). The success of "Treg cell therapy" in solid organ transplantation is subject to confirmation of many clinical trials.

3.2 Induction of tolerance: How far are we?

Manipulating the host immune system to develop antigen-specific immune tolerance leading to graft acceptance is an attractive alternative and is the objective of an increasing number of studies. Two key factors must be considered to induce immune tolerance: firstly, decrease potentially harmful immune effector and memory cells responding to donor tissue, and secondly, increase donor-reactive tolerant cells. The comprehension of how we can harness the immune response towards tolerant cells should permit us to switch the balance from rejection towards long-term tolerance of donor grafts, without the need for immunosuppressive drugs (Long et al., 2009). The evaluation of the impact of therapeutic agents for tolerance is not clearly mastered and understood. Today we know that intense immunosuppressive therapy is not the solution for long term graft survival. Manipulating the immune system by mixed chimerism, monoclonal antibody and tolerogenic cell therapy remains in a clinical trial state because of the lack of knowledge and potential lethal and deleterious effects of these approaches. But all studies try to display the perfect balance between donor cells, recipient effector and regulatory cells and treatments. Unfortunately we still lack tools to identify such perfect tolerance balance. Thus, for the moment no protocol of induction of tolerance is used in routine in clinic.

4. Dissecting the operational tolerance phenotype

Operational tolerance is a state referred as long term graft survival, with a stable function of the graft without immunosuppression in an immunocompetent recipient (Ansari and Sayegh, 2004). Other factors can help to complete the definition of operational tolerance as the lack of anti-donor antibodies, no infiltration of effector cells in graft and a global unresponsiveness against the donor in vitro (Ferh and Sykes 2004). Phenomena of operational tolerance remain very rare in kidney but are real. Indeed, some patients have been tolerant for more than ten years with a stable function of their graft (Roussey-Kesler et al., 2006). The clinical history of these operationally tolerant patients, who stopped IS mostly by incompliance, is not different from kidney recipients (Roussey-Kesler et al., 2006). Moreover these patients do not seem to be immunosuppressed because they do not have more significant opportunistic infections following immunosuppression withdrawal. A small proportion of patient also presents anti-donor class II antibody without showing any signs of graft degradation. Finally, some of them lost their graft decades after transplantation suggesting that this phenomenon of "operational tolerance" is a metastable process that likely corresponds to an absence of "lesional response" in a protective environment.

Although these patients display heterogeneous characteristics, they offer the opportunity (i) to understand mechanisms responsible for tolerance in human kidney transplantation and (ii) to identify molecules that can induce, predict or diagnostic tolerance. Many teams are fundamentally interested in developing a better understanding of the basic processes of operational tolerance in kidney transplantation. They have engaged multiples studies to determine if there is a specific phenotype of tolerance in the blood of patients. The identification of pertinent biomarkers of tolerance is very important to predict and diagnose long term graft survival and potentially adapt therapy in stable patients under immunosuppression.

Whereas studies in animals put on light the role of Tregs in transplantation tolerance, first studies in human kidney transplantation showed no alteration in phenotype and functions of T cells in the blood of tolerant patients compared to healthy volunteers and stable patients under immunosuppressive therapy (Louis et al., 2006). Nevertheless, other studies showed an increase of Tregs in the blood of tolerant patients (Braudeau et al., 2007), a global unresponsiveness against the graft (Brouard et al., 2005) and a decreased expression of Myd88 and TLR4 in the PBMCs (Braudeau et al., 2008) compared to patients with chronic rejection. Moreover, a decrease of perforin and granzyme A, cytotoxic molecules, was reported in the CD8+ CD28- T cell subset in tolerant patients compared to patients with chronic rejection (Baeten et al., 2006) confirming the quiescence of the immune system in tolerant recipients. A study by our team identified by microarray a 49 gene signature of tolerance in operationally tolerant patients (Brouard et al., 2007). This signature can discriminate tolerant recipients from healthy volunteers, stable patients and recipients with chronic rejection. Moreover, this fingerprint of tolerance can predict and classify stable patients as potential tolerant patients, which would permit a progressive diminution of immunosuppressive drugs. It was also shown that tolerant patients display a lower expression of genes involved in effector immune responses confirming the global unresponsiveness against the graft (Brouard et al., 2007). Interestingly, this differential profile was composed of several genes specific of B cells (Brouard et al., 2007, Pallier et al., 2010) that also correlated with an increased number of peripheral B cells in these patients (Louis et al., 2006). We characterized more specifically the phenotype of these B lymphocytes (Pallier et al., 2010) and reported a global inhibitory phenotype of B cell compartment (Pallier et al., 2010). The genetic and B cell signature of these patients was independently verified by the ITN and IOT networks (Newell et al., 2010; Sagoo et al., 2010). It is nowadays a need to validate these biomarkers using larger multicentric cohorts in order to move from potential biomarkers into clinically useful biomarkers. Indeed a combination of several parameters is necessary to predict long-term graft survival. To increase the sensitivity and the specificity of the prediction, the composite score needs to be infusing with immunological parameters. Large cohort of patients has to be enrolled in order to take into account potential confounding factors when evaluating diagnostic or prognostic biomarkers. Finally, it will be necessary to move from snapshot studies into longitudinal studies in order to define the fluctuation of these biomarkers and better evaluate, understand and why not induce tolerance in transplantation.

5. References

Annaick Pallier, Sophie Hillion, Richard Danger et al. Patients with drug-free long-term graft function display increased numbers of peripheral B cells with a memory and inhibitory phenotype. *Kidney international* 2010

Ansari, M.J. and M.H. Sayegh. (2004). Clinical transplantation tolerance: the promise and challenges. *Kidney Int* 65:1560-3.

Atsushi Imai, Tomomi Suzuki, Atsushi Sugitani, TomooItoh, ShinyaUeki, Takeshi Aoyagi, Kenichiro Yamashita, Masahiko Taniguchi, Nobuaki Takahashi, Toru Miura,Tsuyoshi Shimamura, Hiroyuki Furukawa, and Satoru Todo. A Novel Fully Human Anti-CD40 Monoclonal Antibody, 4D11, for Kidney Transplantation in Cynomolgus Monkeys. *Transplantation* 2007; 84, 8.

Baeten, D., S. Louis, C. Braud, C. Braudeau, C. Ballet, F. Moizant, A. Pallier, M. Giral, S. Brouard and J.P. Soulillou. Phenotypically and functionally distinct CD8+

lymphocyte populations in long-term drug-free tolerance and chronic rejection in human kidney graft recipients. 2006 *J AmSoc Nephrol* 17:294-304.

Billingham RE, Brent L, Medawar PB (1953) Actively acquired tolerance of foreign cells. *Nature* 172: 603-606

Bluestone JA. Regulatory T-cell therapy: Is it ready for the clinic? *Nat Rev Immunol* 2005; 5: 343.

Braudeau, C., J. Ashton-Chess, M. Giral, E. Dugast, S. Louis, A. Pallier, C. Braud, A. Moreau,K. Renaudin, J.P. Soulillou and S. Brouard. (2008). Contrasted blood and intragraft toll-like receptor 4 mRNA profiles in operational tolerance versus chronic rejection in kidney transplant recipients. *Transplantation* 86:130-6.

Braudeau, C., M. Racape, M. Giral, S. Louis, A. Moreau, L. Berthelot, M. Heslan, J. Ashton-Chess, J.P. Soulillou and S. Brouard. (2007). Variation in numbers of CD4+CD25highFOXP3+ T cells with normal immuno-regulatory properties in long-term graft outcome. *Transpl Int* 20:845-55.

Brennan DC, Daller JA, Lake KD, Cibrik D, Del Castillo D. Rabbit antithymocyte globulin versusbasiliximab in renal transplantation. *N Engl J Med* 2006 ; 355 : 1967-77.

Calne R, Friend P, Moffatt S, *et al*. Prope tolerance, perioperative campath 1H, and low-dose cyclosporin monotherapy in renal allograft recipients. *Lancet* 1998 ; 351 : 1701-2.

Carole Guillonneau, Venceslas Aubry, Karine Renaudin, Céline Séveno, Claire Usal, Katsunari Tezuka, and Ignacio Anegon. Inhibition of Chronic Rejection and Development of Tolerogenic T Cells after ICOS-ICOSL and CD40-CD40L Co-stimulation Blockade. *Transplantation* 2005 ; 80, 4.

Cho, B.K., V.P. Rao, Q. Ge, H.N. Eisen and J. Chen.(2000). Homeostasis-stimulated proliferation drives

Christensen, L.L.,Grunnet, N., Rudiger, N., Moller, B., and Birkeland, S.A. 1998. Indications of immunological tolerance in kidney transplantation. *Tissue Antigens* 51:637-644.

Ciancio G, Burke GW. Third Alemtuzumab (Campath-1H) in kidney transplantation. *Am J Transplant* 2008 ; 8 :15-20.

Clatworthy MR, Peter JF, Calne RY, Perpetua RU, Hale G, Waldmann H and Christopher J.E. Watson. Alemtuzumab (CAMPATH-1H) for the Treatment of Acute Rejection in Kidney Transplant Recipients: Long-Term Follow-Up. *Transplantation* 2009; 87: 7

Cobbold SP, Martin G, Qin S, Waldmann H. Monoclonal antibodies to promote marrow engraftment and tissue graft tolerance. *Nature* 1986; 323:164–166.

Cobbold SP, Martin G, Waldmann H. Monoclonal antibodies for the prevention of graft-versus-host disease and marrow graft rejection: The depletion of T cell subsets in vitro and in vivo. *Transplantation* 1986; 42:239- 247

Cosimi AB, Colvin RB, Burton RC et al. Use of monoclonal antibodies to T-cell subsets for immunologic monitoring and treatment in recipients of renal allografts. *N Engl J Med* 1981 ; 305 : 308-14.

Fadi Issa, Joanna Hester, Ryoichi Goto, Satish N. Nadig, Tim E. Goodacre and Kathryn Wood. Ex Vivo–Expanded Human Regulatory T Cells Prevent the Rejection of Skin Allografts in a Humanized Mouse Model. *Transplantation* 2010;90: 1321–1327

Fadi Issa, Joanna Hester, Ryoichi Goto, Satish N. Nadig, Tim E. Goodacre, and Kathryn Wood. Ex Vivo–Expanded Human Regulatory T Cells Prevent the Rejection of Skin Allografts in a Humanized Mouse Model. *Transplantation* 2010; 90: 1321–1327

Fehr, T. and M. Sykes (2004). Tolerance induction in clinical transplantation. *Transpl Immunol*13:117-30.

Fishman J. Infection in solid-organ transplantation. *N Engl J Med* 2007; 357: 2601-2614

Flavio Vincenti, Christian Larsen, Antoine Durrbach, Thomas Wekerle, Bjorn Nashan, Gilles Blancho, Philippe Lang, Josep Grinyo, Philip F. Halloran, Kim Solez, David Hagerty, Elliott Levy, Wenjiong Zhou, Kannan Natarajan, and Bernard Charpentier, for the Belatacept Study Group. Costimulation blockade with belatacep in renal transplantation. *N Engl J* Med 2005 353;8

Fuchs EJ and Matzinger P. B cells turn off virgin but not memory T cells. *Science* 1992; 13;258(5085):1156-9

G. Roussey-Kesler, M. Giral, A. Moreau, J.-F. Subrac, C. Legendred, C. Noele, E. Pillebout, S. Brouard and J.-P.Soulillou. Clinical Operational Tolerance after Kidney Transplantation 2006. *Am J transplant* 6: 736–746

Gallon, L., E. Gagliardini, A. Benigni, D. Kaufman, A. Waheed, M. Noris and G. Remuzzi.(2006). Immunophenotypic analysis of cellular infiltrate of renal allograft biopsies in patients with acute rejection after induction with alemtuzumab (Campath-1H). *Clin J Am Soc Nephrol* 1:539-45.

Galon, J., Franchimont, D., Hiroi, N., Frey, G., Boettner, A., Ehrhart-Bornstein, M., O'Shea, J.J., Chrousos, G.P. and Bornstein, S.R. Gene profiling reveals unknown enhancing and suppressive actions of glucocorticoids on immune cells. *FASEB J*. 2002, 16:61-71

Graca L, CobboldSP,Waldmann H. Identification of regulatory T cells in tolerated allografts. *J Exp Med*. 2002; 195:1641-1646.

Hale G, Slavin S, Goldman JM, et al. Alemtuzumab (Campath-1H) for treatment of lymphoid malignancies in the age of nonmyeloablative conditioning? *Bone Marrow Transplant* 2002; 30: 797.

Hara M, Kingsley CI, Niimi M, et al. IL-10 is required for regulatory T cells to mediate tolerance to alloantigens in vivo. *J Immunol*. 2001; 166: 3789-3796.

Hengartner H, Odermatt B, Schneider R, et al. Deletion of self-reactive T cells before entry into the thymus medulla. Nature 1988; 336:388-90.

Hori S, Nomura T, Sakaguchi S. Control of regulatory T cell development by the transcription factor Foxp3 [see comment]. *Science* 2003; 299: 1057.

Ildstad S. T., S. M. Wren, J. A. Bluestone, S. A. Barbaieri, D. Stephany, and D. H. Sachs. 1986. Effect of selective T cell depletion of host and/or donor bone marrow on lymphopoietic repopulation, tolerance, and graft-vs-host disease in mixed allogeneic chimeras (B10+ B10.D2-B10). *J. Immunol*. 136:28.

Ildstad, S. T., S. M. Wren, J. A. Bluestone, S. A. Barbieri, andD. H. Sach. 1985. Characterization of mixed allogeneic chimeras: immunocompetence, in vitro reactivity and genetic specificity of tolerance. J. Exp. Med. 162:231 .and immune response gene phenotype of T-helper cells .*J Exp Med* 153 :1286.

Imai A, Suzuki T, Sugitani A, *et al.* A novel fully human anti-CD40 monoclonal antibody, 4D11, for kidney transplantation in cynomolgus monkeys. *Transplantation* 2007 ; 84 : 1020-8.

J. A. Bluestone, W. Liua,b, J. M. Yabub, Z. G. Laszikc, A. Putnama,b, M. Belingherib, D. M. Grossa,d, R. M. Townsende and F. Vincentib. The Effect of Costimulatory and Interleukin 2 Receptor Blockade on Regulatory T Cells in Renal Transplantation. *Am J Transplant* 2008; 8: 2086–2096

J. Leruta, and A. Sanchez-Fueyo. An Appraisal of Tolerance in Liver Transplantation. *Am J transp* 2006; 6: 1774–1780

Jian Zheng, Yinping Liu, Yu-Lung Lau and Wenwei Tu. CD40-activated B cells are more potent than immature dendritic cells to induce and expand CD4+ regulatory T cells. *Cellular & Molecular Immunology* 2010: 7, 44–50

Kawai T, Andrews D, Colvin RB, et al. Thromboembolic complications after treatment with monoclonal antibody against CD40 ligand. *Nat Med* 2000; 6: 114.

Kawai T, Cosimi AB, Colvin RB et al. Mixed allogeneic chimerism and renal allograft tolerance in cynomolgus monkeys *Transplantation* 1995: 59: 256

Kawai, T., A.B. Cosimi, T.R. Spitzer, N. Tolkoff-Rubin, M. Suthanthiran, S.L. Saidman, J. Shaffer, F.I. Preffer, R. Ding, V. Sharma, J.A. Fishman, B. Dey, D.S. Ko, M. Hertl, N.B. Goes, W. Wong, W.W. Williams, Jr., R.B. Colvin, M. Sykes and D.H. Sachs. (2008). HLA-mismatched renal transplantation without maintenance immunosuppression. *N Engl J Med* 358:353-61.

Kawai, T., et al. HLA-Mismatched Renal Transplantation without Maintenance Immunosuppression. *N Engl J Med; 358: 353-61*

Kenneth A. Newell, Adam Asare, Allan D. Kirk, Trang D. Gisler, Kasia Bourcier, Manikkam Suthanthiran, William J. Burlingham, William H. Marks, Ignacio Sanz, Robert I. Lechler, Maria P. Hernandez-Fuentes, Laurence A. Turka, and Vicki L. Seyfert-Margolis, for the Immune Tolerance Network ST507 Study Group. Identification of a B cell signature associated with renal transplant tolerance in humans. *J Clin Invest.* 2010; 120:1836–1847

Khan, A. et al. (1996) Thymic dependence of loss of tolerance in mixed allogeneic bone marrow chimeras after depletion of donor antigen. Peripheral mechanisms do not contribute to maintenance of tolerance. *Transplantation* 62, 380–387

Kirk AD, Burkly LC, Batty DS, et al. Treatment with humanized monoclonal antibody against CD154 prevents acute renal allograft rejection in nonhuman primates. *Nat Med* 1999; 5: 686.

Kirkman RL, Barret LV, Gaulton GN, Kelley V, Ythier A, Strom TB. Administration of an anti-interleukin 2 receptor monoclonal antibody prolongs cardiac allograft survival in mice. *J Exp Med* 1985; 162: 358-62.

Kohler G, Milstein C. Continuous cultures of fused cells secreting antibody of predefined specificity. Nature 1975; 256:495–497.

Kurtz J., Wekerle T., and Sykes M. Tolerance in mixed chimerism, a role for regulatory cells ? *TRENDS in Immunology* 2004: 25; 10

Larsen CP, Pearson TC, Adams AB et al. Rational development of LEA29Y (belatacept), a high-affinity variant of CTLA4-Ig with potent immunosuppressive properties. *Am J Transplant* 2005; 5:443–453.

Long E, Wood KJ. Regulatory T cells in transplantation: transferring mouse studies to the clinic. *Transplantation* 2009; 88: 1050.

Louis, S., C. Braudeau, M. Giral, A. Dupont, F. Moizant, N. Robillard, A. Moreau, J.P. Soulillou and S.

Brouard. Contrasting CD25hiCD4+T cells/FOXP3 patterns in chronic rejection and operational drug-free tolerance. *Transplantation 2006:* 81:398-407.

MorelliAE,ThomsonAW. Tolerogenic dendritic cells and the quest for transplant tolerance. *Nat Rev Immunol* 2007; 7: 610.

Nadig SN, Wieckiewicz J, Wu DC, et al. In vivo prevention of trans- plant arteriosclerosis by ex vivo-expanded human regulatory T cells. *Nat Med* 2010; 16: 809

Nick D. Jones, Nick C. Fluck, Andrew L. Mellor, Peter J. Morris and Kathryn J. Wood. The induction of transplantation tolerance by intrathymic (i.t.) delivery of alloantigen: a critical relationship between i.t. deletion, thymic export of new T cells and the timing of transplantation. *International Immunology* No.11:1637–1646

Nossal GJ. Negative selection of lymphocytes. Cell 1994; 76:229-39

Ojo A., Held P., Port F., Wolfe R., Leichtman A., Young E. et al. Chronic renal failure after transplantation of non-renal organ. *N Engl J Med* 2003; 349 (10):931-940

Oluwole SF, Chowdhmy NC, Fawwaz RA. Induction of donor- specific unresponsiveness to rat cardiac allografts by pretreatment with intrathymic donor MHC class I antigens. *Transplantation* 1993; 55: 1396-1402.

Ortho Multicenter Transplant Study Group.A randomized clinical trial of OKT3 monoclonal antibody for acute rejection of cadaveric renal transplants. *N Engl J Med* 1985; 313: 337–342

Owens, M.L., Maxwell, J.G., Goodnight, J., and Wolcott, M.W. 1975. Discontinuance of immunosupression in renal patients. *ArchSurg* 110:1450-1451.

Philip F., immunosuppressive drugs for kidney transplantation. *N Engl J Med* 2004; 351: 2715-2729

Posselt et al. Induction of Donor-Specific Unresponsiveness by Intrathymic Islet Transplantation. 1990 *Science*

Qin SX, Cobbold S, Benjamin R,Waldmann H. Induction of classical transplantation tolerance in the adult. *J Exp Med.* 1989; 169:779-794.

Read S, Malmstrom V, Powrie F. Cytotoxic T lymphocyte-associated antigen 4 plays an essential role in the function of CD4+CD25+ regulatory cells that control intestinal inflammation. *J Exp Med.* 2000; 192:295-302.

Remuzzi G, Ferrazzi P, Bontempelli M, Senni M, Glauber M, et al. Preliminary results of intrathymic injection of donor cells to prevent acute rejection in human heart transplantation (1995). *J Am Soc Nephrol* 6: 1291-1294

Remuzzi G, Rossini M, Imberti O, and Perico N. Kidney graft survival in rats without immunosuppressants after intrathymic glomerular transplantation. *The Lancet* 1991

Rosa Bacchetta, Uwe Jansen, Silvia Gregori, MaurilioPonzoni, GiorgiaSerafini, Claudia Sartirana, Carlo TerenzioPaties, Ute Schulz, Katharina Fleischhauer, ElisabettaZino, Stefan Tomiuk, and Maria GraziaRoncarolo. Molecular and functional characterization of allogantigen-specific anergic T cells suitable for cell therapy. *haematologica* 2010; 95(12)

Roussey-Kesler, G., Giral, M., Moreau, A., Subra, F.F., Legendre, C., Noel, C., Pillebout, E., Brouard, S., and Soulillou, J.P. 2006.Clinical operational tolerance after kidney transplantation. *Am J Transplant* 6:736-746.

Sagoo P, et al. Development of a cross-platform bio- marker signature to detect renal transplant tolerance in humans. *J Clin Invest.* 2010; 120:1848–1861

Sakaguchi S, Sakaguchi N, Asano M, et al. Immunologic self-tolerance maintained by activated T cells expressing IL-2 receptor alpha-chains (CD25). Breakdown of a single mechanism of self-tolerance causes various autoimmune diseases. *J Immunol* 1995; 155: 1151.

Sanchez-FueyoA,Weber M, Domenig C, Strom TB, Zheng XX. Tracking the immunoregulatory mechanisms active during allograft tolerance. *J Immunol.* 2002; 168:2274-2281

Sayegh MH, Turka LA. The role of T-cell costimulatory activation pathways in transplant rejection. *N Engl J Med* 1998; 338:1813

Scandling J.D. et al. Tolerance and Chimerism after Renal and Hematopoietic-Cell Transplantation. n *Engl J Med* 2008; 358;4

Schwartz RH. A cell culture model for T lymphocyte clonal anergy. *Science* 1990; 248(4961): 1349.

Scully R, Qin S, CobboldS,Waldmann H. Mechanisms in CD4 antibody-mediated transplantation tolerance: kinetics of induction, antigen dependency and role of regulatory T cells. *Eur J Immunol.* 1994; 24:2383-2392.

Seino, K. I., K. Fukao, K. Muramoto, K. Yanagisawa, Y. Takada, S. Kakuta, Y. Iwakura, L. Van Kaer, K. Takeda, T. Nakayama, et al. Requirement for natural killer T (NKT) cells in the induction of allograft tolerance. *Proc. Natl. Acad. Sci.*2001 98: 2577–2581.

Shapiro ME, Kirkman RL, Reed MH, et al. Monoclonal anti-L2 receptor antibody in primate renal transplantation. *Transplant Proc* 1987; 19: 594-98.

Sharabi Y, Sachs DH Mixed chimerism and permanent specific transplantation tolerance induced by a nonlethal preparative regimen. *J Exp Med* 1989: 169: 493

Shimizu J, Yamazaki S, Takahashi T, Ishida Y, Sakaguchi S. Stimulation of CD25+CD4+ regulatory T cells through GITR breaks immunological self-tolerance. *Nat Immunol.* 2002; 3:135-142.

Sophie Brouard, Elaine Mansfieldb, Christophe Braud, Li Li, Magali Girala, Szu-chuan Hsieh, Dominique Baetena, Meixia Zhangb, Joanna Ashton-Chess, Cecile Braudeau, Frank Hsieh, Alexandre Duponta, Annaik Pallier, Anne Moreau, Stephanie Louis, Catherine Ruiz, Oscar Salvatierra, Jean-Paul Soulillou, and Minnie Sarwa. Identification of a peripheral blood transcriptional biomarker panel associated with operational renal allograft tolerance. *PNAS* 2007; 39:15448–15453

Soulillou JP and Giral M. Controlling the incidence of infection and malignancy by modifying immunosuppression. *Transplantation* 2001; 72: S89-93

Soulillou JP, Cantarovich D, Le Mauff B, et al. Randomized controlled trial of a monoclonal antibody against the interleukin-2 receptor (33B3.1) as compared with rabbit antithymocyte globulin for prophylaxis against rejection of renal allografts. *N Engl J Med* 1990 ; 322 : 1175-82.

Soulillou JP, Peyronnet P, Le Mauff B, *et al.* Prevention of rejection of kidney transplants by monoclonal antibody directed against interleukin 2. *Lancet* 1987 ; 1 : 1339-42.

Stegall MD., Everson GT., Schroter G., Karrer F., Bilir B., Sternberg T. et al. Prednisone withdrawal late after adult liver transplantation reduces diabetes, hypertension and hypercholesterolemia without causing graft loss. *Hepatology* 1997; 25 (1): 173-177

Strober, S., D.L. Modry, R.T. Hoppe, J.L. Pennock, C.P. Bieber, B.I. Holm, S.W. Jamieson, E.B. Stinson, J.Schroder, H. Suomalainen and et al. (1984). Induction of specific unresponsiveness to heart allografts in mongrel dogs treated with total lymphoid irradiation and antithymocyte globulin. *J Immunol* 132:1013-8.

Strober, S., M. Dhillon, M. Schubert, B. Holm, E. Engleman, C. Benike, R. Hoppe, R. Sibley, J.A.Myburgh, G. Collins and et al. (1989). Acquired immune tolerance to cadaveric renal allografts. A study of three patients treated with total lymphoid irradiation. *N Engl J Med* 321:28-33.

Thornton AM, Shevach EM. CD4+CD25+ immunoregulatory T cells suppress polyclonal T cell activation in vitro by inhibiting interleukin 2 production. *J Exp Med.* 1998; 188:287-296.

Uehling, D.T., Hussey, J.L., Weinstein, A.B., Wank, R., and Bach, F.H. 1976. Cessation of immunosuppression after renal transplantation. *Surgery* 79:278-282.

Van Maurik A, HerberM,Wood KJ, Jones ND. Cutting edge: CD4+CD25+ alloantigen-specific immunoregulatory cells that can prevent CD8+ T cell-mediated graft rejection: implications for anti- CD154 immunotherapy. *J Immunol.* 2002; 169: 5401-5404.

Vincenti F, Kirkman R, Light S et al. Interleukin-2-receptor blockade with daclizumab to prevent acute rejection in renal transplantation. *N Engl J Med* 1998; 338: 161–165

Vincenti F, Larsen C, DurrbachA et al. Costimulation blockade with belatacept in renal transplantation.*N Engl J Med* 2005; 353:770–781.

Von Boehmer H, Kisielow P. Self-non-self discrimination by T cells. *Science* 1990; 248:1369-73.

Waldmann H. Reprogramming the immune system. *Immunological Reviews* 2002; 185: 227-235

Webster AC, Pankhurst T, Rinaldi F, *et al.* Monoclonal and polyclonal antibody therapy for treating acute rejection in kidney transplant recipients: a systematic review of randomized trial data. *Transplantation* 2006 ; 81 : 953-65.

Wise MP, Bemelman F, CobboldSP,Waldmann H. Linked suppression of skin graft rejection can operate through indirect recognition. *J Immunol.* 1998; 161:5813-5816

Wu, Z., S.J. Bensinger, J. Zhang, C. Chen, X. Yuan, X. Huang, J.F. Markmann, A. Kassaee, B.R. Rosengard, W.W. Hancock, M.H. Sayegh and L.A. Turka. (2004). Homeostatic proliferation is a barrier to transplantation tolerance. *Nat Med* 10:87-92.

Xia MQ, Hale G, Lifely MR, et al. Structure of the CAMPATH-1 antigen, a glycosylphosphatidylinositol-anchored glycoprotein which is an exceptionally good target for complement lysis. *Biochem J* 1993; 293: 633.

Yang, J., M.O. Brook, M. Carvalho-Gaspar, J. Zhang, H.E. Ramon, M.H. Sayegh, K.J. Wood, L.A. Turka and N.D. Jones. (2007). Allograft rejection mediated by memory T cells is resistant to regulation. *Proc Natl Acad Sci U S A*104:19954-9.

Yukihiro Tomita,Abrar Khan, and Megan Sykes. Role of lntrathymic Clonal Deletion and Peripheral Anergy in Transplantation Tolerance Induced by Bone Marrow Transplantation in Mice Conditioned with a Nonmyeloablative Regimen. *J Immunol* 1994

10

Mechanisms of Tolerance: Role of the Thymus and Persistence of Antigen in Calcineurin-Induced Tolerance of Renal Allografts in MGH Miniature Swine

Joseph R. Scalea, Isabel Hanekamp and Kazuhiko Yamada*
Transplantation Biology Research Center, Massachusetts General Hospital, Harvard Medical School, USA
*(*Address any correspondence to Kazuhiko Yamada)*

1. Introduction

The induction of donor-specific tolerance remains a major goal of clinical transplantation. Partially inbred MGH miniature swine, in which swine leukocyte antigens (SLA) have been defined and fixed, have been utilized extensively as a preclinical model for tolerance induction. This preclinical large-animal model is an invaluable tool for studying the mechanism of transplantation tolerance. Recently, we have investigated the role of the persistence of donor antigen in the maintenance of tolerance and the peripheral regulatory cells' ability to confer tolerance to naïve animals.

Mechanisms of tolerance can be elucidated in part by attempting to interfere with (or "break") the tolerant state. We have previously reported that a short course of calineurin inhibition permits the uniform development of long-term, donor-specific tolerance to renal allografts in juvenile miniature swine. Once tolerant, animals that undergo graft nephrectomy and immediate retransplantation accept donor-MHC matched kidneys while maintaining stable renal function without further immunosuppression.

Utilizing this model we have attempted to break tolerance using several strategies. These have included administration of recombinant IL-2 to provide additional T-cell help, manipulation of the host thymus, and removal of donor grafts. Our data indicate that (1) presence of an intact thymus is essential for the induction, but not for the maintenance of tolerance; (2) the persistence of the donor renal graft is essential for the indefinite continuation of tolerance; and (3) the pathway of donor antigen presentation, in tolerant and previously tolerant animals, is important for preservation or loss of the tolerant state. Although obvious limitations exist with regard to animal studies, our consistently reproducible results using MHC inbred miniature swine provide a unique opportunity to study the mechanisms of transplantation in animals physiologically similar to humans. As we have previously shown, our results are highly suggestive of what will occur in clinical human transplantation protocols.

2. Abbreviations

APC: Antigen Presenting Cell
CTL: Cytotoxic T-Lymphocytes
CyA: Cyclosporine A
FoxP3+: Forkhead Box 3
HSC: Hematopoietic Stem Cells
IL-2: Interleukin 2
MGH: Massachusetts General Hospital
MHC: Major Histocompatibility Complex
PBL: Peripheral Blood Lymphocytes
SLA: swine leukocyte antigens
UNOS: United Network for Organ Sharing

3. Importance of tolerance

According to UNOS, over 110,000 patients are currently awaiting organ transplantation in the United States. However, in 2010 there were only 14,506 donors. Although the benefits of valued organ transplants are substantial, patients must accept the risks of the required immunosuppression. Immunosuppressive protocols generally include T-cell depletion in the perioperative period, followed by initiation of calcineurin inhibition, mycophenolic acid, and steroids. Many centers have been successful in reducing or eliminating the use of chronic steroids, but patients are still susceptible to the morbidity associated with immunosuppression (1,2).

Transplantation tolerance, or immunologic non-responsiveness to donor antigen, would reduce the morbidity observed with immunosuppression (3). Immunosuppression has been associated with malignancy, infection, end-organ damage, and economic burden. As many as 30% of renal transplant recipients develop skin cancer within 10 years of transplantation (4) similar results have been reported in the cardiac transplant patient population (4,5). Furthermore, viral and bacterial infections are more likely to occur in the immunocompromised patient and although death rates from infection have decreased every decade for the last 30 years, patients at the extremes of age are still considered high-risk for infectious complications (6). End-organ failure is also a potential complication of immunosuppression; renal failure, likely due to calcineurin inhibitors, has been associated with chronic immunosuppression (7,8). Additionally, the lifetime economic cost of immunosuppressive drugs alone following kidney transplantation range from $68,000 to $88,000 depending on the selected regimen (9,10).

Tolerance strategies would potentially alleviate the risks of malignancy, organ-failure, and infectious complications as well as the cost associated with anti-rejection medications. Recent clinical successes in inducing tolerance to kidney (11,12) and liver (13) grafts have proven that tolerance strategies are clinically applicable.

4. Antigen presentation of allogeneic antigens and tolerance

Tissue antigens are any proteins which when presented by the major histocompatability complex lead to immunologic responses (14,15). Proof of this MHC restriction earned Zinkernagel and Doherty the Nobel Prize in 1996 for work that was done in the 1970s (15).

In transplantation, these antigens can be presented by either donor or recipient antigen presenting cells (APCs). The presentation of antigen to recipient lymphocytes potentially leads to allosensitization of recipient T-cells. In direct alloantigen presentation, donor tissue antigens are recognized by recipient T-cells in the context of donor MHC molecules. Conversely, indirect antigen presentation occurs when alloantigens are recognized in the setting of recipient MHC. Recently, one group described an additional "semi-direct" mechanism in which the recipient cells acquire the intact MHC from the donor and subsequently present antigen in the context of the newly acquired donor MHC (16).

A comprehensive understanding of antigen presentation is helpful for elucidating both transplantation rejection and tolerance. In allotransplantation, passenger lymphocytes and professional APCs within the transplanted organ present donor antigen to recipient T-cells leading to acute rejection (17,18). Indirect presentation of donor antigen may continue indefinitely and is generally associated with chronic rejection (19). These two pathways, however, are not mutually exclusive as early rejection episodes portend increased risk of future chronic rejection (20). While these alloreactive stimuli are known to play a role in rejection, small and large animal studies of tolerance have also demonstrated the importance of donor antigen presentation in the establishment of a tolerogenic milieu (21-23).

Mechanisms of transplantation tolerance have been broadly categorized as "central" or "peripheral" on the basis of whether T-cells are rendered unresponsive during their maturation in the thymus or after they have left the thymus, respectively (24-26). Deletion is thought to be the mechanism responsible for central tolerance, whereas peripheral tolerance is likely mediated by anergy, suppression, or ignorance (27). Central tolerance can be induced by exposing newly developed T-cells to alloantigens on the progeny of hematopoietic stem cells (HSC) injected either at a very early stage in the development of the immune system, either in utero or in neonates (28,29) or in adult animals following ablation of mature T cells (30-32). This tolerance is deletional and presumably utilizes the same process of negative selection that is responsible for self-tolerance during T-cell maturation in the thymus (29,33). In addition to bone marrow transplantation, another strategy to induce central tolerance is thymic transplantation. We, and others, have demonstrated successful induction of tolerance with donor thymic grafts across allogeneic and xenogeneic barriers in small and large animal models (34-36).

Peripheral tolerance to alloantigens has been induced in many ways, generally by providing alloantigen in a non-stimulatory fashion or at a time when the aggressive alloreactive response has been simultaneously averted. Peripheral tolerance has been ascribed to the same processes as those invoked to explain peripheral tolerance to self - i.e. anergy(37-41), peripheral deletion(42,43), clonal ignorance (32) and regulation (44-49).

Investigation of peripheral cellular suppression began over 40 years ago, though the implications of these findings were not immediately evident. Tada et al. demonstrated that when KLH primed T-lymphocytes were passively transferred to mice prior to immunization with DNP-KLH, antibody formation was inhibited. In contrast, when these cells were transferred after immunization with DNP-KLH, antibody formation was not inhibited. These results demonstrated that a peripheral T-cell response was suppressing immunologic response to immunization (50,51). This phenomenon was studied extensively in the 1970s and 1980s, and Castagnoli et al. found that the supernatant from antigen-specific suppressive thymoma cells was capable of suppressing an alloreactive response to the same antigen. These and other data suggested that the effects of purported T suppressor cells are mediated by one or more soluble factors (52,53). Our understanding of these suppressive cells was broadened further when Sakaguchi et al. demonstrated that the lack of ostensible suppressor cells in nude/nude mice led to severe autoimmune disease, which could be rectified by inoculation with nude/+ thymocyte suspensions. Sakaguchi and his colleagues then successfully phenotyped these suppressor/regulatory cells as $CD4^{+ve}$, $CD25hi^{+ve}$ (and some years later, FoxP3+) and showed that these cells are likely responsible for tolerance of self, and possibly necessary for the maintenance of peripheral tolerance (47,54).

5. Importance of large animal models

While small animal data are valuable for defining mechanisms, large animal studies are imperative for the development of preclinical models (55). Numerous strategies for tolerance induction in rodents have proven fruitful, though few have been successfully translated to humans, non-human primates, or other large animals (55,56). Likely owing to the increased complexity of the immune system in large animals and longer-term exposure to environmental antigens, the results from tolerance induction protocols in large animals have been less successful than rodent studies (55-57). Another possible cause for this difference is that MHC class II expression on endothelial cells that is the first target in the alloreactive response to in solid organs. Murine "resting" endotherial cells do not express MHC class II while swine, whereas primate endothelial cells do (58).

6. MHC inbred MGH miniature swine: A unique large animal model to study mechanisms of acceptance/rejection

Miniature swine have been developed in our laboratory over the past thirty years as a model system for studies of transplantation biology. Swine were chosen for this purpose because they represent one of the few large animal species in which breeding characteristics make genetic experiments possible. Swine have a relatively large litter size (3-10 offspring) and a short gestational cycle (3 months). They reach sexual maturity at approximately 6 months of age, and sows have an estrous cycle every 3 weeks. These breeding characteristics have made it possible to develop MHC homozygous lines of miniature swine in a relatively short time and have also made it possible to isolate new MHC recombinants, to breed them to homozygosity, and to carry out short-term backcross experiments in order to identify and study the segregation of genetic characteristics (59). Our miniature swine thus represent the only large animal model in which MHC genetics can be reproducibly controlled. As such, these animals have been particularly useful in assessing the effects of MHC matching on rejection and/or tolerance induction (60,61).

At present, we maintain swine of three homozygous SLA haplotypes, SLA^a, SLA^c, SLA^d and five lines bearing intra-SLA recombinant haplotypes as illustrated in Fig. 1. All of these lines differ by minor histocompatibility loci, thus providing a model in which most of the transplantation combinations relevant to human transplantation can be mimicked. Thus, for example, transplants within an MHC homozygous herd simulate transplants between HLA identical siblings, while transplants between herds resemble cadaveric or non-matched sibling transplants. Likewise, transplants between pairs of heterozygotes can be chosen to resemble parent into offspring or one-haplotype mismatched sibling transplants (22). In addition, we have chosen one subline of our SLA^{dd} animals for further inbreeding, in order to produce a fully inbred line of miniature swine. This subline reached a coefficient of inbreeding of >96%, leading for the first time to long-term acceptance of reciprocal skin grafts (62). These animals have also made it possible to carry out adoptive transfer experiments for the first time in a large animal model, as reported here (Scalea et al, manuscript in preparation).

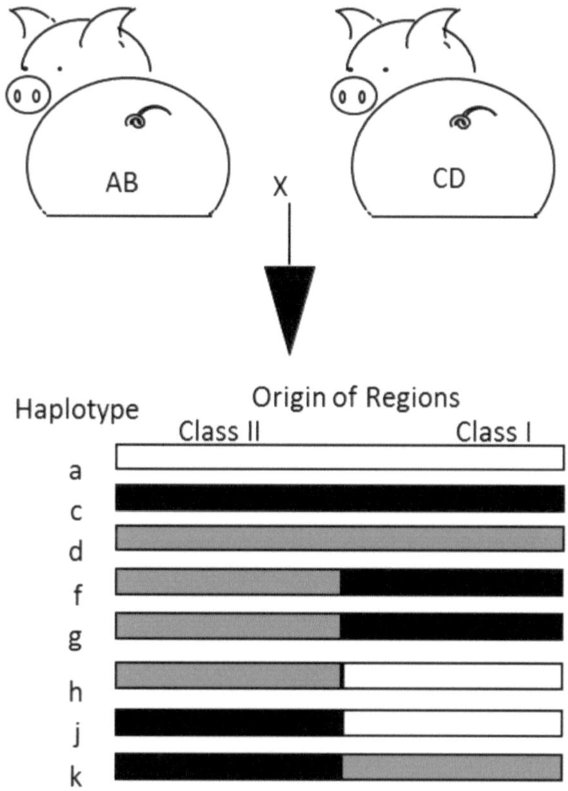

Fig. 1. The serial breeding of MGH swine has led to fixed, defined MHC classes. Transplantation between lines of these swine allows researchers to mimic living-related and cadaveric organ transplantation.

7. Thymic-dependent and antigen-dependent tolerance in MHC miniature swine renal transplant models

7.1 Induction of tolerance with a short course and high dose calcineurin inhibitor in MGH miniature swine

i. **Effects of CyA on renal allograft survival across a selective MHC barrier:** We have attempted to induce tolerance using pharmacological limitation of T cell help. For this purpose, class I mismatched renal transplants were performed using a short course of treatment with Cyclosporin A (CyA) (63,64). We chose to study the effect of CyA across a selective *two-haplotype class I mismatched, class II matched* barrier, since without immunosuppression such recipients uniformly reject renal allografts within three weeks without immunosuppression (Fig. 2). As reported in our initial study of this treatment regimen, a twelve-day course of CyA (10-13 mg/kg/day) induced long-term, specific tolerance in eight of eight *two-haplotype class II matched, class I mismatched* recipients(64). This result has been reproduced subsequently in more than fifty additional CyA-treated animals, 100% of which develop long-term tolerance across a class I disparity. It is important to note that although this dose and the resulting blood levels (400-800 ng/dl) are high with respect to clinically acceptable values, the toxicity caused by such levels clinically is generally reversible if discontinued after a two- week course (65).

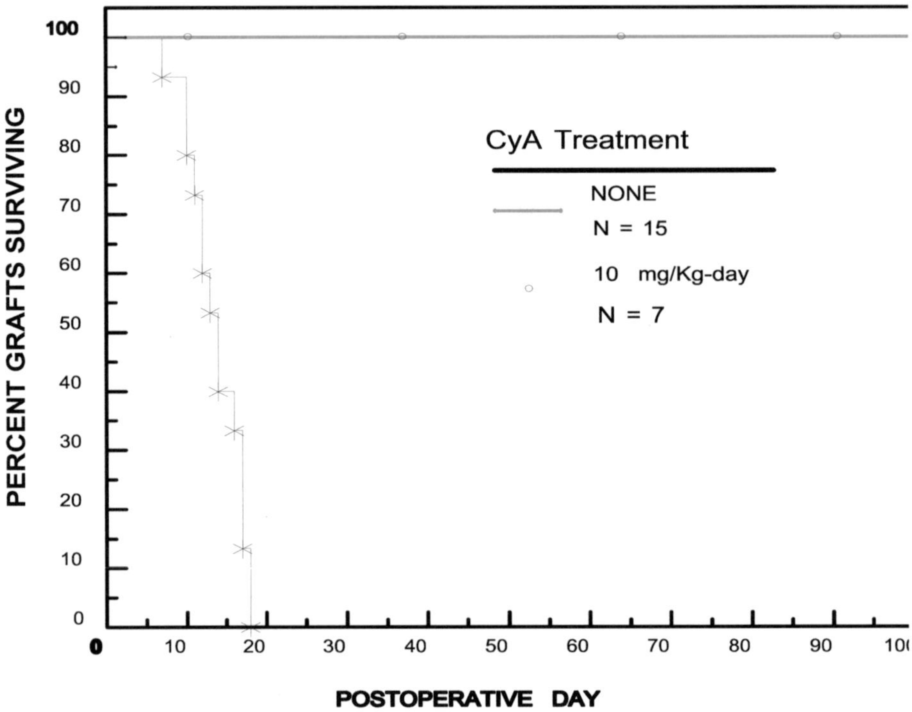

Fig. 2. With a short-course of high-dose Cyclosporine A, tolerance is uniformly established across an MHC class-I mismatch in MGH miniature swine (n>50).

ii. **Effects of CyA on renal allograft survival across other selective MHC barriers:** We have also studied whether tolerance is induced with a 12-day course of CyA therapy across further immunologic disparities. Although the CyA regimen was capable of prolonging renal allograft survival across a full MHC barrier, it did not induce long-term tolerance in any of the animals tested (64). However, since pharmacologic help limitation by CyA should be possible regardless of the MHC disparity, we also tested the effect of the CyA regimen on renal transplants selectively mismatched for class II or for one full haplotype (66,67). Of seven *CyA-treated class I matched, class II mismatched* kidney transplants, five (71%) were accepted long-term, whereas two rejected on days 20 and 39, respectively (68). Similarly, of six CyA-treated recipients of single haplotype mismatched kidney allografts, two rejected (on days 31 and 37), while four (67%) accepted long-term. Thus, tolerance was possible across both class II and single haplotype full mismatches, but with a lower success rate and with a less stable clinical course than across a selective class I mismatch.

iii. **Effects of Tacrolimus on renal allograft survival across other selective MHC barriers** According to the latter hypothesis, increasingly potent immunosuppression of T-cell help would be required for increasing the extent of the MHC disparity (i.e. class I < class II < one full haplotype < two full haplotypes). Our subsequent results using

Tacrolimus corroborate this finding (69). We have demonstrated that Tacrolimus at blood levels between 35 and 80ng/ml facilitates tolerance induction not only across a class I barrier, but also across a two-haplotype full MHC barrier in-vivo (69). However, like CyA-induced tolerance across class I mismatched barrier, thymic-dependent mechanisms are involved in this Tacrolimus-induced tolerance (70). Tolerance was only induced in juvenile hosts (see more details blow).

7.2 Mechanisms of tolerance using high-dose calcineurin inhibitors

To understand better the mechanisms of tolerance induction, both the role of thymus (i.e. aging) and persistence of donor antigens in tolerance induction/maintenance have been studied.

i. *Thymic dependent tolerance:* A series of experiments were performed using aged and thymectomized animals. The data from these studies demonstrated that when aged animals underwent class-I mismatched kidney transplantation followed by 12-days of CyA, tolerance could not be induced. Similarly, thymectomy prior to kidney transplantation interfered with the development of tolerance across the same class-I barrier (71). Interestingly, thymectomy in a maintenance period (beyond 6 weeks after transplantation) did not abrogate tolerance (70). Recent work from this laboratory has also demonstrated thymic dependent mechanisms play important role in tacrolimus induced tolerance in both miniature swine and nonhuman primates (Yamada et al manuscript in preparation). These studies indicated that that 1) tolerance induction is thymus-dependent, whereas tolerance-maintenance is not and 2) an interaction between central and peripheral mechanisms of tolerance is likely occurring in the stably tolerant animal.

ii. *Regulatory mechanisms and stability of tolerance – Class I mismatched kidney transplantation with a 12-day course of CyA:*

   a. In vitro assays suggesting involvement of regulatory mechanisms

Because thymectomy post-transplantation did not lead to the abrogation of tolerance, investigators postulated that a suppressive peripheral regulatory mechanism had developed in class I mismatched tolerant model. When peripheral blood lymphocytes (PBL) from long-term tolerant animals were stimulated with donor PBLs, and re-cultured with naïve SLA matched PBLs plus either donor-PBLs or 3rd party PBLs, we observed suppression of the naïve-SLA anti-donor CTL response and maintenance of naïve-SLA anti-3rd party CTL responses (45). This co-culture assay demonstrated in-vitro that a peripheral cellular mechanism of suppression was present. To study activation and effector function of these purported regulatory cells, we performed co-culture assays in which PBLs taken from a tolerant animal were placed in a transwell culture system such that they were separated from donor PBLs by a permeable membrane (69). In previous co-culture CTL assays performed without the membrane barrier, we observed that naïve-recipient SLA matched PBLs were inhibited by the presence of PBLs taken from a tolerant animal. However, when the cells were separated by a permeable membrane, the cells were no longer suppressive (69,72). This demonstrated that 1) direct cell-to-cell contact is required for activation of the peripheral regulatory mechanism and 2) soluble factors produced by the peripheral regulatory cells are themselves incapable of regulatory effector activation in this class I mismatched kidney model.

   b. Exogenous T-cell help interfered with the induction of tolerance but not maintenance of tolerance

Based on these in-vivo and in-vitro data, we attempted to further define the role of regulatory cells in the MGH miniature swine model, by attempting to abrogate tolerance in animals. Because a lack or T cell help likely plays an essential role in calcineurin-induced tolerance, we administered exogenous IL-2 either 1) during the induction period (Days 8. 9 and 10) or 2) once animals were long-term tolerant (73). Much like our thymectomy experiments, we found that whereas IL-2 administration can prohibit the induction of tolerance if administered perioperatively, treatment with exogenous IL-2 failed to abrogate tolerance in long-term tolerant (LTT) animals (73). To further distill the role of T-cell help required for the anti-donor cellular response in tolerant animals, we challenged LTT animals with skin grafts from class-I donor/class-II third party donors instead of IL-2 (74). We reasoned that the class-II disparate graft may be capable of providing the necessary T-cell help by stimulating the alloreactive CD4+ population. Although recipient animals experienced a brief rejection crisis following skin grafting, they remained tolerant in the long-term (74). Thus, once established, the peripheral mechanism of tolerance is steadily stable, and capable of suppressing further stimulation with donor antigen.

c. Role of graft in maintenance of tolerance

Because 1) removal of the thymus in a tolerant animal did not lead to tolerance abrogation and 2) based on the in-vitro data suggesting that tolerance was mediated by an active cellular process, we next questioned if the graft itself was providing the tolerogenic stimulus for maintenance of tolerance. To test this hypothesis, we designed several experiments in which the tolerated graft was removed and replaced by a donor-MHC matched graft (21) (75). In the first experiment, long-term tolerant animals underwent graft nephrectomy and immediate retransplantation with a donor-MHC matched graft. As previously published, each animal uniformly accepted the retransplanted graft and never experienced rejection. In the next experiments, we introduced a period of "absence-of-donor-antigen" by removing the tolerated kidney from LTT animals and replacing it with a self-MHC matched graft to support the life of the animal. Then, at 1 and 3 months, animals were retransplanted with a donor-MHC matched graft. When animals bearing self-MHC matched grafts underwent retransplantation from actual donors immediately after primary graft nephrectomy, all animal accepted kidney with stable renal function(21). However, we observed a brief rejection crisis followed by uniform acceptance when second kidneys were transplanted at one month after the primary graft nephrectomy. Moreover, as the period of absence-of-donor-antigen was increased to 3 months, retransplantation was followed by significant rejection crisis in two of three animals. One animal completely rejected the retransplanted graft within 2 months and the other had severe rejection episodes (21). Furthermore, when skin grafts from class-I donor/class-II third party donors were transplanted onto animals during absence of donor kidneys, second kidneys transplanted 3 months after primary kidney nephrectomy were uniformly rejected in an accelerated manner (<7 days), indicating a "broken tolerance" (Yamada et al., manuscript in preparation). This series of experiments confirmed that the kidney plays an essential role in the maintenance of tolerance. Because we observed rejection of the retransplanted donor-MHC matched graft following periods without donor antigen present, it is likely that the kidney provides a constant tolerogenic stimulus via a peripheral mechanism which is required for maitenence of T-regulatory cells.

d. Current evidence for the role of T-regulatory cells in peripheral tolerance

The previous experiment clarified our understanding of the role that persistence of donor antigen plays in the maintenance of tolerance and provided indirect evidence that this process was mediated by T-regulatory cells (21,45). We then postulated that, if T-regulatory cells were responsible for maintaining tolerance then removal of T-regulatory cells from a LTT animal, may lead to abrogation. Thus, we next attempted to hasten the onset of rejection by performing an extensive leukapheresis immediately prior to retransplantation of a donor-matched graft following a three month period of absence-of-donor-antigen. In eight of ten animals in this protocol, we observed rejection of a subsequently retransplanted donor-MHC matched graft, and complete or chronic rejection in four of ten animals (Scalea et al, manuscript being submitted). When the leukapheresed cells were evaluated in vitro, we observed that they were capable of suppressing a naïve anti-donor response in a cell mediated lympholysis (CTL) co-culture assay in a donor-specific manner (Scalea et al, manuscript in preparation).

Having determined that these cells were capable of suppressing a naïve response in-vitro (45), we then questioned whether they would be suppressive in-vivo. However, based on our absence-of-donor-antigen and leukapheresis with retransplantation experiments, it appeared that both the kidney and peripheral regulatory cells were important for the continuation of tolerance (21). To resolve the contribution of the circulating cellular compartment versus the kidney itself, we adoptively transferred leukapheresed cells from tolerant donors that were from our most highly-inbred line of miniature swine. We found that when either the LTT kidney was transplanted into a naïve animal, or leukapheresed cells were transferred along with a naïve donor graft, there was prolonged graft survival, but not long-term acceptance (Scalea et al, manuscript in preparation). Conversely, when the leukapheresed cells and kidney were transferred from the same LTT animal, the naïve recipient experienced long-term graft survival. Additionally, these recipients were unresponsive to donor in CML assay as early as day 28, and in one case, as late as 150 days following transplantation (Scalea et al, manuscript being submitted).

8. Summary

In summary, our understanding of the mechanisms of tolerance has blossomed over the last several decades. It is clear that while small animal data has helped elucidate the molecular basis for tolerance, large animal studies are required for the development of preclinical models. While animal models have some limitations, our unique model allows us to model accurately the clinical scenarios of clinical transplantation. Using this model, we have demonstrated the importance of the thymus for tolerance induction and the persistence of donor antigen for the maintenance of tolerance. Recent work in our laboratory has demonstrated that stable peripheral tolerance is mediated by a cellular mechanism that is best explained by the presence of T-regulatory cells.

9. References

[1] Yamani MH, Taylor DO, Czerr J et al. Thymoglobulin induction and steroid avoidance in cardiac transplantation: results of a prospective, randomized, controlled study. Clin Transplant 2008;22: 76-81.

[2] Sarwal MM, Yorgin PD, Alexander S et al. Promising early outcomes with a novel, complete steroid avoidance immunosuppression protocol in pediatric renal transplantation. Transplantation 2001;72: 13-21.

[3] Griesemer AD, Sorenson EC, Hardy MA. The role of the thymus in tolerance. Transplantation 2010;90: 465-474.

[4] Carroll RP, Segundo DS, Hollowood K et al. Immune phenotype predicts risk for posttransplantation squamous cell carcinoma. J Am Soc Nephrol 2010;21: 713-722.

[5] Brewer JD, Colegio OR, Phillips PK et al. Incidence of and risk factors for skin cancer after heart transplant. Arch Dermatol 2009;145: 1391-1396.
[6] George JF, Pamboukian SV, Tallaj JA et al. Balancing rejection and infection with respect to age, race, and gender: clues acquired from 17 years of cardiac transplantation data. J Heart Lung Transplant 2010;29: 966-972.
[7] Scalea JR, Butler CC, Munivenkatappa RB et al. Pancreas transplant alone as an independent risk factor for the development of renal failure: a retrospective study. Transplantation 2008;86: 1789-1794.
[8] Ziolkowski J, Paczek L, Senatorski G et al. Renal function after liver transplantation: calcineurin inhibitor nephrotoxicity. Transplant Proc 2003;35: 2307-2309.
[9] Earnshaw SR, Graham CN, Irish WD, Sato R, Schnitzler MA. Lifetime cost-effectiveness of calcineurin inhibitor withdrawal after de novo renal transplantation. J Am Soc Nephrol 2008;19: 1807-1816.
[10] Yao G, Albon E, Adi Y et al. A systematic review and economic model of the clinical and cost-effectiveness of immunosuppressive therapy for renal transplantation in children. Health Technol Assess 2006;10: iii-xi, 1.
[11] Kawai T, Cosimi AB, Spitzer TR et al. HLA-mismatched renal transplantation without maintenance immunosuppression. N Engl J Med 2008;358: 353-361.
[12] Scandling JD, Busque S, Dejbakhsh-Jones S et al. Tolerance and chimerism after renal and hematopoietic-cell transplantation. N Engl J Med 2008;358: 362-368.
[13] Alexander SI, Smith N, Hu M et al. Chimerism and tolerance in a recipient of a deceased-donor liver transplant. N Engl J Med 2008;358: 369-374.
[14] Zinkernagel RM, Doherty PC. Restriction of in vitro T cell-mediated cytotoxicity in lymphocytic choriomeningitis within a syngeneic or semiallogeneic system. Nature 1974;248: 701-702.
[15] Zinkernagel RM, Doherty PC. Immunological surveillance against altered self components by sensitised T lymphocytes in lymphocytic choriomeningitis. Nature 1974;251: 547-548.
[16] Smyth LA, Herrera OB, Golshayan D, Lombardi G, Lechler RI. A novel pathway of antigen presentation by dendritic and endothelial cells: Implications for allorecognition and infectious diseases. Transplantation 2006;82: S15-S18.
[17] Sayegh MH. Why do we reject a graft? Role of indirect allorecognition in graft rejection. Kidney Int 1999;56: 1967-1979.
[18] Giangrande I, Yamada K, Germana S, Sachs DH, LeGuern C. Tolerant cells infiltrating class I mismatched swine kidney allografts lack the CD4 single positive subset and down regulate TCR gene expression. Transplant Proc 1997;29: 1164.
[19] Kuo E, Maruyama T, Fernandez F, Mohanakumar T. Molecular mechanisms of chronic rejection following transplantation. Immunol Res 2005;32: 179-185.
[20] Pascual M, Theruvath T, Kawai T, Tolkoff-Rubin N, Cosimi AB. Strategies to improve long-term outcomes after renal transplantation. N Engl J Med 2002;346: 580-590.
[21] Okumi M, Fishbein JM, Griesemer AD et al. Role of persistence of antigen and indirect recognition in the maintenance of tolerance to renal allografts. Transplantation 2008;85: 270-280.
[22] Rosengard BR, Ojikutu CA, Fishbein J, Kortz EO, Sachs DH. Selective breeding of miniature swine leads to an increased rate of acceptance of MHC-identical, but not of class-I disparate, renal allografts. J Immunol 1992;149: 1099-1103.

[23] Griesemer AD, LaMattina JC, Okumi M et al. Linked suppression across an MHC-mismatched barrier in a miniature swine kidney transplantation model. J Immunol 2008;181: 4027-4036.
[24] Wekerle T, Kurtz J, Bigenzahn S, Takeuchi Y, Sykes M. Mechanisms of transplant tolerance induction using costimulatory blockade. Curr Opin Immunol 2002;14: 592-600.
[25] Sachs DH. Transplantation tolerance. Transplant Proc 1998;30: 1627-1629.
[26] Sachs DH. Immunologic tolerance to organ transplants. J Gastrointestinal Surgery 1999;3: 105-110.
[27] Sykes M, Sachs DH. Immunobiology of transplantation. In: Dulbecco R, ed. Encyclopedia of Human Biology. San Diego: Academic Press, Inc., 1991: 357-365.
[28] Anderson D, Billingham RE, Lampkin GH, Medawar PB. The use of skin grafting to distinguish between monozygotic and dizygotic twins in cattle. Heredity 1951;5: 379.
[29] Inaba M, Inaba K, Hosono M et al. Distinct mechanisms of neonatal tolerance induced by dendritic cells and thymic B cells. J Exp Med 1991;173: 549-559.
[30] Rayfield LS, Brent L. Tolerance, immunocompetence, and secondary disease in fully allogeneic radiation chimeras. Transplantation 1983;36: 183-189.
[31] Ildstad ST, Sachs DH. Reconstitution with syngeneic plus allogeneic or xenogeneic bone marrow leads to specific acceptance of allografts or xenografts. Nature 1984;307(5947): 168-170.
[32] Tomita Y, Khan A, Sykes M. Role of intrathymic clonal deletion and peripheral anergy in transplantation tolerance induced by bone marrow transplantion in mice conditioned with a non-myeloablative regimen. J Immunol 1994;153: 1087-1098.
[33] Barclay AN, Mayrhofer G. Bone marrow origin of Ia-positive cells in the medulla of rat thymus. J Exp Med 1981;153: 1666.
[34] Zhao Y, Swenson K, Sergio JJ, Arn JS, Sachs DH, Sykes M. Skin graft tolerance across a discordant xenogeneic barrier. Nature Med 1996;2: 1211-1216.
[35] Yamada K, Shimizu A, Utsugi R et al. Thymic transplantation in miniature swine. II. Induction of tolerance by transplantation of composite thymokidneys to thymectomized recipients. J Immunol 2000;164: 3079-3086.
[36] Kamano C, Vagefi PA, Kumagai N et al. Vascularized thymic lobe transplantation in miniature swine: Thymopoiesis and tolerance induction across fully MHC-mismatched barriers. Proc Natl Acad Sci U S A 2004;101: 3827-3832.
[37] Charlton B, Auchincloss H, Jr., Fathman CG. Mechanisms of transplantation tolerance. Annu Rev Immunol 1994;12: 707-734.
[38] Kurtz J, Shaffer J, Lie A, Anosova N, Benichou G, Sykes M. Mechanisms of early peripheral CD4 T-cell tolerance induction by anti-CD154 monoclonal antibody and allogeneic bone marrow transplantation: evidence for anergy and deletion but not regulatory cells. Blood 2004;103: 4336-4343.
[39] Quezada SA, Jarvinen LZ, Lind EF, Noelle RJ. CD40/CD154 interactions at the interface of tolerance and immunity. Annu Rev Immunol 2004;22: 307-328.
[40] Rocha B, Grandien A, Freitas AA. Anergy and exhaustion are independent mechanisms of peripheral T cell tolerance. J Exp Med 1995;181: 993-1003.

[41] Sato K, Yamashita N, Yamashita N, Baba M, Matsuyama T. Regulatory dendritic cells protect mice from murine acute graft-versus-host disease and leukemia relapse. Immunity 2003;18: 367-379.

[42] Charpentier B, Alard P, Hiesse C, Lantz O. Induction of peripheral T cell tolerance and allo/xenoimmunity. Pathol Biol (Paris) 1994;42: 237-240.

[43] Wekerle T, Kurtz J, Sayegh M et al. Peripheral deletion after bone marrow transplantation with costimulatory blockade has features of both activation-induced cell death and passive cell death. J Immunol 2001;166: 2311-2316.

[44] Hara M, Kingsley CI, Niimi M et al. IL-10 is required for regulatory T cells to mediate tolerance to alloantigens in vivo. J Immunol 2001;166: 3789-3796.

[45] Ierino FL, Yamada K, Hatch T, Sachs DH. Preliminary in vitro evidence for regulatory cells in a miniature swine renal allograft model. Transplant Proc 1997;29: 1165.

[46] Sakaguchi S. Regulatory T cells: key controllers of immunologic self-tolerance. Cell 2000;101: 455-458.

[47] Sakaguchi S, Sakaguchi N, Asano M, Itoh M, Toda M. Immunologic self-tolerance maintained by activated T cells expressing IL-2 receptor alpha-chains (CD25). Breakdown of a single mechanism of self-tolerance causes various autoimmune diseases. J Immunol 1995;155: 1151-1164.

[48] Wing K, Onishi Y, Prieto-Martin P et al. CTLA-4 control over Foxp3+ regulatory T cell function. Science 2008;322: 271-275.

[49] Wood KJ, Sakaguchi S. Regulatory T cells in transplantation tolerance. Nat Rev Immunol 2003;3: 199-210.

[50] Tada T, Takemori T. Selective roles of thymus-derived lymphocytes in the antibody response. I. Differential suppressive effect of carrier-primed T cells on hapten-specific IgM and IgG antibody responses. J Exp Med 1974;140: 239-252.

[51] Takemori T, Tada T. Selective roles of thymus-derived lymphocytes in the antibody response. II. Preferential suppression of high-affinity antibody-forming cells by carrier-primed suppressor T cells. J Exp Med 1974;140: 253-266.

[52] Lee ST, Paraskevas F. Soluble factors in immune sera of mice. I. Specific and non-specific suppressive activity. Clin Exp Immunol 1976;24: 177-184.

[53] Ricciardi-Castagnoli P, Doria G, Adorini L. Production of antigen-specific suppressive T cell factor by radiation leukemia virus-transformed suppressor T cells. Proc Natl Acad Sci U S A 1981;78: 3804-3808.

[54] Sakaguchi S, Sakaguchi N, Shimizu J et al. Immunologic tolerance maintained by CD25+ CD4+ regulatory T cells: their common role in controlling autoimmunity, tumor immunity, and transplantation tolerance. Immunol Rev 2001;182:18-32.: 18-32.

[55] Kirk AD. Crossing the bridge: large animal models in translational transplantation research. Immunol Rev 2003;196: 176-196.

[56] Larsen CP, Knechtle SJ, Adams A, Pearson T, Kirk AD. A new look at blockade of T-cell costimulation: a therapeutic strategy for long-term maintenance immunosuppression. Am J Transplant 2006;6: 876-883.

[57] Salama AD, Remuzzi G, Harmon WE, Sayegh MH. Challenges to achieving clinical transplantation tolerance. J Clin Invest 2001;108: 943-948.

[58] Madsen JC, Yamada K, Allan JS et al. Transplantation tolerance prevents cardiac allograft vasculopathy in major histocompatibility complex class I-disparate miniature swine. Transplantation 1998;65: 304-313.
[59] Pennington LR, Flye MW, Kirkman RL, Thistlethwaite JR Jr, Williams GM, Sachs DH. Transplantation in miniature swine. X. Evidence for non-SLA-linked immune response gene(s) controlling rejection of SLA-matched kidney allografts. Transplantation 1981;32: 315-320.
[60] Gianello PR, Yamada K, Fishbein JM et al. Long-term acceptance of primarily vascularized renal allografts in miniature swine. Systemic tolerance versus graft adaptation. Transplantation 1996;61: 503-506.
[61] Fishbein JM, Gianello P, Nickeleit V et al. Interleukin-2 reverses the ability of cyclosporine to induce tolerance to class I disparate kidney allografts in miniature swine. Transplant Proc 1993;25: 322-323.
[62] Mezrich J, Yamada K, Sachs DH, Madsen JC. Regulatory T cells generated by the kidney may mediate the beneficial immune effects of combining kidney with heart transplantation. Surgery 2004;135: 473-478.
[63] Gianello P, Fishbein JM, Sachs DH. Tolerance to primarily vascularized allografts in miniature swine. Immunol Rev 1993;133: 19-44.
[64] Rosengard BR, Ojikutu CA, Guzzetta PC et al. Induction of specific tolerance to class I disparate renal allografts in miniature swine with cyclosporine. Transplantation 1992;54: 490-497.
[65] Radovancevic B, Frazier OH. Treatment of moderate heart allograft rejection with Cyclosporine. J Heart Transplant 1986;5: 307-311.
[66] Gianello PR, Fishbein JF, Rosengard BR et al. Tolerance to class I disparate renal allografts in miniature swine: maintenance of tolerance despite induction of specific antidonor CTL responses. Transplantation 1995;59: 772-777.
[67] Gianello PR, Lorf T, Yamada K et al. Induction of tolerance to renal allografts across single- haplotype MHC disparities in miniature swine. Transplantation 1995;59: 884-890.
[68] Fishbein JM, Rosengard BR, Gianello P et al. Development of tolerance to class II mismatched renal transplants following a short course of cyclosporine therapy in miniature swine. Transplantation 1994;57: 1303-1308.
[69] Utsugi R, Barth RN, Lee RS et al. Induction of transplantation tolerance with a short course of tacrolimus (FK506): I. Rapid and stable tolerance to two-haplotype fully mhc-mismatched kidney allografts in miniature swine. Transplantation 2001;71: 1368-1379.
[70] Vagefi PA, Ierino FL, Gianello PR et al. Role of the thymus in transplantation tolerance in miniature Swine: IV. The thymus is required during the induction phase, but not the maintenance phase, of renal allograft tolerance. Transplantation 2004;77: 979-985.
[71] Yamada K, Vagefi PA, Utsugi R et al. Thymic transplantation in miniature swine: III. Induction of tolerance by transplantation of composite thymokidneys across fully major histocompatibility complex-mismatched barriers. Transplantation 2003;76: 530-536.
[72] Ierino FL, Yamada K, Hatch T, Rembert J, Sachs DH. Peripheral tolerance to class I mismatched renal allografts in miniature swine: donor antigen-activated peripheral

blood lymphocytes from tolerant swine inhibit antidonor CTL reactivity. J Immunol 1999;162: 550-559.
[73] Gianello PR, Blancho G, Fishbein JF et al. Mechanism of cyclosporin-induced tolerance to primarily vascularized allografts in miniature swine. Effect of administration of exogenous IL-2. J Immunol 1994;153: 4788-4797.
[74] Rosengard BR, Kortz EO, Ojikutu CA et al. The failure of skin grafting to break tolerance to class I disparate renal allografts in miniature swine despite inducing marked anti-donor cellular immunity. Transplantation 1991;52: 1044-1052.
[75] Rosengard BR, Fishbein JM, Gianello PR et al. Retransplantation in miniature swine: lack of a requirement for graft adaptation for maintenance of specific renal allograft tolerance. Transplantation 1994;57: 794-799.

11

Operational Tolerance after Renal Transplantation in the Regenerative Medicine Era

Giuseppe Orlando[1], Pierpaolo Di Cocco[2], Lauren Corona[3], Tommaso Maria Manzia[4], Katia Clemente[2], Antonio Famulari[2] and Francesco Pisani[2]

[1]Nuffield Department of Surgery, University of Oxford,
[2]Renal Failure and Transplant Surgery, Department of Surgery, University of L'Aquila
[3]Wayne State University School of Medicine,
[4]Transplant Surgery, Tor Vergata University of Rome,
[1]UK
[3]USA
[2,4]Italy

1. Introduction

An immunosuppression [IS]-free state is the ultimate goal to achieve in solid organ transplantation [SOT] because IS-related toxicity tremendously impact on overall clinical outcome [Orlando, Hematti et al., 2010]. The IS-free state substantiates into what is referred to as clinical operational tolerance [COT], defined as the condition in which a SOT recipient retains stable graft function and lacks histological signs of rejection, after having been completely off all IS for at least 1 year. The patient in question is an immunocompetent host capable of responding to other immune challenges, including infections or transplantation of organs from third party donors [Orlando, Hematti et al., 2010; Orlando et al., 2008]. However, experimental and clinical information collected so far show that COT is extremely difficult to achieve and is organ-dependent. In fact, the majority of cases of COT reported so far relate to liver graft recipients, in reason of the well known immune-privileged status of the liver determined by factors that remain obscure.

In this chapter, we will provide evidence that the achievement of COT after RT remains exceptional and that tolerogenic strategies are not yet available for daily clinical practice. To do so, we will illustrate and discuss the most relevant cases of COT described so far in the English literature. However, by briefly touching the recent outstanding progress achieved in regenerative medicine, we will bring the attention of the reader on the fact that regenerative medicine may offer a valuable approach to generate immediate, stable and durable COT in SOT recipients.

2. Classification

Several classifications have been proposed to categorize all strategies proposed so far to induce COT in RT recipients [Fehr & Sykes, 2004; Orlando et al, 2008; Orlando, Hematti et al, 2010]. Nevertheless, given the interest and enthusiasm generated by recent investigations in the field of stem cell biology, we believe that so-called tolerogenic strategies - namely, protocols implemented to induce COT - may be divided into two new groups, cell-based and non-cell-based, according to whether or not stem cell strains showing some immunomodulatory effect *in vitro* are administered in the preoperative period in addition to standard IS.

2.1 Cell-based approach

2.1.1 Metachronous bone-marrow transplant for hematologic disorders

Bone marrow transplantation [BMT], results in the total replacement of the recipient's bone marrow by the donor's bone marrow hematopoietic cells, a condition referred to as full chimerism [Delis et al, 2004]. If the patient receives an organ from the same bone marrow donor late after BMT, then the reconstituted white cell compartment may recognize the new organ as self; theoretically, no response will be mounted by the host immune system and the new graft will be tolerated without need for any IS. However, despite several cases of BMT plus solid organ transplants [RT included] have been reported [Butcher et al, 1999; Chiang & Lazarus, 2003; Helg et al, 1994; Jacobsen et al, 1994; Light et al, 2002; Sayegh et al, 1991; Sellers et al, 2001; Sorof et al, 1995], yet COT has been an exceptional finding. Importantly, according to what reported by all series, COT developed in patients in which the transplant was performed several years after BMT, but never where BMT and RT were performed simultaneously.

2.1.2 Perioperative infusion of HSC

Somehow, the above reported data conflicted with what described in mice by Monaco and Wood, namely that the addition of donor bone marrow to a strong lymphocyte depleting regimen may result in the long-lasting survival of skin allografts from the same donor, without any maintenance IS [Monaco et al, 1970; Monaco et al, 1976; Monaco et al, 1985]. These experimental findings represented the platform for translational investigations aimed to prove that the peroperative infusion of donor-derived bone marrow cells can prolong allograft survival [Sykes, 2009]. The group at Massachusetts General Hospital adopted such strategy in 7 adult patients with renal failure due to multiple myeloma, who received combined human leukocyte antigen [HLA]-matched kidney and bone marrow transplant after a non-myeloablative conditioning regimen consisting of cyclophosphamide, antithymocyte globulin, and pretransplant thymic irradiation [Buhler et al, 2002; Fudaba et al, 2006; Spitzer et al, 1999; Spitzer et al, 2011]. Maintenance IS consisted of cyclosporine which was discontinued as early as day 73 post-transplant. Patients were followed for a mean of 7.4 (range 4-12) years. Two of them died for relapse of the baseline disease and therapy-related acute myeloid leukemia after 7.7 and 4.2 years, respectively; noteworthy, both were IS-free at the time of death. Of the 5 patients who are still alive [4 of whom with no evidence of myeloma recurrence], 3 are IS-free, and show serum creatinine levels of 0.63, 1.14 and 1.7 mg/dL, respectively. The remaining 2 individuals are receiving either prednisone or tacrolimus for graft-versus-host disease [but no rejection!], and present serum creatinine levels of 0.9 and 1.42 mg/dL.

More recently, the same group reported the short-term results of a seminal trial in which non-cancer patients received renal grafts and bone marrow from HLA haploidentical donors following nonmyeloablative conditioning to induce renal allograft tolerance [Kawai et al,

2008; Porcheray et al, 2009]. Even in this case, cyclosporine was the only immunosuppressant used for maintenance therapy. IS could be successfully weaned in 4 out of 5 patients, whereas the remaining patient experienced acute rejection and lost his graft. Cyclosporine could be withdrawn after 294 (range 240-272) days. However, matters of concern are represented by two major findings. First, the reported most recent mean creatinine clearance (67 ml/min, range 60-75) and serum creatinine levels (1.5 mg/dl, range 1.2-1.8) levels in the 4 IS-free patients were slightly abnormal. Second, 2 of these patients have shown evidence of *de novo* antibodies reactive to donor antigens between 1 and 2 years after the transplant [Porcheray et al, 2009]. Overall, this series demonstrates that B-cell immunity can occur in the context of T-cell tolerance to donor antigens through unknown mechanisms, otherwise said T-cell unresponsiveness is not synonymous of tolerance of both arms of the adaptive immune system. This is consistent with information reported by Nantes. Soulillou et al. extensively studied IS-free RT recipients [Ashton-Chess et al., 2007; Baeten et al., 2006; Ballet et al., 2006; Brouard et al., 2005; Louis et al., 2006; Roussey-Kesler et al., 2006;] and found that COT may occur in the presence of anti-donor class II antibodies, as well as in patients who have previously experienced acute rejection. Moreover, they showed that IS-free RT recipients are more likely to have received grafts from donors younger than 30 years of age, are low-responders to blood transfusion, may develop graft dysfunction at any time after the weaning of IS, and show an incidence of infectious diseases comparable to that in normal individuals.

The Stanford group has implemented a similar strategy in two distinct small series, where patients received a renal graft followed by the infusion of HSC from the same HLA-mismatched (x4) or -matched (x6) donors, respectively [Millan et al., 2002; Scandling et al., 2008]. IS consisted of induction with total lymphoid irradiation and rabbit anti-thymocyte globulin, followed by cyclosporine and prednisone as maintenance therapy. After steroid discontinuation on day 10, mycophenolate mofetil was introduced and administered for 1 month. Intravenous injection of HSC was repeated during the third postoperative week. Results were poor. In the first trial, only one patient could be weaned off IS, while however showing slightly elevated serum creatinine leves (1.4 mg/dL). In the second trial, one individual could be weaned off IS but renal function tests are not shown. Two further patients rejected, while the remaining 3 were still under weaning at the time of publication.

Overall, based on the reported information, the above series show the lack of safety of hematopoietic stem cell-based regimens. Despite this approach may allow minimization of overall IS, however further studies are required to improve safety and effectiveness. Importantly, most of the IS-free patients reported above do not comply with the stringent criteria for COT adopted in the present chapter.

2.1.3 Perioperative infusion of alternative types of immunomodulatory cells

Transplant-acceptance-inducing cells (TAIC) are immunoregulatory macrophages which have shown some capacity of establishing a state of alloantigen-specific partial tolerance of solid organ transplants in renal transplant recipients [Hutchinson, Brem-Exner et al., 2008; Hutchinson, Riquelme et al., 2008; Riquelme P et al., 2009]. TAIC's presumed tolerogenic properties have been tested in two safety trials differing in the method for TAIC preparation, numbers of cells infused, induction IS, and timing of infusions. None of the 17 patients enrolled in either study could be weaned off IS, most of them rejected, 2 dropped out the study for non-immunological causes, while only 2 individuals did well yet under tacrolimus monotherapy at the end of the study. Overall, although these trials demonstrated that the infusion of TAIC is feasible, major concerns remain regarding the efficacy and safety of such an approach. It is unclear whether or not this approach confers any benefit in the establishment of minimal IS in RT patients when compared to the protocols currently adopted, as clearly stated by authors in the discussion. Lastly, the optimal dose and timing of cell infusions, as well as the most appropriate concomitant IS regimen, is yet to be determined.

For their ability for tissue repair and immunomodulation, mesenchymal stem cells (MSCs) are currently being evaluated for a wide variety of clinical applications including the treatment of disorders characterized by a dysfunction of immune regulation, such as graft versus host disease after bone marrow transplantation and rejection after cell or organ transplantation [Crop et al., 2009; Ding et al., 2009; Hematti, 2008; Le Blanc et al., 2008; Le Blanc & Ringden, 2007]. As MSCs seem to be able to promote engraftment of allogeneic cells, tissues and organs, as well as to prevent or treat rejection in pre-clinical models, they provide an exciting opportunity for further research in the field of IS minimization and withdrawal in SOT [Hematti, 2008; Hoogduijn MJ et al., 2010].

It is worth to mention that, in addition to stem cells, the therapeutic properties of various other immune cells like regulatory T cells or dendritic cells are currently being explored for SOT purposes [Issa, Hester et al., 2010; Issa, Schiopu et al., 2010; Orlando, Hematti et al., 2010].

2.2 Non cell-based protocols

2.2.1 Non-adherence to IS

The majority of cases of COT described so far after RT is represented by patients who spontaneously decided to stop IS for non-compliance to treatment [Ashton-Chess et al., 2007; Baeten et al., 2006; Ballet et al., 2006; Brouard et al., 2005; Hussey, 1975; Louis et al., 2006; Najarian, 1975; Newell et al., 2010; Owens et al., 1975; Roussey-Kesler et al., 2006; Sagoo et al., 2010; Uehling et al., 1976; Zoller et al., 1980]. These patients have been the object of numerous investigations conducted at different times by diverse authors with methods presenting dissimilar accuracy. However, we believe that it is worth to report the investigations by Burlingham et al. In an attempt to identify patients who may be weaned off IS at no risk, he recurred to the human-to-mouse trans-vivo delayed-type hypersensitivity assay [Geissler et al., 2001; VanBuskirk et al., 2000]. By observing that 2 renal allograft recipients failed to exhibit donor-reactive delayed type hypersensitivity responses, although they frequently develop donor-reactive alloantibodies, the authors demonstrated that this pattern of immune responses is not due to an absence of allosensitization, but to the development of an immune mechanism that actively inhibits anti-donor delayed-type (i.e., cell-mediated) immune responses. In other words, authors provided evidence that COT develops following the onset of regulatory, rather than suppressing mechanisms.

Of interest is the case of spontaneous interruption of IS by a 24-year old woman who had received a deceased donor RT at the age of 13 for membranoproliferative glomerulonephritis. When the woman found out to be pregnant, she stopped all IS to protect the fetus from any possible IS-induced teratogenic effect [Fischer et al., 1996]. Interestingly, she did not resume any IS after delivery, and no immunological response was observed for 9 years after the withdrawal of IS, while the patient was showing perfectly normal renal function tests.

2.2.2 Molecule-based tolerogenic protocols

A molecule-based tolerogenic regimen was implemented by Starzl a decade ago [Starzl et al., 2003]. The working hypothesis was that the need for continual high dose IS could be avoided in most cases with the use of a strong lymphocyte-depleting regimen prior to engraftment, followed by the administration of low dose tacrolimus monotherapy. The rationale was to remove the non-specific clones of immune cells responsible for rejection before contact with foreign donor antigens occurs. Once the donor antigens are in place after implantation of the new organ, repletion of immune cells occurs, favored by the homeostatic expansion triggered by leukocyte depletion. In addition, minimization of maintenance IS was implemented to further reduce the anti-donor response with just enough treatment to prevent irreversible immune damage to the graft, but not with such heavy treatment that the donor-specific clonal exhaustion-deletion process is precluded.

Broadly reacting rabbit antithymocyte globulins were administered preoperatively, followed by tacrolimus monotherapy, to 82 adult kidney, liver, pancreas, and intestinal transplant recipients. After a mean follow-up time of 18-months, 1-year patient and graft survival rates were 95% and 82% overall, respectively, IS-related morbidity was virtually eliminated, and 48/72 surviving patients were receiving spaced doses of tacrolimus monotherapy. Noteworthy, 25/39 (64%) renal, 12/17 (70%) liver, 5/12 (42%) pancreas, as well as 6/11 (54%) intestinal transplant recipients, resulted on tacrolimus spaced doses at the time of publication. However, IS could not be weaned off in any patient. Other protocols based on a similar strategy – i.e., leukocyte depletion followed by the administration of low dose single-drug IS - have been implemented after RT [Agarwal et al., 2008; Calne et al., 2000; Calne et al., 1999; Calne et al., 1998; Ciancio & Burke, 2008; Clatworthy et al., 2009; Kirk et al., 2003; Kirk et al., 2005; Orlando, Hematti et al., 2010; Trzonkowski et al., 2006; Trzonkowski et al., 2008; Watson et al., 2005] and liver, the organ most capable of developing COT, transplantation [Eason et al., 2005]. However, none of these protocols has proved effective or safe in producing COT nor has they shown any convincing impact on overall outcomes.

2.2.3 Total lymphoid irradiation

Three cases of COT have been described in RT recipients subjected to total lymphoid irradiation, a perioperative course of antithymocyte globulin, and maintenance prednisone that was gradually weaned and eventually stopped [Strober et al., 1989; Strober et al., 2000; Strober et al., 2004]. Two patients remained IS-free for 12 years and 69 months, while the third developed severe urinary tract obstruction 10 months after the IS withdrawal, for which he was eventually retransplanted. Importantly, the complete original series comprised 28 RT recipients, 25 of whom did not develop COT.

2.2.4 COT developed after intentional IS withdrawal for lymphoproliferative disorders

Two cases of COT developing after the intentional withdrawal of IS due to the development of post transplant lymphoproliferative disorders (PTLD) have been described, mainly within a larger series [Roussey-Kesler et al., 2006]. A third case relates to a 21-year-old man who received 2 haplo-identical RTs, the first at age 11 from his mother and the second at age 15 from his father [Christensen et al., 1998]. Three years after the second RT, he developed PTLD. IS was promptly interrupted and the PTLD subsequently resolved. At the time of publication, IS had been withdrawn for 3 years with no rejection.

Classification	Subtype	Center	Type of study	Claimed cases of COT	Length of follow up from the time of the withdrawal of the IS
Cell-based	Previous BMT	Boston, Brigham and Women Hospital [Sayegh et al, 1991]	Case report	2*	7 and 3 years
		Geneva [Helg et al, 1994]	Case report	1	2 years
		Copenhagen [Jacobsen et al, 1994]	Case report	1	1 year
		San Francisco [Sorof et al, 1995]	Case report	1	2 year
		Milwaukee [Bucther et al, 1999]	Case report	3	3, 11, 18 years
		Birmingham, US [Sellers et al, 2001]	Case report	1	7
	HSC	Boston, Massachussetts General Hospital [Spitzer et al, 1999; Buhler et al, 2002; Fudaba et al, 2006; Spitzer et al, 2011]	Prospective, non comparative	3/6	12.1, 7.7, 4, 6.8 years
		Boston, Massachussetts General Hospital [Kawai et al, 2008; Porcheray et al, 2009]	Prospective, non comparative	4/5	4.6, 3.4, 2.2 and 1.2 years
		Stanford [Millan et al, 2002]	Prospective, non comparative	1/4	14 years
		Stanford [Scandling et al, 2008]	Prospective, non comparative	1/3	28 months

Classification	Subtype	Center	Type of study	Claimed cases of COT	Length of follow up from the time of the withdrawal of the IS
		Miami [Ciancio et al, 2004]	Prospective, non randomized, comparative	0/63	-
	TACI	Kiel [Hutchinson et al, 2008]	Prospective, non comparative	0/12	-
		Kiel [Hutchinson et al, 2008]	Prospective, non comparative	0/5	-
Non cell-based	Non-adherence to IS	Columbus-Madison [VanBuskirk et al, 2000; Geissler et al, 2001]	Case report	3	3 years
		Madison [Uehling et al, 1976]	Case report	5, but 4 rejected after few months	5 years
		Los Angeles [Owens et al, 1975]	Case report	4, but eventually 1 rejected after 18 months	17, 23, 52 months
		Minneapolis [Najarian, 1975]	Case report	6, but 5 rejected after few months	NA
		Madison [Hussey, 1975]	Case report	8, but 7 rejected after few months	40
	TBI	Stanford [Strober et al, 1989; Strober et al, 2000]	Prospective	3/28, but 1 rejected after 10 months for non-immunological reasons	144 and 69 months
	Pregnancy	Erlangen-Munster [Fischer et al, 1996]	Case report	1	9 years

Classification	**Subtype**	**Center**	**Type of study**	**Claimed cases of COT**	**Length of follow up from the time of the withdrawal of the IS**
	PTLD	Aarhus [Christensen et a, 1998]	Case report	1	>3 years
	Molecule-based	Pittsburgh [Starzl et al, 2003]	Prospective, non comparative	0/39	-
		Cambridge [Clatworthy et al, 2009; Watson et al, 2005; Calne et al, 2000; Calne et al, 1999; Calne et al, 1998]	Prospective, comparative, non randomized	0/33	-
		Oxford [Trzonkoski et al, 2008]	Prospective, non comparative	0/13	-
		Bethesda [Kirk et al, 2003]	Prospective, non comparative	0/7	-
		Bethesda [Kirk et al, 2005]	Prospective, non comparative	0/5	-
	Surveys	Boston [Zoller et al, 1980]	Descriptive, observational	13	>1 year
		Nantes [Roussey-Kesler et al, 2006]	Descriptive, investigative	10, but 2 rejected after 7 and 13 years	9 years [mean time, range 1-20]
		Nantes [Braud et al, 2008; Sivozhelezov et al, 2008]	Descriptive, investigative	8	>1 year
		Nantes [Bouard et al, 2007]	Descriptive, investigative	17	>1 year
		Los Angeles [Owens et al, 1975]	Descriptive, observational	24, but 22 rejected after few months	9, 36 months

Classification	Subtype	Center	Type of study	Claimed cases of COT	Length of follow up from the time of the withdrawal of the IS
		European Consortium for tolerance [Sagoo et al, 2010]	Descriptive, investigative	11	>1 year
		American network for immune tolerance [Newell et al, 2010]	Descriptive, investigative	25	>1 year

Table 1. Synoptic view of all successful and unsuccessful cases of COT described after RT. The mismatch between the number of cases claimed by numerous authors and the real effectice number of COT calculated according to the definition of COT adopted in the present manuscript is evident [116 vs. 108, respectively].

3. Immune monitoring

As illustrated above, most cases of COT have developed in individuals who have spontaneously terminated IS. When all clinical trials in which a presumed tolerogenic protocol has been implemented are taken into consideration, it is frustrating to observe that COT could be obtained in only 6 out of 248 patients, accounting for a poor, unacceptable success rate of 2.5% [Orlando, Hematti et al , 2010]. As a corollary, the tolerogenic regimens attempted so far in RT recipients are not efficient and, more importantly, lack safety. Ideally, before implementing any of such regimens, investigators should rely on parameters able to predict with high accuracy whether patients would tolerate the weaning process without any risk to reject. Unfortunately, no parameter as such is available for routine practice, not even renal biopsy. For example, Burlingham reported on a late graft rejection in a patient who received a RT 9.5 years earlier from his mother and who had been IS-free for 7 years; a gradual rise in serum creatinine level to 2.0 mg/dl prompted a biopsy that ruled out rejection, yet 10 months later severe cellular rejection arose [Burlingham et al., 2000].
Investigators have obtained promising results in the field of liver transplantation where this problem has been circumvented by the identification of so-called markers of tolerance [Martinez-Llordella et al., 2008; Martinez-Llordella et al., 2007], defined as functional and molecular correlates of immune reactivity whose purpose is to provide clinically useful information for therapeutic decision-making in view of IS withdrawal [Ashton-Chess et al., 2009]. Investigations in tolerant liver transplant recipients resulted in the discovery and validation of a tolerance-associated transcriptional patterns, consisting of several gene signatures and multiple peripheral blood lymphocyte subsets capable of identifying tolerant and non-tolerant recipients with high accuracy. As these data suggested that transcriptional profiling of peripheral blood can be employed to identify recipients who can discontinue immunosuppressive therapy at no risk for rejection, RT researchers are currently exploring a

signature of COT after RT which may allow the selection of those patients who may be more prone to develop an IS-free state with no or quasi no risk for rejection.

The group in Nantes has pioneered investigations aimed to the identification of specific biological signatures of COT [Braud et al., 2008; Brouard et al., 2007; Sivozhelezov et al., 2008]. Brouard et al. identified a set of 49 genes and differentially expressed gene transcripts using gene-expression profiling of peripheral blood from 17 tolerant RT recipients, with tolerance class prediction scores of >90% [Brouard et al., 2007]. This fingerprint is expected to identify patients who might be eligible for a progressive tapering of their immunosuppressive medications and, more importantly, those who instead need to stay on their current IS regimen. The same group has also exploited the capabilities of high throughput microarray technology to study peripheral blood specific gene expression profiles and corresponding molecular pathways associated with operational tolerance [Braud et al., 2008; Sivozhelezov et al., 2008]. Investigations revealed that tolerant patients display a set of 343 differentially expressed genes, mainly immune and defense genes, in their peripheral blood mononuclear cells (PBMC), of which 223 were also different from healthy volunteers. Using the expression pattern of these 343 genes, they were able to correctly classify >80% of the patients in a cross-validation analysis and correctly identified all of the samples over time. All together, this study identified a unique PBMC gene signature associated with human operational tolerance in kidney transplantation [Orlando, Hematti et al., 2010].

Investigations have been conducted in parallel in Europe and the United States. The European Union Indices of Tolerance Network showed that IS-free RT patients present a distinctive expansion of peripheral blood B lymphocytes and natural killer cells and differential expression of several immune-relevant genes in the absence of donor-specific antibodies [Sagoo et al., 2010]. Similar population expansion of B immune cells and selective expression of B cell-related genes in samples obtained from tolerant individuals were noted by the National Institute of Health's Immune Tolerance Network [Newell et al., 2010].

4. The potential of regenerative medicine

The term regenerative medicine refers to that field in the health sciences which aims to replace or regenerate *human cells, tissues, or organs in order to restore or establish normal function* [Mason & Dunnill, 2008; Orlando, Baptista et al., 2010; Orlando et al., 2011]. The process of regenerating body parts can occur *in vivo* or *ex vivo* and may require cells, natural or artificial scaffolding materials, growth factors, or different combinations of all three elements. Instead, the term tissue engineering refers to a field which is narrower in scope and strictly limited to the production of body parts *ex vivo*, by seeding cells either on or into a supporting scaffold [Orlando et al., 2011].

In the last decade, investigators in the field have been able to produce and implant in patients relatively simple hollow organs like skin [Naughton et al., 1999], vessels [Hibino et al., 2010; L'Heureux N et al., 2007; McAllister et al., 2009; Shinoka et al., 2001; Shinoka et al., 2005;], bladders [Atala et al., 2006], windpipes [Macchiarini et al., 2008] and urethras [Raya-Rivera et al., 2011]. Importantly, all constructs were manufactured by either combining autologous cells with scaffolding material, or through the engineering of autologous cells *per se* [Orlando, Baptista et al., 2010; Orlando et al., 2011]. Importantly, none of the patients did require IS at any time after implantation of the bioengineered body part. Therefore,

regenerative medicine has shown the potential to offer a valuable approach to COT. Importantly, as the above mentioned implanted body parts were bioengineered from autologous cells, recipients never required IS and therefore we can conclude that regenerative medicine offers the only possible approach to immediate, stable and durable COT. In fact, as illustrated throughout the whole chapter, all cases of COT reported so far in the English literature developed at least several weeks after the transplants and always required some IS, the exception being RT between identical twins [Orlando, Hematti et al., 2010]. Moreover, in several circumstances, patients who could be weaned off IS eventually rejected and required resumption of IS.
Bioengineering technology has been implemented to manufacture heart [Ott et al., 2008], liver [Badylak et al., 2011; Baptista et al., 2011; Uydun et al., 2010;] and lung [Ott et al., 2010; Petersen et al., 2010;] organoids from rodent organs [Orlando, Baptista et al, 2010; Orlando et al, 2011]. *In extenso,* rat or ferret organs were decellularized with detergents and repopulated with cells from unrelated species, humans included. In the ideal scenario, when and if this technology will be perfected, the cellular compartment will be reconstituted - even in this case - from patient's autologous cells, whereas the supporting scaffold will be represented by an acellular porcine or non-human primate organ depleted of its native cells.

5. Conclusions

When all the above information is taken together, it is clear that, although a wealth of knowledge exists, little progress has been made in developing a sure-fire strategy towards attaining COT. Despite tolerance has been widely investigated for decades, efforts to understand the mechanisms underlying this phenomenon and how to achieve it have thus far been to no avail. In addition to the failure of all molecule-based strategies, we have learned that stem cells do exert some modulatory effect on the immune system but we do not know why and how this occurs. Therefore, we cannot predict when the opportunities for COT to develop in a patient the greatest.
As it stands, with the technology that is currently available, the withdrawal of IS after RT cannot yet be encouraged because it is neither effective nor safe and must be considered as still in an experimental phase. Efforts to identify a peripheral blood transcriptional biomarker panel associated with COT after RT are certainly laudable but, provided the safety for the withdrawal of IS is not guaranteed, any clinical implementation should be banned outside specialized cutting-edge center. The lack of safety of all tolerogenic strategies implemented so far remains their major weakness. Recent revolutionary progress in regenerative medicine has revealed the immense potential of the field pertinent to COT. In a foreseeable future, regenerative medicine will meet the two major needs of SOT, namely that of a potentially inexhaustible source of organs and COT itself [Orlando, 2011].

6. References

Agarwal, A., Shen, LY., & Kirk, AD. (2008). The role of alemtuzumab in facilitating maintenance immunosuppression minimization following solid organ transplantation. *Transplant Immunology,* Vol.20, No.1-2, (November 2008), pp. 6-11, ISSN 0966-3274

Ashton-Chess, J., Giral, M., Soulillou, JP., & Brouard, S. (2009). Can immune monitoring help to minimize immunosuppression in kidney transplantation? *Transplant*

International: official journal of the European Society for Organ Transplantation, Vol.22, No.1, (January 2009), pp. 110-119, ISSN 0934-0874

Ashton-Chess, J., Giral, M., Brouard, S., & Soulillou, JP. (2007). Spontaneous operational tolerance after immunosuppressive drug withdrawal in clinical renal allotransplantation. *Transplantation,* Vol.84, No.10, (November 2007), pp. 1215-1219, ISSN 0041-1337

Atala, A., Bauer, SB., Soker, S., Yoo, JJ., & Retik, AB. 2006. Tissue-engineered autologous bladders for patients needing cystoplasty. *Lancet,* Vol.367, No.9518, (April 2006), pp. 1241-1246, ISSN 0140-6736

Badylak, SF., Zhang, L., Medberry, CJ., Fukumitsu, K., Faulk, D., Jiang, H., Reing, JE., Gramignoli, R., Komori, J., Ross, M., Nagaya, M., Lagasse, E., Beer Stolz, D., Strom, S., & Fox, IJ. (n.d.). A Whole Organ Regenerative Medicine Approach for Liver Replacement. *Tissue Engineering. Part C, Methods,* (March 2011), ISSN 1937-3384

Baeten, D., Louis, S., Braud, C., Braudeau, C., Ballet, C., Moizant, F., Pallier, A., Giral, M., Brouard, S., & Soulillou, JP. (2005). Phenotypically and functionally distinct CD8+ lymphocyte populations in long-term drug-free tolerance and chronic rejection in human kidney graft recipients. *Journal of the American Society of Nephrology: JASN,* Vol.17, No.1, (December 2005), pp. 294-304, ISSN 1046-6673.

Ballet, C., Roussey-Kesler, G., Aubin, JT., Brouard, S., Giral, M., Miqueu, P., Louis, S., Van der Werf, S., & Soulillou, JP. (2006). Humoral and cellular responses to influenza vaccination in human recipients naturally tolerant to a kidney allograft. *American Journal of Transplantation: official journal of the American Society of Transplantation and the American Society of Transplant Surgeons,* Vol.6, No.11, (November 2006), pp. 2796-2801, ISSN 1600-6135

Baptista, PM., Siddiqui, MM., Lozier, G., Rodriguez, SR., Atala, A., & Soker, S. (2011). The use of whole organ decellularization for the generation of a vascularized liver organoid. *Hepatology: official journal of the American Association for the study of Liver Diseases*, Vol.53, No.2, (November 2010), pp. 604-617, ISSN 0270-9139.

Braud, C., Baeten, D., Giral, M., Pallier, A., Ashton-Chess, J., Braudeau, C., Chevalier, C., Lebars, A., Léger, J., Moreau, A., Pechkova, E., Nicolini, C., Soulillou, JP., & Brouard, S. (2008). Immunosuppressive drug-free operational immune tolerance in human kidney transplant recipients: Part I. Blood gene expression statistical analysis. *Journal of cellular biochemistry,* Vol.103, No.6, (April 2008), pp. 1681-1692, ISSN 0730-2312

Brouard, S., Dupont, A., Giral, M., Louis, S., Lair, D., Braudeau, C., Degauque, N., Moizant, F., Pallier, A., Ruiz, C., Guillet, M., Laplaud, D., & Soulillou, JP. (2005). Operationally tolerant and minimally immunosuppressed kidney recipients display strongly altered blood T-cell clonal regulation. *American Journal of Transplantation: official journal of the American Society of Transplantation and the American Society of Transplant Surgeons,* Vol.5, No.2, (February 2005), pp. 330-340, ISSN 1600-6135

Brouard, S., Mansfield, E., Braud, C., Li, L., Giral, M., Hsieh, SC., Baeten, D., Zhang, M., Ashton-Chess, J., Braudeau, C., Hsieh, F., Dupont, A., Pallier, A., Moreau, A., Louis, S., Ruiz, C., Salvatierra, O., Soulillou, JP., & Sarwal, M. (2007). Identification of a peripheral blood transcriptional biomarker panel associated with operational renal allograft tolerance. *Proceedings of the National Academy of Sciences of the United States of America*, Vol.104, No.39, (September 2007), pp. 15448-15453, ISSN 0027-8424

Bühler, LH., Spitzer, TR., Sykes, M., Sachs, DH., Delmonico, FL., Tolkoff-Rubin, N., Saidman, SL., Sackstein, R., McAfee, S., Dey, B., Colby, C., & Cosimi, AB. (2002). Induction of kidney allograft tolerance after transient lymphohematopoietic chimerism in patients with multiple myeloma and end-stage renal disease. *Transplantation*, Vol.74, No.10, (November 2002), pp. 1405-1409, ISSN 0041-1337

Burlingham, WJ., Jankowska-Gan, E., VanBuskirk, A., Orosz, CG., Lee, JH., & Kusaka, S. (2000). Loss of tolerance to a maternal kidney transplant is selective for HLA class II: evidence from trans-vivo DTH and alloantibody analysis. *Human Immunology*, Vol.61, No.12, (December 2000), pp. 1395-1402, ISSN 0198-8859

Butcher, JA., Hariharan, S., Adams, MB., Johnson, CP., Roza, AM., & Cohen, EP. (1999). Renal transplantation for end-stage renal disease following bone marrow transplantation: a report of six cases, with and without immunosuppression. *Clinical Transplantation*, Vol.13, No.4, (August 1999), pp. 330-335, ISSN 0902-0063

Calne, R., Moffatt, SD., Friend, PJ., Jamieson, NV., Bradley, JA., Hale, G., Firth, J., Bradley, J., Smith, KG., & Waldmann, H. (2000). Prope tolerance with induction using Campath 1H and low-dose cyclosporin monotherapy in 31 cadaveric renal allograft recipients. *Nippon Geka Gakkai Zasshi*, Vol.101, No.3, (March 2000), pp. 301-306, ISSN 0301-4894

Calne, R., Moffatt, SD., Friend, PJ., Jamieson, NV., Bradley, JA., Hale, G., Firth, J., Bradley, J., Smith, KG., & Waldmann, H. (1999). Campath IH allows low-dose cyclosporine monotherapy in 31 cadaveric renal allograft recipients. *Transplantation*, Vo.68, No.10, (November 1999), pp.1613-1616, ISSN 0041-1337

Calne, R., Friend, P., Moffatt, S., Bradley, A., Hale, G., Firth, J., Bradley, J., Smith, K., & Waldmann H. (1998). Prope tolerance, perioperative Campath 1H, and low-dose cyclosporin monotherapy in renal allograft recipients. *Lancet*, Vol.351, No.9117, (June 1998), pp. 1701-1702, ISSN 0140-6736

Chiang, KY., & Lazarus, HM. (2003). Should we be performing more combined hematopoietic stem cell plus solid organ transplants? *Bone marrow transplantation*, Vol.31, No.8, (April 2003), pp. 633-642, ISSN 0268-3369

Christensen, LL., Grunnet, N., Rüdiger, N., Møller, B., & Birkeland, SA. (1998). Indications of immunological tolerance in kidney transplantation. *Tissue Antigens*, Vol.51, No.6, (June 1998), pp. 637-644, ISSN 0001-2815

Ciancio, G., & Burke, GW. 3rd. (2007). Alemtuzumab (Campath-1H) in kidney transplantation. *American journal of transplantation: official journal of the American Society of Transplantation and the American Society of Transplant Surgeons*, Vol.8, No.1, (December 2007), pp.15-20, ISSN 1600-6135

Ciancio, G., Burke, GW., Moon, J., Garcia-Morales, R., Rosen, A., Esquenazi, V., Mathew, J., Jin, Y., & Miller, J. (2004). Donor bone marrow infusion in deceased and living donor renal transplantation. *Yonsei medical journal*, Vol.45, No.6, (December 2004), pp. 998-1003, ISSN 0513-5796 2004;45:998-1003.

Clatworthy, MR., Friend, PJ., Calne, RY., Rebello, PR., Hale, G., Waldmann, H., & Watson, CJ. (2009). Alemtuzumab (CAMPATH-1H) for the Treatment of Acute Rejection in Kidney Transplant Recipients: Long-Term Follow-Up. *Transplantation*, Vol.87, No.7, (April 2009), pp.1092-1095, ISSN 0041-1337

Crop, M., Baan, C., Weimar, W., & Hoogduijn, M. (2009). Potential of mesenchymal stem cells as immune therapy in solid-organ transplantation. *Transplant International: official journal of the European Society for Organ Transplantation,* Vol.22, No.4, (April 2009), pp. 365-376, ISSN 0934-0874

Delis, S., Ciancio, G., Burke, GW., Garcia-Morales, G., & Miller, J. (2004). Donor bone marrow transplantation, chimerism and tolerance. (2004). *Transplant Immunology,* Vol.13, No.2, (September-October 2004), pp. 105-115, ISSN 0966-3274

Ding, Y., Xu, D., Feng, G., Bushell, A., Muschel, RJ., & Wood, KJ. (2009). Mesenchymal stem cells prevent the rejection of fully allogenic islet grafts by the immunosuppressive activity of matrix metalloproteinase-2 and -9. *Diabetes,* Vol.58, No.8, (June 2009), pp. 1797-1806, ISSN 0012-1797

Eason, JD., Cohen, AJ., Nair, S., Alcantera, T., & Loss, GE. (2005). Tolerance: is it worth the risk? *Transplantation,* Vol.79, No.9, (May 2005), pp.1157-1159, ISSN 0041-1337

Fehr, T., & Sykes, M. (2004). Tolerance induction in clinical transplantation. *Transplant Immunology,* Vol.13, No.2, (September-October 2004), pp. 117-130, ISSN 0966-3274

Fischer, T., Schobel, H., & Barenbrock, M. (1996). Specific immune tolerance during pregnancy after renal transplantation. *European journal of obstetrics, gynecology, and reproductive* biology, Vol.70, No.2, (December 1996), pp. 217-219, ISSN 0301-2115

Fudaba, Y., Spitzer, TR., Shaffer, J., Kawai, T., Fehr, T., Delmonico, F., Preffer, F., Tolkoff-Rubin, N., Dey, BR., Saidman, SL., Kraus, A., Bonnefoix, T., McAfee, S., Power, K., Kattleman, K., Colvin, RB., Sachs, DH., Cosimi, AB., & Sykes, M. (2006). Myeloma responses and tolerance following combined kidney and nonmyeloablative marrow transplantation: in vivo and in vitro analyses. *American journal of transplantation: official journal of the American Society of Transplantation and the American Society of Transplant Surgeons,* Vol.6, No.9, (September 2006), pp. 2121-2133, ISSN 1600-6135

Geissler, F., Jankowska-Gan, E., DeVito-Haynes, LD., Rhein, T., Kalayoglu, M., Sollinger, HW., & Burlingham, WJ. (2001). Human liver allograft acceptance and the "tolerance assay": in vitro anti-donor T cell assays show hyporeactivity to donor cells, but unlike DTH, fail to detect linked suppression. *Transplantation,* Vol.72, No.4, (August 2001), pp. 571-580, ISSN 0041-1337

Helg, C., Chapuis, B., Bolle ,JF., Morel, P., Salomon, D., Roux, E., Antonioli, V., Jeannet, M., & Leski, M. (1994). Renal transplantation without immunosuppression in a host with tolerance induced by allogeneic bone marrow transplantation. *Transplantation,* Vol.58, No.12, (December 1994), pp. 1420-1422, ISSN 0041-1337

Hutchinson, JA., Brem-Exner, BG., Riquelme, P., Roelen, D., Schulze, M., Ivens, K., Grabensee, B., Witzke, O., Philipp, T., Renders, L., Humpe, A., Sotnikova, A., Matthäi, M., Heumann, A., Gövert, F., Schulte, T., Kabelitz, D., Claas, FH., Geissler, EK., Kunzendorf, U., & Fändrich, F. (2008). A cell-based approach to the minimization of immunosuppression in renal transplantation. *Transplant International: official journal of the European Society for Organ Transplantation,* Vol.21, No.8, (August 2008), pp. 742-54, ISSN 0934-0874

Hutchinson, JA., Riquelme, P., Brem-Exner, BG., Schulze, M., Matthäi, M., Renders, L., Kunzendorf, U., Geissler, EK., & Fändrich, F. (2008). Transplant acceptance-inducing cells as an immune-conditioning therapy in renal transplantation. *Transplant International: official journal of the European Society for Organ Transplantation,* Vol.21, No.8, (August 2008), pp. 728-741, ISSN 0934-0874

Hematti, P. (2008). Role of mesenchymal stromal cells in solid organ transplantation. *Transplantation reviews*, Vol.22, No.4, (October 2008), pp. 262-273, ISSN 0955-470X

Hibino, N., McGillicuddy, E., Matsumura, G., Ichihara, Y., Naito, Y., Breuer, C., & Shinoka, T. (2010). Late-term results of tissue-engineered vascular grafts in humans. *The Journal of thoracic and cardiovascular surgery*, Vol.139, No.2, (Februrary 2010), pp.431-436, 436.e1-2, ISSN 0022-5223

Hoogduijn, MJ., Popp, FC., Grohnert, A., Crop, MJ., van Rhijn, M., Rowshani, AT., Eggenhofer, E., Renner, P., Reinders, ME., Rabelink, TJ., van der Laan, LJ., Dor, FJ., Ijzermans, JN., Genever, PG., Lange, C., Durrbach, A., Houtgraaf, JH., Christ, B., Seifert, M., Shagidulin, M., Donckier, V., Deans, R., Ringden, O., Perico, N., Remuzzi, G., Bartholomew, A., Schlitt, HJ., Weimar, W., Baan, CC., & Dahlke, MH.; MISOT Study Group. (2010). Advancement of mesenchymal stem cell therapy in solid organ transplantation (MISOT). *Transplantation,* Vol.90, No.2, (July 2010), pp. 124-126, ISSN 0934-0874

Hussey, JL. (1976). Letter: Discontinuance of immunosuppression. *Archives of surgery,* Vol.111, No.5, (May 1976), p. 614, ISSN 0272-5533

Issa, F., Hester, J., Goto, R., Nadig, SN., Goodacre, TE., & Wood, K. (2010). Ex vivo-expanded human regulatory T cells prevent the rejection of skin allografts in a humanized mouse model. *Transplantation,* Vol.90, No.12, (December 2010), pp. 1321-1327, ISSN 0934-0874

Issa, F., Schiopu, A., & Wood, KJ.(2010). Role of T cells in graft rejection and transplantation tolerance. *Expert review of clinical immunology*, Vol.6, No.1, (January 2010), pp. 155-169, ISSN 1744-666X

Jacobsen, N., Taaning, E., Ladefoged, J., Kristensen, JK., & Pedersen, FK. (1994). Tolerance to an HLA-B,DR disparate kidney allograft after bone-marrow transplantation from same donor. *Lancet,* Vol.343, No.8900, (March 1994), p. 800, ISSN 0140-6736

Kawai, T., Cosimi, AB., Spitzer, TR., Tolkoff-Rubin, N., Suthanthiran, M., Saidman, SL., Shaffer, J., Preffer, F., Ding, R., Sharma, V., Fishman, JA., Dey, B., Ko, DS., Hertl, M., Goes, NB., Wong, W., Williams, WW. Jr, Colvin, RB., Sykes, M., & Sachs DH. (2008). HLA-mismatched renal transplantation without maintenance immunosuppression. *The New England journal of medicine*, Vol.358, No.4, (January 2008), pp. 353-361, ISSN 0028-4793

Kirk, AD., Mannon, RB., Kleiner, DE., Swanson, JS., Kampen, RL., Cendales, LK., Elster, EA., Wakefield, T., Chamberlain, C., Hoffmann, SC., & Hale, DA. (2005). Results from a human renal allograft tolerance trial evaluating T-cell depletion with alemtuzumab combined with deoxyspergualin. *Transplantation,* Vol.80, No.8, (October 2005), pp. 1051-1059, ISSN 0934-0874

Kirk, AD., Hale, DA., Mannon, RB., Kleiner, DE., Hoffmann, SC., Kampen, RL., Cendales, LK., Tadaki, DK., Harlan, DM., & Swanson, SJ. (2003). Results from a human renal allograft tolerance trial evaluating the humanized CD52-specific monoclonal antibody alemtuzumab (CAMPATH-1H). *Transplantation,* Vol.76, No.1, (July 2003), pp. 120-129, ISSN 0934-0874

Le Blanc, K., Frassoni, F., Ball, L., Locatelli, F., Roelofs, H., Lewis, I., Lanino, E., Sundberg, B., Bernardo, ME., Remberger, M., Dini, G., Egeler, RM., Bacigalupo, A., Fibbe, W., & Ringdén, O.; Developmental Committee of the European Group for Blood and Marrow Transplantation. (2008). Mesenchymal stem cells for treatment of steroid-resistant, severe, acute graft-versus-host disease: a phase II study. *Lancet,* Vol.371, No.9624, (May 2008), pp. 1579-1586, ISSN 0140-6736

Le Blanc, K., & Ringdén, O. (2007). Immunomodulation by mesenchymal stem cells and clinical experience. *Journal of internal medicine,* Vol.262, No.5, (November 2007), pp. 509-525, ISSN 0954-6820

L'Heureux, N., McAllister, TN., & de la Fuente, LM. (2007). Tissue-engineered blood vessel for adult arterial revascularization. *The New England journal of medicine,* Vol.357, No.14, (October 2007), pp. 1451-1453, ISSN 0028-4793

Light, J., Salomon, DR., Diethelm, AG., Alexander, JW., Hunsicker, L., Thistlethwaite, R., Reinsmoen, N., & Stablein, DM. (2007). Bone marrow transfusions in cadaver renal allografts: pilot trials with concurrent controls. Clinical transplantation, Vol.357, No.14, (October 2007), pp.1451-1453, ISSN 0902-0063

Louis, S., Braudeau, C., Giral, M., Dupont, A., Moizant, F., Robillard, N., Moreau, A., Soulillou, JP., & Brouard, S. (2006). Contrasting CD25hiCD4+T cells/FOXP3 patterns in chronic rejection and operational drug-free tolerance. *Transplantation,* Vol.81, No.3, (February 2006), pp. 398-407, ISSN 0934-0874

Macchiarini, P., Jungebluth, P., Go, T., Asnaghi, MA., Rees, LE., Cogan, TA., Dodson, A., Martorell, J., Bellini, S., Parnigotto, PP., Dickinson, SC., Hollander, AP., Mantero, S., Conconi, MT., & Birchall, MA. (2008). Clinical transplantation of a tissue-engineered airway. *Lancet,* Vol.372, No.9655, (December 2008), pp. 2023-2030, ISSN 0140-6736

Martínez-Llordella, M., Lozano, JJ., Puig-Pey, I., Orlando, G., Tisone, G., Lerut, J., Benitez, C., Pons, JA., Parrilla, P., Ramirez, P., Bruguera, M., Rimola, A., & Sánchez-Fueyo, A. (2008). Towards a diagnostic test of operational tolerance in liver transplantation employing transcriptional profiling. *The Journal of clinical investigation,* Vol.118, No.8, (August 2008), pp.2845-2857, ISSN 0021-9738

Martínez-Llordella, M., Puig-Pey, I., Orlando, G., Tisone, G., Ramoni, M., Lerut, J., Rimola, A., Navasa, M., Margarit, C., Bilbao, I., Hernández-Fuentes, M., Soulillou, JP., & Sánchez-Fueyo, A. (2007). Multiparameter immune profiling of operational tolerance in liver transplantation. *American journal of transplantation: official journal of the American Society of Transplantation and the American Society of Transplant Surgeons,* Vol.7, No.2, (February 2007), pp. 309-319, ISSN 1600-6135

Mason, C., & Dunnill, P. (2008). A brief definition of regenerative medicine. *Regenerative medicine,* Vol.3, No.1 (January 2008), pp. 1-5, ISSN 1746-0751

McAllister, TN., Maruszewski, M., Garrido, SA., Wystrychowski, W., Dusserre, N., Marini, A., Zagalski, K., Fiorillo, A., Avila, H., Manglano, X., Antonelli, J., Kocher, A., Zembala, M., Cierpka, L., de la Fuente, LM., & L'heureux, N. (2009). Effectiveness of haemodialysis access with an autologous tissue-engineered vascular graft: a multicentre cohort study. *Lancet,* Vol.373, No.9673, (April 2009), pp. 1440-1446, ISSN 0140-6736

Millan, MT., Shizuru, JA., Hoffmann, P., Dejbakhsh-Jones, S., Scandling, JD., Grumet, FC., Tan, JC., Salvatierra, O., Hoppe, RT., & Strober, S. (2002). Mixed chimerism and immunosuppressive drug withdrawal after HLA-mismatched kidney and hematopoietic progenitor transplantation. *Transplantation,* Vol.73, No.9, (May 2002), pp. 1386-1391, ISSN 0934-0874

Monaco, AP., Wood, ML., Maki, T., Madras, PN., Sahyoun, AI., &Simpson, MA. (1985). Attempt to induce unresponsiveness to human renal allografts with antilymphocyte globulin and donor-specific bone marrow. Transpl Proc 1985;27:1312-1314

Monaco, AP., Clark, AW., Wood, ML., Sahyoun, AI., Codish, SD., & Brown, RW.. (1976). Possible active enhancement of a human cadaver renal allograft with antilymphocyte serum (ALS) and donor bone marrow: case report of an initial attempt. *Surgery*, Vol.79, No.4, (April 1976), pp. 384-392, ISSN 0039-6060

Monaco, AP., & Wood, ML. (1970). Studies on heterologous antilymphocyte serum in mice. VII. Optimal cellular antigen for induction of immunologic tolerance with antilymphocyte serum. *Transplantation proceedings*, Vol.2, No.4, (December 1970), pp. 489-496, ISSN 0041-1345

Najarian, JS (1975). Editorial comment. Arch Surg 1975;110:1451.

Naughton, G. (1999). The Advanced Tissue Sciences story. *Scientific American*, Vol.280, No.4 (April 1999), pp. 84-85, ISSN 0036-8733

Newell, KA., Asare, A., Kirk, AD., Gisler, TD., Bourcier, K., Suthanthiran, M., Burlingham, WJ., Marks, WH., Sanz, I., Lechler, RI., Hernandez-Fuentes, MP., Turka, LA., & Seyfert-Margolis, VL.; Immune Tolerance Network ST507 Study Group. (2010). Identification of a B cell signature associated with renal transplant tolerance in humans. *The Journal of clinical investigation*, Vol.120, No.6, (June 2010), pp. 1836-1847, ISSN 0021-9738

Orlando, G., Wood, KJ., Stratta, RJ., Yoo, J., Atala, A., & Soker, S. (n.d.) Regenerative medicine and organ transplantation: Past, present and future. *Transplantation*, in press, ISSN 0934-0874

Orlando, G. (2011). Transplantation as a subfield of regenerative medicine. An interview by Lauren Constable. *Expert review of clinical immunology*, Vol.7, No.???, (Month 2011), pp. 137-141, ISSN 1744-666X

Orlando, G., Baptista, P., Birchall, M., De Coppi, P., Farney, A., Guimaraes-Souza, NK., Opara, E., Rogers, J., Seliktar, D., Shapira-Schweitzer, K., Stratta, RJ., Atala, A., Wood, KJ., & Soker, S. (2010). Regenerative medicine as applied to solid organ transplantation: current status and future challenges. *Transplant International: official journal of the European Society for Organ Transplantation,* Vol.24, No.3, (March 2011), pp. 223-232, ISSN 0934-0874

Orlando, G., Hematti, P., Stratta, RJ., Burke, GW., Di Cocco, P., Pisani, F., Soker, S., & Wood, KJ. (2010). Clinical operational tolerance after renal transplantation: current status and future challenges. *Annals of surgery*, Vol.252, No.6, (December 2010), pp. 915-928, ISSN 0003-4932

Orlando, G., Soker, S., & Wood, K. (2009). Operational tolerance after liver transplantation. *Journal of hepatology*, Vol.50, No.6, (June 2009), pp. 1247-1257, ISSN 0168-8278

Ott, HC., Clippinger, B., Conrad, C., Schuetz, C., Pomerantseva, I., Ikonomou, L., Kotton, D., & Vacanti, JP. (2010). Regeneration and orthotopic transplantation of a bioartificial lung. *Nature medicine*, Vol.16, No.8, (August 2010), pp. 927-933, ISSN 1078-8956

Ott, HC., Matthiesen, TS., Goh, SK., Black, LD., Kren, SM., Netoff, TI., & Taylor, DA. (2008). Perfusion-decellularized matrix: using nature's platform to engineer a bioartificial heart. *Nature medicine*, Vol.14, No.2, (February 2008), pp.213-221, ISSN 1078-8956

Owens, ML., Maxwell, G., Goodnight, J., & Wolcott, MW. (1975).Discontinuance of immunosuppression in renal transplant patients. *Archives of surgery*, Vol.110, No.12, (December 1975), pp.1450-1451, ISSN 0272-5533

Petersen, TH., Calle, EA., Zhao, L., Lee, EJ., Gui, L., Raredon, MB., Gavrilov, K., Yi, T., Zhuang, ZW., Breuer, C., Herzog, E., & Niklason, LE. (2010). Tissue-Engineered Lungs for in Vivo Implantation. *Science*, Vol.329, No.599`, (July 2010), pp. 538-541, ISSN 0193-4511

Raya-Rivera, A., Esquiliano, DR., Yoo, JJ., Lopez-Bayghen, E., Soker, S., & Atala, A. (2011). Tissue-engineered autologoug urethras for patients who need reconstruction: an observational study. *Lancet*, (n.d.) ISSN 0140-6736

Riquelme, P., Gövert, F., Geissler, EK., Fändrich, F., & Hutchinson, JA. (2009). Human transplant acceptance-inducing cells suppress mitogen-stimulated T cell proliferation. *Transplant immunology*, Vol.21, No.3, (July 2009), pp. 162-165, ISSN 0966-3274

Roussey-Kesler, G., Giral, M., Moreau, A., Subra, JF., Legendre, C., Noel, C., Pillebout, E., Brouard, S., & Soulillou, JP. (2006). Clinical operational tolerance after kidney transplantation. *American journal of transplantation: official journal of the American Society of Transplantation and the American Society of Transplant Surgeons*, Vol.6, No.4, (April 2006), pp. 736-746, ISSN 1600-6135

Sagoo, P., Perucha, E., Sawitzki, B., Tomiuk, S., Stephens, DA., Miqueu, P., Chapman, S., Craciun, L., Sergeant, R., Brouard, S., Rovis, F., Jimenez, E., Ballow, A., Giral, M., Rebollo-Mesa, I., Le Moine, A., Braudeau, C., Hilton, R., Gerstmayer, B., Bourcier, K., Sharif, A., Krajewska, M., Lord, GM., Roberts, I., Goldman, M., Wood, KJ., Newell, K., Seyfert-Margolis, V., Warrens, AN., Janssen, U., Volk, HD., Soulillou, JP., Hernandez-Fuentes, MP., & Lechler, RI. (2010). Development of a cross-platform biomarker signature to detect renal transplant tolerance in humans. *The Journal of clinical investigation*, Vol.120, No.6, (June 2010), pp. 1848-1861, ISSN 0021-9738

Sayegh, MH., Fine, NA., Smith, JL., Rennke, HG., Milford, EL., & Tilney, NL. (1991). Immunologic tolerance to renal allografts after bone marrow transplants from the same donors. *Annals of internal medicine*, Vol.114, No.11, (June 1991), pp. 954-955, ISSN 0003-4819

Scandling, JD., Busque, S., Dejbakhsh-Jones, S., Benike, C., Millan, MT., Shizuru, JA., Hoppe, RT., Lowsky, R., Engleman, EG., & Strober, S. (2008). Tolerance and chimerism after renal and hematopoietic-cell transplantation. *The New England journal of medicine*, Vol.358, No.4, (January 2008), pp. 362-368, ISSN 0028-4793

Sellers, MT., Deierhoi, MH., Curtis, JJ., Gaston, RS., Julian, BA., Lanier, DC. Jr, & Diethelm, AG. (2001). Tolerance in renal transplantation after allogeneic bone marrow transplantation-6-year follow-up. *Transplantation*, Vol.71, No.11, (June 2001), pp. 1681-1683, ISSN 0041-1337

Shinoka, T., Matsumura, G., Hibino, N., Naito, Y., Watanabe, M., Konuma, T., Sakamoto, T., Nagatsu, M., & Kurosawa, H. (2005). Midterm clinical result of tissue-engineered vascular autografts seeded with autologous bone marrow cells. *The Journal of thoracic and cardiovascular surgery*, Vol.129, No.6, (June 2005), pp. 1330-1338, ISSN 0022-5223

Shinoka, T., Imai, Y., & Ikada, Y. (2001). Transplantation of a Tissue-Engineered Pulmonary Artery. *The New England journal of medicine*, Vol.344, No.7, (February 2001), pp. 532-533, ISSN 0028-4793

Sivozhelezov, V., Braud, C., Giacomelli, L., Pechkova, E., Giral, M., Soulillou, JP., Brouard, S., & Nicolini, C. (2008). Immunosuppressive drug-free operational immune tolerance in human kidney transplants recipients. Part II. Non-statistical gene microarray analysis. *Journal of cellular biochemistry*, Vol.103, No.6, (April 2008), pp. 1693-1906, ISSN 0730-2312

Sorof, JM., Koerper, MA., Portale, AA., Potter, D., DeSantes, K., &Cowan, M. (1995). Renal transplantation without chronic immunosuppression after T cell-depleted, HLA-mismatched bone marrow transplantation. *Transplantation*, Vol.59, No.11, (June 1995), pp. 1633-1635, ISSN 0041-1337

Spitzer, TR., Delmonico, F., Tolkoff-Rubin, N., McAfee, S., Sackstein, R., Saidman, S., Colby, C., Sykes, M., Sachs, DH., & Cosimi, AB. (1999). Combined histocompatibility leukocyte antigen-matched donor bone marrow and renal transplantation for multiple myeloma with end stage renal disease: the induction of allograft tolerance through mixed lymphohematopoietic chimerism. *Transplantation*, Vol.68, No.4, (August 1999), pp. 480-484, ISSN 0041-1337

Starzl, TE., Murase, N., Abu-Elmagd, K., Gray, EA., Shapiro, R., Eghtesad, B., Corry, RJ., Jordan, ML., Fontes, P., Gayowski, T., Bond, G., Scantlebury, VP., Potdar, S., Randhawa, P., Wu, T., Zeevi, A., Nalesnik, MA., Woodward, J., Marcos, A., Trucco, M., Demetris, AJ., & Fung, JJ. (2003). Tolerogenic immunosuppression for organ transplantation. *Lancet*, Vol.361, No.9368, (May 2003), pp. 1502-1510, ISSN 0140-6736

Strober, S., Lowsky, RJ., Shizuru, JA., Scandling, JD., & Millan, MT. (2004). Approaches to transplantation tolerance in humans. *Transplantation*, Vol.77, No.6, (March 2004), pp. 932-936, ISSN 0041-1337

Strober, S., Benike, C., Krishnaswamy, S., Engleman, EG., & Grumet, FC. (2000). Clinical transplantation tolerance twelve years after prospective withdrawal of immunosuppressive drugs: studies of chimerism and anti-donor reactivity. *Transplantation*, Vol.69, No.8, (April 2000), pp. 1549-1554, ISSN 0041-1337

Strober, S., Dhillon, M., Schubert, M., Holm, B., Engleman, E., Benike, C., Hoppe, R., Sibley, R., Myburgh, JA., Collins, G., & Levin, B. (1989). Acquired immune tolerance to cadaveric renal allografts. A study of three patients treated with total lymphoid irradiation. *The New England journal of medicine*, Vol.321, No.1, (July 1989), pp. 28-33, ISSN 0028-4793

Sykes, M. (2009). Hematopoietic cell transplantation for tolerance induction: animal models to clinical trials. *Transplantation*, Vol.77, No.6, (February 2009), pp. 932-936, ISSN 0041-1337

Trzonkowski, P., Zilvetti, M., Chapman, S., Wieckiewicz, J., Sutherland, A., Friend, P., & Wood, KJ. (2008). Homeostatic repopulation by CD28-CD8+ T cells in alemtuzumab-depleted kidney transplant recipients treated with reduced immunosuppression. *American journal of transplantation: official journal of the American Society of Transplantation and the American Society of Transplant Surgeons*, Vol.8, No.2, (February 2008), pp. 338-347, ISSN 1600-6135

Uehling, DT., Hussey, JL., Weinstein, AB., Wank, R., & Bach, FH. (1976). Cessation of immunosuppression after renal transplantation. *Surgery*, Vol.79, No.3, (March 1976), pp. 278-282, ISSN 0039-6060

Uygun, BE., Soto-Gutierrez, A., Yagi, H., Izamis, ML., Guzzardi, MA., Shulman, C., Milwid, J., Kobayashi, N., Tilles, A., Berthiaume, F., Hertl, M., Nahmias, Y., Yarmush, ML., & Uygun, K. (2010). Organ reengineering through development of a transplantable recellularized liver graft using decellularized liver matrix. *Nature medicine*, Vol.16, No.7, (July 2010), pp. 814-820, ISSN 1078-8956

VanBuskirk, AM., Burlingham, WJ., Jankowska-Gan, E., Chin, T., Kusaka, S., Geissler, F., Pelletier, RP., & Orosz, CG. (2000). Human allograft acceptance is associated with immune regulation. *The Journal of clinical investigation*, Vol.106, No.1, (July 2000), pp. 145-155, ISSN 0021-9738

Watson, CJ., Bradley, JA., Friend ,PJ., Firth, J., Taylor, CJ., Bradley, JR., Smith, KG., Thiru, S., Jamieson, NV., Hale, G., Waldmann, H., & Calne, R. (2005). Alemtuzumab (CAMPATH 1H) induction therapy in cadaveric kidney transplantation--efficacy and safety at five years. *American journal of transplantation: official journal of the American Society of Transplantation and the American Society of Transplant Surgeons*, Vol.5, No.6, (June 2005), pp. 1347-1353, ISSN 1600-6135

Zoller, KM., Cho, SI., Cohen, JJ., & Harrington, JT. (1980). Cessation of immunosuppressive therapy after successful transplantation: a national survey. *Kidney international*, Vol.18, No.1, (July 1980), pp. 110-114, ISSN 0085-2538

12

Ischemia Reperfusion Injury in Kidney Transplantation

Bulent Gulec
Gulhane Military Medical Academy,
Haydarpaşa Teaching Hospital, Istanbul
Turkey

1. Introduction

Ischemia and reperfusion have been a natural step during kidney transplantation. Impairment of blood flow starts with brain death due to severe hemodynamic disturbances in cadaveric donor. Clamping of renal artery causes an absolute ischemia during harvesting operation. Cold ischemia during allograft kidney storage may also cause additional ischemic damages (Southard et al. 1985; Ploeg et al.1988; Dong & Tilney 2001). On the other hand, allograft kidney transplantation from living related donor is also subjected to warm ischemia beginning from arterial clamping. Following the blood flow reconstruction in kidney transplantation, the final stage of injury occurs during reperfusion –so called reperfusion injury. Ischemia reperfusion injury is actually an immediate nonspecific inflammatory response (Koo & Fuggle 2000). In this response, endothelium is activated by reactive oxygen species and inflammatory cytokines, then adhesion molecules like P-selectin and E-selectin are involved and induce the adherence of platelets to the epithelium. Leukocytes, initially neutrophils then monocytes and macrophages infiltrate into the affected tissue besides T lymphocytes (Koo & Fuggle 2002).

The pathophysiological changes associated with ischemia/reperfusion injury in renal transplantation are not yet well defined although it has been studied extensively (Koo et al 1998). However, it is well known that prolonged cold ischemia is associated with delayed graft function with elevated creatinine levels in addition to inferior graft survival on long term follow up (Homer-Vanniasinkam et al.1997; Land 1999). Animal studies showed that the main mechanisms were related to leukocyte-endothelium interactions, reactive oxygen species, and the complement system (Kurokawa & Takagi 1999). Many interrelated pathways also control these fundamental biological systems. Free radicals appear to mediate tissue injury through lipid peroxidation and the activation of endothelial cells, resulting in functional and structural cell damage. Apoptosis and cell necrosis also take place as a result of injury. The disturbance of microcirculation in the graft besides mitochondria and some other cellular organelles are parts of these changes (Jassem et al. 2002). The main pathological changes are cellular death of affected tissue. Many other factors including the duration of ischemia dictate the magnitude of injury (Massberg et al. 1998; Land 1999; Gulec et al. 2006). The age and types of tissue are strongly correlated to the magnitude of damages in ischemia and reperfusion (Homer-Vanniasinkam et al.1997; Torras et al 1999).

2. Mechanism of ischemia reperfusion injury

Many studies have been employed to explain the damage caused by ischemia reperfusion injury (Land 1999). Blood flow stops and substrates and energy are deprived of so that cellular homeostasis and ionic gradient can not be maintained anymore. This is a stressful state for the affected cells. In the beginning of ischemia, adenosine triphosphate is provided by glycolysis. However, glycogen stocks are limited and soon are emptied meanwhile waste products and toxic metabolites including lactate are accumulated.

By changes in metabolism during ischemia, intracellular pH falls as a result of anaerobic glycolysis and the hydrolysis of adenosine triphosphate. It is surprising that, restoration of a normal pH during reperfusion in ischemic cells accelerates cell killing, a phenomenon called the 'pH paradox'. If ischemic cells are reperfused at acidotic pH or a rise in intracellular pH after reperfusion is inhibited, cell killing is abrogated. In contrast, the rise in intracellular pH during reperfusion provokes cell killing. Reperfusion exacerbates this damage by triggering an inflammatory reaction involving oxygen-free radicals, endothelial factors, and leukocytes (Figure 1). This triggering disrupts the microcirculation with attraction, activation, adhesion, and migration of neutrophils (Massberg & Messmer 1998). Actually, the target site of ischemia reperfusion injury is the vascular endothelium and the microcirculation of the graft.

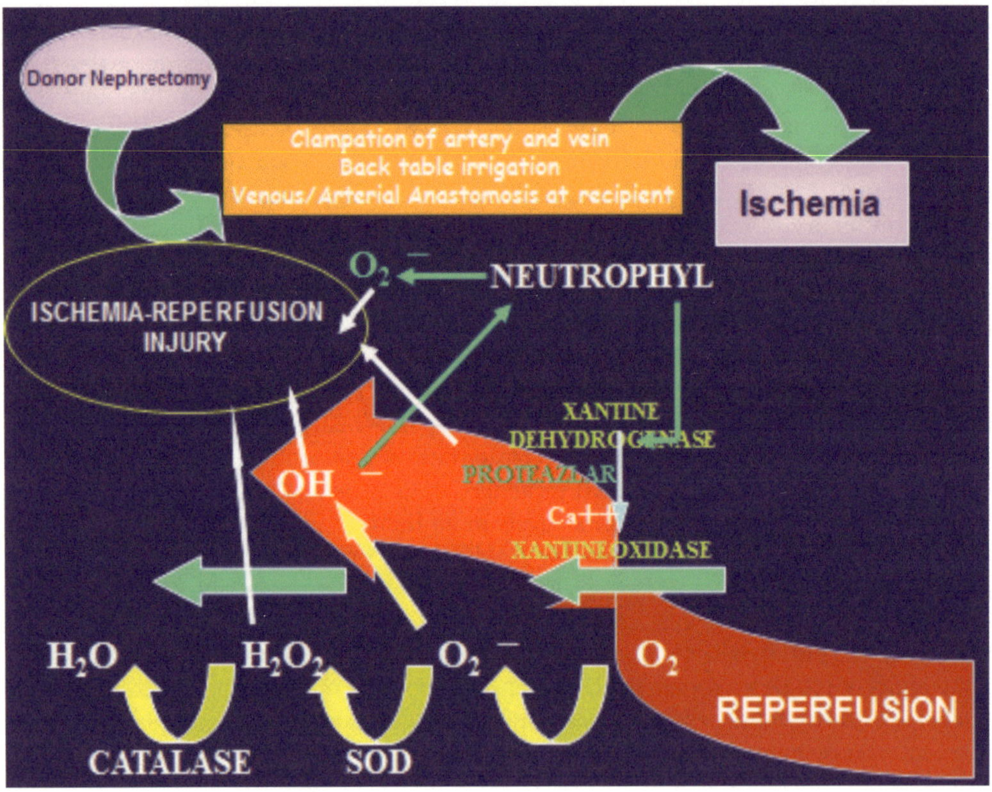

Fig. 1. The ischemia reperfusion injury

In order to understand mechanisms involved in ischemia reperfusion injury, initial and late phases should be evaluated. Activation of leucocytes and interactions between leucocytes and endothelium provoking inflammation take place at initial phase and release of reactive oxygen species from different sources, activation of complements and triggering the innate immunity causing apoptosis and necrosis of the cells are late phase response following ischemia reperfusion injury. Chemotactic mediators during ischemia, activate leucocytes and enzymes like phospholipase A2 which converts cell membrane phospholipids into arachidonic acid, and lysozymes which are proteolytic digesting pathogens and necrotic cells (Figure 2). Arachidonic acid itself is a precursor for inflammatory mediators such as leukotrienes and prostaglandins. By way of lipoxygenase and cyclooxygenase pathways, metabolites of arachidonic acid but mainly the leukotrienes increase the vascular endothelial adhesion of leukocytes and increase the postcapillary permeability. On the other hand, when leukocytes bind to endothelium, adhesion molecules such as P selectin and L selectin besides intercellular adhesion molecule (ICAM) occur and make more leucocytes adhere to the site. It is sure that reperfusion will increase these interactions between leucocytes and epithelium. Actually, leucocytes release some chemotactic agents recruiting much more leucocytes in the area. Leucocytes also release lysozymes and produce reactive oxygen species which are essentials in ischemia reperfusion injury. It has been shown that activated neutrophils also release elastase, cathepsin G, heparanase, collagenase and hydrolytic enzymes that are likely to be directly cytotoxic to hepatocytes (Kang 2002).

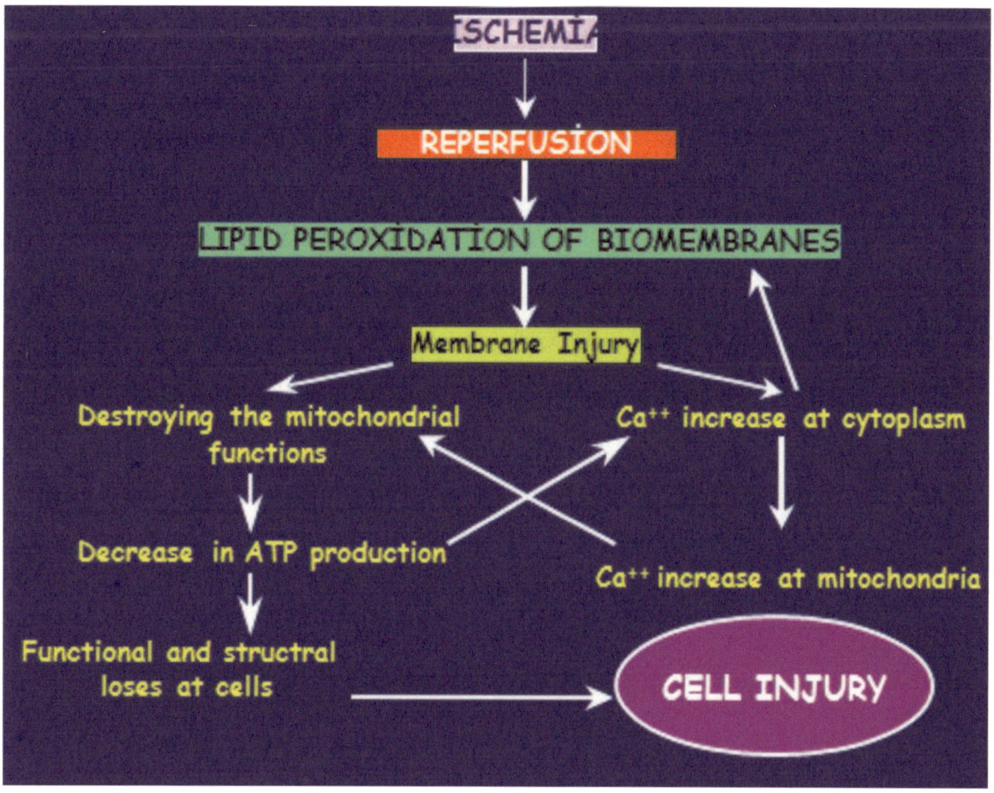

Fig. 2. Lipid peroxidation of biomembranes in ischemia reperfusion injury

Reactive oxygen species as highly unstable oxygen molecules with unpaired electrons are capable of oxidizing many biological molecules, such as proteins, lipids, and DNA. They react with the cell membrane causing lipid peroxidation. Lipid peroxidation affects leucocytes and platelets so that further vasoconstriction and the diminished perfusion occur. The antioxidant activity of glutathione, superoxide dismutase, and catalase in the body control the concentrations of reactive oxygen species. Reactive oxygen species can be released by way of different ways in various tissues like through cytochrome P450 in lung or xanthine oxidase and cyclooxygenase in endothelium or nicotinamide adenine dinucleotide phosphate oxidase in leucocytes (Khalil et al. 2006). In animals with nicotinamide adenine dinucleotide phosphate oxidase deficiency, interestingly enough reperfusion injury is still observed (Hoffmeyer et al. 2000). It suggests that reactive oxygen species are solely not the only contributor to reperfusion injury.

The terminal complement complex and C5a are the complement activation products mainly involved in tissue injury by ischemia reperfusion (Ferraresso et al. 2000). As a part of nonspecific inflammatory response, the deposition of terminal complement components in reperfused tissue has been detected. In contrary, depletion of complements in animals reduces the extent of injury (Amsterdam et al. 1995). It suggests that complement is another key mediator of reperfusion injury by an alternative pathway. The formation of membrane-attack complexes is the end product that damages cells by creating pores in cell membranes. Complement activation releases chemotactic agent (C5a) and anaphylatoxins (C3a, C5a) that induce degranulation of mast cell and the release of chemical mediators like histamine etc. (Lazarus, et al. 2000). It has been suggested that antibody complexes may form during reperfusion injury (Austen et al. 2003). Studies by Williams et al. 1999 and Zhang et al.2004 reported that immunoglobulin M plays a role in pathogenic injury with in situ evidence of immunoglobulin M and C3 and C4 complement deposition in damaged tissue.

The host innate immune system participates in inflammation. As the most potent antigen presenting cells, dendritic cells are also involved in this process. Epithelial and endothelial cells besides dendritic cells express so called toll like receptors which are activated by endogenous ligands. It has been clearly demonstrated that toll-like receptors signaling is involved in the immune recognition of kidney allografts (Obhrai & Goldstein 2006). Further investigation about innate immunity during transplantation will likely improve future therapeutic interventions in this area.

Ischemia reperfusion injury in organ transplantation is mediated as briefly described above by a complex mechanism ending with cell death by apoptosis and necrosis (Thomas et al. 2000). Although apoptosis is a unique and required mechanism to maintain normal physiology, growth, differentiation in a scheduled manner; cell damage in ischemia reperfusion injury can also induce apoptosis. (Thomas et al. 2000; Daemen et al. 2002)

3. Ischemia reperfusion injury during renal transplantation

A better understanding of the underlying mechanisms of ischemia reperfusion injury will help further improvements in graft survival. Post-transplant renal failure has been studied extensively. Almost 30 % of the delayed graft dysfunction following kidney transplantation is attributable to ischemia reperfusion injury (Jassem et al 2002). Apoptosis has been identified as a central mechanism in many aspects of organ and tissue transplantation, rejection, and immune tolerance (Thomas et al 2000). The classical effector enzymes of apoptosis, caspases are able to induce not only apoptosis but also inflammation following ischemia reperfusion injury in experimental models (Daemen et al. 2002). Indeed, ischemia reperfusion injury is one of the most important nonspecific and otherwise nonimmunologic factor affecting both delayed graft function and late allograft dysfunction (Halloran et al. 1988; Womer et al. 2000).

The transplanted kidney may be susceptible to ischemia reperfusion injury at various stages of transplantation. Hemodynamic instability of cadaver donors may also cause repeated in situ warm ischemia attacks of kidneys. Warm ischemia may also be experienced during organ procurement. In situ cooling may be useful to minimize ischemia reperfusion injury during organ retrieval from a cadaveric donor (Koo et al 1998). However, organs from non-heart-beating donors are at risk of much longer periods of warm ischemia before cooling with iced perfusion solution at back table. Cold ischemia is another issue and allograft kidneys are exposed to some degree of cold ischemia during storage of kidneys from cadaveric donors. Although it is relatively short period of time, allograft kidney is subjected to cold ischemia during living related renal transplantation. When blood flow starts again, proinflammatory cytokines were released and innate immunity was activated by the reactive oxygen species mediated injury. This early innate immune response and the ischemic damage will initiate adaptive responses. Repair and regeneration process including cellular apoptosis, autophagy, and necrosis will take place. The final result is directly related to early and late function of the transplanted kidney.

Studies investigating the effects of ischemia reperfusion injury in clinical renal transplantation are limited. It is documented that the length of warm or cold ischemia is proportional to the incidence of delayed graft function in transplanted patients (Koo et al 1998, Mateo et al. 2002). Ischemia reperfusion injury in the allograft kidney provokes renal tubular apoptosis and inflammatory response that may stimulate alloimmunity against the graft (Lieberthal et al 1998; Daemen et al. 2002). Physiologic apoptosis does not provoke an immune response; moreover apoptotic cells may suppress inflammation. However, apoptosis following ischemia reperfusion injury instigate inflammation by way of activated caspases (Daemen et al. 2002). The most important of all, apoptosis requires adenosine triphosphate while necrosis can occur even in adenosine triphosphate depleted conditions.

Greene & Paller 1992, showed that rat proximal tubule epithelial cells produced reactive oxygen species in case of ischemia reperfusion. Glutathione and vitamin E as reactive oxygen species scavengers reduced the magnitude of injury. The role of polimorphonuclear leucocytes in ischemia reperfusion injury is upon revascularization. The adhesion molecules, ICAM-1 and VCAM-1 take place in mediating renal damage during reperfusion injury. Briscoe et al. 1992 showed that circulating ICAM-1 levels and ICAM-1 expression by proximal tubule cells have increased during acute rejection besides over expression of VCAM-1 at sites where T-cells accumulated.

Rainger et al. 1995, showed that reactive oxygen species induce adhesion molecule expression, resulting in activation and increased binding of neutrophils at human umbilical vein endothelial cells. In another experimental study by Shoskes et al. 1990, increased expression of adhesion molecules and neutrophil infiltration within hours of reperfusion, followed by mononuclear cell infiltration and up-regulation of major histocompatibility complex class II expression several days later have been shown following ischemia reperfusion injury of the kidney. These immunogenic changes triggered by the early nonspecific inflammatory events will play a major role in determining the quality of graft function in the long term.

Previous clinical studies on ischemia reperfusion have relied mainly on the measurement of malondialdehyde as a marker of lipid peroxidation, although elevated levels of malondialdehyde in plasma after reperfusion of the graft were not correlated with subsequent graft function (Davenport et al.1995). In the early era of transplantation, postperfusion state biopsy in order to evaluate hyperacute rejection was frequently obtained at an hour after revascularization. Neutrophil infiltration in the glomeruli was assessed as an indicator of hyperacute rejection of the allograft, although a direct correlation between neutrophil infiltrations and either hyperacute rejection or acute rejection episode was not established (Gaber et al. 1992). Due to modern pluripotent immunosupressive agents and improvements in antibody screening and crossmatching, hyperacute rejection has been virtually eliminated. So that there is no need to obtain biopsy at postperfusion state. Gaber et al. 1992, stated that polymorphonuclear leukocytes detected in biopsies from cadaver renal allografts, were associated with long cold-storage times. They observed 4 hyperacute rejection cases of 57 allografts studied and concluded that it was not clear whether these polymorphonuclear leukocytes entered upon reperfusion or were already present within the donor kidney.

4. Remote organ effects of ischemia reperfusion injury following kidney transplantation

Transplantation of an ischemic organ can cause dysfunction in distant organs. Above mentioned various mediators are released into systemic circulation following ischemia reperfusion injury. These circulating mediators may be harmful at distant tissues and organs like native kidneys, lungs, liver and heart. Mediators like TxA2 and LTB4 may cause transient pulmonary hypertension by way of sequestration of leukocytes and increased capillary permeability (Anner et al. 1988). Inhibition of these eicosanoids greatly attenuates pulmonary injury. Electrolyte imbalance including potassium and hydrogen ions besides myoglobin released into the circulation following revascularisation of ischemic limbs can impair renal, cardiac and pulmonary functions. Similarly increased levels of TNF-a, IL-1, and IL-6 occur following hindlimb reperfusion and may influence PMN-mediated remote organ injury. Enhanced lung permeability is prevented by blocking these pathways (Seekamp et al. 1993).

Distant organ injury or multiple organ failure is the end point of remote effects of ischemia reperfusion injury. Pulmonary injury is a major component of all. Leucocyte sequestration in pulmonary tissue was prevented by inactivation of xanthine oxidase in a rat model of intestinal reperfusion (Terada et al. 1992, Poggetti et al. 1992). Both local and systemic tissue injury occurs following reperfusion of ischemic organ. It is now clear that the pathogenesis of remote organ injury is multifactorial including the intracellular signaling pathways which promote these events. Further studies including prevention techniques and will help to prevent remote organ effects of ischemia reperfusion injury following kidney transplantation.

5. Prevention of ischemia reperfusion injury

The renal transplantation is the only definitive treatment for patients with end stage kidney disease. Advances in immunology and success in surgical technique provide almost 95 % graft survival for the first year in living related kidney transplantation. However, the delayed graft dysfunction following kidney transplantation is a main problem affecting long term graft survival (Jassem et al 2002). Ischemia reperfusion injury induces acute renal failure which is very crucial for transplanted kidney survival. At present it is not possible to prevent acute renal failure following transplantation. Success at minimizing ischemic injury should be aimed. The organ shortage worldwide has increased the interest about drugs, perfusion solutions and perfusion methods to minimize ischemia reperfusion injury. Prevention attempts should begin when a potential donor is determined. It is especially important for suboptimal kidney donors.

The fundamental concerns are to keep the donor hemodynamically stable, to prevent the extent of tubular epithelial cell injury of the kidney following an ischemic insult and to improve its recovery if injury occurs.

Any attempt to prevent renal ischemia is required. Many agents including calcium channel blockers like diltiazem, nifedipine or verapamil; prostaglandins like prostacyclin; thyroid hormone; xanthine oxidase inhibitors like allopurinol or oxypurinol; hydroxyl radicals like dimethylthiourea; ATP-$MgCl_2$ can be used either alone or in combination to modify the effects of ischemia reperfusion (Finn 1990).

The harvested kidneys should be preserved using iced perfusion solutions like Eurocollins or University of Wisconsin. Immunosuppression is started perioperatively. Treatment of ischemic reperfusion injury to allografts with the free radical scavenger superoxide dismutase during kidney transplantation significantly reduced the incidence of acute rejection episodes and early immune-mediated graft loss with remarkably improved the long-term graft outcome (Land 2005)

A significant portion of the damage sustained by the ischemic kidney occurs not during the period of ischemia, but rather during and following reperfusion. The major affected site is tubular epithelial cells. The success of agents in minimizing renal injury is not increasing renal blood flow but promoting and preserving cell viability.

Hypothermia drops oxygen consumption in the kidney. At temperatures of 6° C to 10° C—the temperature range at which human cadaveric kidneys are perfused prior to transplantation—metabolism is reduced by 90% to 95% (Finn 1990 as cited as Brown & Brengelmann 1965). Cooling will prevent rapid loss of mitochondrial activity and its ability to transport electrons.

In kidney transplantation, free oxygen radicals promotes inflammation and apoptosis triggering alloimmunity against the allograft. In a prospective randomized double-blind placebo-controlled trial, kidney-transplanted, cyclosporine-treated patients received 200 mg human recombinant superoxide dismutase during surgery to prevent and ablate free oxygen radical-mediated reperfusion injury of the graft. Although early function of renal allografts could not be improved by this method, the incidence of first degree acute rejection episodes and acute irreversible allograft rejection were significantly reduced following allogeneic kidney transplantation.

Superoxide-radical-induced cytotoxicity appears largely to depend on the subsequent production of hydroxyl radical. Histidine, tryptophan, ascorbate, and alphatocopherol are natural hydroxyl radical scavengers. When lipid peroxidation by free radicals occurs, malondialdehyde, conjugated dienes, hydroperoxides, and short alkanes such as methane, ethane, and pentane are formed. The infusion of ATP, ADP, or AMP are equally effective in promoting early recovery, rather than lessening the initial injury (Land 1999).

The mode of action of superoxide dismutase is blocking both radical mediated and radical dependent (via OH, ONOO2, H2O2 generation) pathways leading to cellular injury during reperfusion. Ischemia reperfusion injury to hearts has been almost completely prevented in hSOD1-transgenic mice (Land 1999 as cited Zweier et al. 1994). This can lead to the chance of successful transplantation of organs from DAF-transgenic pigs to patients would be greater if those animals are also transgenic for the human SOD1 (Land 1999).

6. Conclusion

Ischemia and reperfusion have been a natural step during kidney transplantation. Repair and regeneration process including cellular apoptosis, autophagy, and necrosis follows ischemia reperfusion injury. The final result is directly related to early and late function of the transplanted kidney.

Every transplanted kidney is a damaged organ, and drugs can be used either alone or in combination to modify the effects of ischemia reperfusion besides perfusion solutions and perfusion methods. Further investigations are required to eliminate the effects of ischemia reperfusion injury during kidney transplantation.

7. References

Amsterdam EA, Stahl GL, Pan H, Rendig SV, Fletcher MP, Longhurst JC. (1995) Limitation of reperfusion injury by a monoclonal antibody to C5a during myocardial infarction in pigs. Am. J. Physiol. 268: H448-H457. ISSN 1931-857X

Anner H, Kaufman RP Jr, Valeri CR, Shepro D, Hechtman HB. (1988) Reperfusion of ischemic lower limbs increases pulmonary microvascular permeability. J Trauma; 28: 607-610. ISSN 0022-5282

Austen, W. G., Jr., Kobzik, L., Carroll, M., et al. (2003) The role of complement and natural antibody in intestinal ischemiareperfusion injury. Int. J. Immunopathol. Pharmacol. 16: 1. ISNN 0394-6320

Briscoe DM, Pober JS, Harmon WE, Cotran RS. (1992) Expression of vascular cell adhesion molecule-1 in human renal allografts. J Am Soc Nephol 3: 1180-1185. ISSN 1046-6673

Daemen MARC, De Vries B, Buurman WA. (2002) Apoptosis and inflammation in renal reperfusion injury. Transplantation; 73 (11), 1693–1700. ISSN 0041-1337.

Davenport A, Hopton M, Bolton C (1995) Measurement of malondialdehyde as a marker of oxygen free radical production during renal allograft transplantation and the effect on early graft function. Clin Transplant, 9:171–175

Dong VM, Tilney NL. (2001) Reduction of ischemia/reperfusion injury in organ transplants by cytoprotective strategies Current Opinion in Organ Transplantation, 6:69–74. ISSN 1068–9508

Ferraresso M, Macor P, Valente M, Barbera MD, D'Amelio F, Borghi O, Raschi E, Durigutto P, Meroni P, Tedesco F. (2008) Posttransplant Ischemia-Reperfusion Injury In Transplanted Heart Is Prevented By A Minibody to the Fifth Component of Complement. Transplantation; 86: 1445–1451. ISSN 0041-1337

Finn WF. (1990) Prevention of ischemic injury in renal transplantation. Kidney International, 37: 171—182. ISSN 0085 - 2538

Gaber LW, Gaber AO, Tolley EA, Hathaway DK (1992). Prediction by postrevascularization biopsies of cadaveric kidney allografts of rejection, graft loss, and preservation nephropathy. Transplantation, 53: 1219–1225. ISSN 0041-1337

Gulec B, Coskun K, Oner K, Aydin A, Yigitler C, Kozak O, Uzar A, Arslan I. (2006) The effects of perfusion solutions at kidney ischemia reperfusion injury in pigs Transplantation Proceedings, 38 (2): 371-374. ISSN 0041-1345.

Halloran PF, Aprile MA, Farewell V, et al. (1988) Early function as the principal correlate of graft survival. A multivariate analysis of 200 cadaveric renal transplants treated

with a protocol incorporating antilymphocyte globulin and cyclosporine. Transplantation 46: 223 - 228. ISSN 0041-1337
Hoffmeyer MR, Jones SP, Ross C, Sharp B, Grisham MB, Laroux FS, Stalker TJ, Scalia R, Lefer DJ. (2000) Myocardial ischemia/reperfusion injury in NADPH oxidase-deficient mice. Circ. Res. 87: 812 - 817. ISSN: 1524-4571
Homer-Vanniasinkam S, Crinnion JN., Gough MJ. (1997) Post-ischaemic Organ Dysfunction: A Review * Eur J Vasc Endovasc Surg 14: 195-203
Jassem W, Fuggle SV, Rela M, Koo DDH, Heaton ND. (2002) The Role of Mitochondria in Ischemia / Reperfusion Injury. Transplantation 73(4): 493–499. ISSN 0041-1337
Jassem W, Roake JA. (1998) The molecular and cellular basis of reperfusion injury following organ transplantation. Transplant Rev; 12: 14 - 33 ISSN: 0955-470X).
Kang KJ. (2002) Mechanism of Hepatic Ischemia/Reperfusion Injury and Protection Against Reperfusion Injury. Transplantation Proceedings, 34: 2659–2661 ISSN 0041-1345
Khalil AA., Farah AA, Hall JC. (2006) Reperfusion Injury Plastic and Reconstructive Surgery 117 (3): 1024 - 1032 ISSN: 0032-1052
Klausner JM, Paterson IS, Goldman G, Kobzik L, Rodzen C, Lawrence R, Valeri CR, Shepro D, Hechtman HB. (1989) Postischemicrenal injury is mediated by neutrophils and leukotrienes. Am J Physiol; 256: F794-F802. ISSN: 0363-6127
Koo DDH; Welsh KI.; Roake JA.; Morris PJ & Fuggle SV (1998). Ischemia/Reperfusion Injury in Human Kidney Transplantation An Immunohistochemical Analysis of Changes after Reperfusion Am J Pathol, 153:557–566. ISSN:0002-9440
Koo DDH, Fuggle SV. (2000) Impact of ischemia/reperfusion injury and early inflammatory responses in kidney transplantation. Transplant Rev; 14: 210-224
Koo DDH, Fuggle SV. (2002) Chemokines in ischemia/reperfusion injury. Current Opinion in Organ Transplantation, 7:100–106. ISSN 1087–2418
Kurokawa T., Takagi H. (1999) Mechanism and Prevention of Ischemia-Reperfusion Injury. Transplantation Proceedings, 31: 1775–1776. ISSN 0041-1345
Land W. (1999) Postischemic Reperfusion Injury and Allograft Dysfunction: Is Allograft Rejection the Result of a Fateful Confusion by the Immune System of Danger and Benefit? Transplantation Proceedings, 31: 332–336 ISSN 0041-1345
Land WG. (2005) The Role of Postischemic Reperfusion Injury and Other Nonantigen-Dependent Inflammatory Pathways in Transplantation. Transplantation, 79: 505–514. ISSN 0041-1337
Lieberthal W, Koh JS, Levine JS. (1998) Necrosis and apoptosis in acute renal failure. Semin Nephrol; 18: 505 - 518. ISSN 0270-9295
Massberg S, Messmer K. (1998) The Nature of Ischemia/Reperfusion Injury. Transplantation Proceedings, 30, 4217–4223. ISSN 0041-1345
Mateo R, Barr ML, Selby R, Sher L, Jabbour N, Genyk Y. (2002) Donor organ preservation effects on the recipient. Current Opinion in Organ Transplantation, 7: 53–59. ISSN 1087-2418
Obhrai J,Goldstein DR.(2006) The Role of Toll-like Receptors in Solid Organ Transplantation. Transplantation, 81: 497–502. ISSN 0041-1337
Ploeg RJ, Vreugdenhil P, Goossens D, Mcanulty JF, Southard JH, Belzer FO.(1988) Effect of pharmacologic agents on the function of the hypothermically preserved dog kidney during normothermic reperfusion. Surgery 103: 676-683.

Poggetti RS, Moore FA, Moore EE, Koeike K, Banerjee A. (1992) Simultaneous liver and lung injury following gut ischemia is mediated by xanthine oxidase. J Trauma 32: 723-727.

Rainger GE, Fisher A, Shearman C, Nash GB (1995) Adhesion of flowing neutrophils to cultured endothelial cells after hypoxia and reoxygenation in vitro. Am J Physiol, 269:H1398–H1406 ISSN 1931-857X

Shoskes DA, Partrey NA, Halloran PF (1990) Increased major histocompatibility complex antigen expression in unilateral ischemic acute tubular necrosis in the mouse. Transplantation, 49:201–207. ISSN 0041-1337

Southard JH, Rice MJ, Ametani M, Belzer FO: (1985) Effects of short-term hypothermic perfusion and cold storage on function of the isolated-perfused dog kidney. Cryobiology 22: 147-155

Terada LS, Dormish JJ, Shanley PF, Leff JA, Anderson BO, Repıne JE. (1992) Circulating xanthine oxidase mediates lungneutrophil sequestration after intestinal ischemia-reperfusion. Am J. Physiol; 263: L394-L401.

Thomas F, Wu J, Thomas JM. (2000) Apoptosis and organ transplantation Current Opinion in Organ Transplantation, 5:35–41 ISSN 1087–2418

Torras J, Cruzado JM, Grinyo JM. (1999) Ischemia and Reperfusion Injury in Transplantation Transplantation Proceedings, 31, 2217–2218 ISSN 0041-1345

Womer KL, Vella JP, Sayegh MH (2000) Chronic allograft dysfunction: mechanisms and new approaches to therapy. Semin Nephrol, 20:126–147. ISSN 0270-9295

13

Transforming Growth Factor-Beta in Kidney Transplantation: A Double-Edged Sword

Caigan Du
University of British Columbia
Canada

1. Introduction

Transforming growth factor (TGF)-beta consists of three isoforms (TGF-beta 1, TGF-beta 2 and TGF-beta 3) and is synthesized and secreted in nearly every cell type (Massague, 1990), including in the kidneys and kidney transplants (Horvath et al., 1996; Ando et al., 1998). A variety of biological activities of TGF-beta have been demonstrated in different experimental systems, including stimulation of cellular proliferation and cellular differentiation, or oppositely induction of cell apoptosis and anti-proliferation (Siegel and Massague, 2003), suggesting that TGF-beta, particularly TGF-beta 1, is a key regulatory factor for tissue homeostasis. In cultured renal cells, these three TGF-beta isoforms have similar activities (Yu et al., 2003; Qi et al., 2006), but the activities of TGF-beta 2 and TGF-beta 3 may be partially mediated by TGF-beta 1 (Yu et al., 2003).

Kidney transplantation is the best therapy for individuals who unfortunately have end-stage kidney disease; individuals with kidney transplants live longer with a better quality of life compared to those on dialysis (Port et al., 1993; Laupacis et al., 1996; Schnuelle et al., 1998). However, the progressive loss of kidney transplants remains an elusive objective in clinical care of these patients as indicated by 2009 OPTN/SRTR annual report; the unadjusted kidney graft survival for deceased donors was decreased to 95.3% after 3 months, 91.0% after 1 year, 69.3% after 5 years and 43.3% after 10 years, whereas the similar trend was seen for living donors. It has been shown in numerous studies that ischemia-reperfusion injury, acute rejection episodes, chronic rejection and/or nephrotoxicity of immunosuppressive drugs are the risk factors for this problem (Li and Yang, 2009; de Fijter, 2010), and evidence in literature suggests that there is a possible association of up-regulation of TGF-beta expression and its signaling with poor outcomes in kidney transplantation (Pribylova-Hribova et al., 2006; Einecke et al., 2010). In this chapter, the role of TGF-beta in each of these factors in the progression of kidney transplant dysfunction is discussed.

2. The beneficial effects of TGF-beta on kidney transplant survival

2.1 TGF-beta, a growth and survival factor for renal regeneration after ischemia-reperfusion injury

Graft ischemia-reperfusion injury in kidney transplants is an inevitable event that occurs following the disruption of blood supply to a donor kidney when harvested, and reperfusion with recipient's blood after transplanted. Ischemia-reperfusion injury to kidney grafts is associated with delay graft function that has a negative impact on graft survival and worsens both acute and chronic rejection episodes (Peeters et al., 2004; Chapman et al., 2005). The loss of functioning tubular epithelial cells in renal ischemia-reperfusion injury is caused by both apoptosis and necrosis (Savill, 1994; Gobe et al., 1999a). Thus, its severity may depend on the resistance of renal cells to cell death during the injury, and recovery on cellular regeneration after the damage.

A significant up-regulation of TGF-beta 1 expression has been detected in regenerating renal tubules following ischemic injury in the kidneys (Basile et al., 1996), as well as in renal biopsies of kidney transplants from cold ischemic donors or at five days post-transplantation (Lario et al., 2003). However, the role of TGF-beta in cellular process of ischemia-reperfusion injury or its repair is still contradicted. In cultured renal epithelial cells, addition of TGF-beta 1 directly induces cell apoptosis (Bhaskaran et al., 2003) or promotes angiotensin II- or staurosporine-mediated cell death (Bhaskaran et al., 2003; Dai et al., 2003), while in contrast renal protection of TGF-beta 1 has been reported by several recent studies; TGF-beta 1 is required for renal protection of volatile anesthetics in the protection from H_2O_2-induced apoptosis in cultured human proximal tubular epithelial cells (Lee et al., 2007), and reduces cellular necrosis and inflammation in renal ischemia-reperfusion injury (Lee et al., 2004). Our recent study demonstrates that a deficiency in TGF-beta 1 expression worsens the severity of renal ischemia-reperfusion injury in mice, and overexpression of TGF-beta 1 increases the resistance of cultured human tubular epithelial cells to TNF-alpha-mediated apoptosis (Guan et al., 2010).

The renal protection of TGF-beta in renal ischemia-reperfusion injury may be contributed by its two activities: stimulation of cellular growth and induction of anti-apoptosis. It has been known that many growth factors, such as epidermal growth factor (Danielpour et al., 1991), platelet-derived growth factor (Phillips et al., 1995; Di Paolo et al., 1996; Yamabe et al., 2000) and basic fibroblast growth factor (Phillips et al., 1997; Yamabe et al., 2000), stimulate TGF-beta 1 production in various renal cell cultures, and co-upregulated with TGF-beta in the proliferating or regenerating tubular cells during renal ischemia-reperfusion injury (Schaudies et al., 1993; Toubeau et al., 1994; Nakagawa et al., 1999; Villanueva et al., 2006). The treatment with epidermal growth factor or basic fibroblast growth factor or disruption of platelet-derived growth factor signaling indicate that these factors enhances renal tubule cell regeneration or repair and consequently accelerates the recovery of renal function after renal ischemia-reperfusion injury (Humes et al., 1989; Nakagawa et al., 1999; Villanueva et al., 2006). In addition, TGF-beta 1 in renal cells is upregulated by an autoinduction mechanism (Nowak and Schnellmann, 1996; Grande et al., 2002; Dockrell et al., 2009). Data from all these studies simply imply that TGF-beta may be one of key growth factors for renal regeneration or repair post ischemia-reperfusion injury.

In the kidney, anti-apoptotic Bcl-2 may be pivotal for renal cell survival as in fetal kidneys, the distribution of apoptotic cells is inversely correlated with expression of Bcl-2, and augmented metanephric apoptosis occur in Bcl-2–deficient mice (Winyard et al., 1996). In a rat model of renal ischemia-reperfusion injury, Bcl-2 expression markedly increases in the distal tubules and is associated with increased survival of both the distal and adjacent proximal segment at acute phases (0 to 2 days). After renal injury, expression of both TGF-beta 1 and Bcl-2 is enhanced in regenerating proximal tubule cells relining the basement membrane (Gobe et al., 1999b). Our data also indicate that in cultures of renal TECs, TGF-beta 1 induces Bcl-2 expression and prevents TNF-alpha-mediated apoptosis (Guan et al., 2010). All these studies suggest that Bcl-2 may mediate renal protective role or anti-apoptotic activity of TGF-beta in renal ischemia-reperfusion injury.

2.2 TGF-beta, a FOXP3$^+$ Treg cells inducer for suppression of alloimmune response

It has been well-known for a while that TGF-beta is a potent immunosuppressive cytokine with multiple suppressive actions on a variety of immune cells including T cells, B cells, macrophages, and other cells, and acts with some other inhibitory molecules to maintain a state of immune tolerance in peripheral tissues (Prud'homme and Piccirillo, 2000). Mice with homozygous for *Tgfb1* gene mutation die due to a massive multifocal mixed inflammatory cell infiltration and tissue necrosis in numerous organs (Shull et al., 1992; Christ et al., 1994) through autoimmune responses, such as antibody deposit in renal glomeruli (Yaswen et al., 1996). However, the cellular mechanisms by which TGF-beta suppresses immune responses are not fully understood. Recent findings suggest that TGF-beta is required for regulatory T (Treg) cell development; TGF-beta induces FOXP3 (forkhead box P3) expression in nonregulatory $CD4^+CD25^-$ T cells, and consequently converts these cells to $CD4^+CD25^+FOXP3^+$ Treg cells in vitro (Chen et al., 2003), and in vivo is required for expansion of this phenotype of Treg cells (Peng et al., 2004). TGF-beta-dependent FOXP3$^+$ Treg cells, including both CD4$^+$ and CD8$^+$ phenotypes, can induce immune tolerance to allografts in animal models (Cobbold et al., 2004; Kapp et al., 2006). However, it is also suggested that in the presence of IL-6, TGF-beta induces differentiation of naïve CD4$^+$ T cells to effector interleukin (IL)-17-producing Th17 cells (Bettelli et al., 2006; Veldhoen et al., 2006), but the evidence for TGF-beta-dependent Th17 cell development in vivo has not been confirmed yet. Indeed, recent studies suggest that TGF-beta does not directly stimulate Th17 cell differentiation, instead it inhibits Th1 cells development that indirectly favors Th17 cell expansion (Santarlasci et al., 2009), and Th17 cells can be generated in the absence of TGF-beta signaling (Ghoreschi et al., 2010). Thus, TGF-beta may not have any direct effect on effector Th17 cells, and it may only act as an immuno-down regulatory cytokine by its induction of FOXP3$^+$ Treg cell as well as directly and indirectly in the suppression of other types of immune cells.

The positive correlation of TGF-beta expression at early phase of transplantation with kidney transplant survival has reported in literature. A higher level of TGF-beta in the biopsies within 6 months of transplantation or during acute rejection episodes is associated with a decreased risk of chronic rejection development (Eikmans et al., 2002), and better graft function (Ozdemir et al., 2005). In the early antibody-mediated rejection, occurring within the first 3 weeks after transplantation, there is a strong correlation of intrarenal expression of TGF-beta 1 with FOXP3 mRNA, and importantly the low intrarenal TGF-beta 1 and FOXP3 have significantly shorter graft survival, implied by an increased risk for renal graft failure within next 12 months (Viklicky et al., 2010). The beneficial effect of immunoregulatory TGF-beta on early survival of kidney transplants is further supported by a recent experimental study, demonstrating that only the early renal allograft acceptance is associated with TGF-beta-induced immune regulation, both peripherally by splenocytes as well as locally by graft-infiltrating cells (Cook et al., 2008). All these studies may indicate that TGF-beta may benefit kidney transplant survival at the early phase of transplantation by its immunoregulatory activities, including induction of FOXP3-expressing Treg cells.

3. The adverse effects of TGF-beta on kidney transplant survival

3.1 TGF-beta, a fibrotic factor for chronic rejection of kidney transplants

Chronic rejection in kidney transplants is a major cause of long-term graft dysfunction and ultimate failure, and is characterized as a progressive process of interstitial fibrosis, tubular atrophy, and glomerulosclerosis and vascular sclerosis (Racusen et al., 1999; Nankivell et al.,

2003). Although the pathogenesis of chronic rejection is not fully understood, it is proposed that these pathologies may result from chronic repair response towards injurious and inflammatory stimuli. As a result, extracellular matrix (ECM) accumulates in functional tissue leading to successive tissue fibrosis in the vascular (vascular sclerosis), tubulointerstitium (interstitial fibrosis) and glomeruli (glomerulosclerosis), and the excessive interstitial fibrosis progressively consequently leads to tubular atrophy in kidney transplants. It has been reported that much of this ECM is produced by alpha-smooth muscle actin (alpha-SMA)-expressing myofibroblasts (Simonson, 2007; Wynn, 2008), and early presence of alpha-SMA expression predicts the progression toward pathologic changes for chronic rejection in kidney transplants (Badid et al., 2002; Hertig et al., 2008), suggesting that myofibroblasts are the primary effector cells for chronic rejection of kidney transplants.

Numerous studies have reported a significant correlation of the up-regulation of intragraft TGF beta 1 and active plasma TGF-beta 1 with chronic rejection in kidney transplants (Sharma et al., 1996; Ozdemir et al., 2005; Harris et al., 2007; Del Prete et al., 2009) and with cyclosporine A (CsA) toxicity (Ozdemir et al., 2005). In kidney cell cultures, in addition to the growth factors as discussed above, many injury or pro-inflammatory factors (e.g. platelet-activating factor, hydrogen peroxide, IL-1beta and TNF-alpha) and CsA induce TGF-beta 1 expression (Ruiz-Ortega et al., 1997; Iglesias-De La Cruz et al., 2001; Vesey et al., 2002a; Vesey et al., 2002b; Slattery et al., 2005; Guan et al., 2010). Thus, TGF-beta has been considered as a fibrogenic cytokine, involved in fibrosis or chronic rejection of kidney transplants (Morris-Stiff, 2005), and has been proposed as a therapeutic target for this problem (Mannon, 2006). However, the pathways of fibrotic activity of TGF-beta in chronic rejection of kidney transplants are not completely understood.

TGF-beta is a pivotal factor for the normal process of tissue homeostasis in every part of our body (Siegel and Massague, 2003). Hence, it is easy to understand why TGF-beta is up-regulated and involved in chronic tissue repair when kidney transplants are exposed to chronic inflammation/injury as well as nephrotoxicity of immunosuppressive drugs, but how TGF-beta-mediated chronic repair responses leads to the pathologic changes of chronic rejection in kidney transplants is not exactly known. It has been documented that epithelial-to-mesenchymal transition (EMT) can be induced by TGF-beta and is considered as a continuous supply to myofibroblast population during the progression of renal fibrosis (Iwano, 2010). Indeed, EMT has been detected in kidney transplant biopsies with chronic rejection but not in those with stable function (Vongwiwatana et al., 2005). However, recent experimental studies demonstrates that in the kidneys with unilateral ureteral obstruction a large majority of myofibroblasts for kidney fibrosis actually comes from the phenotypic transition of existing normal interstitial fibroblasts, whereas there is no evidence indicating that epithelial cells migrate outside of the tubular basement membrane and differentiate into interstitial myofibroblasts or EMT (Humphreys et al., 2010), and overexpression of TGF-beta 1 in renal TECs induces fibrosis in the kidney that is associated with interstitial fibroblast proliferation but not with EMT (Koesters et al., 2010). This notion may be also applied to the chronic rejection of kidney transplants that remains further elusive. At the molecular level, TGF-beta stimulates ECM production and/or inhibits ECM degradation in various kidney cells including TECs, interstitial fibroblasts and mesanglial cells (Ruiz-Ortega et al., 1997; Iglesias-De La Cruz et al., 2001; Bottinger and Bitzer, 2002; Vesey et al., 2002a; Vesey et al., 2002b; Tian et al., 2006; Huang et al., 2008). All these data suggest that the fibrotic effect of TGF-beta in the chronic rejection of kidney transplants may be mediated simply by its stimulation of fibroblast growth and ECM remodeling leading to ECM accumulation or fibrosis.

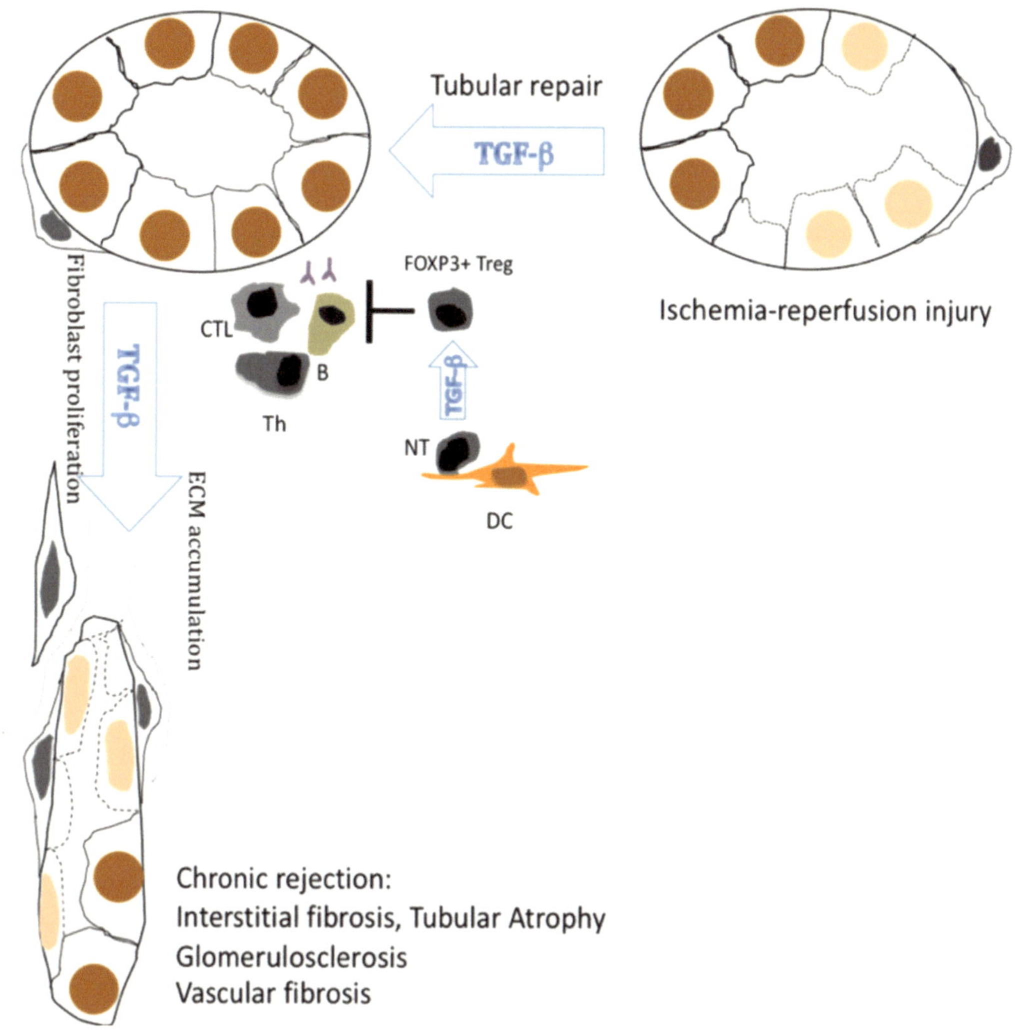

Fig. 1. A simple scheme for cellular pathways of TGF-beta in renal repair/regeneration, immune-modulation and renal fibrosis in kidney transplants.

Following ischemia-reperfusion injury, renal tubular epithelial cells and other types of renal cells are programmed to death (apoptosis and necrosis). TGF-beta may protect cells from apoptosis and stimulate proliferation of surviving renal cells to repair or regenerate the damaged tissue of kidney transplants. When naïve T cells are primed by alloantigens from the kidney transplants, TGF-beta may induce the development of $FOXP3^{+}$ Treg cells that suppress alloimmunity against the kidney transplants. However, chronic up-regulation of TGF-beta production in the kidney transplants may induce ECM-producing myofibroblasts and chronic stimulation of cell growth of myofibroblasts in the tubulointerstitium, glomeruli and vascular tissue may result in chronic rejection, indicated by interstitial fibrosis, tubular atrophy, glomerulosclerosis, and vascular fibrosis. DC: dendritic cells; NT: naïve T cells; Th: T helper cells; B: B and plasma cells; CTL: CD8+ cytotoxic T cells.

4. Conclusion

TGF-beta affects kidney transplant survival in many ways; it is a growth factor for tissue regeneration and tissue remodeling when kidney transplants are damaged, and is an immunosuppressive factor when cellular immune response to kidney transplants is activated. At the beginning of transplantation, when kidney transplants are damaged by ischemia-reperfusion injury and recipient's immune response is activated, TGF-beta may repair kidney transplants by stimulation of tissue regeneration, protection of renal cells from apoptosis and negatively regulates cellular immune response to kidney transplants by induction of $FOXP3^{+}$ Treg cells. Later on, when kidney transplants are attacked by chronic inflammation including drug-resistant immune response and virus infection, and nephrotoxicity of immune suppressive drugs, the chronic repair response of TGF-beta may induce tissue remodeling of kidney transplants leading to chronic rejection (Figure 1). Thus, despite of the short-term beneficial effects of tubule-repairing and immune-down-regulation immediately posttransplantation, the long-term effects of TGF-beta on kidney transplant survival under current immune therapies seem to be negative as increased expression of TGF-beta1 promotes growth of fibroblasts and ECM accumulation leading to tissue remodeling in the tubulointerstitium, vascular tissue and glomeruli or chronic rejection.

5. Acknowledgment

The author wants to apologize to those authors whose important contributions to this field are not mentioned in this review.
This work has been supported by the Kidney Foundation of Canada, the Canadian Institutes of Health Research, the Centres of Excellence for Commercialization and Research (Canada) and the Natural Sciences and Engineering Council of Canada.

6. References

Ando, T.; Okuda, S.; Yanagida, T. & Fujishima, M. (1998). Localization of TGF-beta and its receptors in the kidney. *Mineral and Electrolyte Metabolism,* Vol.24, No.2-3, pp. 149-153

Badid, C.; Desmouliere, A.; Babici, D.; Hadj-Aissa, A.; McGregor, B.; Lefrancois, N.; Touraine, J. L. & Laville, M. (2002). Interstitial expression of alpha-SMA: an early marker of chronic renal allograft dysfunction. *Nephrology Dialysis Transplantation,* Vol.17, No.11, (November 2002), pp. 1993-1998

Basile, D. P.; Rovak, J. M.; Martin, D. R. & Hammerman, M. R. (1996). Increased transforming growth factor-beta 1 expression in regenerating rat renal tubules following ischemic injury. *American Journal of Physiology,* Vol.270, No.3 Pt 2, (March 1996), pp. F500-509

Bettelli, E.; Carrier, Y.; Gao, W.; Korn, T.; Strom, T. B.; Oukka, M.; Weiner, H. L. & Kuchroo, V. K. (2006). Reciprocal developmental pathways for the generation of pathogenic effector TH17 and regulatory T cells. *Nature,* Vol.441, No.7090, (May 2006), pp. 235-238

Bhaskaran, M.; Reddy, K.; Radhakrishanan, N.; Franki, N.; Ding, G. & Singhal, P. C. (2003). Angiotensin II induces apoptosis in renal proximal tubular cells. *American Journal Physiolology - Renal Physiololgy,* Vol.284, No.5, (May 2003), pp. F955-965

Bottinger, E. P. & Bitzer, M. (2002). TGF-beta signaling in renal disease. *Journal of American Society of Nephrology*, Vol.13, No.10, (October 2002), pp. 2600-2610

Chapman, J. R.; O'Connell, P. J. & Nankivell, B. J. (2005). Chronic renal allograft dysfunction. *Journal of American Society of Nephrology*, Vol.16, No.10, (October 2005), pp. 3015-3026

Chen, W.; Jin, W.; Hardegen, N.; Lei, K. J.; Li, L.; Marinos, N.; McGrady, G. & Wahl, S. M. (2003). Conversion of peripheral $CD4^{+}CD25^{-}$ naive T cells to $CD4^{+}CD25^{+}$ regulatory T cells by TGF-beta induction of transcription factor Foxp3. *Journal of Experimental Medicine*, Vol.198, No.12, (December, 2003), pp. 1875-1886

Christ, M.; McCartney-Francis, N. L.; Kulkarni, A. B.; Ward, J. M.; Mizel, D. E.; Mackall, C. L.; Gress, R. E.; Hines, K. L.; Tian, H.; Karlsson, S. et al. (1994). Immune dysregulation in TGF-beta 1-deficient mice. *Journal of Immunology*, Vol.153, No.5, (September 2004), pp. 1936-1946

Cobbold, S. P.; Castejon, R.; Adams, E.; Zelenika, D.; Graca, L.; Humm, S. & Waldmann, H. (2004). Induction of $FOXP3^{+}$ regulatory T cells in the periphery of T cell receptor transgenic mice tolerized to transplants. *Journal of Immunology*, Vol.172, No.10, (May 2004), pp. 6003-6010

Cook, C. H.; Bickerstaff, A. A.; Wang, J. J.; Nadasdy, T.; Della Pelle, P.; Colvin, R. B. & Orosz, C. G. (2008). Spontaneous renal allograft acceptance associated with "regulatory" dendritic cells and IDO. *Journal of Immunology*, Vol.180, No.5 (March 2008), pp. 3103-3112

Dai, C.; Yang, J. & Liu, Y. (2003). Transforming growth factor-beta1 potentiates renal tubular epithelial cell death by a mechanism independent of Smad signaling. *Journal of Biological Chemistry*, Vol.278, No.14, (April 2003), pp. 12537-12545

Danielpour, D.; Kim, K. Y.; Winokur, T. S. & Sporn, M. B. (1991). Differential regulation of the expression of transforming growth factor-beta s 1 and 2 by retinoic acid, epidermal growth factor, and dexamethasone in NRK-49F and A549 cells. *Journal of Cellular Physiology*, Vol.148, No.2, (August 1991), pp. 235-244

de Fijter, J. W. (2010). Rejection and function and chronic allograft dysfunction. *Kidney International*, Supplements, No.119, (December, 2010), pp. S38-41

Del Prete, D.; Ceol, M.; Anglani, F.; Vianello, D.; Tiralongo, E.; Valente, M.; Graziotto, R.; Bonfante, L.; Scaparrotta, G.; Furian, L.; Rigotti, P.; Gambaro, G. & D'Angelo, A. (2009). Early activation of fibrogenesis in transplanted kidneys: a study on serial renal biopsies. *Experimental and Molecular Pathology*, Vol.87, No.2, (October 2009), pp. 141-145

Di Paolo, S.; Gesualdo, L.; Ranieri, E.; Grandaliano, G & Schena, F. P. (1996). High glucose concentration induces the overexpression of transforming growth factor-beta through the activation of a platelet-derived growth factor loop in human mesangial cells. *American Journal Pathology*, Vol.149, No.6, (December 1996), pp. 2095-2106

Dockrell, M. E.; Phanish, M. K. & Hendry, B. M. (2009). TGF-beta auto-induction and connective tissue growth factor expression in human renal tubule epithelial cells requires N-ras. *Nephron Experimental Nephrology*, Vol.112, No.3, pp. e71-79

Eikmans, M.; Sijpkens, Y. W.; Baelde, H. J.; de Heer, E.; Paul, L. C. & Bruijn, J. A. (2002). High transforming growth factor-beta and extracellular matrix mRNA response in renal allografts during early acute rejection is associated with absence of chronic rejection. *Transplantation*, Vol.73, No.4, (February 2002), pp. 573-579

Einecke, G.; Reeve, J.; Sis, B.; Mengel, M.; Hidalgo, L.; Famulski, K. S.; Matas, A.; Kasiske, B.; Kaplan, B. & Halloran, P. F. (2010). A molecular classifier for predicting future graft loss in late kidney transplant biopsies. *Journal of Clinical Investigation*, Vol.120, No.6, (June 2010), pp. 1862-1872

Ghoreschi, K.; Laurence, A.; Yang, X. P.; Tato, C. M.; McGeachy, M. J.; Konkel, J. E.; Ramos, H. L.; Wei, L.; Davidson, T. S.; Bouladoux, N.; Grainger, J. R.; Chen, Q.; Kanno, Y.; Watford, W. T.; Sun, H. W.; Eberl, G.; Shevach, E. M.; Belkaid, Y.; Cua, D. J.; Chen, W. & O'Shea, J. J. (2010). Generation of pathogenic Th17 cells in the absence of TGF-beta signalling. *Nature*, Vol.467, No.7318, (October 2010), pp. 967-971

Gobe, G.; Willgoss, D.; Hogg, N.; Schoch, E. & Endre, Z. (1999a). Cell survival or death in renal tubular epithelium after ischemia-reperfusion injury. *Kidney International*, Vol.56, No.4, (October 1999), pp. 1299-1304

Gobe, G.; Zhang, X. J.; Cuttle, L.; Pat, B.; Willgoss, D.; Hancock, J.; Barnard, R. & Endre, R B. (1999b). Bcl-2 genes and growth factors in the pathology of ischaemic acute renal failure. *Immunology & Cell Biology*, Vol.77, No.3, (June 1999), pp. 279-286

Grande, J. P.; Warner, G. M.; Walker, H. J.; Yusufi, A. N.; Cheng, J.; Gray, C. E.; Kopp, J. B. & Nath, K. A. (2002). TGF-beta1 is an autocrine mediator of renal tubular epithelial cell growth and collagen IV production. *Experimental Biology and Medicine* (Maywood), Vol.227, No.3, (March 2002), pp. 171-181

Guan, Q.; Nguan, C. Y. & Du, C. (2010). Expression of transforming growth factor-beta1 limits renal ischemia-reperfusion injury. *Transplantation*, Vol.89, No.11, (June 2010), pp. 1320-1327

Harris, S.; Coupes, B. M.; Roberts, S. A.; Roberts, I. S.; Short, C. D. & Brenchley, P. E. (2007). TGF-beta1 in chronic allograft nephropathy following renal transplantation. *Journal of Nephrology*, Vol.20, No.2, (March-April 2007), pp. 177-185

Hertig, A.; Anglicheau, D.; Verine, J.; Pallet, N.; Touzot, M.; Ancel, P. Y.; Mesnard, L.; Brousse, N.; Baugey, E.; Glotz, D.; Legendre, C.; Rondeau, E. & Xu-Dubois, Y. C. (2008). Early epithelial phenotypic changes predict graft fibrosis. *Journal of American Society of Nephrology*, Vol.19, No.8, (August 2008), pp. 1584-1591

Horvath, L. Z.; Friess, H.; Schilling, M.; Borisch, B.; Deflorin, J.; Gold, L. I.; Korc, M. & Buchler, M. W. (1996). Altered expression of transforming growth factor-beta S in chronic renal rejection. *Kidney International*, Vol.50, No.2, (August 1996), pp. 489-498

Huang, W.; Xu, C.; Kahng, K. W.; Noble, N. A.; Border, W. A. & Huang, Y. (2008). Aldosterone and TGF-beta1 synergistically increase PAI-1 and decrease matrix degradation in rat renal mesangial and fibroblast cells. *American Journal of Physiology - Renal Physiology*, Vol.294, No.6, (June 2008), pp. F1287-1295

Humes, H. D.; Cieslinski, D. A.; Coimbra, T. M.; Messana, J. M. & Galvao, C. (1989). Epidermal growth factor enhances renal tubule cell regeneration and repair and accelerates the recovery of renal function in postischemic acute renal failure. *Journal of Clinical Investigation*, Vol.84, No.6, (December 1989), pp. 1757-1761

Humphreys, B. D.; Lin, S. L.; Kobayashi, A.; Hudson, T. E.; Nowlin, B. T.; Bonventre, J. V.; Valerius, M. T.; McMahon, A. P. & Duffield, J. S. (2010). Fate tracing reveals the pericyte and not epithelial origin of myofibroblasts in kidney fibrosis. *American Journal of Pathology*, Vol.176, No.1, (January 2010), pp. 85-97

Iglesias-De La Cruz, M. C.; Ruiz-Torres, P.; Alcami, J.; Diez-Marques, L.; Ortega-Velazquez, R.; Chen, S.; Rodriguez-Puyol, M.; Ziyadeh, F. N. & Rodriguez-Puyol, D. (2001).

Hydrogen peroxide increases extracellular matrix mRNA through TGF-beta in human mesangial cells. *Kidney International*, Vol.59, No.1 (January 2001), pp. 87-95

Iwano, M. (2010). EMT and TGF-beta in renal fibrosis. *Frontiers in Bioscience* (Scholar Edition), Vol.2, No.2, pp. 229-238

Kapp, J. A.; Honjo, K.; Kapp, L. M.; Xu, X.; Cozier, A. & Bucy, R. P. (2006). TCR transgenic $CD8^+$ T cells activated in the presence of TGF beta express FoxP3 and mediate linked suppression of primary immune responses and cardiac allograft rejection. *International Immunology*, Vol.18, No.11, (November 2006), pp. 1549-1562

Koesters, R.; Kaissling, B.; Lehir, M.; Picard, N.; Theilig, F.; Gebhardt, R.; Glick, A. B.; Hahnel, B.; Hosser, H.; Grone, H. J. & Kriz, W. (2010). Tubular overexpression of transforming growth factor-beta1 induces autophagy and fibrosis but not mesenchymal transition of renal epithelial cells. *American Journal of Pathology*, Vol.177, No.2, (August 2010), pp. 632-643

Lario, S.; Mendes, D.; Bescos, M.; Inigo, P.; Campos, B.; Alvarez, R.; Alcaraz, A.; Rivera-Fillat, F. & Campistol, J. M. (2003). Expression of transforming growth factor-beta1 and hypoxia-inducible factor-1alpha in an experimental model of kidney transplantation. *Transplantation*, Vol.75, No.10, (May 2003), pp. 1647-1654

Laupacis, A.; Keown, P.; Pus, N.; Krueger, H.; Ferguson, B.; Wong, C. & Muirhead, N. (1996). A study of the quality of life and cost-utility of renal transplantation. *Kidney International*, Vol.50, No.1, (July 1996), pp. 235-242

Lee, H. T.; Kim, M.; Kim, J.; Kim, N. & Emala, C. W. (2007). TGF-beta1 release by volatile anesthetics mediates protection against renal proximal tubule cell necrosis. *American Journal of Nephrology*, Vol.27, No.4, pp. 416-424

Lee, H. T.; Ota-Setlik, A.; Fu, Y.; Nasr, S. H. & Emala, C. W. (2004). Differential protective effects of volatile anesthetics against renal ischemia-reperfusion injury in vivo. *Anesthesiology*, Vol.101, No.6, (December 2004), pp. 1313-1324

Li, C. & Yang, C. W. (2009). The pathogenesis and treatment of chronic allograft nephropathy. *Nature Reviews Nephrology*, Vol.5, No.9, (September 2009), pp. 513-519

Mannon, R. B. (2006). Therapeutic targets in the treatment of allograft fibrosis. *American Journal of Transplantation*, Vol.6, No.5 Pt 1, (May 2006), pp. 867-875

Massague, J. (1990). The transforming growth factor-beta family. *Annual Review of Cell Biology*, Vol.6, pp. 597-641

Morris-Stiff, G. (2005). TGF beta-1 and the development of chronic graft nephropathy: relative roles of gene, mRNA and protein. *Annals of The Royal College of Surgeons of England*, Vol.87, No.5, (September 2005), pp. 326-330

Nakagawa, T.; Sasahara, M.; Haneda, M.; Kataoka, H.; Nakagawa, H.; Yagi, M.; Kikkawa, R. & Hazama, F. (1999). Role of PDGF B-chain and PDGF receptors in rat tubular regeneration after acute injury. *American Journal of Pathology*, Vol.155, No.5, (November 1999), pp. 1689-1699

Nankivell, B. J.; Borrows, R. J.; Fung, C. L.; O'Connell, P. J.; Allen, R. D. & Chapman, J. R. (2003). The natural history of chronic allograft nephropathy. *New England Journal of Medicine*, Vol.349, No.24, (December 2003), pp. 2326-2333

Nowak, G. & Schnellmann, R. G. (1996). Autocrine production and TGF-beta 1-mediated effects on metabolism and viability in renal cells. *American Journal of Physiology*, Vol.271, No.3 Pt 2, (September 1996), pp. F689-697

Ozdemir, B. H.; Ozdemir, F. N.; Demirhan, B. & Haberal, M. (2005). TGF-beta1 expression in renal allograft rejection and cyclosporine A toxicity. *Transplantation*, Vol.80, No.12, (December 2005), pp. 1681-1685

Peeters, P.; Terryn, W.; Vanholder, R. & Lameire, N. (2004). Delayed graft function in renal transplantation. *Current Opinion in Critical Care*, Vol.10, No.6, (December 2004), pp. 489-498

Peng, Y.; Laouar, Y.; Li, M. O.; Green, E. A. & Flavell, R. A. (2004). TGF-beta regulates in vivo expansion of Foxp3-expressing $CD4^{+}CD25^{+}$ regulatory T cells responsible for protection against diabetes. *Proceedings of the National Academy of Sciences of the United States of America*, Vol.101, No.13, (March 2004), pp. 4572-4577

Phillips, A. O.; Steadman, R.; Topley, N. & Williams, J. D. (1995). Elevated D-glucose concentrations modulate TGF-beta 1 synthesis by human cultured renal proximal tubular cells. The permissive role of platelet-derived growth factor. *American Journal of Pathology*, Vol.147, No.2, (August 1995), pp. 362-374

Phillips, A. O.; Topley, N.; Morrisey, K.; Williams, J. D. & Steadman, R. (1997). Basic fibroblast growth factor stimulates the release of preformed transforming growth factor beta 1 from human proximal tubular cells in the absence of de novo gene transcription or mRNA translation. *Laboratory Investigation*, Vol.76, No.4, (April 1997), pp. 591-600

Port, F. K.; Wolfe, R. A.; Mauger, E. A.; Berling, D. P. & Jiang, K. (1993). Comparison of survival probabilities for dialysis patients vs cadaveric renal transplant recipients. *Journal of the American Medical Association*, Vol.270, No.11, (September 1993), pp. 1339-1343

Pribylova-Hribova, P.; Kotsch, K.; Lodererova, A.; Viklicky, O.; Vitko, S.; Volk, H. D. & Lacha, J. (2006). TGF-beta1 mRNA upregulation influences chronic renal allograft dysfunction. *Kidney International*, Vol.69, No.10, (May 2006), pp. 1872-1879

Prud'homme, G. J. & Piccirillo, C. A. (2000). The inhibitory effects of transforming growth factor-beta-1 (TGF-beta1) in autoimmune diseases. *Journal of Autoimmunity*, Vol.14, No.1, (February 2000), pp. 23-42

Qi, W.; Chen, X.; Holian, J.; Mreich, E.; Twigg, S.; Gilbert, R. E. & Pollock, C. A. (2006). Transforming growth factor-beta1 differentially mediates fibronectin and inflammatory cytokine expression in kidney tubular cells. *American Journal of Physiology - Renal Physiology*, Vol.291, No.5, (November 2006), pp. F1070-1077

Racusen, L. C.; Solez, K.; Colvin, R. B.; Bonsib, S. M.; Castro, M. C.; Cavallo, T.; Croker, B. P.; Demetris, A. J.; Drachenberg, C. B.; Fogo, A. B.; Furness, P.; Gaber, L. W.; Gibson, I. W.; Glotz, D.; Goldberg, J. C.; Grande, J.; Halloran, P. F.; Hansen, H. E.; Hartley, B.; Hayry, P. J.; Hill, C. M.; Hoffman, E. O.; Hunsicker, L. G.; Lindblad, A. S.; Yamaguchi, Y. et al. (1999). The Banff 97 working classification of renal allograft pathology. *Kidney International*, Vol.55, No.2, (February 1999), pp. 713-723

Ruiz-Ortega, M.; Largo, R.; Bustos, C.; Gomez-Garre, D. & Egido, J. (1997). Platelet-activating factor stimulates gene expression and synthesis of matrix proteins in cultured rat and human mesangial cells: role of TGF-beta. *Journal of American Society of Nephrology*, Vol.8, No.8, (August 1997), pp. 1266-1275

Santarlasci, V.; Maggi, L.; Capone, M.; Frosali, F.; Querci, V.; De Palma, R.; Liotta, F.; Cosmi, L.; Maggi, E.; Romagnani, S. & Annunziato, F. (2009). TGF-beta indirectly favors the development of human Th17 cells by inhibiting Th1 cells. *European Journal of Immunology*, Vol.39, No.1, (January 2009), pp. 207-215

Savill, J. (1994). Apoptosis and the kidney. *Journal of American Society of Nephrology*, Vol.5, No.1, (July 1994), pp. 12-21

Schaudies, R. P.; Nonclercq, D.; Nelson, L.; Toubeau, G.; Zanen, J.; Heuson-Stiennon, J. A. & Laurent, G. (1993). Endogenous EGF as a potential renotrophic factor in ischemia-induced acute renal failure. *American Journal of Physiology*, Vol.265, No.3 Pt 2, (September 1993), pp. F425-434.

Schnuelle, P.; Lorenz, D.; Trede, M. & Van Der Woude, F. J. (1998). Impact of renal cadaveric transplantation on survival in end-stage renal failure: evidence for reduced mortality risk compared with hemodialysis during long-term follow-up. *Journal of American Society of Nephrology*, Vol.9, No.11, (November 1998), pp. 2135-2141

Sharma, V. K.; Bologa, R. M.; Xu, G. P.; Li, B.; Mouradian, J.; Wang, J.; Serur, D.; Rao, V. & Suthanthiran, M. (1996). Intragraft TGF-beta 1 mRNA: a correlate of interstitial fibrosis and chronic allograft nephropathy. *Kidney International*, Vol.49, No.5, (May 1996), pp. 1297-1303

Shull, M. M.; Ormsby, I.; Kier, A. B.; Pawlowski, S.; Diebold, R. J.; Yin, M.; Allen, R.; Sidman, C.; Proetzel, G.; Calvin, D.; et al. (1992). Targeted disruption of the mouse transforming growth factor-beta 1 gene results in multifocal inflammatory disease. *Nature*, Vol.359, No.6397, (October 1992), pp. 693-699

Siegel, P. M. & Massague, J. (2003). Cytostatic and apoptotic actions of TGF-beta in homeostasis and cancer. *Nature Reviews Cancer*, Vol.3, No.11, (November 2003), pp. 807-821

Simonson, M. S. (2007). Phenotypic transitions and fibrosis in diabetic nephropathy. *Kidney International*. Vol.71, No.9, (May 2007), pp. 846-854

Slattery, C.; Campbell, E.; McMorrow, T. & Ryan, M. P. (2005). Cyclosporine A-induced renal fibrosis: a role for epithelial-mesenchymal transition. *American Journal of Pathology*, Vol.167, No.2, (August 2005), pp. 395-407

Tian, Y. C.; Chen, Y. C.; Hung, C. C.; Chang, C. T.; Wu, M. S.; Phillips, A. O. & Yang, C. W. (2006). Leptospiral outer membrane protein induces extracellular matrix accumulation through a TGF-beta1/Smad-dependent pathway. *Journal of American Society of Nephrology*, Vol.17, No.10, (October 2006), pp. 2792-2798

Toubeau, G.; Nonclercq, D.; Zanen, J.; Laurent, G.; Schaudies, P. R. & Heuson-Stiennon, J. A. (1994). Renal tissue expression of EGF and EGF receptor after ischaemic tubular injury: an immunohistochemical study. *Experimental Nephrology*, Vol.2, No.4, (July-August 1994), pp. 229-239

Veldhoen, M. Hocking, R. J.; Atkins, C. J.; Locksley, R. M. & Stockinger, B. (2006). TGF beta in the context of an inflammatory cytokine milieu supports de novo differentiation of IL-17-producing T cells. *Immunity*, Vol.24, No.2, (February 2006), pp. 179-189

Vesey, D. A.; Cheung, C.; Cuttle, L.; Endre, Z.; Gobe, G. & Johnson, D. W. (2002a). Interleukin-1beta stimulates human renal fibroblast proliferation and matrix protein production by means of a transforming growth factor-beta-dependent mechanism. *Journal of Laboratory and Clinical Medicine*, Vol.140, No.5, (November 2002), pp. 342-350

Vesey, D. A.; Cheung, C. W.; Cuttle, L.; Endre, Z. A.; Gobe, G. & Johnson, D. W. (2002b). Interleukin-1beta induces human proximal tubule cell injury, alpha-smooth muscle actin expression and fibronectin production. *Kidney International*, Vol.62, No.1, (July 2002), pp. 31-40

Viklicky, O.; Hribova, P.; Volk, H. D.; Slatinska, J.; Petrasek, J.; Bandur, S.; Honsova, E. & Reinke, P. (2010). Molecular phenotypes of acute rejection predict kidney graft prognosis. *Journal of American Society of Nephrology*, Vol.21, No.1, (January 2010), pp. 173-180

Villanueva, S.; Cespedes, C.; Gonzalez, A. & Vio, C. P. (2006). bFGF induces an earlier expression of nephrogenic proteins after ischemic acute renal failure. *American Journal of Physiology – Regulatory, Integrative and Comparative Physiology*, Vol.291, No.6, (December 2006), pp. R1677-1687

Vongwiwatana, A.; Tasanarong, A.; Rayner, D. C.; Melk, A & Halloran, P. F. (2005). Epithelial to mesenchymal transition during late deterioration of human kidney transplants: the role of tubular cells in fibrogenesis. *American Journal of Transplantation*, Vol.5, No.6, (June 2005), pp. 1367-1374

Winyard, P. J.; Nauta, J.; Lirenman, D. S.; Hardman, P.; Sams, V. R.; Risdon, R. A. & Woolf, A. S. (1996). Deregulation of cell survival in cystic and dysplastic renal development. *Kidney International*, Vol.49, No.1, (January 1996), pp. 135-146

Wynn, T. A. (2008). Cellular and molecular mechanisms of fibrosis. *Journal of Pathology*, Vol.214, No.2, (January 1996), pp. 199-210

Yamabe, H.; Osawa, H.; Kaizuka, M.; Tsunoda, S.; Shirato, K.; Tateyama, F. & Okumura, K. (2000). Platelet-derived growth factor, basic fibroblast growth factor, and interferon gamma increase type IV collagen production in human fetal mesangial cells via a transforming growth factor-beta-dependent mechanism. *Nephrology Dialysis Transplantation* Vol.15, No.6, (June 2000), pp. 872-876

Yaswen, L.; Kulkarni, A. B.; Fredrickson, T.; Mittleman, B.; Schiffman, R.; Payne, S.; Longenecker, G.; Mozes, E. & Karlsson, S. (1996). Autoimmune manifestations in the transforming growth factor-beta 1 knockout mouse. *Blood*, Vol.87, No.4, (February 1996), pp. 1439-1445

Yu, L.; Border, W. A.; Huang, Y. & Noble, N. A. (2003). TGF-beta isoforms in renal fibrogenesis. *Kidney International*, Vol.64, No.3, pp. 844-856

14

The Impact of Ischemia and Reperfusion Injury in Kidney Allograft Outcome

Valquiria Bueno
UNIFESP – Federal University of São Paulo
Brazil

1. Introduction

Acute kidney injury (AKI) is characterized by a relatively sudden decrease in the production, processing, and excretion of ultrafiltrate by the kidney (decrease in glomerular filtration rate - GFR). Acute kidney injury (AKI) caused by ischemia and reperfusion injury (IRI) is a common event in transplantation and 20% to 80% of kidneys from deceased donors can present delayed graft function (DGF) depending on the injury extent (Perico et al., 2004). After transplantation it could be expected immediate renal function, slow recovery function, non-oliguric acute tubular necrosis (ATN), total anuria. Delayed graft function (DGF) is defined by transplant centers as: the need of dialysis (at least one session) during the first week post-transplantation (Koning et al., 1997), early urine output lower than 1200mL/day or no decrease in serum creatinine within 48h (Shoskes et al., 2001), creatinine clearance lower than 10mL/min (Giral-Classe et al., 1998), creatinine at day 10 higher than 221μmol/L (Cosio et al., 1997).

Delayed graft function has been considered an independent predictor of graft loss since multivariate analysis showed a relative risk of graft loss 2.9 times greater for DGF than for kidneys with immediate function (Halloran et al., 1988). The US Renal Data System (37,000 primary cadaver transplants) showed a relative risk of 1.53 for 5-year graft loss in association with DGF (Ojo et al., 1997). In cadaver transplants (1994-1998 in USA) the half-life of kidneys with DGF was 7.2 years whereas in kidneys with immediate function it was 11.5 years (Halloran et al., 2001). In the presence of rejection DGF's effect is even stronger and kidney graft half-life decreases from 9.4 to 6.2 years (Shoskes et al., 1998). Kyllönen et al. (2000) showed in a follow-up of 1047 cadaveric kidney transplants performed at University of Helsinki that 5-years graft survival was 60% in patients presenting DGF and rejection, 73% in patients with rejection, 77% in patients with DGF and 88% in patients without both risk factors. They concluded that DGF was a significant factor affecting long-term graft survival, both through and independent of acute rejection. In 10-years of transplantation follow-up Troppman et al. (1999) observed 64% of graft survival in patients without DGF or rejection episodes, 44% in patients with DGF, 36% in patients with rejection, and 15% in patients presenting both risk factors.

A range of factors could lead to DGF such as organ procurement (i.e. kidneys from non-heart-beating donors), donor characteristics (i.e. donors older than 55 years), period of ischemia, recipient historic (i.e. number of recipient's previous transplants), renal toxicity, ureteral obstruction, among others. Since DGF is considered an independent risk for graft loss and one of the factors inducing DGF is ischemia and reperfusion we will focus this chapter on the impact of ischemia and reperfusion in kidney allograft outcome.

2. Ischemia and reperfusion injury

Nankivell & Chapman (2006) conclude in their review that kidney damage after transplantation is mediated by alloimune, ischemic and inflammatory stimuli causing tubular injury in association with profibrotic healing response. In addition to the changes in kidney histology be multifactor post-transplantation, the underestimation of this organ injury by serum creatinine measurement make complex the dissection of the steps during kidney damage. Therefore, biopsy histology is still the gold standard technique to evaluate clinical kidney damage after transplantation. Sequential studies of biopsies show early tubulointerstitial damage followed by later microvascular and glomerular changes with progressive fibrosis and atrophy (Solez et al., 1998; Kuypers et al., 1999, Cosio et al., 1999).

Tubulointerstitial damage begins soon after transplantation due to ischemia-reperfusion injury and the resolution of this process is crucial for kidney outcome. The tubulointerstitium is an essential component of a functioning kidney as it accounts for 95% of a kidney by weight, performs almost all of the metabolic work, and is responsible for salt and water balance, potassium excretion, acid-base control, small protein catabolism, and hormone production such as erythropoietin (Nankivell et al., 2003).

The major events affecting the tubulointerstitium are listed as it follows:

- Oxygen deprivation due to ischemia induces early ATP depletion which stops ATP-dependent transport pumps, resulting in mitochondrial swelling. Mitochondrial swelling results in outer membrane rupture, with release of mitochondrial intermembrane proteins. Caspase 1 or interleukin-1 converting enzyme (ICE) cleaves interleukin (IL)-1b. IL-1b is a pro-inflammatory cytokine, and can induce renal tubular epithelial cells to secrete chemokines such as keratinocyte-induced chemoattractant (KC), macrophage inflammatory protein (MIP)-1a, or RANTES (Furuichi et al., 2002).
- Hypoxia inducible factor (HIF-1, HIF-2, HIF-3), HIF-3 may be a negative regulator of hypoxia-inducible genes expressed by HIF-1 and HIF-2 (Nangaku et al., 2008). HIF-1 is unstable under normal conditions but it is stable and works under hypoxic conditions (Huang et al., 1996; Salceda & Caro, 1997). Many genes encoding for cytokines and growth factors are induced by HIF-1 activation (El Awad B et al., 2000; Zhou & Brune, 2006).
- Oxygen-derived free radicals and in particular hydrogen peroxide, which is a source of oxygen-derived free radicals after IR injury, has been reported to induce TNF-α production by activating p38 mitogen-activated protein kinase (MAPK) (Meldrum et al, 1998).

Ischemia injury begins with the cessation of arterial blood flow and immediate oxygen deprivation in cells (i.e., hypoxia with accumulation of metabolic products). In the kidney, decreased blood supply is associated with flow diversion from cortex to medulla which preserves oxygenation of the metabolically vulnerable medulla at the expense of cortical perfusion and glomerular filtration (Woolfson et al., 1994). Sensitivity to hypoxia or ischemia has been demonstrated in both proximal tubules (Shanley et al., 1986) and their thick ascending limbs (Brezis et al., 1985).

Severe reduction of renal blood flow causes cell damage both by the high-energy phosphate depletion and the subsequent failure to maintain physiological ion gradients across the cell membrane. However, the major injury to the ischemic organ occurs during the reperfusion phase in which the blood flow returns to the ischemic tissue. Reperfusion is associated with free radical generation leading to lipid peroxidation, polysaccharide depolymerization and deoxyribonucleotide degradation. Injured endothelial cells fail to vasodilate underlying vascular smooth muscle, release potent vasoconstrictors and swell which leads to increased permeability (Woolfson et al., 1994).

Following kidney IRI, the coordinated action of cytokines/chemokines, reactive oxygen intermediates and adhesion molecules causes a cascade of events leading to endothelial cell dysfunction, tubular epithelial cell injury and activation of both tissue-resident and kidney infiltrating leukocytes (Bonventre & Weinberg, 2003; Li & Okusa, 2006).

2.1 Kidney-resident cells can express markers of activation and thus generate inflammatory responses

Toll-like receptors (TLRs) are a family of transmembrane proteins expressed in monocytes, macrophages, dendritic cells, T-and B cells, and neutrophils. TLRs expression by primary culture of mouse cortical renal epithelial cells was first reported by Tsuboi et al. (2002). Renal tubule cells from mouse, rat, and human have been shown to express TLR2 and TLR4 (Wolfs et al., 2002; Yang et al., 2006; Chowdhury et al., 2006; Chassin et al., 2006; Shigeoka et al., 2007; El-Achkar et al., 2006; Bäckhed et al., 2001; Samuelsson et al., 2004). The activation of TLRs can be initiated by pathogens and also by a "sterile" inflammatory process mediated by DAMPs (damage associated molecular pattern molecules). DAMPs are endogenous constituents released by damaged/necrotic cells (heat shock proteins, high mobility group box 1 - HMGB1, fibronectin, heparan sulfate, hyaluronic acid) and components of the extracellular matrix released by proteases to which TLR2 and TLR4 bind.

TLR2 and TLR4 constitutively expressed in resident kidney cells are upregulated after IRI (Wolfs et al., 2002; Kim et al., 2005). TLR cell surface activation triggers an intracellular cascade of events resulting in the release of NF-κB from IκB, allowing NF-κB to translocate from cytoplasm to the nucleus and mediate an increase in inflammatory genes expression which leads to pro-inflammatory responses (Liew et al. 2005; O'Neill, 2006).

Lassen et al. (2010) propose that ischemia reperfusion-induced reactive oxygen species (ROS) activates tubular epithelial cells to release DAMPs which activate TLRs signaling and the subsequent production of proinflammatory cytokines and chemokines either by intrinsic renal cells and intrarenal antigen presenting cells (APCs). As a consequence leukocytes are attracted to the kidney, accumulate in this site, get activated and produce pro-inflammatory cytokines. (Li et al., 2007; Kelly et al., 1996; Wu et al., 2007; Kielar et al., 2005).

IRI causes damages in endothelial cells which in turn increase vascular permeability (Sutton et al., 2003; Brodsky et al., 2002) and the expression of adhesion molecules (Kelly et al., 1996) contributing thus for leukocyte migration to the kidney. Both E-selectin and intercellular adhesion molecule-1 (ICAM-1) on peritubular capillary cells play crucial roles in IRI.

Mice submitted to 32 minutes of bilateral renal pedicles clamp showed a maximum kidney E-selectin expression 24 hours later when renal tissue was evaluated by Western blot. Moreover, the immunostaining localized E-selectin in the endothelium of the peritubular capillary plexus. Administration of anti-E-selectin or use of E-selectin deficient mice was associated with lower creatinine concentrations at 24 hours indicating a potential therapeutic perspective for this molecule (Singbartl & Ley, 2000).

The evaluation of 49 renal transplant patients with mean cold ischemia time of 27 hours showed that 3 minutes after kidney graft reperfusion the renal vein presented concentrations of E-selectin, VCAM and ICAM which correlated positively with hypoxanthine concentrations. This correlation may be associated with the release of hypoxanthine by the graft as an ischemia marker reflecting metabolic changes in renal tissue during reperfusion (Domanski et al., 2009).

The inflammatory microenvironment in the kidney is closely associated with the functional and structural renal changes occurring in this organ after IRI.

2.2 Cells associated with IRI

2.2.1 Dendritic cells

Dendritic cells (DCs - $CD11c^{+}$) and class II major histocompatibility complex (MHC Class $II)^{+}$ DCs are the most abundant leukocyte subset residing in the normal mouse kidney (Li et al., 2008; Soos et al., 2006) suggesting an important role in renal immunity and inflammation. TNF-α, IL-6, MCP-1 and RANTES (pro-inflammatory cytokines/chemokines) are produced by renal DCs after IRI, and depletion of DCs prior to IRI significantly reduced the kidney levels of TNF-α (Dong et al., 2007).

2.2.2 Neutrophils

Neutrophils inhibition has been shown in some studies to attenuate renal injury after IRI (Kelly et al., 1996), whereas other studies failed to find a protective effect of neutrophil blockade or depletion (Thornton et al., 1989). Many factors affecting neutrophil infiltration or activation including neutrophil elastase, tissue-type plasminogen activator, hepatocyte growth factor, and CD44 have been suggested to contribute for the renal damage following IRI (Hayama et al., 2006; Roelofs et al., 2006; Mizuno et al., 2005; Rouschop et al., 2005). Despite discrepancies in data provided by different research groups, it is likely that neutrophils participate in inducing renal injury by plugging renal microvasculature and releasing oxygen-free radicals and proteases.

2.2.3 Macrophages

Macrophages infiltrate the injured kidney early within 1 hour of reperfusion, and this infiltration is mediated by CCR2 and CX_3CR1 signaling pathways (Oh et al., 2008; Li et al., 2008). Analysis of kidney infiltrating macrophages by flow cytometry demonstrated that these leukocytes are significant producers of the cytokines IL-1α, IL-6, IL-12p40/70 and TNF-α (Li et al., 2008).

2.2.4 Natural Killer

Natural Killer (NK) cells have recently been reported to infiltrate the post-ischemic kidney by 4 hours of reperfusion. IRI induced the expression of an NK cell-activating ligand (Rae-1) on tubule epithelial cells (TECs) and *in vitro* studies demonstrated that the interaction of the NKG2D receptor on NK cells with Rae-1 on TECs causes perforin-dependent lysis of cultured kidney cells. Antibody-mediated depletion of NK cells inhibited IRI in wild-type (WT) mice and adoptive transfer of WT, but not perforin KO, NK cells into a T, B and NK cell-deficient mouse enhanced IRI (Zhang et al., 2008).

2.2.5 Invariant Natural Killer T

Invariant Natural Killer T (iNKT) cells are a unique subset of T lymphocytes with surface receptors and functional properties shared with conventional T cells and NK cells. In contrast to conventional T cells, iNKT cells are activated by endogenously released glycolipid antigens. A recent finding is that the number of IFN-γ-producing iNKT cells in the kidney is significantly increased by 3 hours of reperfusion compared to sham-operated mice. Also, blockade of NKT cell activation with the anti-CD1d mAb, NKT cell depletion with an anti-NK1.1 mAb in WT mice, or use of iNKT cell deficient mice ($J\alpha 18^{-/-}$) inhibited the accumulation of IFN-γ-producing neutrophils after IRI and prevented AKI (Li et al., 2007).

2.2.6 T lymphocytes

In the early stage of IRI, T cells may become activated through antigen-independent mechanisms by inflammatory cytokines and reactive oxygen intermediates (Bacon et al., 1995). T cell trafficking was observed as early as 1 h after IRI and decreased at 24 h following IRI (Noiri et al., 2009; Ascon et al., 2006). T cell recruitment influences proinflammatory cytokine production, neutrophil trafficking, and progression to fibrosis (Burne et al., 2001). Moreover, T cells also influence vascular permeability in early ischemic AKI (Saito et al., 2009). Increased numbers of activated and effector-memory T cells were found in the postischemic kidneys as late as 6 weeks after IRI, suggesting that T cells are also involved in long term structural changes of postischemic kidneys (Ascon et al., 2008).

2.3 Histology changes in kidney after IRI

IRI is associated with several complexes events such as negative impact in capillary density (Basile et al., 2001) and increase of the vascular permeability which interferes with the protective barrier among circulating elements and parenchyma cells. These factors induce the no-reflow phenomenon and leads to inflammation (Cicco et al., 2005; Sutton TA, 2009).

Jayle et al. (2007) showed that in pig kidney autotransplant model the development of chronic fibrosis and subsequent renal failure were associated with the severity of IRI with more damage occurring in kidneys submitted to 60 or 90 minutes of IRI than to 45 minutes. Using the same model Thuillier et al. (2010) evaluated 60 minutes of renal pedicle clamping, kidney removal and preservation for 24 hours in UW solution followed by autotransplantation and showed that 3 months later the GFR was still significantly lower and the proteinuria was increased. Grafts presented a significant amount of interstitial fibrosis and tubular atrophy besides of T and ED1+ cells infiltration. Authors concluded that IRI has the ability to induce chronic adaptive inflammation response, even in autologous grafts. Moreover, even 6 weeks later of prolonged ischemia (unilateral renal pedicle clamp for 60 minutes) in the absence of transplantation it was possible to observe kidney shrunken in size with loss of tubular architecture (dilatation of tubules and cyst formation). It was also found infiltration of phagocytes, neutrophils and T cells suggesting long-term kidney inflammation (Burne-Taney et al., 2005).

Williams et al. (1997) showed that rats submitted to 45 minutes of bilateral renal pedicle clamp presented a peak of increased serum creatinine 24 hours later which was in accordance with the highest renal myeloperoxidase activity (and indicator of neutrophil infiltration) and massive amount of proximal convoluted tubule cells necrosis. Despite the return of creatinine to normal levels at 1 week later, atrophic tubules and focal fibrosis were still observed suggesting permanent tubular loss.

It has been shown that hypoxic stress induces apoptosis of renal proximal tubular cells via mitochondria-dependent and -independent pathways, partly by activation of caspase-3 (Edelstein et al., 1999). Clinical and experimental models demonstrate that immunosuppressive drugs can impair tubular cells proliferation in replacement to those in apoptosis.

Lui et al. (2006) observed that mice treated with Rapamycin from day -1 and submitted to 45 minutes of bilateral renal pedicles clamping presented 24 hours later significantly increased levels of creatinine. Moreover, renal tubular cells showed generalized swelling and vascuolization besides of very low numbers of PCNA-positive nuclei cells. These factors were normalized on day 3 except for PCNA which increased only on day 7 suggesting that early after IR Rapamycin impairs renal function and retards the proliferative response of the renal tubular cells.

Sirolimus exposure in recipients of cadaveric kidneys (mean of cold ischemia time = 20 hours) experiencing DGF showed strong association with prolonged time for the recovery of the graft function. This finding indicates that sirolimus impairs the kidney's ability to recovery from injury (McTaggart et al., 2003).

Novick et al. (1986) showed that cadaveric transplants with mean preservation time of 37 hours presented one-year actuarial graft survival of 78% in ALG (azathioprine – prednisone - antilymphocyte globulin) versus 48% in CsA (prednisone- cyclosporine) immunosuppressive protocol. The difference was attributed to the large number of primary nonfunctioning grafts in CsA group probably due to the effect of CsA's nephrotoxicity superimposed on renal ischemia incurred prior to transplantation.

2.4 Ischemic acute kidney injury (AKI) influences the choice of the immunosuppressive therapy after transplantation

Nankivell et al. (2003) evaluated biopsies of 120 patients maintained on Cyclosporine-based immunosuppression 5 years post-transplantation and found that 66% of them presented moderate-to-severe interstitial fibrosis and 90.3% presented arteriolar hyalinosis. Authors proposed two phases of chronic allograft nephropathy: an early fibrogenic phase attributed to ischemia-reperfusion injury and a late phase with fibrosis and arteriolar hyalianosis generated by cyclosporine (CsA) toxicity. On the other hand, Stegall et al. (2010) showed in 296 biopsies that the prevalence of moderate/severe histology changes at both 1 and 5 years post-transplantation was less than 20% including fibrosis and hyalinosis in recipients treated with a triple therapy (Tacrolimus, MMF and Azatioprine, or Sirolimus in the CNI-free protocol). Authors also found that the most important variable associated with moderate/severe fibrosis at 5 years was delayed graft function (DGF).

Despite of the controversy in how significant is the hazard added by the immunosuppression (past immunosuppressive protocols versus new immunosuppressive era) to the kidney function and histology it seems to be a consensus that DGF is an independent risk at any of the immunosuppressive protocols evaluated. This has been confirmed recently by Snoeijs et al. (2011) in MMF or SRL protocols when 8 recipients of kidneys from deceased donors with ischemia and reperfusion injury (DCD) were compared with 8 recipients of kidneys from living donors with minimal ischemic injury (LD). Delayed graft function was 70% in recipients of DCD kidneys whereas 100% of patients receiving LD kidneys showed immediate graft function. Creatinine clearance was significantly lower in recipients of DCD kidneys than in recipients of LD kidneys whereas the fractional excretion of sodium was higher in DCD group. In addition, kidneys from DCD donors presented post-transplantation early necrotic tubular epithelial cell death and systemic immune response activation.

Boratynska et al. (2008) showed that patients receiving kidney transplants with cold ischemia time longer than 24 hours and treated with a SRL (SRL + CsA + Prednisone, n=23) or CsA (Azathioprine + CsA + Prednisone, n=23) protocol presented DGF in 39% and 35% of cases respectively. Moreover, the duration of DGF and the decrease in serum creatinine were prolonged in the SRL protocol whereas biopsies from both groups presented loss of the brush border in tubular epithelial cells. One and 5-year graft survival were 100% and 87% in SRL and 95% and 74% in CsA protocols showing improved renal graft survival in patients treated with SRL. Serum creatinine level at the 12th month was higher in patients with DGF independent of the immunosuppressive protocol.

Experimental models have contributed extensively to the better knowledge in IRI, immunosuppressive regimen and kidney damage. Moreover, clinical findings are in line with experimental models as it follows:

Ninova et al. (2004) showed in a rat model that at early time point (14 days) few signs of nephrotoxicity developed when unilateral nephrectomy was performed and animals were treated with Tacrolimus or Sirolimus. However, when kidneys were submitted to IRI due to transplantation, there was increase in serum creatinine, interstitial fibrosis, vacuolization and inflammation. It was also found, intragraft expression of TGF-β and α-SMA indicating a profibrotic environment. These results suggest that IRI plays a significant role in drug-induced nephrotoxicity.

Delbridge et al. showed that rats submitted to monolateral renal clamp for 45 minutes and nephrectomy of the contrateral kidney presented 30 days later a serum creatinine (SCr) still significantly higher than control rats. The treatment with FTY720 alone (1mg/kd) decreased SCr to control levels while CsA (15mg/kg) potentiated the increase in SCr. However, the decrease in SCr was observed when FTY720 was administered in association with CsA suggesting a protective effect for the treatment with FTY720. The same was observed for proteinuria, kidney fibrosis and levels of serum TGF-β1 (Delbridge et al., 2007). Using the same model and treating rats with MMF (20mg/kg/d) Sabbatini et al. (2010) showed 6 months after IRI that the glomerular filtration rate (GFR) was similar when non-treated animals (GFR=0.50) were compared with those treated with MMF (GFR=0.49) which was significantly lower than in normal uninephrectomized animals (GFR=0.87). Even though MMF significantly reduced the early kidney inflammatory process, renal histology in treated rats was similar to that of untreated animals showing 28% and 34% respectively of tubular necrotic cells.

3. Conclusion

Ischemia reperfusion injury is a common event in kidney cadaveric transplantation and leads to delayed graft function. The choice of the immunosuppressive protocol should consider that the early administration of drugs such as CNIs and Sirolimus could retard the recovery of kidney function and structure.

4. Acknowledgements

Financial support FAPESP and CNPQ

5. References

Ascon M, Ascon DB, Liu M et al. (2008). Renal ischemia–reperfusion leads to long term infiltration of activated and effector-memory T lymphocytes. *Kidney International* 75:pp.526–535, ISSN 0085-2538

Ascon DB, Lopez-Briones S, Liu M, Ascon M, Savransky V, Colvin RB, et al. (2006). Phenotypic and functional characterization of kidney-infiltrating lymphocytes in renal ischemia reperfusion injury. *The Journal of Immunology* 177:pp. 3380–3387, ISSN 1550-6606

Bäckhed F, Söderhäll M, Ekman P, Normark S, Richter-Dahlfors A. (2001). Induction of innate immune responses by Escherichia coli and purified lipopolysaccharide correlate with organ- and cell-specific expression of toll-like receptors within the human urinary tract. *Cell Microbiology* 3: pp. 153-158, ISSN 1462-5822

Bacon KB, Premack BA, Gardner P, Schall TJ. (1985). Activation of dual T cell signaling pathways by the chemokine RANTES. *Science* 269: pp. 1727–1730, ISSN 1095-9203

Basile DP, Donoheo D, Roethe K, et al. (2001). Renal ischemic injury results in permanent damage to peritubular capillaries and influences long-term function. *American Journal of Physiology Renal Physiology* 281: pp. F887-F899, ISSN 1522-1466

Blydt-Hansen TD, Gibson IW, Birk PE. (2010). Histological progression of chronic renal allograft injury comparing sirolimus and mycophenolate mofetil-based protocols. A single-center, prospective, randomized, controlled study. *Pediatric Transplantation* 14: pp. 909-918, ISSN 1397-3142

Bonventre JV, Weinberg JM. (2003). Recent advances in the pathophysiology of ischemic acute renal failure. *The Journal of American Society of Nephrology* 14: pp. 2199–2210, ISSN 1533-3450

Boratynska M, Banasik M, Patrzalek D, Klinger M. (2008). Impact of sirolimus treatment in kidney allograft recipients with prolonged cold ischemia times: 5-year outocomes. *Experimental and Clinical Transplantation* 6: pp. 59-66, ISSN 1304-0855

Brezis M, Shanley P, Silva P et al. (1985). Disparate mechanisms for hypoxic injury in different nephron segments. Studies in the isolated perfused rat kidney. *Journal of Clinical Investigation* 76: pp. 1796-1806, ISSN 0021-9738

Brodsky SV, Yamamoto T, Tada T, Kim B, Chen J, Kajiya f, Goligorsky MS. (2002). Endothelial dysfunction in ischemic acute renal failure: rescue by transplanted endothelial cells. *American Journal of Physiology Renal Physiology* 282: pp. F1140-F1149, ISSN 1522-1466

Burne-Taney MJ, Yokota N, Rabb H. (2005). Persistent renal and extrarenal immune changes after severe ischemic injury. *Kidney International* 67: pp. 1002-1009, ISSN 0085-2538

Burne MJ, Daniels F, El Ghandour A, Mauiyyedi S, Colvin RB, O'Donnell MP, et al. (2001). Identification of the CD4 T cell as a major pathogenic factor in ischemic acute renal failure. *Journal of Clinical Investigation* 108: pp. 1283–1290, ISSN 0021-9738

Chassin C, Goujon HM, Darche S, du Merle L, Bens M, Cluzeaud F, Werts C, Ogier-Denis E, Le Bouguénec C, Buzoni-Gatel D, Vandewalle A. (2006). Renal collecting duct epithelial cells react to pyelonephritis-associated Escherichia coli by activating distinct TLR4-dependent and –independent inflammatory pathways. *The Journal of Immunology* 177: pp. 4773-4784, ISSN 1550-6606

Chowdhury P, Sacks SH, Sheerin NS. (2006). Toll-like receptors TLR2 and TLR4 initiate the innate immune response of the renal tubular epithelium to bacterial products. *Clinical Experimental Immunology* 145: pp. 346-356, ISSN 1365-2249

Cicco G, Panzera PC, Catalano G, et al. (2005). Microcirculation and reperfusion injury in organ transplantation. *Advances in Experimental Medicine and Biology* 566: pp. 363-373, ISSN 0065-2598

Cosio FG, Pelletier RP, Falkenhain ME, et al. (1997). Impact of acute rejection and early allograft function on renal allograft survival. *Transplantation* 63: pp. 1611-1615, ISSN 1534-0608

Cosio FG, Pelletier RP, Sedmak DD, et al. (1999). Pathologic classification of chronic allograft nephropathy: pathogenic and prognostic implications. *Transplantation* 67: pp. 690-696, ISSN 1534-0608

Delbridge MS, Shrestha BM, Raftery AT, El Nahas AM, Haylor J. (2007). FTY720 reduces extracellular matrix expansion associated with ischemia-reperfusion induced injury. *Transplantation Proceedings* pp. 39: 2992-2996, ISSN 0041-1345

Domanski L, Pawlik A, Safranow K, Gryczman M, Sulikowski T, Jabubowska K, Olszewska M, Dziedziejko V, Ostrowski M, Chlubek D, Ciechanowski K. (2009). Circulating adhesion molecules and purine nucleotides during kidney allograft reperfusion. *Transplantation Proceedings* 41: pp. 40-43, ISSN 0041-1345

Dong X, Swaminathan S, Bachman LA, Croatt AJ, Nath KA, Griffin MD. (2007). Resident dendritic cells are the predominant TNF-secreting cell in early renal ischemia-reperfusion injury. *Kidney International* 71: pp. 619–628, ISSN 0085-2538

Edelstein CL, Shi Y, Schrier RW. (1999). Role of caspases in hypoxia-induced necrosis of rat renal proximal tubules. *Journal of American Society of Nephrology* 10: pp. 1940-1949, ISSN 1533-3450

El-Achkar TM, Huang X, Plotkin Z, Sandoval RM, Rhodes GJ, Dagher PC. (2006). Sepsis induces changes in the expression and distribution of toll-like receptor 4 in the rat kidney. *The American Journal of Physiology Renal Physiology* 290: pp. F1034-F1043, ISSN 1522-1466

El Awad B, Kreft B, Wolber EM, Hellwig-Burgel T, Metzen E, Fandrey J, et al. (2000). Hypoxia and interleukin-1beta stimulate vascular endothelial growth factor production in human proximal tubular cells. *Kidney International* 58: pp. 43–50, ISSN 0085-2538

Furuichi K, Wada T, Iwata Y, Sakai N, Yoshimoto K, Kobayashi Ki K, et al. (2002). Administration of FR167653, a new anti-inflammatory compound, prevents renal ischaemia/reperfusion injury in mice. Nephrology Dialysis and *Transplantation* 17: pp. 399–407, ISSN 0931-0509

Giral-Classe M, Hourmant M, Cantarovich D, et al. (1998). Delayed graft function of more than six days strongly decreases long-term survival of transplanted kidneys. *Kidney International* 54: pp. 972-978, ISSN 0085-2538

Hayama T, Matsuyama M, Funao K et al. (2006). Beneficial effect of neutrophil elastase inhibitor on renal warm ischemia- reperfusion injury in the rat. *Transplantation Proceedings* 38: pp. 2201–2202, ISSN 0041-1345

Halloran PF, Aprile MA, Farewell V, et al. (1988). Early function as the principal correlate of graft survival: a multivariate analysis at 200 cadaveric renal transplants treated with a protocol incorporating antilymphocyte globulin and cyclosporine. *Transplantation* 46: pp. 223-228, ISSN 1534-0608

Halloran PF, Hunsicker LG. (2001). Delayed graft function: stat of the art. *The American Journal of Transplantation* 1: pp. 115-120, ISSN 1600-6143

Huang LE, Arany Z, Livingston DM, Bunn HF. (1996). Activation of hypoxia-inducible transcription factor depends primarily upon redox-sensitive stabilization of its alpha subunit. *The Journal of Biological Chemistry* 271: 32253–32259, ISSN 1083-351X

Jayle C, Favreau F, Zhang K, et al. (2007). Comparison of protective effects of trimetazidine against experimental warm ischemia of different durations: early and long-term effects in a pig kidney model. *American Journal of Physiology Renal Physiology* 292: pp. F1082-1093, ISSN 1522-1466

Kelly KJ, Williams WW Jr. Colvin RB, Meehan SM, Springer TA, Gutierrez-Ramos JC, Bonventre JV. (1996). Intercellular adhesion molecule-1-deficient mice are protected against ischemic renal injury. *The Journal of Clinical Investigation* 97: pp. 1056-1063, ISSN 0021-9738

Kielar ML, John R, Bennett M, Richardson JA, Shelton JM, Chen L, Jeyarajah DR, Zhou XJ, Zhou H, Chiquett B, Nagami GT, Lu CY. (2005). Maladaptive role of IL-6 in ischemic acute renal failure. *Journal of the American Society of Nephrology* 16: pp. 3315-3325, ISSN 1533-3450

Kim BS, Lim SW, Li C, Kim JS, Sun BK, Ahn KO, Han SW, Kim J, Yand CW. (2005). Ischemia-reperfusion injury activates innate immunity in rat kidneys. *Transplantation* 79: pp. 1370-1377, ISSN 1534-0608

Koning OHJ, Ploeg RJ, Van Bockel JH, et al. (1997). Risk factors for delayed graft function in cadaveric kidney transplantation. *Transplantation* 63: pp. 1620-1638, ISSN 1534-0608

Kuypers DR, Chapman JR, O'Connell PJ, et al. (1999). Predictors of renal transplant histology at three months. *Transplantation* 67: pp. 1222-1230, ISSN 1534-0608

Kyllönen LE, Salmela KT, Eklund BH, Halme LE, Höckerstedt KA, Isoniemi HM, Mäkisalo HJ, Ahonen J. (2000). Long-term results of 1047 cadaveric kidney transplantations with special emphasis on initial graft function and rejection. *Transplant International* 13: pp. 122-128, ISSN 1432-2277

Lassen S, Lech M, Römmele C, Mittruecker HW, MaK TW, Anders HJ. (2010). Ischemia reperfusion induces IFN regulatory factor 4 in renal dendritic cells, which suppresses postischemic inflammation and prevents acute renal failure. *The Journal of Immunology* 185: pp. 1976-1983, ISSN 1550-6606

Li L, Huang L, Sung SS, Vergis AL, Rosin DL, Rose CE, Jr, et al. (2008). The chemokine receptors CCR2 and CX3CR1 mediate monocyte/macrophage trafficking in kidney ischemia-reperfusion injury. *Kidney International* 74: pp. 1526–1537, ISSN 0085-2538

Li L, Huang L, Sung SS, Lobo PI, Brown MG, Gregg RK, Engelhard VH, Okusa MD. (2007). NKT cell activation mediates neutrophil IFN-gamma production and renal ischemia-reperfusion injury. *The Journal of Immunology* 178: pp. 5899-5911, ISSN 1550-6606

Li L, Okusa MD. (2006). Blocking the Immune response in ischemic acute kidney injury: the role of adenosine 2A agonists. *Nature Clinical Practice Nephrology* 2: pp. 432–444, ISSN 1745-8331

Liew FY, Xu D, Brint EK, O'Neill LAJ. (2005). Negative regulation of Toll-like receptor-mediated immune responses. *Nature Reviews Immunology* 5(6): pp. 446–458, ISSN 1474-1733.

Lui SL, Chan KW, Tsang R, Yung S, Lai KN, Chan TM. (2006). Effect of rapamycin on renal ischemia-reperfusion injury in mice. *Transplant International* 19: pp. 834-839, ISSN 1432-2277

McTaggart RA, Gottlieb D, Brooks J, et al. (2003). Sirolimus prolongs recovery from delayed graft function after cadaveric renal transplantation. *American Journal of Transplantation* 3: pp. 416-423, ISSN 1600-6143

Meldrum DR, Dinarello CA, Cleveland JC Jr, Cain BS, Shames BD, Meng X, et al. (1998). Hydrogen peroxide induces tumor necrosis factor alpha-mediated cardiac injury by a P38 mitogen-activated protein kinase-dependent mechanism. *Surgery* 124: pp. 291–296, ISSN 1365-2168

Mizuno S, Nakamura T. (2005). Prevention of neutrophil extravasation by hepatocyte growth factor leads to attenuations of tubular apoptosis and renal dysfunction in mouse ischemic kidneys. *American Journal of Pathology* 166: pp. 1895–1905, ISSN 0002-9440

Nangaku M, Inagi R, Miyata T, Fujita T. (2008). Hypoxia and hypoxia inducible factor in renal disease. *Nephron Experimental Nephrology* 110: pp. e1–7, ISSN 1660-2129

Nankivel BJ, Borrows RJ, Fung C L-S, O'Connell PJ, Allean RDM, Chapman JR. (2003). The natural history of chronic allograft nephropathy. *The New England Journal of Medicine* 349: pp. 2326-2331, ISSN 1533-4406

Nankivell BJ, Chapman JR. (2006). Chronic allograft nephropathy: current concepts and future directions. *Transplantation* 81: pp. 643-654, ISSN 1534-0608

Ninova D, Covarrubias M, Rea DJ, Park WD, Grand JP, Stegall MD. (2004). Acute nephrotoxocity of tacrolimus and sirolimus in renal isografts: differential intragraft expression of transforming growth factor-beta 1 and alpha-smooth muscle actin. *Transplantation* 78: pp. 338-344, ISSN 1534-0608.

Noiri E, Doi K, Inagi R, Nangaku M, Fujita T. (2009). Contribution of T lymphocytes to rat renal ischemia/reperfusion injury. *Clinical Experimental Nephrology* 13: pp. 25–32, ISSN 1437-7799

Novick AC, Hwei HH, Steinmuller D, et al. (1986). Detrimental effect of cyclosporine on initial function of cadaver renal allografts following extended preservation: results of randomized prospective study. *Transplantation* 42: pp. 154-158, ISSN 1534-0608

Oh DJ, Dursun B, He Z, Lu L, Hoke TS, Ljubanovic D, et al. (2008). Fractalkine receptor (CX3CR1) inhibition is protective against ischemic acute renal failure in mice. *The American Journal of Physiology Renal Physiology* 294: pp. F264–271, ISSN 1522-1466

Ojo AO, Wolfe RA, Held P, Port FK, Schmouder RL. (1997). Delayed graft function: risk factors and implications for renal allograft survival. *Transplantation* 63: pp. 968-974, ISSN 1534-0608

O'Neill LAJ. How Toll-like receptors signal: what we know and what we don't know. Current Opinion in Immunology 2006; 18(1): pp. 3–9, ISSN 0952-7915

Perico N, Cattaneo D, Sayegh MH, Remuzzi G. (2004). Delayed graft function in kidney transplantation. *Lancet* 364: pp. 1814-1827, ISSN 1474-547X

Roelofs JJ, Rouschop KM, Leemans JC et al. (2006). Tissue-type plasminogen activator modulates inflammatory responses and renal function in ischemia reperfusion injury. *The Journal of American Society of Nephrology* 17: pp. 131–140, ISSN 1533-3450

Rouschop KM, Roelofs JJ, Claessen N et al. (2005). Protection against renal ischemia reperfusion injury by CD44 disruption. *The Journal of American Society of Nephrology* 16: pp. 2034–2043, ISSN 1533-3450

Sabbatini M, Uccello F, Serio V, Troncone G, Varone V, Andreucci M, Faga T, Pisani A. (2010). Effects of mycophenolate mofetil on acute ischemia-reperfusion injury in rats and its consequences in the long term. *Nephrology Dialysis and Transplantation* 25: pp. 1443-1450, ISSN 0931-0509

Saito H, Kitamoto M, Kato K, Liu N, Kitamura H, Uemura K, et al. (2009). Tissue factor and factor V involvement in rat peritoneal fibrosis. *Peritoneal Dialysis International* 29: pp. 340–351, ISSN 1718-4304

Salceda S, Caro J. (1997). Hypoxia-inducible factor 1alpha (HIF-1alpha) protein is rapidly degraded by the ubiquitin-proteasome system under normoxic conditions. Its stabilization by hypoxia depends on redox-induced changes. *The Journal of Biological Chemistry* 272: pp. 22642–22647, ISSN 1083-351X

Samuelsson P, Hang L, Wullt B, Irjala H, Svandborg C. (2004). Toll-like receptor 4 expression and cytokine responses in the human urinary tract mucosa. *Infection and Immunity* 72: pp. 3179-3186, ISSN 1098-5522

Shanley P, Brezis M, Spokes K, Silva P, Epstein F, Rosen S. (1986). Hypoxic injury in the proximal tubule of the isolated perfused rat kidney. *Kidney International* 29: 1021-1032, ISSN 0085-2538

Shigeoka AA, Holscher TD, King AJ, Hall FW, Kiosses WB, Tobias PS, Mackman N, McKay DB. (2007). TLR2 is constitutively expressed within the kidney and participates in ischemic renal injury through both MyD88-dependent and –independent pathways. *The Journal of Immunology* 178: pp. 6252-6258, ISSN 1550-6606

Shoskes DA, Shahed AR, Kim S. (2001). Delayed graft function. Influence on outcome and strategies for prevention. *The Urologic Clinics of North America* 28: pp. 721-732, ISSN 0094-0143

Shoskes DA, Cecka M. (1998). Deleterious effects of delayed graft function in cadaveric renal transplant recipients independent of acute rejection. *Transplantation* 66: pp. 1697-1701, ISSN 1534-0608

Singbartl K, Ley K. (2000). Protection from ischemia-reperfusion induced severe acute renal failure by blocking E-selectin. *Critical Care Medicine* 28: pp. 2507-2514, ISSN 1530-0293

Snoejis MJ, van Bijnen A, Swennen E, Haenen GR, Roberts LJ 2nd, Christiaans MH, Peppelenbosh AG, Buurman WA, Ernest van Heurn LW. (2011). Tubular epithelial injury and inflammation after ischemia and reperfusion in human kidney transplantation. *Annals of Surgery* 253: pp. 598-604, ISSN 1528-1140

Solez K, Vincenti F, Filo RS. (1998). Histopathologic findings from 2-year protocol biopsies from a US multicenter kidney transplant trial comparing tacrolimus versus cyclosporine: a report of the FK506 kidney transplant study group. *Transplantation* 66: pp. 1736-1740, ISSN 1534-0608

Soos TJ, Sims TN, Barisoni L, Lin K, Littman DR, Dustin ML, et al. (2006). CX3CR1+ interstitial dendritic cells form a contiguous network throughout the entire kidney. *Kidney International* 70: pp. 591–596, ISSN 0085-2538

Stegall MD, Park WD, Larson TS, Gloor JM, Cornell LD, Sethi S, Dean PG, Prieto M, Amer H, Textor S, Schwab T, Cosio FG. (2010). The histology of solitary renal allografts at 1 and 5 years after transplantation. *The American Journal of Transplantation* 10: pp. 1-10, ISSN 1600-6143

Sutton TA, Mang HE, Camps SB, Sandoval RM, Yoder MC, Molitoris BA. (2003). Injury of the renal microvascular endothelium alters barrier function after ischemia. *American Journal of Physiology Renal Physiology* 285: pp. F191-F198, ISSN 1522-1466

Sutton TA. (2009). Alteration of microvascular permeability in acute kidney injury. *Microvascular research* 77: pp. 4-7, ISSN 0026-2862

Thuillier R, Favreaus F, Celhay O, Macchi L, Milin S, Hauet T. (2010) Thrombin inhibition during kidney ischemia-reperfusion reduces chronic graft inflammation and tubular atrophy. *Transplantation* 90: pp. 612-621, ISSN 1534-0608

Troppman C, Gruessner AC, Gillingham KJ, Sutherland DER, Matas AJ, Gruessner RWG. (1999). Impact of delayed graft function on long-term graft survival after solid organ transplantation. *Transplantation Proceedings* 31: pp. 1290-1292, ISSN 0041-1345

Thornton MA, Winn R, Alpers CE, Zager RA. (1989). An evaluation of the neutrophil as a mediator of in vivo renal ischemic–reperfusion injury. *American Journal of Pathology* 135: pp. 509–515, ISSN 1943-7722

Tsuboi N, Yoshikai Y, Matsuo S, Kikuchi T, Iwami K, Nagai Y, Takeuchi O, Akira S, Matsuguchi T. (2002). Roles of toll-like receptors in C-C chemokine production by renal tubular epithelial cells. *The Journal of Immunology* 169: pp. 2026-2033, ISSN 1550-6606

Yang CW, Hung CC, Wu MS, Tian YC, Chang CT, Pan MJ, Vandewalle A. (2006). Toll-like receptor 2 mediates early inflammation by leptospiral outer membrane proteins in proximal tubule cells. *Kidney International* 69: pp. 815-822, ISSN 0085-2538

Zhang ZX, Wang S, Huang X, Min WP, Sun H, Liu W, et al. (2008). NK cells induce apoptosis in tubular epithelial cells and contribute to renal ischemia-reperfusion injury. *The Journal of Immunology* 181: pp. 7489–7498 ISSN 1550-6606

Zhou J, Brune B. (2006). Cytokines and hormones in the regulation of hypoxia inducible factor-1alpha (HIF-1alpha). *Cardiovascular and Hematological Agents in Medicinal Chemistry* 4: pp. 189–197, ISSN 1871-5257

Williams P, Lopes H, Britt D, Chan C, Ezrin A, Hottendorf R. (1997). Characterization of renal ischemia-reperfusion injury in rats. *Journal of Pharmacological and Toxicological Methods* 37: pp. 1-7, ISSN 1056-8719

Wolfs TG, Buurman WA, van Schadewijk A, de Vries B, Daemen MA, Hiemstra PS, van't Veer C. (2002). In vivo expression of toll-like receptor 2 and 4 by renal epithelial cells: IFN-gamma and TNF-alpha mediated up-regulation during inflammation. *The Journal of Immunology* 168: pp. 1286-1293, ISSN 1550-6606

Woolfson RG, Millar CGM, Neild GH. (1994). Ischaemia and reperfusion injury in the kidney: current status and future direction. *Nephrology Dialysis and Transplantation* 9(11): pp. 1529-1531, ISSN 0931-0509

Wu H, Chen G, Wyburn KR, Yin J, Bertolino P, Eris JM, Alexander SI, Sharland AF, Chadban SJ. (2007). TLR4 activation mediates kidney ischemia/reperfusion injury. *The Journal of Clinical Investigation* 117: pp. 2847-2859, ISSN 0021-9738

15

ROCK Inhibition – A New Therapeutic Avenue in Kidney Protection

Stefan Reuter, Dominik Kentrup and Eckhart Büssemaker
Department of Medicine D, University of Münster, Münster
Germany

1. Introduction

Chronic allograft nephropathy (CAN) remains the main cause of renal transplant loss besides the death of patients with a functioning graft. Its prevention and treatment still lacks any significant breakthrough since many years (Meier-Kriesche *et al.* 2004; Pascual *et al.* 2002). Pathological manifestations of CAN include interstitial fibrosis, tubular atrophy, vascular occlusive changes, glomerulosclerosis and a progressive renal dysfunction accompanied by hypertension and proteinuria (Joosten *et al.* 2005; Racusen *et al.* 1999). This histopathologic constellation is now more formally and descriptively referred to as interstitial fibrosis and tubular atrophy (IF/TA) without evidence of any specific aetiology (Solez *et al.* 2007). IF/TA or CAN describe the common final path of different injuries causing renal damage, whereas their precise pathogenesis is complex and only incompletely understood (Joosten *et al.* 2005). The process encompasses multifactorial aetiologies including alloantigen-dependent as well as alloantigen-independent factors (Gottmann *et al.* 2003; Joosten *et al.* 2005; Kerjaschki *et al.* 2006; Nankivell *et al.* 2003; Reuter *et al.* 2010; Tullius & Tilney, 1995). Hence, an effective treatment is not available so far.

Rho effectors Rho-associated, coiled-coil containing protein kinases (ROCK) and their associated signaling pathways have emerged as important players in cardiovascular and renal pathophysiology. Recently, it has been shown that ROCK inhibition is protective in diabetic and obstructive nephropathy, hypertensive nephrosclerosis, ischemia reperfusion injury, and chronic allograft nephropathy (Kanda *et al.* 2003a; Kentrup D. *et al.* 10 A.D.; Kentrup D. *et al.* 2010; Komers *et al.* 2011a; Komers *et al.* 2011b; Liu *et al.* 2009; Nagatoya *et al.* 2002; Nishikimi *et al.* 2004a; Satoh *et al.* 2002; Song *et al.* 2008; Versteilen *et al.* 2011).

ROCKs have been initially identified as downstream targets of the small GTP binding protein Rho. Members of the Rho family include Rho (isoforms A–E, and G), Rac (isoforms 1 and 2), Cdc42 and TC10 (Nobes & Hall, 1994). After translocation to the plasma membrane, GTP-RhoA activates its effectors, including the two isoforms of ROCK, ROCK1 (ROKβ, p160ROCK) and ROCK2 (ROKα, Rho kinase) (Nakagawa *et al.* 1996). Although, ROCK1 and 2 can be differentially regulated under distinct circumstances there is no evidence that ROCK1 and ROCK2 have different functions at present (Nobes & Hall, 1994). ROCKs are protein serine/threonine kinases belonging to the AGC (PKA/PKG/PKC) family (Ishizaki *et al.* 1996; Leung *et al.* 1995; Matsui *et al.* 1996). ROCK activity is involved in actin cytoskeletal organization, stress fiber formation, and cell contraction thereby controlling vascular smooth muscle contraction, endothelial barrier and leukocyte functions (e.g., cellular motility, migration, adhesion and transmigration) (Loirand, Guerin & Pacaud, 2006; Riento & Ridley, 2003). Both isoforms of ROCK can be the target of effective inhibitors such as TAT-C3, HMG-CoA reductase inhibitors, mTOR inhibitors, angiotensin II antagonists, Rad GTPase, dominant-negative ROCK, and the specific ROCK inhibitors fasudil, hydroxyfasudil, and Y-27632 (Liao, Seto & Noma, 2007; Oka *et al.* 2008). We herein discuss favourable effects of ROCK inhibitors in kidney transplantation-related diseases, and highlight their potential impact on novel therapeutic strategies to improve long-term renal graft survival.

1.1 Rock Inhibition in Diabetic nephropathy

Diabetic nephropathy (DN) is the most common cause of chronic kidney disease (CKD) with a considerable risk of progression to end stage renal disease (ESRD) (Zimmet, Alberti & Shaw, 2001). Thus, it is not surprising that DN is the main cause of patients entering permanent renal replacement programs (dialysis/transplantation) worldwide (Rugg, 2003). When dialysis is initiated, the survival of patients with DN is inferior when compared with other renal diseases. Despite an inferior survival of diabetics, which is primarily due to cardiovascular disease generally present prior to transplantation, kidney transplantation has been established as the renal replacement therapy of choice for these patients (Cosio *et al.* 2008). Because longer waiting times on dialysis negatively impact post-transplant graft survival (Meier-Kriesche *et al.* 2000) and successful transplantation was shown to confess a substantial survival benefit to patients with diabetic-ESRD, transplantation should be performed early (Becker *et al.* 2006; Hirschl, 1996; Son *et al.* 2010; Wolfe *et al.* 1999). As diabetes persists (or occurs, e.g. post-transplant diabetes (Rodrigo *et al.* 2006)) after renal transplantation it contributes to delayed graft function and long-term (re-)graft loss (Arnol *et al.* 2008; Fellstrom *et al.* 2005; Khalkhali *et al.* 2010; Parekh, Bostrom & Feng, 2010; Wilkinson *et al.* 2005). Interestingly, in a study by Wiesbauer et al. maximal glucose, HbA1c, or diabetes treatment did not influence death-censored functional graft survival but mortality (Wiesbauer *et al.* 2010). However, there is evidence that DN can re-occur after transplantation and that reversal or stabilization of the course of DN (still difficult to achieve) may slower the progress to ESRD again (Bhalla *et al.* 2003; Osterby *et al.* 1991; Salifu *et al.* 2004; Wojciechowski, Onozato & Gonin, 2009).

What happens in DN? The mechanistic driving force of DN still remains undetermined. Only 30-50% of people with diabetes develop overt nephropathy over a lifetime. This suggests that other factors besides diabetes are required to share in for the progression of DN (Nakagawa *et al.* 2011; Rugg, 2003). One important parameter for the development of DN identified is glomerular hypertension due to (intra renal) vascular alterations (Johnston *et al.* 1998). Vascular damage of the glomerular capillaries causes leakage of albumin and other proteins across the filter into the urine. It was postulated that the degree of DN correlates to the amount of urinary albumin excretion. However, others have found that DN is an independent risk factor for the development of microalbuminuria (Chang *et al.* 2011a). In contrast, progressive renal failure in diabetics can also occur in the absence of proteinuria even though histology present with typical signs of DN (Caramori, Fioretto & Mauer, 2003). Thus, it was questioned whether the decline of renal function is linked to proteinuria or whether both simply appear in parallel (Perkins *et al.* 2007) (reviewed in (Jefferson, Shankland & Pichler, 2008)). Because classical cardiovascular risk factors like hyperglycemia, hypertension, and hyperlipidemia are well-described to promote DN it would stand to reason that mechanisms causing vascular damage, such as endothelial dysfunction, oxidative stress, advanced glycation end products

(AGEs), and angiogenesis, are involved in the pathogenesis of DN (Brownlee, 2001; Chang *et al.* 2011b; Jansson, 2007). It was suggested that hyperglycemia accelerates the polyol and the hexosamine pathway, activates protein kinase C (PKC), and induces nonenzymatic glycosylation AGEs (Brownlee, 2001; Schena & Gesualdo, 2005). Especially AGEs lead to fibrosis via accumulation of interstitial collagens. AGEs also induce oxidative stress which activates NF-kappa b. NF-kappa b and PKC-activation are associated with the release of (proinflammatory) cytokines and growth factors such as vascular endothelial growth factor (VEGF), tumor necrosis factor a (TNFa), fibroblast growth factor (FGF), tissue factor, transforming growth factor-beta (TGF-ß), Interleukin 1 (IL-1), IL-6 and IL-18 (Brownlee, 2001; Johnston *et al.* 1998). PKC activation is also related to hemodynamic changes (predominantly through the activation of the renin-angiotensin aldosterone system (RAAS) which in term promotes hypertension, oxidative stress, and fibrosis.

Therefore, current renoprotective treatment strategies for DN are rather classical and include the control of blood glucose, blood pressure, lipids (notably, many cholesterol-independent or "pleiotropic" effects of statins are mediated by ROCK inhibition (Liao, 2007)) and body weight as well as RAAS blockade and physical training (Alicic & Tuttle, 2010; Van Buren & Toto, 2011). The interest emerged on ROCK inhibitors when it was observed that Rho/ROCK play important roles in hypertension/cardiovascular system and in the kidney in models of diabetes (Arita *et al.* 2009; Gojo *et al.* 2007; Kawamura *et al.* 2004; Kolavennu *et al.* 2008; Miao *et al.* 2002; Peng *et al.* 2008; Rikitake & Liao, 2005). Besides hyperglycemia, further factors of the diabetic milieu, such as reactive oxygen species (ROS), oxidized LDL, acceleration of the hexosamine pathway, and AGEs, can activate the Rho/ROCK pathway in vascular and renal cells (Komers, 2011). Interestingly, among other actions AGEs can increase endothelial permeability/hyperpermeability of vessels through the RAGE/Rho signaling pathway which can be inhibited by application of Y-27632 (Hirose *et al.* 2010). Moreover, Rho/ROCK have been identified as key mediators of VEGF-induced endothelial cell hyperpermeability (Zeng *et al.* 2005). As mentioned above, VEGF expression is increased in response to hyperglycemia. Because albuminuria, due to glomerular leakage, is a common feature of DN, ROCK activity might be a mechanism involved in renal proteinuria in these patients. In addition, the Rho/ROCK pathway can be activated by hormones or cytokines involved in DN pathophysiology, like AngII, aldosterone, TGF-ß, and VEGF (Komers, 2011). It was stated that this activation of ROCK-dependent pathways, e.g. due to production of osteopontin, plasminogen activator inhibitor 1, or extracellular matrix, is involved in the pathogenesis of DN. Cell culture studies by Peng et al. and Kolavennu et al. supported these findings. They observed that the activity of Rho/ROCK in mesangial cells increased by glucose treatment. This caused reorganization of cytoskeleton and increased production of fibronectin, collagen IV, VEGF and AP-1, a transcription factor promoting the expression of e.g. TGF-ß. Inhibition of the Rho/ROCK pathway saved the cells from these changes (Kolavennu *et al.* 2008; Peng *et al.* 2008). Moreover, glomerular hypertension is a well described factor participating in the progression of DN. Hypertension causes mechanical stress which activates Rho (see below). In congruence, Komers et al. described improved renal hemodynamics after ROCK inhibition in diabetic rats (Komers *et al.* 2011a). In addition, there is some evidence that Rho is involved in the actions of endothelin 1 (ET-1), a potent vasoconstrictor, which is upregulated in diabetics (Yousif, 2006).

Because of this and comparable evidence from other studies it was assumed that ROCK inhibition is advantageous in diabetes. Komers, Peng and Gojo et al. treated diabetic rats (diabetes type 1 model) with the orally administered ROCK-inhibitor fasudil (Gojo *et al.*

2007; Komers *et al.* 2011b; Peng *et al.* 2008). Their diabetic rats rapidly developed albuminuria, glomerulosclerosis, and renal interstitial fibrosis, as well as decreased glomerular filtration rates (GFR), and increased expression of molecular markers of DN. Sustained ROCK inhibition reduced diabetes-related kidney damage (as confirmed by histology and urinalysis) in the kidney and expression of the molecular markers (including markers of epithelial–mesenchymal transition (EMT)) in association with a slight anti-proteinuric effect (including beneficial effects of fasudil on podocyte foot process effacement) which was independent of blood pressure or glucose control. So far, all long-term studies evidenced nephroprotective effects of ROCK inhibitors being independent from systemic blood pressure. In contrast, Kikuchi et al. failed to suppress the progression of nephropathy by fasudil application (but ameliorated some features of DN) in a rat model of type 2 diabetes (Kikuchi *et al.* 2007) but Kolavennu et al. found ROCK inhibition being kidney protective in type 2 diabetes mice (Kolavennu *et al.* 2008). Interestingly, Peng observed that fasudil and ACE-inhibitors had a comparable effectiveness preventing DN while Komers et al. noted that the combination of fasudil and losartan was not more effective than losartan alone (Komers *et al.* 2011b; Peng *et al.* 2008). ACE-inhibitors and AT1-blockers are well known agents used for kidney protection in (proteinuric) DN for many years. Interestingly, RAAS blockade was effective to inhibit Rho/ROCK activity in several studies suggesting that ROCK activation might follow AT1 activation under certain conditions (Higuchi *et al.* 2007; Komers *et al.* 2011b; Ohtsu *et al.* 2006). Thus, the effects of RAAS blockade partly rely on ROCK inhibition: Angiotensin II (AngII) mediated vasoconstriction (via myosin light chain phosphorylation), proinflammatory effects (via PAI-1 and monocyte chemoattractant protein-1 (MCP-1) induction) and JNK-dependent hypertrophy/cell migration. They can be attributed to Rho activity and are therefore within the therapeutic target range of ROCK inhibitors (Higuchi *et al.* 2007; Ohtsu *et al.* 2006). More evidence comes from Rikitake et al. who showed in ROCK1$^{+/-}$ haploinsufficient mice that perivascular fibrosis induced by AngII was significantly lower than in wild type individuals (Rikitake *et al.* 2005b). In the context of diabetes it is of note that AngII-dependent activation of the Rho/ROCK pathway is partly mediated by NADPH oxidase-dependent ROS (Jin *et al.* 2006). As mentioned above, ROS are present in the hyperglycemic milieu in excess probably promoting AngII effects in diabetics.

1.2 Rock Inhibition in Urethral obstruction

Urethral obstruction (UO) is a typical cause of ESRD in children. In this patient group, UO is responsible for approximately 15 to 25% of kidney failures (Koo *et al.* 1999). This is even a problem after renal transplantation, because obstruction-related side effects influence the success of transplantation. Allograft function and survival are often limited due to urinary tract infection or surgical complications, implying deleterious actions of chronic elevated intravesical pressure (Cairns *et al.* 1991; Churchill *et al.* 1988; Sheldon *et al.* 1994). However, more recent studies claim that patients with severe lower urinary tract abnormalities and ESRD may receive a kidney transplant with comparable safeness and success to patients without abnormalities (Broniszczak *et al.* 2010; Nahas & David-Neto, 2009; Rigamonti *et al.* 2005).

In experimental settings, UO is commonly employed as a normotensive, non-proteinuric and non-hyperlipidemic model of tubulointerstitial fibrosis without any toxic renal insult (Nagatoya *et al.* 2002). Fibrosis is of major interest, not only because it is a common final path of different injuries causing renal damage, but, as a substantial part of IF/TA, also related to the renal (graft) prognosis (Couser & Johnson, 1994; Meier-Kriesche *et al.* 2004; Morgan *et al.* 2011; Nath, 1992; Pascual *et al.* 2002). Depending on the side where it mainly occurs, fibrosis is classified as glomerulosclerosis or tubulointerstitial fibrosis. Nevertheless, in most situations fibrosis is detected in both compartments, hinting towards a not yet fully understood cross-talk in between (Klein *et al.* 2011). Briefly, examples of fibrosis initiating factors are: increased intravascular pressure (hypertension), increased pressure in the tubular lumen (due to obstruction of the urinary tract), hyperglycemia (diabetes), increased urinary albumin concentrations (proteinuria), and toxic substances (puromycin or adriamycin). After ignition of the process due to different stimuli the pathways converge independently of the activator. Signaling includes induction of cytokines and chemokines, like TGF-β, platelet-derived growth factor (PDGF), FGF, ET-1, and osteopontin, leading to renal inflammation (predominant cell types are monocytes and macrophage (Mphi)) and cell activation.

It was suggested that Mphi are central players in the fibroproliferative response (Vernon, Mylonas & Hughes, 2010). They release profibrogenic growth factors i.e., TGF-β, PDGF and FGF, which activate/recruit myofibroblasts and stimulate resident interstitial fibroblasts. These fibroblasts are the main source of interstitial ECM (e.g., collagens and fibronectin, and expression of factors interfering with ECM crosslinking (transglutaminases, high glucose-induced AGEs) and/or turnover (matrix metalloproteinases, plasminogen activator, and their inhibitors) (well summarized in (Klein *et al.* 2011)) that cause fibrosis. In congruence, we and others observed e.g., that the level of L-Plastin, a cytoskeletal protein mainly expressed in interstitial fibroblasts, is increased in IF/TA (Reuter *et al.* 2010). Recently, it was reported that Rho/ROCK are central to differentiation, migration, and contractility of myofibroblasts (Mack *et al.* 2001; Parizi, Howard & Tomasek, 2000). Thus, ROCK inhibition might suppress the destructive activity of myofibroblasts. If not applied, the fibrotic process continues. Blocking of Mphi recruitment and activation ameliorates renal inflammation and fibrosis (Vielhauer *et al.* 2010). As ROCK is essential for Mphi migration its blockade can protect from fibrosis in UO (Nagatoya *et al.* 2002; Satoh *et al.* 2002). In renal graft recipients TGF-ß expression was analyzed in protocol biopsies (performed 3, 6, and 12 months after kidney transplantation). An increased level of TGF-ß was associated with a larger extent of interstitial fibrosis (Baboolal *et al.* 2002). Interestingly, when ROCK is inhibited in vivo the tissue level of the fibrogenic TGF-ß is lower than in control kidneys (Nagatoya *et al.* 2002).

Besides, TGF-ß promotes EMT, a process related to the development of renal fibrosis (Zavadil & Bottinger, 2005). As mentioned before, Rho/ROCK are important players in the (re-)organisation of the cytoskeleton. This implies that they are key mediators/effectors of epithelial plasticity and EMT induced by TGF-ß (Patel *et al.* 2005; Rodrigues-Diez *et al.* 2008; Zavadil & Bottinger, 2005). In summary, kidney protection due to ROCK inhibition can be achieved in UO because Rho/ROCK is involved in different key mechanisms in renal fibrosis.

1.3 Rock Inhibition in Hypertensive Nephrosclerosis

Increased blood pressure is an important health problem and a major risk factor for cardiovascular morbidity and mortality throughout the world (Staessen *et al.* 2003). To date, both the pathogenesis of arterial hypertension and the molecular mechanisms involved in blood pressure control remain poorly understood. Hypertension is characterized by high arterial pressure resulting from increased peripheral vascular resistance that can be attributed to both enhanced contractility of vascular smooth muscle cells and arterial wall remodeling. Increased activity of the Rho/ROCK pathway has been proposed to play an important role in the development and maintenance of hypertension. In various animal models of experimental hypertension a role of RhoA and ROCK has been demonstrated. Blocking ROCK activity with Y-27632 has blood pressure lowering effects in spontaneously hypertensive rats (SHR), deoxycorticosterone-acetate (DOCA)/salt-treated and renal hypertensive rats (Uehata *et al.* 1997). Similarly, oral administration of fasudil to SHR rats significantly lowered blood pressure (Mukai *et al.* 2001). In addition, several studies have addressed changes in RhoA activity in isolated vascular segments from hypertensive animals suggesting that increased RhoA activity is responsible for enhanced ROCK function in the pathology of hypertension. In mesenteric and cerebral arteries from SHR and normotensive rats the relaxation induced by treatment with Y-27632 was markedly higher in arteries from SHR rats (Asano & Nomura, 2003; Chrissobolis & Sobey, 2001). This has also been shown for mesenteric arteries from DOCA/salt-treated rats (Weber & Webb, 2001). In animals treated with L-NAME, an inhibitor of NO-synthase, oral administration of Y-27632 lowered blood pressure and the level of active, GTP-bound RhoA was markedly increased in vessels from L-NAME treated rats (Weber & Webb, 2001). Similarly, direct evidence for increased amounts of active RhoA have been found in stroke-prone SHR, DOCA/salt- and renal hypertensive rats (Moriki *et al.* 2004; Seasholtz *et al.* 2001; Seko *et al.* 2003). Analysis of the expression levels of RhoA has led to controversial results with some studies showing an increased expression of RhoA under hypertensive conditions (Seasholtz *et al.* 2001) whereas in other reports no differences in the expression profile of proteins from the RhoA/ROCK pathway have been detected (Seko *et al.* 2003).

Impaired endothelial function and decreased NO-production have been implicated in the etiology of hypertension. Decreased expression of endothelial nitric oxide synthase (eNOS) is found in aortae from SHR rats (Chou *et al.* 1998) and eNOS-deficient mice have an elevated blood pressure (Huang *et al.* 1995). Interestingly, there seems to be extensive crosstalk between NO and RhoA/ROCK-signaling. There is compelling evidence that the NO/cGK pathway leads to an inhibition of RhoA/ROCK signaling (Carter, Begaye & Kanagy, 2002; Chitaley & Webb, 2002; Sauzeau *et al.* 2000). On the other hand, the RhoA/ROCK cascade seems to reciprocally influence NO-signaling. The mechanism by which ROCK influences NO production seems to be the regulation of eNOS mRNA stability (Eto *et al.* 2001; Rikitake *et al.* 2005a; Takemoto *et al.* 2002).

Chronic hypertension leads to end organ damage in a substantial number of patients. Hypertensive nephrosclerosis is a disorder that is usually associated with chronic hypertension. Histologically it is characterized by vascular, glomerular, and tubulointerstitial changes. The vascular pathology consists of intimal thickening and luminal narrowing of the large and small renal arteries and the glomerular arterioles. Two different processes appear to contribute to the development of the vascular lesions: A hypertrophic response to chronic hypertension evident by medial hypertrophy and fibroblastic intimal thickening, resulting in narrowing of the vascular lumen (Zucchelli & Zuccala, 1994). In the beginning this process is adaptive by minimizing the degree to which the rise in systemic pressure is transmitted to the downstream arterioles and capillaries (Zucchelli & Zuccala, 1994). The other process contributing to the vascular pathology is the deposition of hyaline-like material (plasma protein constituents, such as inactive C3b, part of the third component of complement) into the damaged, more permeable arteriolar wall (Zucchelli & Zuccala, 1994). Arterial hypertension may lead to focal global (involving the whole glomerulus) or focal segemental glomerulosclerosis (Marcantoni *et al.* 2002; Zucchelli & Zuccala, 1994). Global sclerosis is thought to reflect ischemic injury, leading to nephron loss (Marcantoni *et al.* 2002). Focal segmental sclerosis is typically associated with glomerular enlargement, which is probably a compensatory response to nephron loss (Harvey *et al.* 1992). The vascular and glomerular alterations are associated with an often severe interstitial nephritis. Its etiology is incompletely understood. At least in part immunologic processes may be involved. They are probably started by ischemia-induced alterations in antigen expression on the surface of the tubular epithelial cells (Truong *et al.* 1992). Nephrosclerosis is seen with aging but is clearly exacerbated in arterial hypertension (Lindeman, Tobin & Shock, 1984; Rule *et al.* 2010). The incidence of progressive renal disease in hypertensive nephrosclerosis is low, however, three groups of patients are at increased risk to develop progressive kidney function deterioration: patients with more marked elevations in blood pressure, afro-american patients (they have an approximate eight-fold elevation in the risk of hypertension-induced ESRD(Toto, 2003); this increase in risk may persist even with "adequate" blood pressure control) and patients with underlying chronic kidney disease, especially diabetics. Patients with nephrosclerosis typically present with a long history of hypertension. If present, decline in kidney function is slow in progression as indicated by serum-creatinine and blood-urea-nitrogen. Urinalysis is typically benign without appearance of cast or dsymorph erythrocytes. Urinary protein excretion is typically mildly elevated (less than 1 gram per day). Concerning the incidence of renal failure in hypertensive nephrosclerosis there seems to be a clinical paradox as among patients (especially considering afro-americans) entering the chronic hemodialysis program. Hypertensive nephrosclerosis is one of the most common diagnoses, whereas the risk for a hypertensive patient to develop ESRD is rather small. However, at least three large trials might explain this paradox: the number of hypertensive patients is so large that even a small percentage of patients at risk gives a large number; the rate of progression might be so slow that trials that mostly run over 5-7 years might not detect patients at risk (Freedman, Iskandar & Appel, 1995; Madhavan *et al.* 1995). Recent work has shed some light on the importance of the Rho/ROCK pathway in kidney disease. ROCK is constitutionally active in the renal circulation. Studies on glomerular hemodynamics demonstrated that ROCK inhibition by Y-27632 and fasudil dilates the basal tone of afferent and efferent arterioles (Cavarape *et al.* 2003; Nakamura *et al.* 2003). Importantly, both inihibitors reverse angiotensin II-induced vasoconstriction of efferent and afferent arterioles (Nakamura *et al.* 2003). Thus, ROCK inhibition might protect against deleterious hemodynamic effects in kidney disease. In addition, to its critical role for the renal microvasculature the Rho/ROCK pathway is an important regulator of several cell function including proliferation, migration and apoptosis as already stated above (diabetic nephropathy). Of importance for the development of glomerulosclerosis, as a key feature of hypertensive nephrosclerosis, it has been demonstrated that Rho regulates the formation of stress fibers, focal adhesions and peripheral bundles through reorganization of the actin cytoskeleton in a renal epithelial cell line (Nakano *et al.* 1999). Renal epithelial cells are able to transform to mesenchymal-like cells via EMT. These changes have been observed in renal tubulointerstitial fibrosis, another hallmark of hypertensive nephrosclerosis. Mesangial cells reside in the renal glomeruli and produce ECM. Its increased accumulation causes glomerulosclerosis, where TGF-ß has been shown as a causative factor (Nakano *et al.* 1999). As mentioned above Rho/ROCK are key mediators/effectors of epithelial plasticity and EMT induced by TGF-ß (Patel *et al.* 2005; Rodrigues-Diez *et al.* 2008; Zavadil & Bottinger, 2005). Finally, in mesangial cells, mechanical stress, which is considered to cause glomerular hypertension and glomerulosclerosis, enhances mitogen-activated protein kinase (MAP kinase) activity, stress fiber formation, and cellular proliferation (Bruijn *et al.* 1994). In this process of disease the Rho/ROCK pathway plays a pivotal role, acting as a modulator of MAP kinase and the downstream cellular impact. Taken together, these data strengthen an important role of the Rho/ROCK pathway in the development of glomerulosclerotic disease.

Podocytes are highly differentiated cells that are located in the renal glomerulus. Cytoskeleton rearrangement is closely associated with podocyte shape changes and dysfunction in various renal diseases (Zucchelli & Zuccala, 1994). Using the ROCK-inhibitor Y-27632 Endlich et al. could inhibit the reorganization of the cytoskeleton induced by mechanical stress in podocytes. Moreover, inhibition of ROCK prevents TGF-ß-induced increase in CTGF accumulation in fibroblast cells (Heusinger-Ribeiro *et al.* 2001). All these observation strongly suggest a pivotal role of the Rho/ROCK pathway in the progression of renal injury. To date, the body of evidence given by in vivo studies is growing. As the Rho/ROCK pathway regulates glomerular hemodynamics and has profound effects on mesangial cell proliferation and matrix production, ROCK-inhibitors are candidates to serve as therapeutic tools to treat glomerulosclerotic disease. Thus, it has been demonstrated that Y-27632 and fasudil prevent tubulointerstitial fibrosis in a model of unilateral ureteral obstruction [for detail see section on ureteral obstruction]. In 5/6 nephrectomized spontaneously hypertensive rats (SHR), a model of hypertensive glomerulosclerosis, the Rho/ROCK pathway was activated. Treatment with fasudil reduced urinary protein excretion, improved glomerular and tubulointerstitial injury score, and reduced the infiltration of ED-1 positive cells and proliferating cell nuclear antigen positive cells in the kidney of SHR treated by 5/6 nephrectomy. Interestingly, these effects were obtained without lowering blood pressure, indicating blood pressure-independent effects of ROCK (Kanda *et al.* 2003b). Fasudil up-regulated the expression of p27kip1, a cyclin-dependent kinase inhibitor, and increased the p27kip1 immunopositive cells in both glomeruli and tubulointerstitium, indicating inhibition of cell proliferation and macrophage recruitment under fasudil treatment. Another group reported similar beneficial effects in Dahl salt-sensitive rats. In these animals, fasudil improved renal function, proteinuria, and histological findings without changes in blood pressure (Nishikimi *et al.* 2004b). These beneficial effects were most likely accompanied by decreased expression of TGF-ß, collagen-I, and collagen-III mRNA in the renal cortex. In salt-loaded spontaneously hypertensive stroke-prone rats serving as a model of severe hypertension fasudil improved kidney function, proteinuria, histological findings and decreased expression of genes encoding for extracellular matrix, oxidative stress, adhesion molecules and antifibrinolysis. Of note, these effects were independent of the blood pressure-lowering activity of fasudil (Nishikimi *et al.* 2004b). As stated above there is compelling evidence for an extensive crosstalk between NO and RhoA/ROCK-signaling. Indeed, in SHR fasudil partly reversed the progressive nephrosclerosis initiated by administration of the nitric oxide-synthase inhibitor nitro-L-arginine methyl ester (Koshikawa *et al.* 2008).

Although multiple factors contribute to the development and progression of chronic renal disease, the renin-angiotensin-aldosterone system seems to be of major importance. Angiotensin II is considered to be the main mediator of this system. It is a potent vasoconstrictor acting directly on vascular smooth muscle cells, thereby regulating the vascular tone. Besides it alters renal sodium and water absorption by stimulating synthesis and secretion of aldosterone. Further, it is involved in the generation of thirst and the excretion of vasopressin. Hence, it has a pivotal role in acute and chronic regulation of blood

pressure. Studies in chronic renal disease have shown that angII contributes to deterioration of renal function even if blood pressure is unaltered (Anderson, Rennke & Brenner, 1986). In this view it is important to keep in mind that angII activates ROCK in vascular smooth muscle cells (Yamakawa *et al.* 2000). In rats infused with angII, treatment with Y-27632 reduced renal inflammatory cell infiltration and tubular damage. AngII activated nuclear factor-kappaB and initiated overexpression of proinflammatory factors, including TNF-alpha and monocyte chemotactic protein-1 (MCP-1), and of CTGF. Treatment of angII-infused rats with Y-27632 reduced the upregulation of these proinflammatory and profibrotic mediators (Ruperez *et al.* 2005).
Taken together these studies imply that blockade of the Rho/ROCK pathway might prove beneficial in hypertensive nephrosclerosis.

1.4 Rock Inhibition in Ischemia Reperfusion Injury

Renal ischemia-reperfusion (IR) injury (IRI) is a common and important trigger of acute renal injury (AKI). It occurs in a broad spectrum of clinical settings including (transplantation) surgery, trauma, dehydration or sepsis leading to renal hypoperfusion, acute tubular necrosis (ATN), and functional disturbances - namely AKI. Inevitably linked to renal transplantation it is a well known risk factor for delayed graft function associated with prolonged hospitalization, elevated costs, and increased complexity of immunosuppressive drug management. Moreover, by reducing the overall number of nephrons and increasing the risk of acute rejection episodes, IRI might cause a significantly reduced graft survival. Involving both, the innate and the adaptive immune response, causing subsequent sterile inflammation, IRI is composed of a complex cascade of events including the generation of reactive oxygen and nitrogen species, chemotaxis, and phagocytosis. All of which are functional properties of the key effectors of the inflammatory cascade, neutrophiles, the most abundant leukocyte population in circulation, which accumulate as early as 30 minutes after IR particularly in the peritubular capillary network of the outer medulla (Li *et al.* 2008). Attracted leukocytes subsequently transmigrate into the interstitium. This is associated with increased vascular permeability and loss of endothelial and tubular epithelial cell integrity (Awad *et al.* 2009) due to degranulation of neutrophils. Upon activation these neutrophils release proteases, myeloperoxidase, cytokines, and generate reactive species leading to aggravation of injury and damage of endothelial and epithelial cells especially in the outer medulla (Bolisetty & Agarwal, 2009; Jang & Rabb, 2009; Li & Okusa, 2006; Okusa *et al.* 2000). In regard to this, it has recently been shown that ROCK) and their associated signaling pathways play pivotal roles in the development of (experimental) IRI. ROCK-inhibitors such as fasudil or Y-27632 have been shown to provide beneficial effects concerning different ischemic events such as renal (Kentrup D. *et al.* 10 A.D.; Kentrup D. *et al.* 2010; Prakash *et al.* 2008; Teraishi *et al.* 2004; Versteilen *et al.* 2006; Versteilen *et al.* 2011) myocardial (Bao *et al.* 2004; Hamid, Bower & Baxter, 2007; Wolfrum *et al.* 2004), cerebral (Satoh *et al.* 2008; Toshima *et al.* 2000), hepatic (Du & Hannon, 2004; Ikeda *et al.* 2003; Takeda *et al.* 2003), and gastrointestinal (Santen *et al.* 2010) ischemia. However, the exact mechanisms involved remain to be fully elucidated.
In the context of IRI it seems to be of interest that ROCKs are involved in the regulation of leukocyte cellular motility, migration, adhesion, and transmigration (Alblas *et al.* 2001; Honing *et al.* 2004; Lee *et al.* 2004; Samaniego *et al.* 2007; Takesono *et al.* 2010; Vemula *et al.* 2010; Worthylake *et al.* 2001; Worthylake & Burridge, 2003) Regarding this, Teraishi et al. were the first group to test the effectiveness of ROCK-inhibitors in an animal model of renal

IRI. For this, male Sprague-Dawley rats underwent unilateral nephrectomy of the right kidney two weeks before inducing 45 min of warm ischemia in the remaining kidney by clamping the left renal artery and vein. Y-27632 was hereby applied 5 min pre ischemia or 5 min post ischemia. They observed a protective effect for both treatments (i.e. improved renal function, less histological damage) which was based according to them on reduced infiltration by neutrophils as shown by myeloperoxidase assays. However, even though the latter is a non specific detection method and the data regarding the cell types typically involved varies, (e.g. due to the models used (Rabb *et al.* 2003; Thornton *et al.* 1989) or due to non specific detection methods, e.g. myeloperoxidase, naphthol chloroacetate esterase, or HIS-48 staining (Ysebaert *et al.* 2000)), it is well known that the increased influx of neutrophiles, T- and B-lymphocytes as well as macrophages/monocytes significantly contributes to the pathogenesis of AKI (Kinsey, Li & Okusa, 2008). This first study is also in congruence with later work by Versteilen et al.. By pre-treating male Wistar rats with Y-27632 they could show that leukocyte accumulation (60-70% neutrophils) was markedly reduced by ROCK-inhibitor treatment in the microvasculature of the corticomedullary junction and medulla (Versteilen *et al.* 2011). They hypothesize that this may be partly due to NO-mediated effects via activated endothelial cells (i.e. limited expression of adhesion molecules and cytokines leading to attenuation of leukocyte accumulation), eNOS mediated alterations of the renal blood flow (Versteilen *et al.* 2006) and direct effects on the leukocytes. Further, Prakash et al. also applied the ROCK-inhibitor Y-27632 in a rat model of renal ischemia, but used a Y-27632-lysozyme conjugate (Prakash *et al.* 2008). Thus, they tried to guarantee a renal-specific uptake into proximal tubular cells via megalin receptors. In unison with the aforementioned data they describe substantially attenuated tubular damage as indicated by reduced expression of dedifferentiation markers kidney injury molecule 1 (KIM-1) and vimentin. Additionally, they observed reduced fibrosis and inflammation as determined by reduced gene expressions of MCP-1, procollagen Iα1, TGF-β1, tissue inhibitor of metalloproteinase 1 and α-smooth muscle actin, as well as reduced immunohistochemical staining of macrophage infiltration, α-smooth muscle actin, collagen I, collagen III and fibronection compared to untreated animals. However, in contrast to the previous data, they describe adverse systemic effects (e.g. leucopenia) when animals were treated with the unconjugated Y-27632, as performed by others groups. An effect, which cannot easily be explained due to the fact that the beneficial effects of ROCK-inhibitors have not only been shown for the kidney but for other organs as well.

Although and apart from the above described effects, it has recently been shown by Kroening et al. that, in some cases, ROCK inhibition may not adversely influence the migratory capabilities of specific cell types as it has been repeatedly shown. Instead, at least in the case of tubular epithelial cells the migratory capacity may actually be promoted and thus ROCK inhibition may favor repair processes in renal tubules (Kroening *et al.* 2010). The beneficial effects of ROCK inhibition are further supported by work published by Unbekandt et al. who could show that transient ROCK inhibition allows cells from disaggregated embryonic kidneys to form ureteric bud and nephron epithelia (Unbekandt & Davies, 2010). Moreover, one last positive effect of ROCK inhibition related to the prevention of IRI mentioned might be that ROCK inhibition promotes cell survival in human stem cells (Watanabe *et al.* 2007) and is able to reduce apoptosis in conventional embryonic kidney culture (Meyer *et al.* 2006).

1.5 Rock Inhibition in Chronic Allograft Nephropathy

Compared to hemodialysis kidney transplantation significantly reduces mortality when it is applied to the appropriate patient (Wolfe *et al.* 1999). However, even after renal transplantation mortality of transplant recipients is still increased when compared to the general population. This is mainly due to death from cardiovascular disease with a functioning graft as well as immunological and non-immunological factors resulting in graft loss. Despite introduction of new immunosuppressive drugs within the last two decades a substantial increase in graft survival was not achieved. Consequently prevention of graft loss and treatment still lack any significant breakthrough since many years (Gjertson, 1991; Lamb, Lodhi & Meier-Kriesche, 2011; Meier-Kriesche *et al.* 2004; Meier-Kriesche, Schold & Kaplan, 2004). The pathological manifestations seen in chronic graft loss were summarized as chronic allograft nephropathy. In the recent Banff-classification ("Banff `05") which gives a classification of the different pathological features seen in chronic graft loss, the term chronic allograft nephropathy does no longer occur (Solez *et al.* 2007). The rationale for this update of the Banff schema was the misusage of CAN as a generic term for all causes of chronic renal allograft dysfunction with fibrosis that inhibits the accurate diagnosis and appropriate therapy. Thus, the authors of the Banff-classification aimed to present a pathological classification that specifies the underlying disease to facilitate causal treatment. Pathological manifestations of chronic allograft injury include interstitial fibrosis, tubular atrophy, vascular occlusive changes, glomerulosclerosis and a progressive renal dysfunction accompanied by hypertension and proteinuria (Cornell & Colvin, 2005). This histopathologic constellation is now more formally and descriptively referred to as interstitial fibrosis and tubular atrophy (IF/TA) without evidence of any specific aetiology (Solez *et al.* 2007). IF/TA or CAN describe the common final path of different injuries causing renal damage, whereas their precise pathogenesis is complex and only incompletely understood. The process encompasses multifactorial aetiologies including alloantigen-dependent as well as alloantigen-independent factors (Cornell & Colvin, 2005). The latter mainly comprise arterial hypertension, chronic obstruction and calcineurin-inhibitor toxicity (Busauschina, Schnuelle & van der Woude, 2004; Klahr & Morrissey, 2003; Mihatsch, Ryffel & Gudat, 1995; Morozumi *et al.* 2004). Besides, chronic polyoma virus nephrotixicity can lead to IF/TA (Drachenberg *et al.* 2005). Recurrent and de novo glomerular or vascular diseases can also lead to glomerulosclerosis and IF/TA, both early and late post-transplant. It is important to mention that de novo diabetic changes are becoming more common in allografts. As mentioned chronic alloimmune injury is an important cause of IF/TA in kidney grafts. Data on alloantibodies and C4d, a product of the complement cascade in chronically failing grafts, hint at a pathogenic role for humoral immunity in chronic allograft injury. In a prospective study de novo appearance of donor-specific HLA-antibodies was associated with increased graft failure at one year (Terasaki & Ozawa, 2004). These data are consistent with the importance of immunological factors in chronic graft injury.

The Rho/ROCK pathway is potentially crucial in mediating immunological as well as non-immunological injury in chronic graft loss as it is involved in adhesion, migration, proliferation, and cytokine release (Amano *et al.* 1997; Chihara *et al.* 1997; Tharaux *et al.* 2003). The activation of T-cells is involved in alloimmune responses. Here the Rho/ROCK pathway plays a pivotal role in T-cell activation during cellular immune responses by promoting structural rearrangements that are critical for T-cell signaling (Tharaux *et al.* 2003). Besides, a role for Rho/ROCK in HLA class I signaling pathways that have been implicated in the process of chronic rejection has been shown. Ligation of HLA class I molecules by anti-HLA-antibodies resulted in activation of Rho/ROCK and increased stress fiber formation. Inhibitors of Rho-GTPase and ROCK blocked HLA class I-mediated posphorylation of paxillin and FAK, both central elements of the focal adhesion signaling complex (Lepin *et al.* 2004). As stated above not only immunological factors but also non-immunological factors, such as arterial hypertension, are responsible for chronic graft injury. Recent data also show relevance of the Rho/ROCK pathway for the regulation of hemodynamics and arterial hypertension. In 1997 it was shown that the Rho/ROCK pathway is involved in the generation of arterial hypertension in different animal models of hypertension (Uehata *et al.* 1997). Interestingly, these data were confirmed in hypertensive patients showing involvement of Rho/ROCK in the generation of the increased vascular tone in these patients (Masumoto *et al.* 2001). As already stated above there is a close interaction between the RAAS and the Rho/ROCK pathway. Activation of the RAAS in arterial hypertension and vascular disease is associated with increased activation of Rho/ROCK (Higashi *et al.* 2003; Yamakawa *et al.* 2000). Taken together accumulating data suggest a role of the Rho/ROCK pathway in chronic allograft dysfunction. Recent studies in animal models of allograft dysfunction strongly support this view. In a well established model of kidney transplantation Lewis rats acted as kidney graft recipients and Fisher rats as donors. Cyclosporine A was given for immunosuppression. One group of animals additionally received the specific ROCK-inhibitor Y-27632. Renal function deteriorated progressively in the group that received cyclosporine A alone and histology revealed the typical features of IF/TA. ROCK inhibition by Y-27632 significantly prevented the deterioration of kidney function, reduced proteinuria and preserved renal function. These effects were accompanied by down-regulation of the expression of tubular MCP-1, RANTES, and phosphorylated NF-kB. The profibrotic TGF-ß1 and α-SMA, a marker of EMT, were downregulated by the treatment with Y-27632. These data indicated that the Rho/ROCK pathway is critically involved in renal interstitial inflammation and fibrosis, thus efficiently retarding the development of chronic allograft failure (Liu *et al.* 2009). The same group reported that atorvastatin, an inhibitor of the 3-hydroxy-3-methylglutaryl-coenzyme A reductase, exerted protective effects in CAN (Zhang *et al.* 2007). Because 3-hydroxy-3-methylglutaryl-coenzyme A reductase interferes with isoprenylation and activation of Rho, these data support the view that inhibition of the Rho/ROCK pathway could be attractive in prevention of allograft nephropathy. Of note, these data confirmed what was seen earlier in a model of cardiac allograft vasculopathy in mice. Here, coronary remodeling in the allografts characterized by intimal thickening and perivascular fibrosis was dose-dependently suppressed by the ROCK-inhibitor fasudil. These data were strengthened as gene transfer of dominant-negative ROCK mimicked the effects of fasudil. Vascular inflammation and expression of profibrotic mediators were significantly reduced in this model (Hattori *et al.* 2004). Song et al. observed expression of RhoA and ROCK1 mRNA and protein in measangial and tubular cells in the Fisher-to-Lewis model of CAN. Interestingly, they found a negative correlation between RhoA/ROCK1 mRNA and the Banff score. MMF, a potent immunosuppressive drug used in solid organ transplantation attenuated CAN by downregulating the expression of RhoA/ROCK1 (Song *et al.* 2008).

The data available suggest an important role of the Rho/ROCK pathway in chronic allograft dysfunction. Further studies also in humans are needed to support this view and possibly add a new therapeutic strategy to the nephrologist´s therapeutic options in preserving graft function.

2. Conclusion

Recent experimental data provide promising data that kidney protection in diabetic nephropathy, urethral obstruction, hypertensive nephrosclerosis and chronic allograft nephropathy can be brought about by inhibition of the Rho/ROCK pathway. As reviewed above ROCK activity is involved in actin cytoskeletal organization, stress fiber formation, and cell contraction thereby controlling vascular smooth muscle contraction, endothelial barrier and leukocyte functions (e.g., cellular motility, migration, adhesion and transmigration). All of these aspects are important in the pathogenesis of the renal diseases discussed here. However, clinical trials are needed to develop future strategies and transfer new treatment options by ROCK-inhibition from bench to bedside.

3. References

Alblas, J., Ulfman, L., Hordijk, P. & Koenderman, L. (2001). Activation of Rhoa and ROCK are essential for detachment of migrating leukocytes. *Mol.Biol.Cell* 12(7):2137-2145.

Alicic, R.Z. & Tuttle, K.R. (2010). Management of the diabetic patient with advanced chronic kidney disease. *Semin.Dial.* 23(2):140-147.

Amano, M., Chihara, K., Kimura, K., Fukata, Y., Nakamura, N., Matsuura, Y. & Kaibuchi, K. (1997). Formation of actin stress fibers and focal adhesions enhanced by Rho-kinase. *Science* 275(5304):1308-1311.

Anderson, S., Rennke, H.G. & Brenner, B.M. (1986). Therapeutic advantage of converting enzyme inhibitors in arresting progressive renal disease associated with systemic hypertension in the rat. *J.Clin.Invest* 77(6):1993-2000.

Arita, R., Hata, Y., Nakao, S., Kita, T., Miura, M., Kawahara, S., Zandi, S., Almulki, L., Tayyari, F., Shimokawa, H., Hafezi-Moghadam, A. & Ishibashi, T. (2009). Rho kinase inhibition by fasudil ameliorates diabetes-induced microvascular damage. *Diabetes* 58(1):215-226.

Arnol, M., Prather, J.C., Mittalhenkle, A., Barry, J.M. & Norman, D.J. (2008). Long-term kidney regraft survival from deceased donors: risk factors and outcomes in a single center. *Transplantation* 86(8):1084-1089.

Asano, M. & Nomura, Y. (2003). Comparison of inhibitory effects of Y-27632, a Rho kinase inhibitor, in strips of small and large mesenteric arteries from spontaneously hypertensive and normotensive Wistar-Kyoto rats. *Hypertens.Res.* 26(1):97-106.

Awad, A.S., Rouse, M., Huang, L., Vergis, A.L., Reutershan, J., Cathro, H.P., Linden, J. & Okusa, M.D. (2009). Compartmentalization of neutrophils in the kidney and lung following acute ischemic kidney injury. *Kidney Int.* 75(7):689-698.

Baboolal, K., Jones, G.A., Janezic, A., Griffiths, D.R. & Jurewicz, W.A. (2002). Molecular and structural consequences of early renal allograft injury. *Kidney Int.* 61(2):686-696.

Bao, W., Hu, E., Tao, L., Boyce, R., Mirabile, R., Thudium, D.T., Ma, X.L., Willette, R.N. & Yue, T.L. (2004). Inhibition of Rho-kinase protects the heart against ischemia/reperfusion injury. *Cardiovasc.Res.* 61(3):548-558.

Becker, B.N., Rush, S.H., Dykstra, D.M., Becker, Y.T. & Port, F.K. (2006). Preemptive transplantation for patients with diabetes-related kidney disease. *Arch.Intern.Med.* 166(1):44-48.

Bhalla, V., Nast, C.C., Stollenwerk, N., Tran, S., Barba, L., Kamil, E.S., Danovitch, G. & Adler, S.G. (2003). Recurrent and de novo diabetic nephropathy in renal allografts. *Transplantation* 75(1):66-71.

Bolisetty, S. & Agarwal, A. (2009). Neutrophils in acute kidney injury: not neutral any more. *Kidney Int.* 75(7):674-676.

Broniszczak, D., Ismail, H., Nachulewicz, P., Szymczak, M., Drewniak, T., Markiewicz-Kijewska, M., Kowalski, A., Jobs, K., Smirska, E., Rubik, J., Skobejko-Wlodarska, L., Gastol, P., Mikolajczyk, A. & Kalicinski, P. (2010). Kidney transplantation in children with bladder augmentation or ileal conduit diversion. *Eur.J.Pediatr.Surg.* 20(1):5-10.

Brownlee, M. (2001). Biochemistry and molecular cell biology of diabetic complications. *Nature* 414(6865):813-820.

Bruijn, J.A., Roos, A., de, G.B. & de, H.E. (1994). Transforming growth factor-beta and the glomerular extracellular matrix in renal pathology. *J.Lab Clin.Med.* 123(1):34-47.

Busauschina, A., Schnuelle, P. & van der Woude, F.J. (2004). Cyclosporine nephrotoxicity. *Transplant Proc.* 36(2 Suppl):229S-233S.

Cairns, H.S., Leaker, B., Woodhouse, C.R., Rudge, C.J. & Neild, G.H. (1991). Renal transplantation into abnormal lower urinary tract. *Lancet* 338(8779):1376-1379.

Caramori, M.L., Fioretto, P. & Mauer, M. (2003). Low glomerular filtration rate in normoalbuminuric type 1 diabetic patients: an indicator of more advanced glomerular lesions. *Diabetes* 52(4):1036-1040.

Carter, R.W., Begaye, M. & Kanagy, N.L. (2002). Acute and chronic NOS inhibition enhances alpha(2)- adrenoreceptor-stimulated RhoA and Rho kinase in rat aorta. *Am.J.Physiol Heart Circ.Physiol* 283(4):H1361-H1369.

Cavarape, A., Endlich, N., Assaloni, R., Bartoli, E., Steinhausen, M., Parekh, N. & Endlich, K. (2003). Rho-kinase inhibition blunts renal vasoconstriction induced by distinct signaling pathways in vivo. *J.Am.Soc.Nephrol.* 14(1):37-45.

Chang, T.I., Park, J.T., Kim, J.K., Kim, S.J., Oh, H.J., Yoo, D.E., Han, S.H., Yoo, T.H. & Kang, S.W. (2011a). Renal outcomes in patients with type 2 diabetes with or without coexisting non-diabetic renal disease. *Diabetes Res.Clin.Pract.*

Chang, T.I., Park, J.T., Kim, J.K., Kim, S.J., Oh, H.J., Yoo, D.E., Han, S.H., Yoo, T.H. & Kang, S.W. (2011b). Renal outcomes in patients with type 2 diabetes with or without coexisting non-diabetic renal disease. *Diabetes Res.Clin.Pract.*

Chihara, K., Amano, M., Nakamura, N., Yano, T., Shibata, M., Tokui, T., Ichikawa, H., Ikebe, R., Ikebe, M. & Kaibuchi, K. (1997). Cytoskeletal rearrangements and transcriptional activation of c-fos serum response element by Rho-kinase. *J.Biol.Chem.* 272(40):25121-25127.

Chitaley, K. & Webb, R.C. (2002). Nitric oxide induces dilation of rat aorta via inhibition of rho-kinase signaling. *Hypertension* 39(2 Pt 2):438-442.

Chou, T.C., Yen, M.H., Li, C.Y. & Ding, Y.A. (1998). Alterations of nitric oxide synthase expression with aging and hypertension in rats. *Hypertension* 31(2):643-648.

Chrissobolis, S. & Sobey, C.G. (2001). Evidence that Rho-kinase activity contributes to cerebral vascular tone in vivo and is enhanced during chronic hypertension: comparison with protein kinase C. *Circ.Res.* 88(8):774-779.

Churchill, B.M., Sheldon, C.A., McLorie, G.A. & Arbus, G.S. (1988). Factors influencing patient and graft survival in 300 cadaveric pediatric renal transplants. *J.Urol.* 140(5 Pt 2):1129-1133.

Cornell, L.D. & Colvin, R.B. (2005). Chronic allograft nephropathy. *Curr.Opin.Nephrol.Hypertens.* 14(3):229-234.

Cosio, F.G., Hickson, L.J., Griffin, M.D., Stegall, M.D. & Kudva, Y. (2008). Patient survival and cardiovascular risk after kidney transplantation: the challenge of diabetes. *Am.J.Transplant.* 8(3):593-599.

Couser, W.G. & Johnson, R.J. (1994). Mechanisms of progressive renal disease in glomerulonephritis. *Am.J.Kidney Dis.* 23(2):193-198.

Drachenberg, C.B., Hirsch, H.H., Ramos, E. & Papadimitriou, J.C. (2005). Polyomavirus disease in renal transplantation: review of pathological findings and diagnostic methods. *Hum.Pathol.* 36(12):1245-1255.

Du, J. & Hannon, G.J. (2004). Suppression of p160ROCK bypasses cell cycle arrest after Aurora-A/STK15 depletion. *Proc.Natl.Acad.Sci.U.S.A* 101(24):8975-8980.

Eto, M., Barandier, C., Rathgeb, L., Kozai, T., Joch, H., Yang, Z. & Luscher, T.F. (2001). Thrombin suppresses endothelial nitric oxide synthase and upregulates endothelin-converting enzyme-1 expression by distinct pathways: role of Rho/ROCK and mitogen-activated protein kinase. *Circ.Res.* 89(7):583-590.

Fellstrom, B., Holdaas, H., Jardine, A.G., Nyberg, G., Gronhagen-Riska, C., Madsen, S., Neumayer, H.H., Cole, E., Maes, B., Ambuhl, P., Olsson, A.G., Staffler, B. & Pedersen, T.R. (2005). Risk factors for reaching renal endpoints in the assessment of Lescol in renal transplantation (ALERT) trial. *Transplantation* 79(2):205-212.

Freedman, B.I., Iskandar, S.S. & Appel, R.G. (1995). The link between hypertension and nephrosclerosis. *Am.J.Kidney Dis.* 25(2):207-221.

Gjertson, D.W. (1991). Survival trends in long-term first cadaver-donor kidney transplants. *Clin.Transpl.* 225-235.

Gojo, A., Utsunomiya, K., Taniguchi, K., Yokota, T., Ishizawa, S., Kanazawa, Y., Kurata, H. & Tajima, N. (2007). The Rho-kinase inhibitor, fasudil, attenuates diabetic nephropathy in streptozotocin-induced diabetic rats. *Eur.J.Pharmacol.* 568(1-3):242-247.

Gottmann, U., Oltersdorf, J., Schaub, M., Knoll, T., Back, W.E., van der Woude, F.J. & Braun, C. (2003). Oxidative stress in chronic renal allograft nephropathy in rats: effects of long-term treatment with carvedilol, BM 91.0228, or alpha-tocopherol. *J.Cardiovasc.Pharmacol.* 42(3):442-450.

Hamid, S.A., Bower, H.S. & Baxter, G.F. (2007). Rho kinase activation plays a major role as a mediator of irreversible injury in reperfused myocardium. *Am.J.Physiol Heart Circ.Physiol* 292(6):H2598-H2606.

Harvey, J.M., Howie, A.J., Lee, S.J., Newbold, K.M., Adu, D., Michael, J. & Beevers, D.G. (1992). Renal biopsy findings in hypertensive patients with proteinuria. *Lancet* 340(8833):1435-1436.

Hattori, T., Shimokawa, H., Higashi, M., Hiroki, J., Mukai, Y., Kaibuchi, K. & Takeshita, A. (2004). Long-term treatment with a specific Rho-kinase inhibitor suppresses cardiac allograft vasculopathy in mice. *Circ.Res.* 94(1):46-52.

Heusinger-Ribeiro, J., Eberlein, M., Wahab, N.A. & Goppelt-Struebe, M. (2001). Expression of connective tissue growth factor in human renal fibroblasts: regulatory roles of RhoA and cAMP. *J.Am.Soc.Nephrol.* 12(9):1853-1861.

Higashi, M., Shimokawa, H., Hattori, T., Hiroki, J., Mukai, Y., Morikawa, K., Ichiki, T., Takahashi, S. & Takeshita, A. (2003). Long-term inhibition of Rho-kinase suppresses angiotensin II-induced cardiovascular hypertrophy in rats in vivo: effect on endothelial NAD(P)H oxidase system. *Circ.Res.* 93(8):767-775.

Higuchi, S., Ohtsu, H., Suzuki, H., Shirai, H., Frank, G.D. & Eguchi, S. (2007). Angiotensin II signal transduction through the AT1 receptor: novel insights into mechanisms and pathophysiology. *Clin.Sci.(Lond)* 112(8):417-428.

Hirose, A., Tanikawa, T., Mori, H., Okada, Y. & Tanaka, Y. (2010). Advanced glycation end products increase endothelial permeability through the RAGE/Rho signaling pathway. *FEBS Lett.* 584(1):61-66.

Hirschl, M.M. (1996). Type II diabetes mellitus and chronic renal insufficiency: renal transplantation or haemodialysis treatment? *Nephrol.Dial.Transplant.* 11 Suppl 9:98-99.

Honing, H., van den Berg, T.K., van der Pol, S.M., Dijkstra, C.D., van der Kammen, R.A., Collard, J.G. & de Vries, H.E. (2004). RhoA activation promotes transendothelial migration of monocytes via ROCK. *J.Leukoc.Biol.* 75(3):523-528.

Huang, P.L., Huang, Z., Mashimo, H., Bloch, K.D., Moskowitz, M.A., Bevan, J.A. & Fishman, M.C. (1995). Hypertension in mice lacking the gene for endothelial nitric oxide synthase. *Nature* 377(6546):239-242.

Ikeda, F., Terajima, H., Shimahara, Y., Kondo, T. & Yamaoka, Y. (2003). Reduction of hepatic ischemia/reperfusion-induced injury by a specific ROCK/Rho kinase inhibitor Y-27632. *J.Surg.Res.* 109(2):155-160.

Ishizaki, T., Maekawa, M., Fujisawa, K., Okawa, K., Iwamatsu, A., Fujita, A., Watanabe, N., Saito, Y., Kakizuka, A., Morii, N. & Narumiya, S. (1996). The small GTP-binding protein Rho binds to and activates a 160 kDa Ser/Thr protein kinase homologous to myotonic dystrophy kinase. *EMBO J.* 15(8):1885-1893.

Jang, H.R. & Rabb, H. (2009). The innate immune response in ischemic acute kidney injury. *Clin.Immunol.* 130(1):41-50.

Jansson, P.A. (2007). Endothelial dysfunction in insulin resistance and type 2 diabetes. *J.Intern.Med.* 262(2):173-183.

Jefferson, J.A., Shankland, S.J. & Pichler, R.H. (2008). Proteinuria in diabetic kidney disease: a mechanistic viewpoint. *Kidney Int.* 74(1):22-36.

Jin, L., Ying, Z., Hilgers, R.H., Yin, J., Zhao, X., Imig, J.D. & Webb, R.C. (2006). Increased RhoA/Rho-kinase signaling mediates spontaneous tone in aorta from angiotensin II-induced hypertensive rats. *J.Pharmacol.Exp.Ther.* 318(1):288-295.

Johnston, C.I., Risvanis, J., Naitoh, M. & Tikkanen, I. (1998). Mechanism of progression of renal disease: current hemodynamic concepts. *J.Hypertens.Suppl* 16(4):S3-S7.

Joosten, S.A., Sijpkens, Y.W., van, K.C. & Paul, L.C. (2005). Chronic renal allograft rejection: pathophysiologic considerations. *Kidney Int.* 68(1):1-13.

Kanda, T., Wakino, S., Hayashi, K., Homma, K., Ozawa, Y. & Saruta, T. (2003a). Effect of fasudil on Rho-kinase and nephropathy in subtotally nephrectomized spontaneously hypertensive rats. *Kidney Int.* 64(6):2009-2019.

Kanda, T., Wakino, S., Hayashi, K., Homma, K., Ozawa, Y. & Saruta, T. (2003b). Effect of fasudil on Rho-kinase and nephropathy in subtotally nephrectomized spontaneously hypertensive rats. *Kidney Int.* 64(6):2009-2019.

Kawamura, H., Yokote, K., Asaumi, S., Kobayashi, K., Fujimoto, M., Maezawa, Y., Saito, Y. & Mori, S. (2004). High glucose-induced upregulation of osteopontin is mediated via Rho/Rho kinase pathway in cultured rat aortic smooth muscle cells. *Arterioscler.Thromb.Vasc.Biol.* 24(2):276-281.

Kentrup D., Reuter, S., Schnöckel, U., Edemir, B., Grabner, A., Pavenstädt, H., Schlatter, E. & Büssemaker, E. (2010) Alterations in gene expression profile associated with renal ischemia-reperfusion injury are attenuated by hydroxyfasudil mediated Rho-kinase inhibition in a rat model of acute renal failure. *Transpl Int* 23, 50(Abstract)

Kentrup D., Reuter, S., Schnöckel, U., Klokkers, J., Edemir, B., Pavenstädt, H., Schäfers, M., Schlatter, E. & Büssemaker, E. (10 A.D.) ROCK-Inhibition by Hydroxyfasudil Significantly Improves Kidney Function and Attenuates Pro-Inflammatory Infiltration in a Rat Model of Acute Renal Ischemia. *Am.J.Transplant.* 10, 429(Abstract)

Kerjaschki, D., Huttary, N., Raab, I., Regele, H., Bojarski-Nagy, K., Bartel, G., Krober, S.M., Greinix, H., Rosenmaier, A., Karlhofer, F., Wick, N. & Mazal, P.R. (2006). Lymphatic endothelial progenitor cells contribute to de novo lymphangiogenesis in human renal transplants. *Nat.Med.* 12(2):230-234.

Khalkhali, H.R., Ghafari, A., Hajizadeh, E. & Kazemnejad, A. (2010). Risk factors of long-term graft loss in renal transplant recipients with chronic allograft dysfunction. *Exp.Clin.Transplant.* 8(4):277-282.

Kikuchi, Y., Yamada, M., Imakiire, T., Kushiyama, T., Higashi, K., Hyodo, N., Yamamoto, K., Oda, T., Suzuki, S. & Miura, S. (2007). A Rho-kinase inhibitor, fasudil, prevents development of diabetes and nephropathy in insulin-resistant diabetic rats. *J.Endocrinol.* 192(3):595-603.

Kinsey, G.R., Li, L. & Okusa, M.D. (2008). Inflammation in acute kidney injury. *Nephron Exp.Nephrol.* 109(4):e102-e107.

Klahr, S. & Morrissey, J. (2003). Obstructive nephropathy and renal fibrosis: The role of bone morphogenic protein-7 and hepatocyte growth factor. *Kidney Int.Suppl* (87):S105-S112.

Klein, J., Kavvadas, P., Prakoura, N., Karagianni, F., Schanstra, J.P., Bascands, J.L. & Charonis, A. (2011). Renal fibrosis: Insight from proteomics in animal models and human disease. *Proteomics.* 11(4):805-815.

Kolavennu, V., Zeng, L., Peng, H., Wang, Y. & Danesh, F.R. (2008). Targeting of RhoA/ROCK signaling ameliorates progression of diabetic nephropathy independent of glucose control. *Diabetes* 57(3):714-723.

Komers, R. (2011). Rho kinase inhibition in diabetic nephropathy. *Curr. Opin. Nephrol. Hypertens.* 20(1):77-83.

Komers, R., Oyama, T.T., Beard, D.R. & Anderson, S. (2011a). Effects of systemic inhibition of Rho kinase on blood pressure and renal haemodynamics in diabetic rats. *Br.J.Pharmacol.* 162(1):163-174.

Komers, R., Oyama, T.T., Beard, D.R., Tikellis, C., Xu, B., Lotspeich, D.F. & Anderson, S. (2011b). Rho kinase inhibition protects kidneys from diabetic nephropathy without reducing blood pressure. *Kidney Int.* 79(4):432-442.

Koo, H.P., Bunchman, T.E., Flynn, J.T., Punch, J.D., Schwartz, A.C. & Bloom, D.A. (1999). Renal transplantation in children with severe lower urinary tract dysfunction. *J.Urol.* 161(1):240-245.

Koshikawa, S., Nishikimi, T., Inaba, C., Akimoto, K. & Matsuoka, H. (2008). Fasudil, a Rho-kinase inhibitor, reverses L-NAME exacerbated severe nephrosclerosis in spontaneously hypertensive rats. *J.Hypertens.* 26(9):1837-1848.

Kroening, S., Stix, J., Keller, C., Streiff, C. & Goppelt-Struebe, M. (2010). Matrix-independent stimulation of human tubular epithelial cell migration by Rho kinase inhibitors. *J.Cell Physiol* 223(3):703-712.

Lamb, K.E., Lodhi, S. & Meier-Kriesche, H.U. (2011). Long-term renal allograft survival in the United States: a critical reappraisal. *Am.J.Transplant* 11(3):450-462.

Lee, J.H., Katakai, T., Hara, T., Gonda, H., Sugai, M. & Shimizu, A. (2004). Roles of p-ERM and Rho-ROCK signaling in lymphocyte polarity and uropod formation. *J.Cell Biol.* 167(2):327-337.

Lepin, E.J., Jin, Y.P., Barwe, S.P., Rozengurt, E. & Reed, E.F. (2004). HLA class I signal transduction is dependent on Rho GTPase and ROK. *Biochem.Biophys.Res.Commun.* 323(1):213-217.

Leung, T., Manser, E., Tan, L. & Lim, L. (1995). A novel serine/threonine kinase binding the Ras-related RhoA GTPase which translocates the kinase to peripheral membranes. *J.Biol.Chem.* 270(49):29051-29054.

Li, L., Huang, L., Sung, S.S., Vergis, A.L., Rosin, D.L., Rose, C.E., Jr., Lobo, P.I. & Okusa, M.D. (2008). The chemokine receptors CCR2 and CX3CR1 mediate monocyte/macrophage trafficking in kidney ischemia-reperfusion injury. *Kidney Int.* 74(12):1526-1537.

Li, L. & Okusa, M.D. (2006). Blocking the immune response in ischemic acute kidney injury: the role of adenosine 2A agonists. *Nat.Clin.Pract.Nephrol.* 2(8):432-444.

Liao, J.K. (2007). Does it matter whether or not a lipid-lowering agent inhibits Rho kinase? *Curr.Atheroscler.Rep.* 9(5):384-388.

Liao, J.K., Seto, M. & Noma, K. (2007). Rho kinase (ROCK) inhibitors. *J.Cardiovasc.Pharmacol.* 50(1):17-24.

Lindeman, R.D., Tobin, J.D. & Shock, N.W. (1984). Association between blood pressure and the rate of decline in renal function with age. *Kidney Int.* 26(6):861-868.

Liu, M., Gu, M., Wu, Y., Zhu, P., Zhang, W., Yin, C. & Zhang, W.J. (2009). Therapeutic effect of Y-27632 on chronic allograft nephropathy in rats. *J.Surg.Res.* 157(1):e117-e127.

Loirand, G., Guerin, P. & Pacaud, P. (2006). Rho kinases in cardiovascular physiology and pathophysiology. *Circ.Res.* 98(3):322-334.

Mack, C.P., Somlyo, A.V., Hautmann, M., Somlyo, A.P. & Owens, G.K. (2001). Smooth muscle differentiation marker gene expression is regulated by RhoA-mediated actin polymerization. *J.Biol.Chem.* 276(1):341-347.

Madhavan, S., Stockwell, D., Cohen, H. & Alderman, M.H. (1995). Renal function during antihypertensive treatment. *Lancet* 345(8952):749-751.

Marcantoni, C., Ma, L.J., Federspiel, C. & Fogo, A.B. (2002). Hypertensive nephrosclerosis in African Americans versus Caucasians. *Kidney Int.* 62(1):172-180.

Masumoto, A., Hirooka, Y., Shimokawa, H., Hironaga, K., Setoguchi, S. & Takeshita, A. (2001). Possible involvement of Rho-kinase in the pathogenesis of hypertension in humans. *Hypertension* 38(6):1307-1310.

Matsui, T., Amano, M., Yamamoto, T., Chihara, K., Nakafuku, M., Ito, M., Nakano, T., Okawa, K., Iwamatsu, A. & Kaibuchi, K. (1996). Rho-associated kinase, a novel serine/threonine kinase, as a putative target for small GTP binding protein Rho. *EMBO J.* 15(9):2208-2216.

Meier-Kriesche, H.U., Port, F.K., Ojo, A.O., Rudich, S.M., Hanson, J.A., Cibrik, D.M., Leichtman, A.B. & Kaplan, B. (2000). Effect of waiting time on renal transplant outcome. *Kidney Int.* 58(3):1311-1317.

Meier-Kriesche, H.U., Schold, J.D. & Kaplan, B. (2004). Long-term renal allograft survival: have we made significant progress or is it time to rethink our analytic and therapeutic strategies? *Am.J.Transplant* 4(8):1289-1295.

Meier-Kriesche, H.U., Schold, J.D., Srinivas, T.R. & Kaplan, B. (2004). Lack of improvement in renal allograft survival despite a marked decrease in acute rejection rates over the most recent era. *Am.J.Transplant.* 4(3):378-383.

Meyer, T.N., Schwesinger, C., Sampogna, R.V., Vaughn, D.A., Stuart, R.O., Steer, D.L., Bush, K.T. & Nigam, S.K. (2006). Rho kinase acts at separate steps in ureteric bud and metanephric mesenchyme morphogenesis during kidney development. *Differentiation* 74(9-10):638-647.

Miao, L., Calvert, J.W., Tang, J. & Zhang, J.H. (2002). Upregulation of small GTPase RhoA in the basilar artery from diabetic (mellitus) rats. *Life Sci.* 71(10):1175-1185.

Mihatsch, M.J., Ryffel, B. & Gudat, F. (1995). The differential diagnosis between rejection and cyclosporine toxicity. *Kidney Int.Suppl* 52:S63-S69.

Morgan, C., Sis, B., Pinsk, M. & Yiu, V. (2011). Renal interstitial fibrosis in children treated with FK506 for nephrotic syndrome. *Nephrol.Dial.Transplant.*

Moriki, N., Ito, M., Seko, T., Kureishi, Y., Okamoto, R., Nakakuki, T., Kongo, M., Isaka, N., Kaibuchi, K. & Nakano, T. (2004). RhoA activation in vascular smooth muscle cells from stroke-prone spontaneously hypertensive rats. *Hypertens.Res.* 27(4):263-270.

Morozumi, K., Takeda, A., Uchida, K. & Mihatsch, M.J. (2004). Cyclosporine nephrotoxicity: how does it affect renal allograft function and transplant morphology? *Transplant Proc.* 36(2 Suppl):251S-256S.

Mukai, Y., Shimokawa, H., Matoba, T., Kandabashi, T., Satoh, S., Hiroki, J., Kaibuchi, K. & Takeshita, A. (2001). Involvement of Rho-kinase in hypertensive vascular disease: a novel therapeutic target in hypertension. *FASEB J.* 15(6):1062-1064.

Nagatoya, K., Moriyama, T., Kawada, N., Takeji, M., Oseto, S., Murozono, T., Ando, A., Imai, E. & Hori, M. (2002). Y-27632 prevents tubulointerstitial fibrosis in mouse kidneys with unilateral ureteral obstruction. *Kidney Int.* 61(5):1684-1695.

Nahas, W.C. & David-Neto, E. (2009). Strategies to treat children with end-stage renal dysfunction and severe lower urinary tract anomalies for receiving a kidney transplant. *Pediatr.Transplant.* 13(5):524-535.

Nakagawa, O., Fujisawa, K., Ishizaki, T., Saito, Y., Nakao, K. & Narumiya, S. (1996). ROCK-I and ROCK-II, two isoforms of Rho-associated coiled-coil forming protein serine/threonine kinase in mice. *FEBS Lett.* 392(2):189-193.

Nakagawa, T., Tanabe, K., Croker, B.P., Johnson, R.J., Grant, M.B., Kosugi, T. & Li, Q. (2011). Endothelial dysfunction as a potential contributor in diabetic nephropathy. *Nat.Rev.Nephrol.* 7(1):36-44.

Nakamura, A., Hayashi, K., Ozawa, Y., Fujiwara, K., Okubo, K., Kanda, T., Wakino, S. & Saruta, T. (2003). Vessel- and vasoconstrictor-dependent role of rho/rho-kinase in renal microvascular tone. *J.Vasc.Res.* 40(3):244-251.

Nakano, K., Takaishi, K., Kodama, A., Mammoto, A., Shiozaki, H., Monden, M. & Takai, Y. (1999). Distinct actions and cooperative roles of ROCK and mDia in Rho small G protein-induced reorganization of the actin cytoskeleton in Madin-Darby canine kidney cells. *Mol.Biol.Cell* 10(8):2481-2491.

Nankivell, B.J., Borrows, R.J., Fung, C.L., O'Connell, P.J., Allen, R.D. & Chapman, J.R. (2003). The natural history of chronic allograft nephropathy. *N.Engl.J.Med.* 349(24):2326-2333.

Nath, K.A. (1992). Tubulointerstitial changes as a major determinant in the progression of renal damage. *Am.J.Kidney Dis.* 20(1):1-17.

Nishikimi, T., Akimoto, K., Wang, X., Mori, Y., Tadokoro, K., Ishikawa, Y., Shimokawa, H., Ono, H. & Matsuoka, H. (2004a). Fasudil, a Rho-kinase inhibitor, attenuates glomerulosclerosis in Dahl salt-sensitive rats. *J.Hypertens.* 22(9):1787-1796.

Nishikimi, T., Akimoto, K., Wang, X., Mori, Y., Tadokoro, K., Ishikawa, Y., Shimokawa, H., Ono, H. & Matsuoka, H. (2004b). Fasudil, a Rho-kinase inhibitor, attenuates glomerulosclerosis in Dahl salt-sensitive rats. *J.Hypertens.* 22(9):1787-1796.

Nobes, C. & Hall, A. (1994). Regulation and function of the Rho subfamily of small GTPases. *Curr.Opin.Genet.Dev.* 4(1):77-81.

Ohtsu, H., Suzuki, H., Nakashima, H., Dhobale, S., Frank, G.D., Motley, E.D. & Eguchi, S. (2006). Angiotensin II signal transduction through small GTP-binding proteins: mechanism and significance in vascular smooth muscle cells. *Hypertension* 48(4):534-540.

Oka, M., Fagan, K.A., Jones, P.L. & McMurtry, I.F. (2008). Therapeutic potential of RhoA/Rho kinase inhibitors in pulmonary hypertension. *Br.J.Pharmacol.* 155(4):444-454.

Okusa, M.D., Linden, J., Huang, L., Rieger, J.M., Macdonald, T.L. & Huynh, L.P. (2000). A(2A) adenosine receptor-mediated inhibition of renal injury and neutrophil adhesion. *Am.J.Physiol Renal Physiol* 279(5):F809-F818.

Osterby, R., Nyberg, G., Hedman, L., Karlberg, I., Persson, H. & Svalander, C. (1991). Kidney transplantation in type 1 (insulin-dependent) diabetic patients. Early glomerulopathy. *Diabetologia* 34(9):668-674.

Parekh, J., Bostrom, A. & Feng, S. (2010). Diabetes mellitus: a risk factor for delayed graft function after deceased donor kidney transplantation. *Am.J.Transplant.* 10(2):298-303.

Parizi, M., Howard, E.W. & Tomasek, J.J. (2000). Regulation of LPA-promoted myofibroblast contraction: role of Rho, myosin light chain kinase, and myosin light chain phosphatase. *Exp.Cell Res.* 254(2):210-220.

Pascual, M., Theruvath, T., Kawai, T., Tolkoff-Rubin, N. & Cosimi, A.B. (2002). Strategies to improve long-term outcomes after renal transplantation. *N.Engl.J.Med.* 346(8):580-590.

Patel, S., Takagi, K.I., Suzuki, J., Imaizumi, A., Kimura, T., Mason, R.M., Kamimura, T. & Zhang, Z. (2005). RhoGTPase activation is a key step in renal epithelial mesenchymal transdifferentiation. *J.Am.Soc.Nephrol.* 16(7):1977-1984.

Peng, F., Wu, D., Gao, B., Ingram, A.J., Zhang, B., Chorneyko, K., McKenzie, R. & Krepinsky, J.C. (2008). RhoA/Rho-kinase contribute to the pathogenesis of diabetic renal disease. *Diabetes* 57(6):1683-1692.

Perkins, B.A., Ficociello, L.H., Ostrander, B.E., Silva, K.H., Weinberg, J., Warram, J.H. & Krolewski, A.S. (2007). Microalbuminuria and the risk for early progressive renal function decline in type 1 diabetes. *J.Am.Soc.Nephrol.* 18(4):1353-1361.

Prakash, J., de Borst, M.H., Lacombe, M., Opdam, F., Klok, P.A., van, G.H., Meijer, D.K., Moolenaar, F., Poelstra, K. & Kok, R.J. (2008). Inhibition of Renal Rho Kinase Attenuates Ischemia/Reperfusion-Induced Injury. *J.Am.Soc.Nephrol.*

Rabb, H., Wang, Z., Nemoto, T., Hotchkiss, J., Yokota, N. & Soleimani, M. (2003). Acute renal failure leads to dysregulation of lung salt and water channels. *Kidney Int.* 63(2):600-606.

Racusen, L.C., Solez, K., Colvin, R.B., Bonsib, S.M., Castro, M.C., Cavallo, T., Croker, B.P., Demetris, A.J., Drachenberg, C.B., Fogo, A.B., Furness, P., Gaber, L.W., Gibson, I.W., Glotz, D., Goldberg, J.C., Grande, J., Halloran, P.F., Hansen, H.E., Hartley, B., Hayry, P.J., Hill, C.M., Hoffman, E.O., Hunsicker, L.G., Lindblad, A.S., Yamaguchi, Y. & . (1999). The Banff 97 working classification of renal allograft pathology. *Kidney Int.* 55(2):713-723.

Reuter, S., Reiermann, S., Worner, R., Schroter, R., Edemir, B., Buck, F., Henning, S., Peter-Katalinic, J., Vollenbroker, B., Amann, K., Pavenstadt, H., Schlatter, E. & Gabriels, G. (2010). IF/TA-related metabolic changes--proteome analysis of rat renal allografts. *Nephrol.Dial.Transplant.* 25(8):2492-2501.

Riento, K. & Ridley, A.J. (2003). Rocks: multifunctional kinases in cell behaviour. *Nat.Rev.Mol.Cell Biol.* 4(6):446-456.

Rigamonti, W., Capizzi, A., Zacchello, G., Capizzi, V., Zanon, G.F., Montini, G., Murer, L. & Glazel, G.P. (2005). Kidney transplantation into bladder augmentation or urinary diversion: long-term results. *Transplantation* 80(10):1435-1440.

Rikitake, Y., Kim, H.H., Huang, Z., Seto, M., Yano, K., Asano, T., Moskowitz, M.A. & Liao, J.K. (2005a). Inhibition of Rho kinase (ROCK) leads to increased cerebral blood flow and stroke protection. *Stroke* 36(10):2251-2257.

Rikitake, Y. & Liao, J.K. (2005). Rho-kinase mediates hyperglycemia-induced plasminogen activator inhibitor-1 expression in vascular endothelial cells. *Circulation* 111(24):3261-3268.

Rikitake, Y., Oyama, N., Wang, C.Y., Noma, K., Satoh, M., Kim, H.H. & Liao, J.K. (2005b). Decreased perivascular fibrosis but not cardiac hypertrophy in ROCK1+/- haploinsufficient mice. *Circulation* 112(19):2959-2965.

Rodrigo, E., Fernandez-Fresnedo, G., Valero, R., Ruiz, J.C., Pinera, C., Palomar, R., Gonzalez-Cotorruelo, J., Gomez-Alamillo, C. & Arias, M. (2006). New-onset diabetes after kidney transplantation: risk factors. *J.Am.Soc.Nephrol.* 17(12 Suppl 3):S291-S295.

Rodrigues-Diez, R., Carvajal-Gonzalez, G., Sanchez-Lopez, E., Rodriguez-Vita, J., Rodrigues, D.R., Selgas, R., Ortiz, A., Egido, J., Mezzano, S. & Ruiz-Ortega, M. (2008). Pharmacological modulation of epithelial mesenchymal transition caused by angiotensin II. Role of ROCK and MAPK pathways. *Pharm.Res.* 25(10):2447-2461.

Rugg, V. Diabetes and kidney disease: time to Act. International Diabetes Federation and the International Society of Nephrology . 2003. 20-2-2011. (GENERIC)

Ref Type: Electronic Citation

Rule, A.D., Amer, H., Cornell, L.D., Taler, S.J., Cosio, F.G., Kremers, W.K., Textor, S.C. & Stegall, M.D. (2010). The association between age and nephrosclerosis on renal biopsy among healthy adults. *Ann.Intern.Med.* 152(9):561-567.

Ruperez, M., Sanchez-Lopez, E., Blanco-Colio, L.M., Esteban, V., Rodriguez-Vita, J., Plaza, J.J., Egido, J. & Ruiz-Ortega, M. (2005). The Rho-kinase pathway regulates angiotensin II-induced renal damage. *Kidney Int.Suppl* (99):S39-S45.

Salifu, M.O., Nicastri, A.D., Markell, M.S., Ghali, H., Sommer, B.G. & Friedman, E.A. (2004). Allograft diabetic nephropathy may progress to end-stage renal disease. *Pediatr.Transplant.* 8(4):351-356.

Samaniego, R., Sanchez-Martin, L., Estecha, A. & Sanchez-Mateos, P. (2007). Rho/ROCK and myosin II control the polarized distribution of endocytic clathrin structures at the uropod of moving T lymphocytes. *J.Cell Sci.* 120(Pt 20):3534-3543.

Santen, S., Wang, Y., Laschke, M.W., Menger, M.D., Jeppsson, B. & Thorlacius, H. (2010). Rho-kinase signalling regulates CXC chemokine formation and leukocyte recruitment in colonic ischemia-reperfusion. *Int.J.Colorectal Dis.* 25(9):1063-1070.

Satoh, S., Toshima, Y., Hitomi, A., Ikegaki, I., Seto, M. & Asano, T. (2008). Wide therapeutic time window for Rho-kinase inhibition therapy in ischemic brain damage in a rat cerebral thrombosis model. *Brain Res.* 1193:102-108.

Satoh, S., Yamaguchi, T., Hitomi, A., Sato, N., Shiraiwa, K., Ikegaki, I., Asano, T. & Shimokawa, H. (2002). Fasudil attenuates interstitial fibrosis in rat kidneys with unilateral ureteral obstruction. *Eur.J.Pharmacol.* 455(2-3):169-174.

Sauzeau, V., Le, J.H., Cario-Toumaniantz, C., Smolenski, A., Lohmann, S.M., Bertoglio, J., Chardin, P., Pacaud, P. & Loirand, G. (2000). Cyclic GMP-dependent protein kinase signaling pathway inhibits RhoA-induced Ca2+ sensitization of contraction in vascular smooth muscle. *J.Biol.Chem.* 275(28):21722-21729.

Schena, F.P. & Gesualdo, L. (2005). Pathogenetic mechanisms of diabetic nephropathy. *J.Am.Soc.Nephrol.* 16 Suppl 1:S30-S33.

Seasholtz, T.M., Zhang, T., Morissette, M.R., Howes, A.L., Yang, A.H. & Brown, J.H. (2001). Increased expression and activity of RhoA are associated with increased DNA synthesis and reduced p27(Kip1) expression in the vasculature of hypertensive rats. *Circ.Res.* 89(6):488-495.

Seko, T., Ito, M., Kureishi, Y., Okamoto, R., Moriki, N., Onishi, K., Isaka, N., Hartshorne, D.J. & Nakano, T. (2003). Activation of RhoA and inhibition of myosin phosphatase as important components in hypertension in vascular smooth muscle. *Circ.Res.* 92(4):411-418.

Sheldon, C.A., Gonzalez, R., Burns, M.W., Gilbert, A., Buson, H. & Mitchell, M.E. (1994). Renal transplantation into the dysfunctional bladder: the role of adjunctive bladder reconstruction. *J.Urol.* 152(3):972-975.

Solez, K., Colvin, R.B., Racusen, L.C., Sis, B., Halloran, P.F., Birk, P.E., Campbell, P.M., Cascalho, M., Collins, A.B., Demetris, A.J., Drachenberg, C.B., Gibson, I.W., Grimm, P.C., Haas, M., Lerut, E., Liapis, H., Mannon, R.B., Marcus, P.B., Mengel, M., Mihatsch, M.J., Nankivell, B.J., Nickeleit, V., Papadimitriou, J.C., Platt, J.L., Randhawa, P., Roberts, I., Salinas-Madriga, L., Salomon, D.R., Seron, D., Sheaff, M. & Weening, J.J. (2007). Banff '05 Meeting Report: differential diagnosis of chronic allograft injury and elimination of chronic allograft nephropathy ('CAN'). *Am.J.Transplant.* 7(3):518-526.

Son, Y.K., Oh, J.S., Kim, S.M., Jeon, J.M., Shin, Y.H. & Kim, J.K. (2010). Clinical outcome of preemptive kidney transplantation in patients with diabetes mellitus. *Transplant.Proc.* 42(9):3497-3502.

Song, J., Lu, Y.P., Luo, G.H., Yang, L., Ma, X., Xia, Q.J., Shi, Y.J. & Li, Y.P. (2008). Effects of mycophenolate mofetil on chronic allograft nephropathy by affecting RHO/ROCK signal pathways. *Transplant.Proc.* 40(8):2790-2794.

Staessen, J.A., Wang, J., Bianchi, G. & Birkenhager, W.H. (2003). Essential hypertension. *Lancet* 361(9369):1629-1641.

Takeda, K., Jin, M.B., Fujita, M., Fukai, M., Sakurai, T., Nakayama, M., Taniguchi, M., Suzuki, T., Shimamura, T., Furukawa, H. & Todo, S. (2003). A novel inhibitor of Rho-associated protein kinase, Y-27632, ameliorates hepatic ischemia and reperfusion injury in rats. *Surgery* 133(2):197-206.

Takemoto, M., Sun, J., Hiroki, J., Shimokawa, H. & Liao, J.K. (2002). Rho-kinase mediates hypoxia-induced downregulation of endothelial nitric oxide synthase. *Circulation* 106(1):57-62.

Takesono, A., Heasman, S.J., Wojciak-Stothard, B., Garg, R. & Ridley, A.J. (2010). Microtubules regulate migratory polarity through Rho/ROCK signaling in T cells. *PLoS.ONE.* 5(1):e8774.

Teraishi, K., Kurata, H., Nakajima, A., Takaoka, M. & Matsumura, Y. (2004). Preventive effect of Y-27632, a selective Rho-kinase inhibitor, on ischemia/reperfusion-induced acute renal failure in rats. *Eur.J.Pharmacol.* 505(1-3):205-211.

Terasaki, P.I. & Ozawa, M. (2004). Predicting kidney graft failure by HLA antibodies: a prospective trial. *Am.J.Transplant* 4(3):438-443.

Tharaux, P.L., Bukoski, R.C., Rocha, P.N., Crowley, S.D., Ruiz, P., Nataraj, C., Howell, D.N., Kaibuchi, K., Spurney, R.F. & Coffman, T.M. (2003). Rho kinase promotes alloimmune responses by regulating the proliferation and structure of T cells. *J.Immunol.* 171(1):96-105.

Thornton, M.A., Winn, R., Alpers, C.E. & Zager, R.A. (1989). An evaluation of the neutrophil as a mediator of in vivo renal ischemic-reperfusion injury. *Am.J.Pathol.* 135(3):509-515.

Toshima, Y., Satoh, S., Ikegaki, I. & Asano, T. (2000). A new model of cerebral microthrombosis in rats and the neuroprotective effect of a Rho-kinase inhibitor. *Stroke* 31(9):2245-2250.

Toto, R.B. (2003). Hypertensive nephrosclerosis in African Americans. *Kidney Int.* 64(6):2331-2341.

Truong, L.D., Farhood, A., Tasby, J. & Gillum, D. (1992). Experimental chronic renal ischemia: morphologic and immunologic studies. *Kidney Int.* 41(6):1676-1689.

Tullius, S.G. & Tilney, N.L. (1995). Both alloantigen-dependent and -independent factors influence chronic allograft rejection. *Transplantation* 59(3):313-318.

Uehata, M., Ishizaki, T., Satoh, H., Ono, T., Kawahara, T., Morishita, T., Tamakawa, H., Yamagami, K., Inui, J., Maekawa, M. & Narumiya, S. (1997). Calcium sensitization of smooth muscle mediated by a Rho-associated protein kinase in hypertension. *Nature* 389(6654):990-994.

Unbekandt, M. & Davies, J.A. (2010). Dissociation of embryonic kidneys followed by reaggregation allows the formation of renal tissues. *Kidney Int.* 77(5):407-416.

Van Buren, P.N. & Toto, R. (2011). Hypertension in diabetic nephropathy: epidemiology, mechanisms, and management. *Adv.Chronic.Kidney Dis.* 18(1):28-41.

Vemula, S., Shi, J., Hanneman, P., Wei, L. & Kapur, R. (2010). ROCK1 functions as a suppressor of inflammatory cell migration by regulating PTEN phosphorylation and stability. *Blood* 115(9):1785-1796.

Vernon, M.A., Mylonas, K.J. & Hughes, J. (2010). Macrophages and renal fibrosis. *Semin.Nephrol.* 30(3):302-317.

Versteilen, A.M., Blaauw, N., Di, M.F., Groeneveld, A.B., Sipkema, P., Musters, R.J. & Tangelder, G.J. (2011). Rho-Kinase Inhibition Reduces Early Microvascular Leukocyte Accumulation in the Rat Kidney following Ischemia-Reperfusion Injury: Roles of Nitric Oxide and Blood Flow. *Nephron Exp.Nephrol.* 118(4):e79-e86.

Versteilen, A.M., Korstjens, I.J., Musters, R.J., Groeneveld, A.B. & Sipkema, P. (2006). Rho kinase regulates renal blood flow by modulating eNOS activity in ischemia-reperfusion of the rat kidney. *Am.J.Physiol Renal Physiol* 291(3):F606-F611.

Vielhauer, V., Kulkarni, O., Reichel, C.A. & Anders, H.J. (2010). Targeting the recruitment of monocytes and macrophages in renal disease. *Semin.Nephrol.* 30(3):318-333.

Watanabe, K., Ueno, M., Kamiya, D., Nishiyama, A., Matsumura, M., Wataya, T., Takahashi, J.B., Nishikawa, S., Nishikawa, S., Muguruma, K. & Sasai, Y. (2007). A ROCK inhibitor permits survival of dissociated human embryonic stem cells. *Nat.Biotechnol.* 25(6):681-686.

Weber, D.S. & Webb, R.C. (2001). Enhanced relaxation to the rho-kinase inhibitor Y-27632 in mesenteric arteries from mineralocorticoid hypertensive rats. *Pharmacology* 63(3):129-133.

Wiesbauer, F., Heinze, G., Regele, H., Horl, W.H., Schernthaner, G.H., Schwarz, C., Kainz, A., Kramar, R. & Oberbauer, R. (2010). Glucose control is associated with patient survival in diabetic patients after renal transplantation. *Transplantation* 89(5):612-619.

Wilkinson, A., Davidson, J., Dotta, F., Home, P.D., Keown, P., Kiberd, B., Jardine, A., Levitt, N., Marchetti, P., Markell, M., Naicker, S., O'Connell, P., Schnitzler, M., Standl, E., Torregosa, J.V., Uchida, K., Valantine, H., Villamil, F., Vincenti, F. & Wissing, M. (2005). Guidelines for the treatment and management of new-onset diabetes after transplantation. *Clin.Transplant.* 19(3):291-298.

Wojciechowski, D., Onozato, M.L. & Gonin, J. (2009). Rapid onset of diabetic nephropathy in three renal allografts despite normoglycemia. *Clin.Nephrol.* 71(6):719-724.

Wolfe, R.A., Ashby, V.B., Milford, E.L., Ojo, A.O., Ettenger, R.E., Agodoa, L.Y., Held, P.J. & Port, F.K. (1999). Comparison of mortality in all patients on dialysis, patients on dialysis awaiting transplantation, and recipients of a first cadaveric transplant. *N.Engl.J.Med.* 341(23):1725-1730.

Wolfrum, S., Dendorfer, A., Rikitake, Y., Stalker, T.J., Gong, Y., Scalia, R., Dominiak, P. & Liao, J.K. (2004). Inhibition of Rho-kinase leads to rapid activation of phosphatidylinositol 3-kinase/protein kinase Akt and cardiovascular protection. *Arterioscler.Thromb.Vasc.Biol.* 24(10):1842-1847.

Worthylake, R.A. & Burridge, K. (2003). RhoA and ROCK promote migration by limiting membrane protrusions. *J.Biol.Chem.* 278(15):13578-13584.

Worthylake, R.A., Lemoine, S., Watson, J.M. & Burridge, K. (2001). RhoA is required for monocyte tail retraction during transendothelial migration. *J.Cell Biol.* 154(1):147-160.

Yamakawa, T., Tanaka, S., Numaguchi, K., Yamakawa, Y., Motley, E.D., Ichihara, S. & Inagami, T. (2000). Involvement of Rho-kinase in angiotensin II-induced hypertrophy of rat vascular smooth muscle cells. *Hypertension* 35(1 Pt 2):313-318.

Yousif, M.H. (2006). Role of protein kinases in mediating diabetes-induced augmented vasoconstriction to endothelin-1 in the renal arteries of STZ-diabetic rats. *Cell Biochem.Funct.* 24(5):397-405.

Ysebaert, D.K., De Greef, K.E., Vercauteren, S.R., Ghielli, M., Verpooten, G.A., Eyskens, E.J. & De Broe, M.E. (2000). Identification and kinetics of leukocytes after severe ischaemia/reperfusion renal injury. *Nephrol.Dial.Transplant.* 15(10):1562-1574.

Zavadil, J. & Bottinger, E.P. (2005). TGF-beta and epithelial-to-mesenchymal transitions. *Oncogene* 24(37):5764-5774.

Zeng, L., Xu, H., Chew, T.L., Eng, E., Sadeghi, M.M., Adler, S., Kanwar, Y.S. & Danesh, F.R. (2005). HMG CoA reductase inhibition modulates VEGF-induced endothelial cell hyperpermeability by preventing RhoA activation and myosin regulatory light chain phosphorylation. *FASEB J.* 19(13):1845-1847.

Zhang, W., Liu, M., Wu, Y., Zhu, P., Yin, C., Zhang, W. & Gu, M. (2007). Protective effects of atorvastatin on chronic allograft nephropathy in rats. *J.Surg.Res.* 143(2):428-436.

Zimmet, P., Alberti, K.G. & Shaw, J. (2001). Global and societal implications of the diabetes epidemic. *Nature* 414(6865):782-787.

Zucchelli, P. & Zuccala, A. (1994). Primary hypertension--how does it cause renal failure? *Nephrol.Dial.Transplant.* 9(3):223-225.

16

Post-Tx Renal Monitoring with B-Flow Ultrasonography

Paride De Rosa, Enrico Russo and Vincenzo Cerbone
A.O.U. "OO.RR. San Giovanni di Dio e Ruggi d'Aragona, Salerno
Italy

1. Introduction

The examination of blood vessels and the study of arterial districts have been already revolutionized by the introduction of B-mode ultrasonography, widely used to evaluate the blood flow. The lumen and vessel wall together with microscopic characteristics, can be clearly evidenced with this method thanks to the use of Color Doppler Flow Ultrasounds (CDFU) (Wescott 2000). This methodic is able to show the flow direction and the velocity of red blood cells as well as vascular structures. The color signals and generated angiography-like visualization of the vascular lumen surface can be shown by the integration with the Power Doppler Ultrasounds (PDU). Consequently, CDFU and PDU give not an approximate estimation but a precise measure of the residual lumen of the vessels more reliable than with conventional B-mode imaging in case of stenosis (Wescott 2000).
Recently a new technology for the detection of blood circulation has been developed by using digitally encoded sonography to boost blood echoes and to preferentially suppress non-moving tissue signals. This method is known as the B-Flow Ultrasonography (BFU) and it has higher spatial and temporal resolution than Doppler imaging because of the clearer definition of the vessel lumen (Henry 2000). BFU allows the direct visualization of blood reflectors without the limitations of Doppler technology such as aliasing, signal dropout at orthogonal detection angles and wall filter limitations. B-flow visualizes real-time hemodynamic flow in relation to stationary tissue (Jung 2007, Wachsberg 2007).
We evaluated the efficacy of BFU in examining the arterial and venous anastomoses, the cortical flow and other parameters of the graft in patients who underwent kidney transplantation for chronic renal disease.

2. Historical background

When color Doppler sonography was originally introduced, sinologists hoped that the new technology would provide reliable noninvasive mapping of blood flow. Although color Doppler sonography remains an essential technology for noninvasive vascular imaging, it is prone to various artifacts and limitations, resulting in some instances in which true flow is not detected and other instances where Doppler sonography falsely depicts blood flow (Middleton 1998).
The first studies about B-Flow imaging were conducted by vascular surgeon to investigate cerebral circulation in order to improve the detection of carotids stenosis. Toole and

Castaldo (Toole&Castaldo 1994) reported that a more hemodynamically disturbed flow has a greater propensity for distal cerebrovascular events. Different studies (Benefit 1998, Beneficial 1991 trials) demonstrated better outcomes in patients with symptomatic moderate (50%-69%) and highgrade (70%-99%) internal carotid arterial (ICA) stenoses (ICAS) after carotid endarterectomy, as compared with those treated medically. Even in patients with asymptomatic ICAS of 60%-99%, an absolute risk reduction of 5.9% for stroke has been reported at 5 years (ACASC Study 1995).

These studies gave rise to discussions and kindled the interest in and necessity of accurate measurement of arterial stenosis (Staikov 2000). Selective intraarterial angiography of artery is still seen as the reference standard but is an invasive method with a morbidity rate of 1%-4% that bears a 1% risk of periinterventional stroke. Color duplex flow ultrasonography (US) has become the most widely used noninvasive method of assessing arterial occlusive disease (Padayachee 1997) because it avoids the expense and risk of routine arteriography (Bell 1995). Stenotic lesions are identified and quantified by analyzing Doppler US velocity spectra in combination with real-time B-mode and color-flow images (Carpenter 1996).

Despite its broad use, several disadvantages of color duplex flow US have been described. Different studies (Carpenter 1996, Alexandrov 1997) have shown considerable variation in estimating the degree of stenosis, and even with use of similar equipment, rigid velocity criteria do not have the same validity and predictive values for grading an arterial stenoses in different laboratories. It is well recognized that duplex US results are highly dependent on the experience of the operator, which emphasizes the importance of individual evaluation and quality control for each institution (Kruskal 2004). There are also different technical limitations of US depiction of blood flow. Color duplex flow US is very sensitive to flow signals and can yield quantitative velocity and/or power information, but the price is decreased spatial resolution and frame rate, as well as high angle dependency.

Because the color duplex flow US image is presented as an overlay to the B-flow image, any large tissue motion may register as a color flash artifact that can overshadow the true flow data. Conversely, maximizing the color fill-in of vessels will almost always result in some overwriting of the vessel walls on the B-flow image, which can mask any subtle lesion in the vessel under study (GE Ultrasound Europe 1999).

3. B-Flow imaging

A technique for displaying flow information called B-flow imaging was introduced several years ago (Wescott 2000). This is a non-Doppler technology that directly displays flowing intravascular echoes during real-time gray-scale sonography. Flow information is derived by digitally encoding the outgoing ultrasound beam, then decoding and filtering the returning beam so as to amplify echoes generated by the particulate constituents of flowing blood.

The real-time B-flow imaging appearance of blood flow consists of mobile intravascular echoes that simulate a conventional contrast angiogram, similar to the appearance seen during infusion of a sonographic IV contrast agent. The images are particularly impressive when viewed during real-time sonography or on recorded movie clips. The technique is relatively simple to learn and operate, with fewer parameters to manipulate than color Doppler sonography. B-flow imaging was first introduced on linear transducers for vascular imaging and subsequently became available on curved transducers suitable for general abdominopelvic imaging as well.

Recent investigations have documented the value of B-flow imaging for evaluation of flow in superficial vascular structures, in particular carotid arteries and hemodialysis fistulas (Yucel 2005). B-flow imaging is a recently introduced flow technology that extends B-mode imaging capabilities to blood flow, including high frame rate and high-spatial-, high-temporal-, and high contrast-resolution imaging (Wescott 2000). It directly depicts blood echoes in a gray-scale presentation, while simultaneously depicting surrounding anatomy, but without the need for overlays. This explains the unobstructed view of the vessel lumen. These attributes of B-flow imaging promise this technique to be an important additional tool in the evaluation of arterial status. Our experience with B flow imaging has shown that in the poststenotic area, vessel stenoses produce a region of higher gray-scale intensity that we call the *jet stream*. The rationale for this jet stream seems to be that pixel brightness at B-flow imaging is determined by blood-echo strength and velocity, and both factors are influenced by the grade of vessel stenosis (Wescott 2000). However, the literature reveals scant interest in exploring abdominopelvic applications of B-flow imaging. A MEDLINE search of the English-language literature using the term "Bflow imaging" conducted on August 28, 2006, identified one preliminary report on abdominal applications of B-flow imaging published in 2003 and two investigations of B-flow imaging for evaluating fetal cardiovascular anomalies (Wachsberg 2003). In our experience, B-flow imaging is a powerful technique for noninvasive flow evaluation of the transplanted kidney. We performed this prospective pilot trial to assess the interobserver variability of different jet stream parameters and their role in the evaluation of renal stenosis.This article illustrates various advantages of B-flow imaging as a complementary technique to color Doppler sonography of the kidney vasculature.

4. Technical background

4.1 Basics

B-flow images are generated by using digitally encoded US technology consisting of a transmit encoder and a receive decoder in a digital beam former that provides electronic array focusing (Fig. 1). A small number of digitally encoded wideband pulses are transmitted into the body for each scan line. Unlike color imaging techniques, in which the typical packet size is 10–12, B-flow imaging uses a packet size as small as 2-4. Directly after receiving the reversed pulses, the decoder performs pulse-length compression ("coded excitation") on the acoustic data and then performs clutter suppression filtering. The rest of the processing is essentially the same as in conventional Bflow mode (GE Ultrasound Europe 1999).

4.2 Coded excitation

Coded excitation is a technique that increases the transmission energy by as much as one order of magnitude without compromising transverse resolution and is therefore especially suited for high-spatial- and high-temporal resolution imaging of echo sources that are simply weak (such as red blood cells). Through the digital encoder the scanner transmits not one, but a sequence of N wideband pulses in accordance with a specific pattern referred to as a *code*; a decoder on the receiving side is used to effectively compress the returning echo back into a single pulse that has nearly the same resolution but N times more energy (Fig. 2). If the received coded sequence and the sent code are exactly matched, the response is a

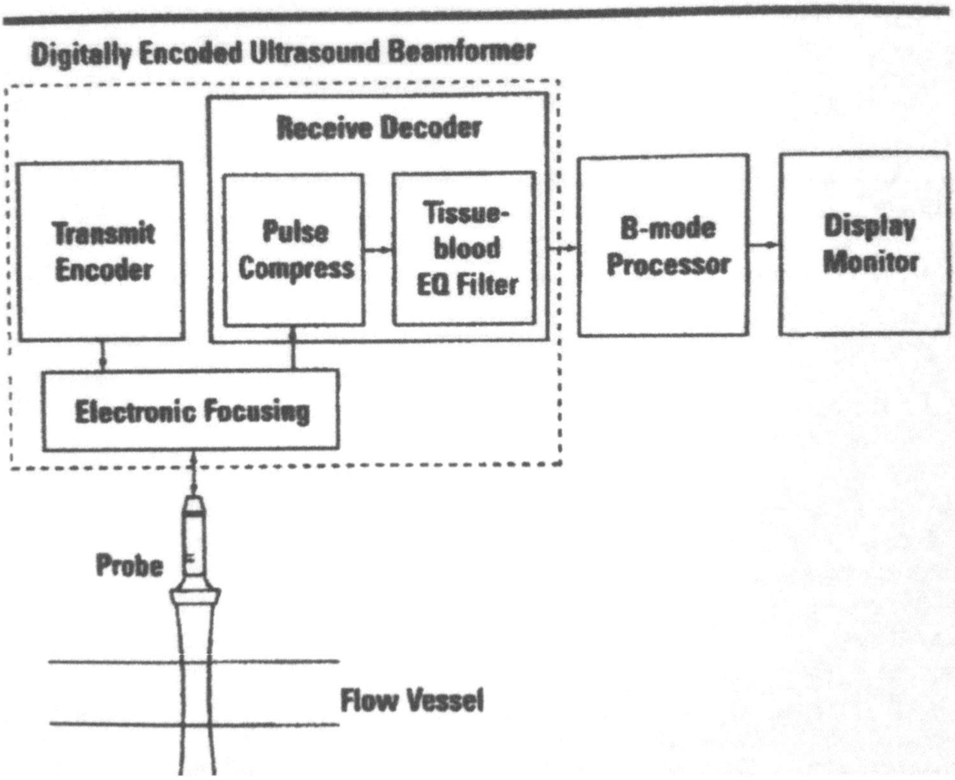

Fig. 1. Digitally Encoded Ultrasound Beamformer

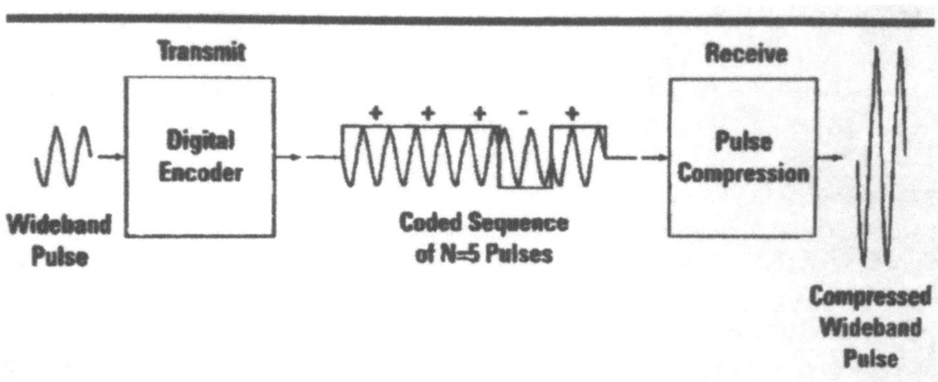

Fig. 2. Compression of wideband pulse

pulse of amplitude N times greater than a single uncoded pulse. At in vivo scanning, the returning signal represents a sum of reflections from multiple sources in body tissue, so that the output of the sum should equal the sum of outputs from individual contributing reflectors (GE Ultrasound Europe 1999).

4.3 Clutter suppression filtering

For each of the coded transmissions, a stream of acoustic backscatter data from the insonated anatomy is received and coded. These data are stored in a buffer in the equalization filter, which then subtracts a fraction of the second transmission from the first transmission. This process suppresses any large and slow-moving tissue clutter component relative to any moving blood-echo component (GE Ultrasound Europe 1999).

5. Comparison between B-Flow Imaging and color-doppler ultrasounds

Doppler sonography uses a high-pass filter to suppress low-amplitude frequency shifts caused by physiologic movement of soft-tissue structures. Unfortunately, this filter also obliterates Doppler shifts produced by slowly flowing blood and may cause a false diagnosis of vascular occlusion. This pitfall does not apply to B-flow imaging, which excellently depicts slow blood flow. Doppler sonography is also prone to artifactual depiction of flow signals within nonvascular hypoechoic structures, whereas B-flow imaging is not plagued by such factitious flow.

The usual practice for optimizing color Doppler sonography is to increase the color gain setting as high as possible until noise develops; then lower the gain slightly to eliminate the noise (Kruskal 2004. However, this practice can exaggerate the spatial location of true flow signal, a phenomenon called "oversaturation," resulting in flow signals that are not confined to the patent lumen (Wachsberg 2003). This pitfall can cause thrombus to be overlooked or improperly characterized and can prompt a false diagnosis of vascular disease. Because of oversaturation, the spatial distribution of color signals can substantially exceed the true dimensions of a vascular structure, whereas the high spatial resolution of B-flow imaging enables excellent display of even complex vasculature. Soft-tissue vibration associated with an arteriovenous fistula, known as "perivascular color bruit," is a phenomenon that can significantly exaggerate the apparent dimensions of a vascular fistula on Doppler sonography, whereas Bflow imaging correctly displays the true dimensions. Vascular stenosis is typically diagnosed when Doppler sonography reveals a localized flow jet.

However, turbulence and other factors can also cause localized acceleration of flow unassociated with anatomic narrowing. B-flow imaging is very helpful at distinguishing between a falsepositive diagnosis of vascular stenosis and a truepositive case.

Noninvasive evaluation of transjugular intrahepatic portosystemic shunts (TIPS) function with Doppler sonography is complex and fraught with pitfalls that can potentially yield misleading findings. In our experience, B-flow imaging is very helpful in supplementing the Doppler sonography TIPS evaluation. The applications illustrated in this article should not be misinterpreted as suggesting that color Doppler sonography has been or will be eclipsed by B-flow imaging. B-flow imaging does not provide information regarding flow velocity and directionality, and its current iteration has other limitations that require improvement. We anticipate that color Doppler sonography will continue to be the primary technique for noninvasive flow mapping, with B-flow imaging as a complementary technique for use in situations where color Doppler sonography findings are ambiguous or otherwise uncertain.

6. Our experience

6.1 Methods

Between June 2006 and May, 2010, 55 consecutive patients with ESRD, 37 men (67.3%) and 18 women (32.7%); mean age 47.8 (ranged between 16 to 60 years) underwent kidney transplantation from cadaveric donor. All the patients has been studied preoperatively with evaluation of principal arterial and venous axis by using Color-Power doppler. All the patients were submitted to ultrasonography check already immediately in the postoperative time . The study consisted of daily controls with a comparative evaluation of both techniques, that is Color and Power Doppler (CDFU+PDU) and B-flow imaging (BFU).
The arterial and venous anastomoses, Cortical blood flow with evaluation of R.I. (resistance index), $V._{max}$ (blood velocity arterial peek) were examined in all patients using LOGIQ 700 ultrasound device (GE Medical Systems) with a 12 or 7 MHz probe focusing on the level around the iliac-graft anastomosis. Routine B-mode, blood flow images by PDI and B-flow were obtained and compared each other. Sequential parallel longitudinal views of flow were displayed. We closely watched vessel walls and hemodynamic flow simultaneously. In the follow-up period we submitted patients to monthly checks, focusing our attention on the detection of particular signs, such as cortical "spots" as well as defects in graft vascularization.

6.2 Results

In our study we observed that the analysis of parameters dropped out from an ultrasonographic study, made of the combination of standard methodics and B-flow imaging, brought to a better estimation of vascular complications after transplantation. In 25 patients (45.5%) we can assert to visualize a clearer cortical blood flow than the standard techniques (Fig. 3,4,5,6,7). Consequently the parameters of intra and extra-renal circulation resulted very easy to measure. We also noticed that in one patient occurred a reduction of blood flow through the renal artery with a sensible increase of V_{max} and R.I. (Fig. 8) during the first 24 hours after the transplantation. This conditions leaded to thing to an arterial stenosis but it could not certainly be included among these after CDU+PDU evaluation. In this case the B-Flow methodic enable us to characterize it as a post-operative arterial spasm (Fig. 9,10).
In this patient we didn't appreciate any reverberation both on cortical flow and on parameters of graft function. The vision of cortical vasculature by using b-flow mode allows a better
In another patient we observed some cortical "spots" that coincided with a reduction of renal function in the first week after transplantation. The functional situation solved after administration of steroids but ecographic signs persists also after some months.

6.3 Discussion

B-flow enabled simultaneous imaging of tissue and real-time blood flow in all patients. Flow pattern was shown in gray-scale imaging. Compared with PDU, B-flow provided higher spatial resolution and frame rate hemodynamic imaging without information on velocity and direction (Volpe 2007).
Consequently, clear definition of the vessel lumen without overlay was obtained . However, resolution of vessel wall tissue was inferior to that of the conventional B-mode and PDU methods. B-flow provided clearer definition of the vessel lumen even in the renal stenosis. PDU tended to overestimate the normal vessel lumen and underestimate that of the severely stenotic portion. B-flow technology was achieved by General Electric's digitally encoded ultrasound (Park 2007).

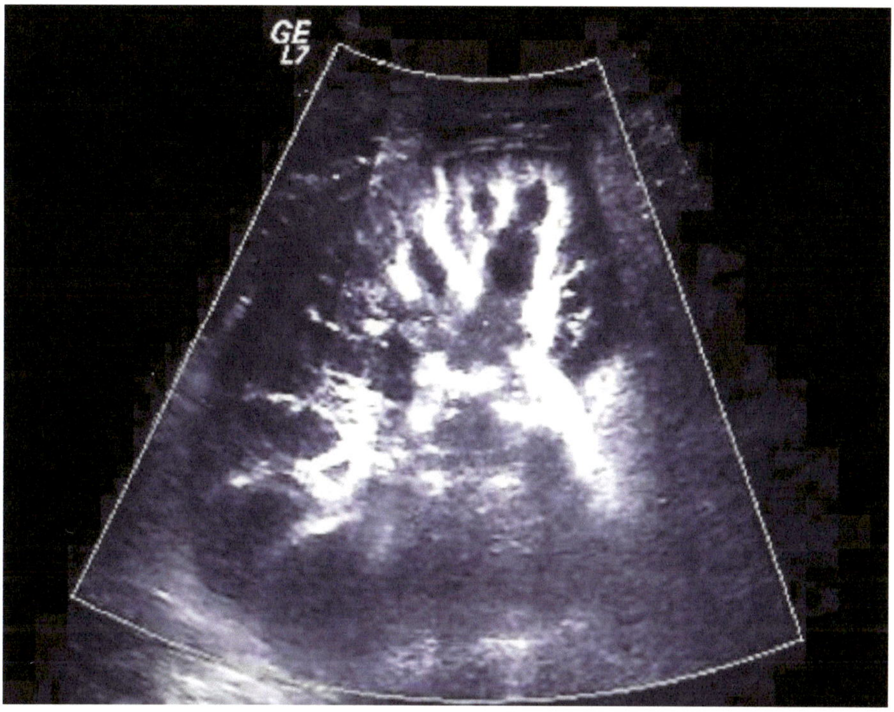

Fig. 3. B-Flow Imaging

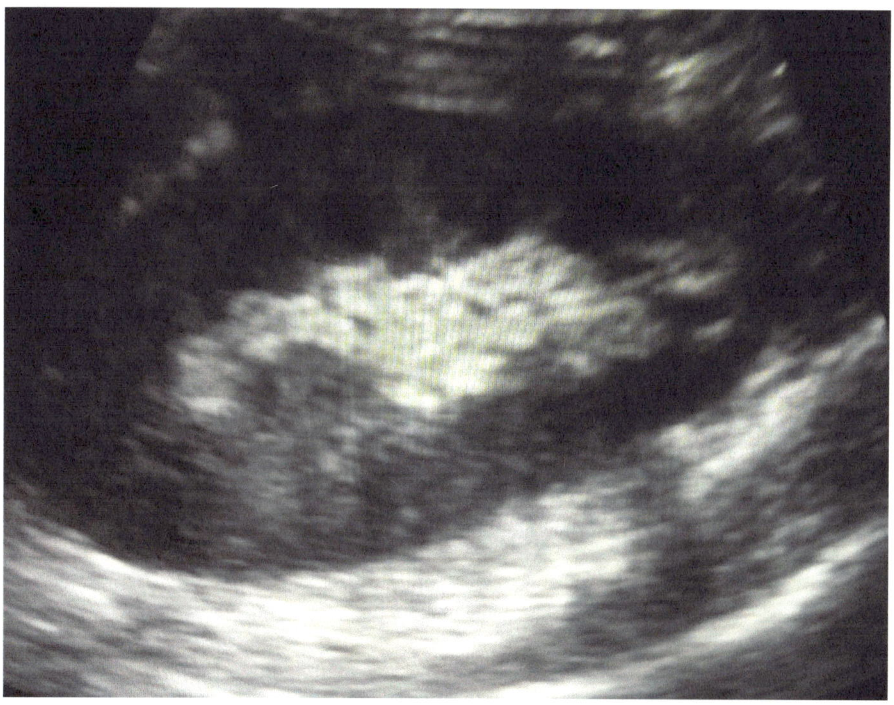

Fig. 4. B-Mode: Transplanted kidney reveiled in b-mode ultrasonography

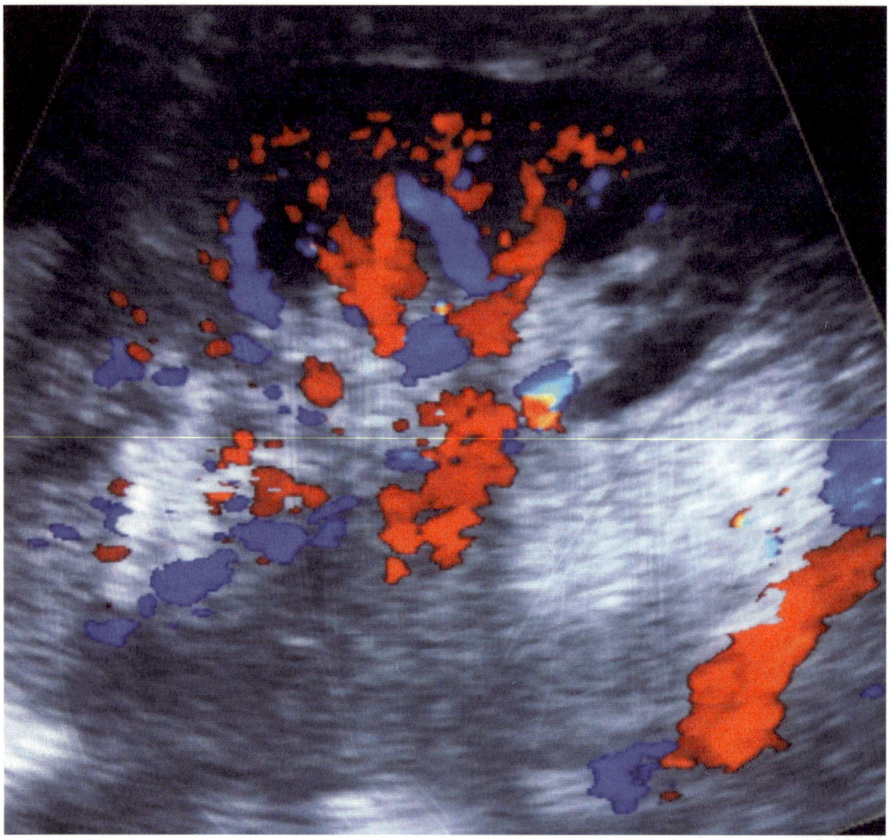

Fig. 5. The same transplanted kidney observed in classic color-power mode

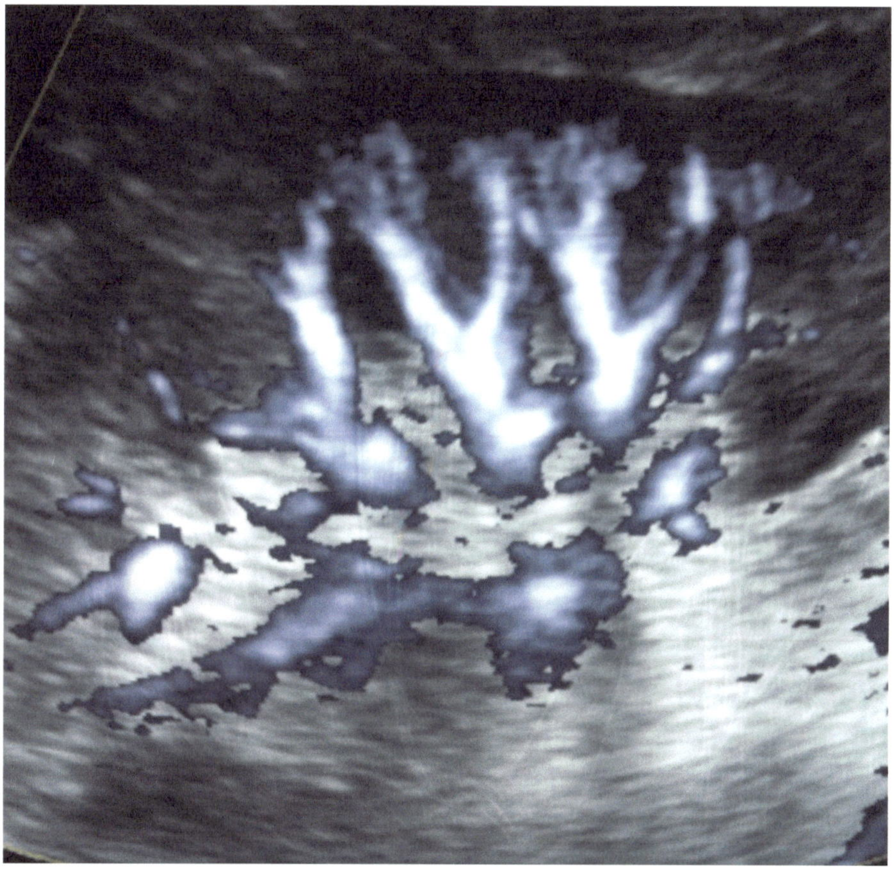

Fig. 6. B-flow vision of the precious transplanted kidney

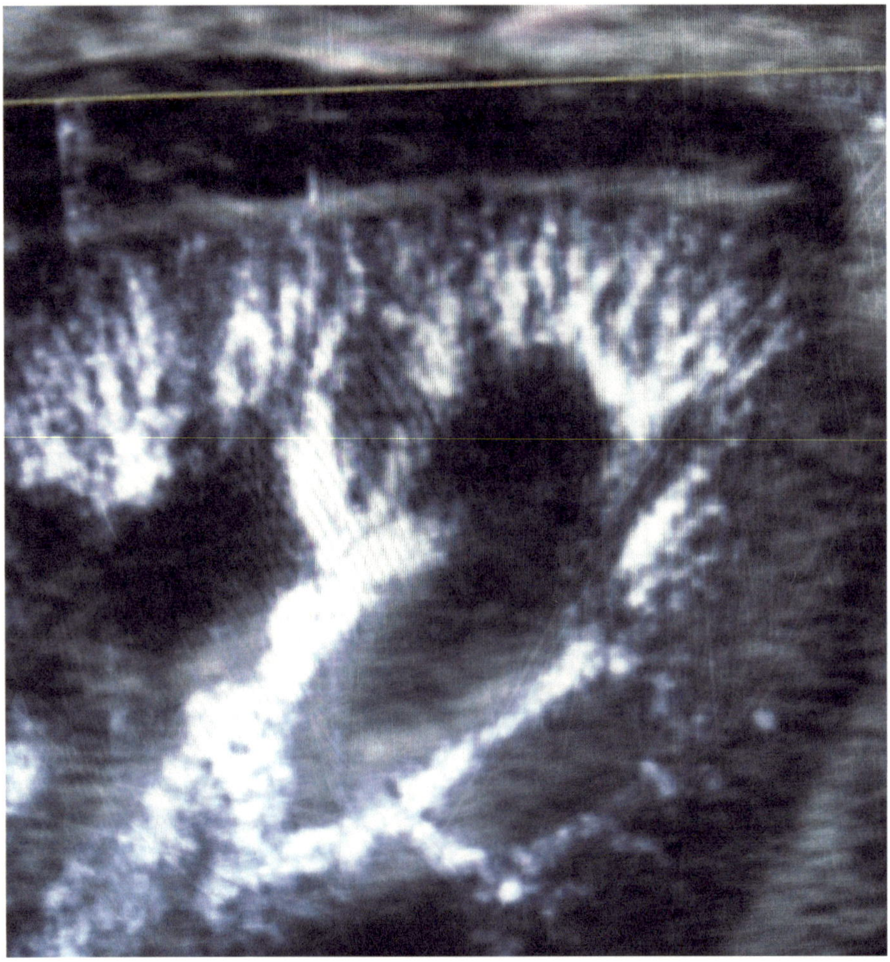

Fig. 7. Cortical vasculature: an extracapsular collection can be observed

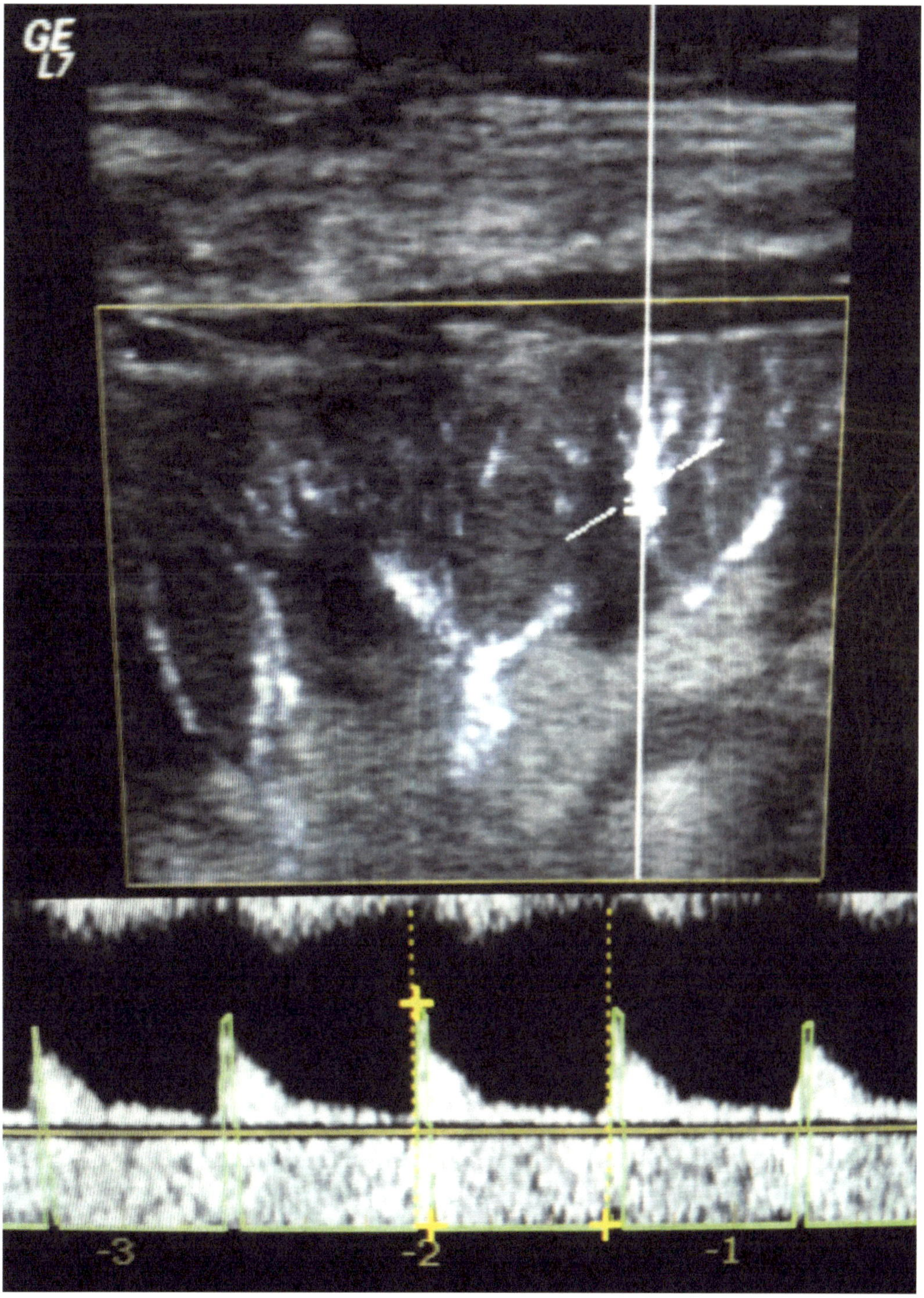

Fig. 8. R.I (Resistance Index) measurement by using b-flow mode

Coded sound waves are transmitted into the body and vasculature, and the returning signals are then decoded and displayed, as in B-mode. This technology enables boosting of weak flow reflector signals from blood reflectors and suppresses unwanted signals and frequencies from tissue. Consequently, B-flow can visualize real-time hemodynamic flow in relation to stationary tissue. In fact, B-flow provided higher spatial resolution for demonstrations of vessel anatomy and higher frame rate hemodynamic imaging than PDU (Clevert 2008).

This result is due to clearer definition of the vessel lumen without the overwriting seen with B-flow. In PDU, overestimation of the normal vessel lumen is caused by overwriting, and underestimation of the stenotic vessel lumen is caused by limitations in detecting flow (Buresley 2008). BFU examination does not require separate equipment and can be implemented by using the same Doppler equipment that has the necessary hardware by adding some software. BFU also has some limitations: A significant technical limitation of direct BFU measurement of renal stenosis arises in the presence of extensive plaque calcification in the iliac artery. Calcification interferes with the ability to achieve a clear sonographic window to the renal artery. In cases in which BFU measurement cannot be made because of calcification, changing the angle and position of the probe on the patient's abdomen usually can provide a sonographic window that is clear enough to measure velocities (Clevert 2008).

Another is that sensitivity in BFU is decreased with increasing depth because of strong dependence on signal intensity strength. This limitation is especially significant in evaluation of iliac vessels, because they are more deeply rooted (Buresley 2008). Finally, the remaining two limitations are background flash and difficulty in showing slow flow. Slow flow limitation, especially in high degree stenosis, may reduce flow velocity at distal normal renal artery and may cause difficulty in imaging of lumen and measurement of diameter. It must be emphasized that B-flow provides a detailed hemodynamic image of phenomena such as bloodstream swirl. Visualization of such a complex flow pattern has not been achieved by CDFU or PDU. Our experience suggests that the use of B-flow ultrasonography may improve the identification of precocious signals of chronic allograft failure that is the finding of cortical spots (Santangelo&De Rosa 2007). Careful analysis of flow patterns at the renal anastomoses relation to the pathogenesis of ischemic graft disfunction disease will be the subject of further study.

Doppler US velocity spectra in combination with real-time B-mode and color duplex flow images of the arteries are used to quantify stenotic lesions. Several teams have evaluated the correlation of different velocity parameters of color duplex flow US with those of angiography, proving sensitivity rates of 85%–87% and specificity rates of 89%–97%, with high interobserver correlation (Staikov 2000). Corresponding results, with excellent correlation between the results of angiography and color duplex flow US, were observed in our experience. On the other hand, clinicians caring for patients with transplanted kidney circulation problems should be aware that the duplex US criteria used for noninvasive estimation of the extent of arterial stenosis may vary considerably (Henri 2000).

Disadvantages of color duplex flow US are limited frame rate, high angle dependency, limited spatial resolution along the beam direction, and "overwriting" of the vessel walls by the color overlay (the so-called blooming artifact), which can mask subtle lesions (Park 2007).

For these reasons, we evaluated B-flow imaging in the evaluation of renal artery condition. Advantages of this recently introduced technique are simultaneous imaging of tissue and

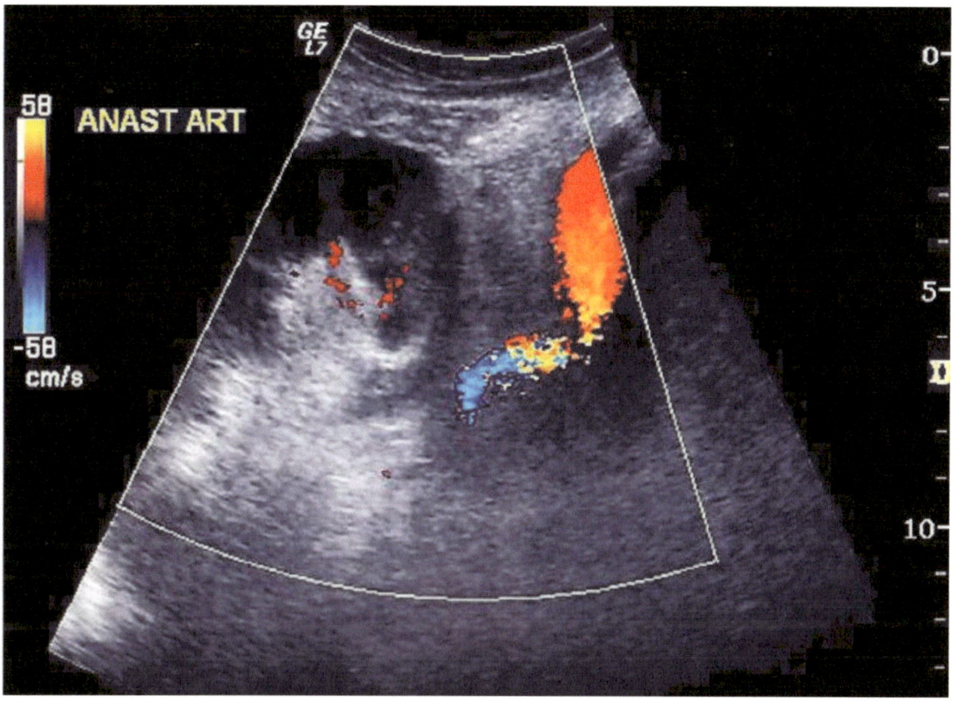

Fig. 9. Color-doppler vision of renal artery spasm

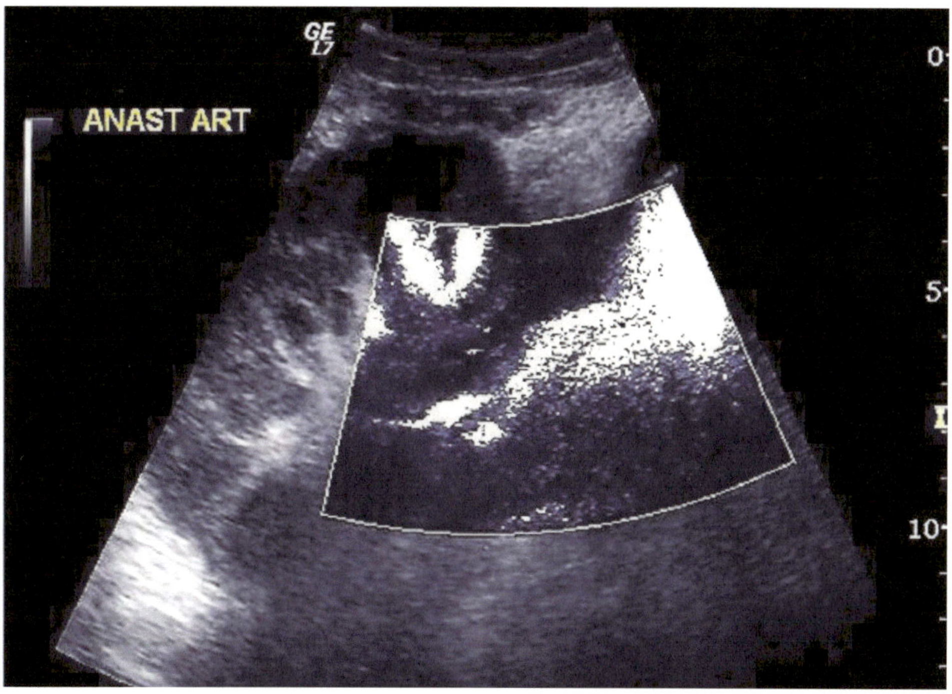

Fig. 10. The same condition in B-Flow mode

blood-echo information, so that blooming artifacts are not possible. A high frame rate is possible, as well as high spatial and transverse resolution, so that imaging of complex flow phenomena becomes possible. A further advantage is that plaque contours or intraluminal structures can be imaged in more detail, as compared with that at color duplex flow US, so there arises the possibility of qualitative description of blood flow, as well as of plaque morphology. The absence of angle dependency in B-flow imaging enables exact planimetric evaluation of the stenosis, which promises high correlation between angiography and B-flow imaging. A limitation of B-flow imaging is that excessive pulsations of the vessel lead to movement of the surrounding structures, so that the vessel wall is sometimes ill defined. Further disadvantages are an inability to obtain signals after plaque calcification (a problem with all US techniques) and decreased sensitivity of B-flow imaging with increasing depth, because of the strong dependence of signal strength (Jung 2007).
On the basis of our experience that high-grade stenosis produces a poststenotic region of higher gray-scale intensity (the jet stream) and the fact that pixel brightness or intensity, with almost no angle dependency, is determined by blood-echo strength and blood velocity (19), we evaluated B-flow imaging in the grading of transplanted kidney artery, as compared with color duplex flow US. Our study revealed no correlation between the investigated B-flow and color duplex flow US parameters. Neither the grayscale intensity nor the length and area of the jet stream yielded any hemodynamic information. Two reasons were suspected for the data mismatch but have been disproved with further statistical analysis: *(a)* the difficulty of clearly defining the points with maximum gray-scale intensity and the start and end points of the jet streams; however, interobserver variability was excellent (or at least almost excellent for the length of the jet stream) for all parameters; and *(b)* the quality of conditions for US assessment; however, no significant influence of this factor on B-flow parameters was identified. Scanning properties were fixed in all patients to exclude a possible influence on our results. The only exception concerned gain, but we calculated an additional gray-scale ratio to exclude possible bias.
As our study population correlates well with our "standard" patient population with regard to age, sex, conditions for assessment of stenosis, and color duplex flow US parameters, we believe that our results are representative, although we included only a small number of patients in the study. On the basis of these initial results, we will not use a larger patient series for the current objective.
Objectives of further clinical B-flow studies will concern the accuracy of planimetric evaluation of artery stenosis or spasm, as compared with that of angiography and plaque morphology.

7. Conclusion

We can say that B-flow imaging is an exciting, relatively new non-Doppler technology for noninvasive flow imaging. Our experience exploring hepatic B-flow imaging indicates that this currently underused technology has the potential to substantially improve noninvasive blood flow evaluation. As the imaging community becomes increasingly aware of abdominopelvic applications of B-flow imaging, it is hoped that manufacturers will advance the capabilities of this technology. Advantages of the method, such as angle independence, absence of blooming artifacts, and high spatial and transverse resolution, allow imaging of complex flow phenomena, as well as detailed examination of plaque morphology. Therefore, B-flow imaging has the potential to be used as an additional tool for this indication.

B-flow is highly effective in visualizing hemodynamic flow and in detecting stenotic lesions in the renal artery. Combined with conventional B-mode technique, B-flow seems to be useful in evaluating renal and anasthomotic stenosis, especially in patients with vascular disease.

8. References

Middleton WD. (1998). *Color Doppler: image interpretation and optimization*, Ultrasound Q; 14:194-208

Weskott HP. (2000). B-flow: a new method for detecting blood flow [in German]. *Ultraschall Med*; 21:59-65

Yucel C, Oktar SO, Erten Y, (2005). *B-flow sonographic evaluation of hemodialysis fistulas: a comparison with low- and high-pulse repetition frequency color and power Doppler sonography*, J Ultrasound Med; 24:1503-1508

Goncalves LF, Espinoza J, Lee W (2005). *A new approach to fetal echocardiography: digital casts of the fetal cardiac chambers and great vessels for detection of congenital heart disease*, J Ultrasound Med; 24:415-424

Kruskal JB, Newman PA, Sammons BA (2004). *Optimizing Doppler and color flow ultrasound.* RadioGraphics; 24:657-675

Machi J, Sigel B, Roberts AB (1994). *Oversaturation of color may obscure small intraluminal partial occlusions in color Doppler imaging*, J Ultrasound Med; 13:735-741

Wachsberg RH. (2003). *Doppler ultrasound evaluation of transjugular intrahepatic portosystemic shunt function: pitfalls and artifacts*, Ultrasound Q; 19:139-148

Toole JF, Castaldo JE. (1994). *Accurate measurement of carotid stenosis*, J Neuroimaging; 4:222-230.

Beneficial (1991) *effect of carotid endarterectomy in symptomatic patients with high-grade carotid stenosis.* North American Symptomatic Carotid Endarterectomy Trial Collaborators. N Engl J Med; 325:445-453.

Benefit (1998) *of carotid endarterectomy in patients with symptomatic moderate or severe stenosis.* North American Symptomatic Carotid Endarterectomy Trial Collaborators. N Engl J Med; 339:1415-1425.

EACAS *(1995). Endarterectomy for asymptomatic carotid artery stenosis.* Asymptomatic Carotid Atherosclerosis Study Collaborators. JAMA; 273:1421-1428.

Staikov IN, Arnold M, Mattle HP. (2000). *Comparison of the ECST, CC and NASCET grading methods and ultrasound for assessing carotid stenosis*, J Neurol; 247:681-686.

Padayachee TS, Cox TCS, Modaresi KB. (1997). *The measurement of internal carotid artery stenosis: comparison of duplex with digital subtraction angiography*, Eur J Vasc Endovasc Surg; 13:180-185.

Bell PR. (1995). *Carotid endarterectomy: preoperative angiography is outdated (letter).* BMJ; 310:1136.

Carpenter JP, Lexa FJ, Davis JT. (1995). *Determination of sixty percent or greater carotid artery stenosis by duplex Doppler ultrasonography*, J Vasc Surg 1995; 22:697-703; discussion 703-705.

Alexandrov AV, Vital D, Brodie DS. (1997). *Grading carotid stenosis with ultrasound. An interlaboratory comparison*, Stroke; 28:1208-1210.

GE Ultrasound Europe. (1999). *B-Flow: a new way of visualizing blood flow – ultrasound technology update*, Solingen, Germany: GE Ultrasound Europe.

Henri P, Tranquart F. (2000). *B-flow ultrasonographic imaging of circulating blood,* J Radiol.;81:465–467.

Jung EM, Kubale R, Clevert DA. (2007). *B-flow and B-flow with 3D and SRI postprocessing before intervention and monitoring after stenting of the internal carotid artery,* Clin Hemorheol Microcirc.;36(1):35-46.

Wachsberg RH. (2007). *B-flow imaging of the hepatic vasculature: correlation with color Doppler sonography,* AJR Am J Roentgenol. Jun;188(6):W522-33. Review.

Park SB, Kim JK, Cho KS. (2007). *Complications of renal transplantation: ultrasonographic evaluation,* J Ultrasound Med. May;26(5):615-33.

Volpe A, Caramaschi P, Marchetta A, (2008). *B-flow ultrasound in a case of giant cell arteritis.* Clin Rheumatol. Nov;26(11):1955-7. Epub 2007 Feb 17.

Clevert DA, Jung EM, Kubale R, (2008). *Value of vascular ultrasound in the evaluation of hemodialysis fistulas.* Radiology. Mar; 48(3):272-80. Review.

Buresley S, Samhan M, Moniri S. (2008). *Postrenal transplantation urologic complications.* Transplant Proc. Sep;40(7):2345-6.

Santangelo M., De Rosa P., (2007). *The Finding of Vascular and Urinary Anomalies in the Harvested Kidney for Transplantation,* Transplantation Proceedings, 39, 1797–1799

17

Immune Gene Polymorphisms Associate with Outcome in Kidney Transplantation

Katri Haimila, Noora Alakulppi and Jukka Partanen
Finnish Red Cross Blood Service
Finland

1. Introduction

A short cold ischemic time, an optimal HLA match and other pre-transplant factors are in a key role in the success of kidney transplantation. Over the past decades, the acute rejection rate of kidney transplants has fallen dramatically and the 1-year graft survival rate has increased to 90% in transplantations with deceased donors and 95% with living related donors. This increase in graft survival is largely due to advances in immunosuppressant medication (Yates & Nicholson, 2006). But, due to undesired side effects usually associated with immunosuppressive regimens, reduced immunosuppression is warranted whenever possible.

Acute rejection has been the most common end point of genetic association studies. This is natural as acute rejection predicts decreased long-term allograft survival. Despite progress in immunosuppression, the long-term graft survival has not increased in patients suffering acute rejection episodes (Meier-Kriesche et al., 2004). In many genetic studies, chronic allograft nephropathy and subsequent graft loss have been the endpoints with which genetic variation has been compared.

1.1 Genetic polymorphisms affect on outcome of kidney transplantation

Although *human leukocyte antigen* (*HLA*) genes are the major genetic factors in the immunological acceptance of the graft, also other, non-*HLA* gene variants may predict outcome of kidney transplantation. Identification of genetic factors determining, for example, the strength of immunological response against the graft, or metabolism or side effects of drugs, could lead to more accurate risk assessments or more tailored immunosupressive regimens for patients.

1.1.1 Immune genes are interesting candidates

Immune genes, i.e. the genes encoding for molecules regulating or affecting immune responses, are involved in the etiopathology of autoimmune diseases and probably also in the outcome of organ transplantation. Polymorphisms in immune genes may induce functional or quantitative differences in immune responsiveness between patients, resulting in for example high and low cytokine producers. Single nucleotide polymorphisms (SNPs) can have an effect on gene expression, not only the SNPs located in exons, possibly changing amino acids, or in promoter regions, possibly changing the crucial regulatory sequences, but also polymorphisms in introns have been shown to be of importance in genetic susceptibility studies. Thus, although functional variants are the most relevant to study, all polymorphisms are potentially interesting. Immune genes encode, for example, cytokines, chemokines, growth factors and T cell co-activation molecules.

1.1.2 Cytokines are major regulators of the immune response

Most genetic association studies in kidney transplantation have focussed on the genes encoding cytokines. Variations in the cytokine genes may lead to differences in the levels of their production or signalling, which in turn may modulate the strength of the immune response. Thus, they are potential candidate genes related to organ transplantation as they may predict the overall immunological responsiveness of the patient toward the graft.
Cytokines can be classified on the basis of their function to the pro-inflammatory cytokines, such as tumor necrosis factor (TNF), interleukin (IL)1β, interferon (IFN) γ, IL6, IL12, IL17 and IL18, and to the anti-inflammatory cytokines, including IL4, IL10, IL13, IFNα and transforming growth factor (TGF) β. However, it is of note that the effect of any single cytokine may depend on the exact environment it is acting in. The balance between pro- and anti-inflammatory cytokines partially determines the level or strength of the immune response (Dinarello, 1997). Below, we present a few examples from the wide variety of cytokines.

1.1.2.1 Tumor necrosis factor

Perhaps the most actively studied cytokine in genetic studies is the tumor necrosis factor (TNF), which has multiple roles in innate immunity, apoptosis and metabolism. TNF stimulates neutrophil and macrophage function and is a key mediator of inflammation. Production of TNF leads to massive inflammatory reactions in response to several immunological challenges (Hehlgans & Pfeffer, 2005). TNF and its receptors could be useful biomarkers for organ rejection, as TNF is not detectable in healthy individuals, but elevated serum levels are found in kidney transplant recipients (Maury & Teppo, 1987).
The *TNF* gene is located on chromosome 6 in the *HLA* class III region and is in linkage disequilibrium with classical *HLA* genes (Low et al., 2002). The -308G>A promoter variant of the *TNF* gene influences the expression of the TNF protein (Abraham & Kroeger, 1999).

1.1.2.2 Transforming growth factor β 1

Mammals have three isoforms of transforming growth factor β (TGFβ-1, TGFβ-2 and TGFβ-3) (Derynck et al., 1985). TGFβ-1 is the most abundant and most studied of the isoforms. It is a strong anti-inflammatory cytokine that regulates proliferation, apoptosis and differentiation of many cell types. TGFβ-1 affects T cell survival and Th differentiation for example regulating the development of effector cells and induction of Treg cells (Rubtsov & Rudensky, 2007). TGFβ-1 activates a profibrotic process and its increased expression has been associated with chronic rejection (Campistol et al., 2001).
The *TGFB1* gene lies on the chromosome region 19q13.2 and encodes a protein of 390 amino acids. A few polymorphisms have been identified in the gene and three of them (Leu10Pro, Arg25Pro and Thr263Ile) change an amino acid.

1.1.2.3 Interleukin 10

Interleukin 10 (IL10) promotes the Th2-type immune response and B-cell mediated functions leading to antibody production. Besides, it inhibits the Th1-type immune response by suppressing the expression of proinflammatory cytokines, hence being anti-inflammatory. IL10 also inhibits antigen presenting cells by downregulating the expression of HLA class II molecules (Ding et al., 1993).

The *IL10* gene, located in 1q32.2, is 4892 bases long and encodes a protein of 178 amino acids. There are several polymorphisms in the promoter region of *IL10*; they are in strong linkage disequilibrium (Turner et al., 1997) and thus, form haplotypes (Lin et al., 2003).

1.1.2.4 Interferon γ

IFNγ is a proinflammatory cytokine produced by activated T cells. IFNγ has several roles in the immune response: it activates macrophages, mediates the lytic effect, potentiates the actions of other interferons and it also inhibits intracellular microorganisms other than viruses (Dianzani & Baron, 1996). IFNγ acts both as an anti-rejection and pro-rejection cytokine, e.g. by inducing microvascularisation in the grafted organ and up-regulating the expression of HLA molecules. The predominant effect mainly depends on the secretion time after transplantation, being protective early on and then later becoming antagonistic (Hidalgo & Halloran, 2002).

The *IFNG* gene lies in 12q15 and encodes a protein of 166 amino acids. The most studied *IFNG* polymorphisms are the SNP +874T>A in the intron 1 and the short tandem repeat CA (rs3138557). These have been associated with acute rejection and chronic allograft nephropathy.

1.1.3 Co-stimulatory receptors mediate T cell activation

Besides cytokine genes, another interesting gene group is those coding for T cell co-stimulatory receptors. Co-stimulatory signals are essential for the activation of naïve T cells and productive immune response. For activation, naïve T cells must receive an antigen-specific signal through the T cell receptor and additionally a signal by co-stimulatory receptors. Without the co-stimulatory signal the T cell turns anergic. In addition, the co-stimulatory signal can be negative, that is, inhibitory after the initial activation. The fine balance between the positive and negative signals determines the outcome of an immune response.

1.1.3.1 CD28 is an essential co-stimulator

The CD28 pathway is crucial for T cell activation; signalling through CD28 increases cytokine production in T cells, by enhancing transcriptional activity and stabilizing messenger RNA (Thompson et al., 1989). CD28 ligation also reduces the number of engaged TCRs that are needed for proliferation or effective cytokine production, thereby lowering the threshold for T cell activation (Viola & Lanzavecchia, 1996). CD28 is expressed constitutively on T cells and it binds to ligands B7-1 (CD80) and B7-2 (CD86) found primarily on antigen presenting cells. These ligands have distinct but overlapping functions; B7-2 may mediate initial T cell activation, while B7-1 may be more important for maintaining the immune response (Vincenti & Luggen, 2007). Antigen specific signal without CD28 mediated signal turns T cells anergic.

Located on chromosome 2q33, the *CD28* gene was identified in the late 1980s (Aruffo & Seed, 1987). The gene contains one microsatellite and at least 50 SNPs, which, however but they are not associated with organ transplantation.

1.1.3.2 CTLA4 has an inhibitory function

Cytotoxic T lymphocyte associated antigen 4 (CTLA4) mediates a critical inhibitory signal for T cell activation. CTLA4 binds with higher affinity, to the same B7 ligands as CD28. It is induced on T cells after their activation, and functions in the downregulation of T cell activation; CTLA4 ligation raises the activation threshold for T cells. CTLA4 decreases interleukin 2 (IL2) and IL2 receptor expression and arrests T cells at the G1 phase of the cell cycle (Vincenti & Luggen, 2007). The CTLA4 pathway may have an important role in peripheral T cell tolerance (Yamada et al., 2002). Principal evidence for an inhibitory function of CTLA4 was obtained from CTLA4 knockout mice. These CTLA4 deficient (CTLA4-/-) mice develop a fatal lymphoproliferative disorder with multiorgan autoimmune disease (Tivol et al., 1995; Waterhouse et al., 1995).

CTLA4 is located adjacent to *CD28*. *CTLA4* includes one microsatellite and four SNPs, of which +49A/G is in a coding region and leads to a change of amino acid (Ala-Thr). Genetic variation in *CTLA4* is associated with several autoimmune diseases including coeliac disease, type 1 diabetes, autoimmune hypothyroidism and Grave's disease (Duffy, 2007).

1.1.3.3 ICOS induces cytokine expression

Inducible co-stimulator (ICOS) plays a critical, independent role in T cell activation, in a manner that is synergistic with CD28 signalling. ICOS augments effector T cell cytokine responses; in particular, it appears to superinduce production of the anti-inflammatory cytokine IL10 (Hutloff et al., 1999). ICOS expression is enhanced on activated T cells by CD28 co-stimulation (Beier et al., 2000). ICOS binds B7 related protein 1, (B7RP-1) which is expressed constitutively by B cells and macrophages (Yoshinaga et al., 1999) but can also be induced on non-lymphoid cells by inflammatory stimuli (Swallow et al., 1999). ICOS knockout mice have reduced CD4+ T cell responses (Dong et al., 2001) as well as defects in immunoglobulin (Ig) class switching (McAdam et al., 2001).

ICOS is located in very close proximity to *CD28* and *CTLA4* on the 2q33 region (Hutloff et al., 1999). The remarkable homology (over 20 %) between the costimulatory receptor genes (Harper et al., 1991; Ling et al., 1999) strongly suggests that the genes belong to the same gene family, which is the result of gene duplications. *ICOS* contains two microsatellites in intron 4 and over 30 SNPs, but so far it has been included in only one genetic association study on solid organ transplantation.

1.1.3.4 Therapeutic potential of co-stimulatory receptors

Blockade of the CD28 co-stimulatory pathway provides a promising therapeutic strategy for transplantation. CTLA4-Ig is a fusion protein which consists of the extracellular binding domain of CTLA4 linked to a modified Fc domain of human antibody IgG. The Fc domain mediates complement activation and interacts with Fc cell surface receptors. The CTLA4 fragment defines the specific targets of the fusion antibody, which are the B7 ligands. It was developed to selectively interrupt full T cell activation by blocking the interaction of CD28 and B7 ligands (Vincenti & Luggen, 2007). The use of CTLA4-Ig is effective in inducing long-term allograft survival in solid organ transplantation in mouse, rat and primate models (Snanoudj et al., 2006). The first clinical trial with CTLA4-Ig in human renal transplantation showed promise although immunosuppressive drug cyclosporine was still more effective in preventing acute rejection (Vincenti, 2005).

The impact of the ICOS co-stimulation pathway on emerging rejection episodes has been demonstrated by anti-ICOS therapy (Özkaynak et al., 2001). Anti-ICOS antibody treatment has also been studied together with anti-CD40L and CTLA4-Ig in animal models of transplantation; the animals displayed fewer signs of chronic rejection (Snanoudj et al., 2006).

2. Accumulated literature of immune gene studies

In this review, we aim to examine all the published association studies of potential candidate genes of cytokines and co-stimulatory receptors. We did a systematic search for literature in the PubMed database (National Library of Medicine, Bethesda, MD, US; www.ncbi.nlm.nih.gov/pubmed). We used search terms renal transplant, renal transplantation, kidney transplant or kidney transplantation and gene*, polymorphism or SNP. Literature addressing genetic association studies related to cytokines and co-stimulatory receptors was selected. Articles not reported in English were excluded; otherwise no limitations were set on the publishing manner.

3. Results

We found 85 original articles which are listed in Tables 1 and 2. Most genetic association studies in kidney transplantation focus on cytokine genes. Despite the number of reported positive associations with cytokine genes, the results are confusing because different studies report differing variants as demonstrating the strongest association. All the genetic associations are listed in the Tables 1 and 2 as they have been published although most of them are just nominally significant, and only in a few studies, the correction for multiple testing is performed appropriately.

3.1 Cytokine genes associate with poor outcome of kidney transplantation

The *TNF* gene is one of the most frequently studied cytokine genes and variation in this gene has been shown to have functional effects (Wilson et al., 1997). The most interesting -308 variant of the gene has a potential functional effect, being associated with elevated TNF levels (Elahi et al., 2009). One of the first large genetic association studies containing cytokine gene polymorphisms was done by Mytilineos et al (2004). A total of 2,298 first and 1,901 repeat kidney recipients were included in the study involving 73 transplant centres. An association was found between the high TNF producer genotype -308A and lower graft survival (P=0.0116 after Bonferroni correction) in retransplant patients (Mytilineos et al., 2004). Other parameters than graft survival were not analysed due to difficulties in getting standardized clinical variables from different centres in the retrospective study. The *TNF* gene, albeit in organ donors, is also associated with acute rejection (Alakulppi et al., 2004; Lee et al., 2004) and delayed graft function (Israni et al., 2008). In a relatively large study by Israni et al (2008), in addition to 965 kidney recipients, also 512 deceased donors were genotyped. The G allele of TNF +851 in donors was found to be associated with delayed graft function (Israni et al., 2008).

The variants of the *IL10* gene have been reported to be associated with acute rejection either by increasing risk or by being protective, depending on the polymorphism and related genotype. The haplotypes containing the promoter region SNPs -1082A>G, -819C>T and -592C>A have been reported to correlate with IL10 production, leading to high (GCC/GCC), intermediate (GCC/ACC or GCC/ATA) and low producers (ATA/ATA) (Koss et al., 2000). In a meta-analysis, combining the data of 1,087 patients from eight studies, a suggestive association was found between a poor outcome (meaning graft failure, acute or chronic rejection and chronic allograft nephropathy) and the *IL10* haplotype -1082A, -819C, -592C (Thakkinstian et al., 2008). The number of cases was high (approximately 300 depending on genetic variant analysed) but the authors had to accept compromises while pooling the data, which may be the reason for the insufficient power in statistical tests.

A total of 237 kidney transplantation patients were included in a multicentre study by Grinyo et al (2008), in which associations were found between the *IL10* and *TNF* gene polymorphisms (P=0.024 and 0.03) and acute rejection (Grinyo et al., 2008). The results were not corrected for multiple testing and would not have been statistically significant after correction. A sufficient number of infrequent genotypes and acute rejection episodes could not be found among 237 patients and thus, some of the groups compared were too small to give adequate power for analysis. The same cytokine genes, *IL10* and *TNF*, were reported to associate with cardiovascular disease after renal transplantation in a cohort of 798 of Italian patients (La Manna et al., 2010). On the other hand, a Czech single centre study did not confirm the association with *TNF, TGFB1* or *IFNG* although the authors had collected samples of 436 kidney recipients, of whom 122 had chronic allograft nephropathy and 190 had acute rejection (Brabcova et al., 2007).

In a recent study by Israni et al (2010), altogether 2,724 SNPs were genotyped in a total of 990 kidney recipients. They found several SNPs to be associated with acute rejection and its severity, among them a polymorphism in the gene of the cytokine IL15 receptor. An interesting finding to arise from this multicentre study was the significant difference (P<0.0001) in rates of acute rejection (0-30%) between different transplantation centres. The data was stratified by centres, thus associations were not masked by the centre to centre variation. This stratification could also be recommended for other multicentre studies. The authors speculated that the variation between transplantation centres can explain why associations are so difficult to repeat in other patient cohorts from different transplantation centres (Israni et al., 2010).

3.2 Co-stimulator receptor genes may predispose to the poor outcome of transplantation

Two of the genetic variants of *CD28* were included in three different association studies but no association was found (Haimila et al., 2009b; Krichen et al., 2009; Kusztal et al., 2010).

CTLA4 gene polymorphisms have been examined in relation to kidney transplantation in a few studies (Table2). An association with outcome of kidney transplantation was reported in seven genetic studies (Slavcheva et al., 2001; Gendzekhadze et al., 2006; Wisniewski et al., 2006; Gorgi et al., 2006; Kusztal et al., 2007, 2010; Kim et al., 2010). On the other hand, four studies did not succeed in replicating the association with *CTLA4* (Dmitrienko et al., 2005; Haimila et al., 2009b; Krichen et al., 2009, 2010). The SNP CTLA4+49 A/G (rs231775) is the most frequently studied variant and most often found to be associated. For example Kim et al studied 325 Korean renal patients for a haplotype of three *CTLA4* markers and reported an association (P=0.039 after Bonferroni correction) with late acute rejection (Kim et al., 2010). The microsatellite CTLA4(AT)n was included in two studies, both reporting an association (Slavcheva et al., 2001; Kusztal et al., 2010). A high number of AT repeats predisposed to acute rejection (Slavcheva et al., 2001) and decreased long-term allograft function (Kusztal et al., 2010).

Variants of the *ICOS* gene are found to predispose to the delayed graft function and the decreased graft survival in kidney transplantation patients (Haimila et al., 2009b). A total of 678 kidney transplantation patients, all from a single transplantation centre, were genotyped for 13 markers across the whole *CD28-CTLA4-ICOS* gene region. A statistically significant association between the *ICOS* marker rs10932037 and graft survival (P= 0.026) was found, in addition to an association with delayed functioning or non-functioning, of the graft with the *ICOS* markers rs10183087 and rs4404254 (P=0.020, OR=5.8 and P=0.019, OR=5.8). This is to date the only study to examine the association of the *ICOS* gene in relation to kidney transplantation.

The distance between the genetic markers used and the actual risk factor may be long due to the strong LD in the region (Holopainen & Partanen, 2001). A thorough examination of polymorphisms within the 2q33 region is necessary for the reliable identification of the primary variant. The association analyses of the published co-stimulator gene studies are solely limited to a few markers in the *CTLA4* gene, unfortunately leaving out the neighbouring *ICOS* and *CD28* genes. In our previous study, we examined genetic markers through the entire chromosome region and the results suggested that *ICOS*, rather than *CTLA4*, is the genetic factor affecting the outcome of kidney transplantation (Haimila et al., 2009b).

Gene polymorphism	**dbSNP rs number**	**Citation Association**	**Citation No association**
TNF -308G>A	rs1800629	Sankaran et al., 1999; Pelletier et al., 2000; Poli et al., 2000; Hahn et al., 2001; Reviron et al., 2001; Wramner et al., 2004; Park et al., 2004; Alakulppi et al., 2004; Grinyo et al., 2008; Pawlik et al., 2005; Tinckam et al., 2005; Lacha et al., 2005; Canossi et al., 2007; Coppo et al., 2007; Manchanda et al., 2008; Manchanda & Mittal, 2008; Mendoza-Carrera et al., 2008; Nikolova et al., 2008; Pawlik et al., 2008; Grenda et al., 2009; La Manna et al., 2010; donor: Nikolova et al., 2008	Hutchings et al., 2002; Marshall et al., 2000; Cartwright et al., 2001; George et al., 2001; Muller-Steinhardt et al., 2002; Weimer et al., 2003; McDaniel et al., 2003; Uboldi de Capei et al., 2004; Ligeiro et al., 2004; Dmitrienko et al., 2005; Gendzekhadze et al., 2006; Azarpira et al., 2006; Brabcova et al., 2007; Breulmann et al., 2007; Satoh et al., 2007; Rodrigo et al., 2007; Alakulppi et al., 2008; Azarpira et al., 2009; Kao et al., 2010; Jacobson et al., 2010; Khan et al., 2010; Omrani et al., 2010; Israni et al., 2010; Kocierz et al., 2011; donor: Sankaran et al., 1999; Poole et al., 2001; Marshall et al., 2001; Hoffmann et al., 2004; Alakulppi et al., 2004; Ligeiro et al., 2004; Israni et al., 2008; Manchanda & Mittal; 2008; Mendoza-Carrera et al., 2008; ; Azarpira et al., 2009; Lobashevsky et al., 2009
TNF -238G>A	rs361525		Rodrigo et al., 2007; Satoh et al., 2007; Lobashevsky et al., 2009; Kao et al., 2010; Khan et al., 2010
TNF +123G>A	rs1800610		Israni et al., 2010; Jacobson et al., 2010

Gene polymorphism	dbSNP rs number	Citation Association	Citation No association
TNF +851G>A	rs3093662		Israni et al., 2010; Jacobson et al., 2010; donor: Israni et al., 2008
TNF +3512G>A	rs1800628		donor: Israni et al., 2008
TGFB1 +869T>C and +915C>G	rs1800470, (rs1982073), rs1800471	McDaniel et al., 2003; Alakulppi et al., 2004; Park et al., 2004; Dmitrienko et al., 2005; Tinckam et al., 2005; Lacha et al., 2005; Hueso et al., 2006; Amirzargar et al., 2007; Manchanda et al., 2008; Nikolova et al., 2008; Kocierz et al., 2011; donor: Park et al., 2004; Ligeiro et al., 2004; Hoffmann et al., 2004; Lacha et al., 2005; Canossi et al., 2007; Nikolova et al., 2008	Pelletier et al., 2000; Marshall et al., 2000; Hutchings et al., 2002; Muller-Steinhardt et al., 2002; Ligeiro et al., 2004; Uboldi de Capei et al., 2004; Mytilineos et al., 2004; Gendzekhadze et al., 2006; Brabcova et al., 2007; Coppo et al., 2007; Satoh et al., 2007; Rodrigo et al., 2007; Manchanda & Mittal, 2008; Grinyo et al., 2008; Mendoza-Carrera et al., 2008; Cho et al., 2008; Khan et al., 2010; Jacobson et al., 2010; Israni et al., 2010; Omrani et al., 2010; Lobashevsky et al., 2009; La Manna et al., 2010; Kozak et al., 2011; donor: Poole et al., 2001; Marshall et al., 2001; Alakulppi et al., 2004; Israni et al., 2008; Manchanda & Mittal, 2008; Mendoza-Carrera et al., 2008
TGFB1 exon 5 (713-8delC)	rs8179182	Manchanda et al., 2008	Manchanda & Mittal, 2008; donor: Manchanda & Mittal, 2008
TGFB1 -509C>T	rs1800469		Satoh et al., 2007; Cho et al., 2008; Grenda et al., 2009; Kozak et al., 2011
TGFB1 +11929C>T	rs1800472		donor: Israni et al., 2008
TGFB1 -800G>A	rs1800468		Kozak et al., 2011
IL10 -1082G>A	rs1800896	Sankaran et al., 1999; George et al., 2001; Hutchings et al., 2002; McDaniel et al., 2003; Uboldi de Capei et al., 2004; Alakulppi et al., 2004; Tinckam et al., 2005; Lacha et al., 2005; Canossi et al., 2007; Coppo et al., 2007;	Pelletier et al., 2000; Cartwright et al., 2000; Marshall et al., 2000; Hahn et al., 2001; Poole et al., 2001; Cartwright et al., 2001; Asderakis et al., 2001; Muller-Steinhardt et al., 2002; Weimer et al., 2003; Plothow et al., 2003; Mytilineos et al., 2004;

Gene polymorphism	dbSNP rs number	Citation Association	Citation No association
		Nikolova et al., 2008; Khan et al., 2010; Amirzargar et al., 2007; La Manna et al., 2010; donor: Nikolova et al., 2008	Ligeiro et al., 2004; Dmitrienko et al., 2005; Loucaidou et al., 2005; Azarpira et al., 2006; Rodrigo et al., 2007; Breulmann et al., 2007; Grinyo et al., 2008; Gendzekhadze et al., 2006; Manchanda & Mittal, 2008; Mendoza-Carrera et al., 2008; Alakulppi et al., 2008; Grenda et al., 2009; Lobashevsky et al., 2009; Azarpira et al., 2009; Jacobson et al., 2010; Omrani et al., 2010; Kocierz et al., 2011; Israni et al., 2010; donor: Sankaran et al., 1999; Poole et al., 2001; Marshall et al., 2001; Alakulppi et al., 2004; Hoffmann et al., 2004; Ligeiro et al., 2004; Lacha et al., 2005; Loucaidou et al., 2005; Manchanda & Mittal, 2008; Mendoza-Carrera et al., 2008; Azarpira et al., 2009
IL10 -819C>T and -592C>A	rs1800871 rs1800872	McDaniel et al., 2003; Alakulppi et al., 2004; Ligeiro et al., 2004; Tinckam et al., 2005; Lacha et al., 2005; Coppo et al., 2007; Amirzargar et al., 2007; Nikolova et al., 2008; Grinyó 2008; Khan et al., 2010; La Manna et al., 2010; donor: Alakulppi et al., 2004; Nikolova et al., 2008	Cartwright et al., 2000; Marshall et al., 2000; Cartwright et al., 2001; Muller-Steinhardt et al., 2002; Weimer et al., 2003; Plothow et al., 2003; Mytilineos et al., 2004; Uboldi de Capei et al., 2004; Loucaidou et al., 2005; Gendzekhadze et al., 2006; Rodrigo et al., 2007; Satoh et al., 2007; Manchanda & Mittal, 2008; Alakulppi et al., 2008; Mendoza-Carrera et al., 2008; Lobashevsky et al., 2009; Jacobson et al., 2010; Israni et al., 2010; Kocierz et al., 2011; donor: Marshall et al., 2001; Ligeiro et al., 2004; Hoffmann et al., 2004; Loucaidou et al., 2005; Lacha et al., 2005; Manchanda & Mittal, 2008; Mendoza-Carrera et al., 2008

Gene polymorphism	dbSNP rs number	Citation Association	Citation No association
IL10 -851C>T	rs1800894		Grinyo et al., 2008
IL10 +4259A>G	rs3024498		donor: Israni et al., 2008
IL10 +434C>T	rs2222202		donor: Israni et al., 2008
IL10 IVS3-112A>G	rs3024494		donor: Israni et al., 2008
IL10 IVS3-474C>G	rs1878672		donor: Israni et al., 2008
IL10 gIVS3+284G>T	rs3024493		donor: Israni et al., 2008
IL10 IVS3+19T>C	rs1554286		donor: Israni et al., 2008
IL10 IVS1-192A>C	rs3021094		donor: Israni et al., 2008
IL6 -174G>C	rs1800795	Hahn et al., 2001; Reviron et al., 2001; Muller-Steinhardt et al., 2002; Lacha et al., 2005; Nikolova et al., 2008; Pawlik et al., 2008; Kocierz et al., 2011; donor: Marshall et al., 2001; Ligeiro et al., 2004; Canossi et al., 2007; Nikolova et al., 2008	Cartwright et al., 2000; Cartwright et al., 2001; Marshall et al., 2001; Hutchings et al., 2002; McDaniel et al., 2003; Ligeiro et al., 2004; Uboldi de Capei et al., 2004;Alakulppi et al., 2004; Hoffmann et al., 2004; Loucaidou et al., 2005; Tinckam et al., 2005; Gendzekhadze et al., 2006; ; Coppo et al., 2007; Breulmann et al., 2007; Satoh et al., 2007; Rodrigo et al., 2007; Alakulppi et al., 2008; Manchanda et al., 2008; Manchanda & Mittal; 2008; Grenda et al., 2009; Martin et al., 2009; Kruger et al., 2009; Lobashevsky et al., 2009; Khan et al., 2010; Jacobson et al., 2010; Sanchez-Velasco et al., 2010; La Manna et al., 2010; Israni et al., 2010; donor: Alakulppi et al., 2004; Loucaidou et al., 2005; Lacha et al., 2005; Manchanda & Mittal, 2008; Martin et al., 2009; Krajewska et al., 2009
IL6 +565>A	rs1800797		Rodrigo et al., 2007; Lobashevsky et al., 2009

Gene polymorphism	dbSNP rs number	Citation Association	Citation No association
IL6 +1888G>T	rs1554606		Kruger et al., 2009
IL6 Pro32Ser	rs2069830		Kruger et al., 2009
IL6 Asp162Val	rs2069860		Kruger et al., 2009
IFNG +874T>A	rs2430561	McDaniel et al., 2003; Tinckam et al., 2005; Mendoza-Carrera et al., 2008; Nikolova et al., 2008; Lobashevsky et al., 2009; Zibar et al., 2011; donor: Hoffmann et al., 2004; Canossi et al., 2007; Nikolova et al., 2008	Hahn et al., 2001; Hutchings et al., 2002; Muller-Steinhardt et al., 2002; Ligeiro et al., 2004; Alakulppi et al., 2004; Uboldi de Capei et al., 2004; Azarpira et al., 2006; Gendzekhadze et al., 2006; Brabcova et al., 2007; Coppo et al., 2007; Rodrigo et al., 2007; Satoh et al., 2007; Azarpira et al., 2009; Singh et al., 2009; Khan et al., 2010; Omrani et al., 2010; Crispim et al., 2010; La Manna et al., 2010; Kocierz et al., 2011; donor: Alakulppi et al., 2004; Ligeiro et al., 2004; Mendoza-Carrera et al., 2008; Azarpira et al., 2009
IFNG (CA)n	rs2234688	Mendoza-Carrera et al., 2008	donor: Mendoza-Carrera et al., 2008
IL1A -889T>C	rs1800587	Jin & Ruiz, 2008; donor: Jin & Ruiz, 2008	Rodrigo et al., 2007; Lobashevsky et al., 2009; Khan et al., 2010
IL1B -31C>T	rs1143627		Grenda et al., 2009
IL1B -511C>T	rs16944	Rodrigo et al., 2007, Jin & Ruiz, 2008; donor: Jin & Ruiz, 2008	Manchanda & Mittal, 2008; Khan et al., 2010; donor: Manchanda & Mittal, 2008
IL1B +3962C>T	rs1143634	Manchanda & Mittal, 2008; Jin & Ruiz, 2008; donor: Jin & Ruiz, 2008	Rodrigo et al., 2007; Manchanda & Mittal, 2008; Lobashevsky et al., 2009; Khan et al., 2010; donor: Manchanda & Mittal, 2008; Krajewska et al., 2009; Khan et al., 2010
IL1R +1970C>T	rs2234650		Rodrigo et al., 2007; Lobashevsky et al., 2009
IL1RA +11100 T>C	rs315952		Rodrigo et al., 2007; Lobashevsky et al., 2009; Khan et al., 2010,
IL1RN VNTR	rs2234663	Jin & Ruiz, 2008; donor: Jin & Ruiz, 2008	Manchanda & Mittal, 2008; Grenda et al., 2009; donor: Manchanda & Mittal, 2008

Gene polymorphism	dbSNP rs number	Citation Association	Citation No association
IL2 -330T>G	rs2069762	Satoh et al., 2007	Rodrigo et al., 2007; Grinyo et al., 2008; Manchanda et al., 2008; Manchanda & Mittal, 2008; Pawlik et al., 2008; Lobashevsky et al., 2009; donor: Manchanda & Mittal, 2008
IL2 +166G>T	rs2069763		Rodrigo et al., 2007; Grinyo et al., 2008; Lobashevsky et al., 2009
IL3 +132C>T	rs40401	Lee et al., 2010	
IL3 -1107G>A	rs181781	Lee et al., 2010	
IL3 -1484G>A	rs2073506	Lee et al., 2010	
IL4 VNTR intron 3	rs8179190	Manchanda et al., 2008	Manchanda & Mittal, 2008; donor: Manchanda & Mittal, 2008
IL4 -1098T>G	rs2243248		Rodrigo et al., 2007; Lobashevsky et al., 2009
IL4 -590T>C	rs2243250		Rodrigo et al., 2007, Satoh et al., 2007; Pawlik et al., 2008; Lobashevsky et al., 2009
IL4 -33T>C	rs2070874		Rodrigo et al., 2007; Lobashevsky et al., 2009
IL4R +1902G>A	rs1801275	Lobashevsky et al., 2009	Rodrigo et al., 2007
IL8 -251A>T	rs4073	Singh et al., 2009	La Manna et al., 2010; Ro et al., 2010; donor: Ro et al., 2010
IL12 -1188C>A	rs3212227	Rodrigo et al., 2007; Hoffmann et al., 2008; Lobashevsky et al., 2009	
IL12A +8685G>A	rs568408	Jacobson et al., 2010	Israni et al., 2010
IL12B -1188C>A	rs3212227		Kolesar et al., 2007; Satoh et al., 2007; Chin et al., 2008; Khan et al., 2010
IL18 -137G>C	rs187238	Kim et al., 2008; Mittal et al., 2011	donor: Mittal et al., 2011
IL18 -607A>C	rs1946518	Kolesar et al., 2007	Mittal et al., 2011; donor: Mittal et al., 2011
IL23R +2199A>C	rs10889677	Tsai et al., 2011	

Table 1. All the published genetic association studies related to cytokines listed according to the polymorphisms examined.

3.3 Kidney transplantation is a challenging study subject

During the last decade, a number of genetic association studies focusing on the outcome in kidney transplantation have been published. The results as a whole are contradictory and the effect of genetic variation on the outcome of transplantation still requires confirmation. It might be that the results of genetic studies are not reproduced due to a high level of genetic and environmental heterogeneity, both certainly relevant in kidney transplantation. There is growing evidence that certain genes or gene loci, such as *CTLA4–CD28–ICOS* cluster, regulate the immune response as their variation is associated with both susceptibility to autoimmunity and the outcome of transplantation. However, the same genes may also indirectly predispose to the underlying disease and its progression, or to the need for transplantation. Non-genetic, confounding factors are numerous: the original disease causing the need for kidney replacement, donor matching, surgical aspects, condition of the donor organ prior to transplantation etc. Besides, immunosuppressive drugs are highly effective and their administration can mask the genetic effect on the variance in immune response. Furthermore, it is essential to consider the effects of immunosuppressive drugs: gene variants regulating e.g. T cell response may not be detectable in patients receiving immunosuppressants affecting the T cell response.

As the current immunosuppressive regimens are very effective, the patients who still develop rejection, or some other complication, can be assumed to belong to the extreme high-responder end of patients. In genetic analysis this can be regarded as strength -we know we are studying the patients with a very strong tendency to develop immunological problems in kidney transplantation.

The problems related to the environmental factors can be reduced by a careful study design, such as attention to the precise definition of outcome phenotypes. Recruitment of sufficient numbers of patients would naturally improve the quality of studies. Prospective studies, if possible in a single centre single-centre would also be preferable, as many environmental factors could then be controllable but the number of cases available may remain relatively modest. Most studies have focused on allograft recipients, but evaluating also donors or even donor-recipient pairs, would give a new point of view.

Genetic variants should be carefully chosen instead of settling for a few most studied single nucleotide polymorphisms. Strong linkage disequilibrium (LD) influences association studies. It is currently assumed that our chromosomes are composed of haplotypic blocks that are relatively well conserved, in other words the genetic markers are said to be in linkage disequilibrium with each other. LD may help genetic studies as certain informative markers can be used as tags for a preliminary screening of haplotype blocks. On the other hand, the conserved structure of the blocks may be a hurdle in pinpointing the actual causative polymorphism. Exceptionally strong LD throughout the *HLA* region is well known. This fact also affects the interpretation of the role of *TNF* as it is located within the *HLA* block and hence *HLA* compatibility or matching leads to *TNF* matching as well. There is also strong LD on the 2q33 region (Holopainen & Partanen, 2001); not only within co-stimulatory receptor genes but also between them. *CD28* and the 5'end of *ICOS* exist in their own LD blocks, and between them, *CTLA4* and the 3' part of *ICOS* are within the same LD block (Ueda et al., 2003). Conservative haplotypes containing variants of both *CTLA4* and *ICOS* genes are found (Haimila et al., 2009a) and thus, the haplotypes must be taken in consideration when making conclusions from association results. Once good candidate polymorphisms with detectable and confirmed genetic effects are found, it is essential to start looking for functional differences. This has turned out to be problematic but not impossible. For example certain genetic variations in the *CTLA4–CD28-ICOS* cluster appear to affect the gene expression level or change the alternative splicing preferences of the genes (Ueda et al., 2003; Kaartinen et al., 2007).

More complex statistical analyses of many genetic and environmental variants simultaneously are required to test joint contributions to the risk and adjustment for potential confounders. Multivariate analyses have more power to detect minor impacts of single variables. Besides, correction of multiple comparisons is required due to a high probability of false positives (type 1 error) when several polymorphisms related to several outcomes are tested. A particular statistical challenge in the transplantation settings, which has not been tackled so far, is the fact that we are studying donor - recipient pairs instead of merely patients versus non-affected.

Gene polymorphism	**dbSNP rs number**	**Citation Association**	**Citation No association**
CD28-594A>G	rs35593994		Haimila et al., 2009b
CD28ivs3+17C >T	rs3116496		Krichen et al., 2010; Kusztal et al., 2010
CTLA4-1722A>G	rs733618		Gendzekhadze et al., 2006
CTLA4-1661G>A	rs553808		Gendzekhadze et al., 2006; Haimila et al., 2009b
CTLA4-1147C>T	rs16840252		Wisniewski et al., 2006; Kim et al., 2010
CTLA4-318C>T	rs5742909	Wisniewski et al., 2006; Gorgi et al., 2006; Kusztal et al., 2007	Dmitrienko et al., 2005; Gendzekhadze et al., 2006; Haimila et al., 2009b; Kim et al., 2010; Kusztal et al., 2010
CTLA4+49A>G	rs231775	Gendzekhadze et al., 2006; Gorgi et al., 2006; Kusztal et al., 2007; Kim et al., 2010; Kusztal et al., 2010	Slavcheva et al., 2001; Dmitrienko et al., 2005; Wisniewski et al., 2006; Haimila et al., 2009b
CTLA4(AT)n		Slavcheva et al., 2001; Kusztal et al., 2010	Krichen et al., 2010
CT60G>A	rs3087243		Haimila et al., 2009b
ICOSivs+173T>C	rs10932029		Haimila et al., 2009b
ICOSc602A>C	rs10183087	Haimila et al., 2009b	
ICOSc1564C>T	rs4404254	Haimila et al., 2009b	
ICOSc1624C>T	rs10932037	Haimila et al., 2009b	
ICOSc2373G>C	rs4675379		Haimila et al., 2009b

Table 2. All the published genetic association studies related to T cell co-stimulatory receptors listed according to the polymorphisms examined.

Although genome-wide association studies are simple to conduct and commonly used in other complex trait studies, none have been carried out in organ transplantation. In a typical genome-wide association study, up to a million genetic markers covering a significant portion of the common variation are simultaneously tested. The two main characteristics of genome wide studies are the large number of SNPs and the unbiased selection of these SNPs. Another approach, already demonstrated to be effective in bone marrow transplantation (McCarroll et al., 2009), is the systematic screening of gene deletions in the genome. Homozygous deletion of a gene in a recipient leads to immunological recognition of the encoded molecule if the graft can express the molecule. The results demonstrate that deletions are surprisingly common in our genome.

4. Conclusions

The identification of genetic factors that can modulate severity of acute rejection episodes may help to improve long-term graft survival. Functional variation in the gene regions of cytokines and/or T cell co-stimulatory receptors may affect the immune responsiveness of a graft recipient and thus, may predispose to the poor outcome of kidney transplantation. Technological advances in high-throughput genotyping methods would allow more intense genotyping of patients before transplantation. On the basis of genetic information, an amount of immunosuppressants could be set to a right level to avoid graft loss, on one hand, and undesired side effects of drugs, on the other hand.

The genes of cytokines and T cell co-stimulatory receptors are highly interesting but the final evidence for their role in renal transplantation still remains to be found. Genetic risk may not be due to a polymorphism in a single gene but rather a few haplotypes carrying a pattern of variations that act together. The combinatory effect may allow classification of patients into low- and high-responders. The involvement of several polymorphisms as well as confounding non-genetic factors, in particular differences in immunosuppression would explain the conflicting association reports from different populations. Larger studies are, however, still required. Even more importantly, true disease risk variants must be confirmed by functional assays. In addition, implementation of genome-wide association studies is necessary. Besides SNPs, the effect of structural variants, such as insertion/deletion and copy number variations should also be scrutinized in organ transplantation.

The major problem with genetic association studies is the small size of study populations (Hattersley & McCarthy, 2005). Although the sizes have increased in the more recent studies, the number of endpoint cases is still small and thus, the power of analysis is inadequate. The median rate of acute rejection was 18% in the recent multicentre study by Israni et al (2010). This means that thousands of patients need to be enrolled to the study before the number of acute rejection (or another endpoint) cases is sufficient for detecting the real underlying genetic variants, each of which may only have a weak individual effect.

Despite improved immunosuppressive medicaments, new organ preservation techniques, and decreased rejection rates, the improvement in long-term kidney allograft survival has been modest. There is growing interest in immunogenetics: if genetic factors determining the level of the immune response are combined with knowledge on effects of gene variation on drug metabolism, more personalized immunosuppression regimes for the patients can be developed.

5. References

Abraham, L.J. and Kroeger, K.M. (1999). Impact of the -308 TNF promoter polymorphism on the transcriptional regulation of the TNF gene: relevance to disease. *J Leukoc.Biol*, Vol.66, No.0741-5400; 4, pp. 562-6

Alakulppi, N.S.; Kyllönen, L.E.; Jäntti, V.T.; Matinlauri, I.H.; Partanen, J.; Salmela, K.T. & Laine, J.T. (2004). Cytokine gene polymorphisms and risks of acute rejection and delayed graft function after kidney transplantation. *Transplantation,* Vol.78, No.0041-1337; 10, pp. 1422-8

Alakulppi, N.S.; Kyllonen, L.E.; Partanen, J.; Salmela, K.T. & Laine, J.T. (2008). Lack of association between thrombosis-associated and cytokine candidate gene polymorphisms and acute rejection or vascular complications after kidney transplantation. *Nephrology, dialysis, transplantation : official publication of the European Dialysis and Transplant Association - European Renal Association,* Vol.23, No.1, pp. 364-8, ISSN 0931-0509

Amirzargar, M.; Yavangi, M.; Basiri, A.; Moghadam, S.H.; Khosravi, F.; Solgi, G.; Gholiaf, M.; Khoshkho, F.; Dadaras, F.; Mahmmodi, M.; Ansaripour, B.; Amirzargar, A. & Nikbin, B. (2007). Genetic Association of Interleukin-4, Interleukin-10, and Transforming Growth Factor-beta Gene Polymorphism With Allograft Function in Renal Transplant Patients. *Transplant Proc.,* Vol.39, No.0041-1345; 4, pp. 954-7

Aruffo, A. and Seed, B. (1987). Molecular cloning of a CD28 cDNA by a high-efficiency COS cell expression system. *Proceedings of the National Academy of Sciences of the United States of America,* Vol.84, No.23, pp. 8573-7, ISSN 0027-8424

Asderakis, A.; Sankaran, D.; Dyer, P.; Johnson, R.W.; Pravica, V.; Sinnott, P.J.; Roberts, I. & Hutchinson, I.V. (2001). Association of polymorphisms in the human interferon-gamma and interleukin-10 gene with acute and chronic kidney transplant outcome: the cytokine effect on transplantation. *Transplantation,* Vol.71, No.0041-1337; 5, pp. 674-7

Azarpira, N.; Aghdai, M.H.; Raisjalali, G.A.; Darai, M. & Tarahi, M.J. (2009). Influence of recipient and donor IL-10, TNFA and INFG genotypes on the incidence of acute renal allograft rejection. *Molecular biology reports,* Vol.36, No.6, pp. 1621-6, ISSN 1573-4978

Azarpira, N.; Aghdaie, M.; Geramizadeh, B.; Behzadi, S.; Nikeghbalian, S.; Sagheb, F.; Rahsaz, M.; Behzad-Behbahanie, A.; Ayatollahi, M.; Darai, M.; Azarpira, M.; Banihashemie, M. & Tabei, S. (2006). Cytokine gene polymorphisms in renal transplant recipients. *Exp.Clin Transplant,* Vol.4, No.1304-0855; 2, pp. 528-31

Beier, K.C.; Hutloff, A.; Dittrich, A.M.; Heuck, C.; Rauch, A.; Buchner, K.; Ludewig, B.; Ochs, H.D.; Mages, H.W. & Kroczek, R.A. (2000). Induction, binding specificity and function of human ICOS. *European journal of immunology,* Vol.30, No.12, pp. 3707-17, ISSN 0014-2980

Brabcova, I.; Petrasek, J.; Hribova, P.; Hyklova, K.; Bartosova, K.; Lacha, J. & Viklicky, O. (2007). Genetic variability of major inflammatory mediators has no impact on the outcome of kidney transplantation. *Transplantation,* Vol.84, No.8, pp. 1037-44, ISSN 0041-1337

Breulmann, B.; Bantis, C.; Siekierka, M.; Blume, C.; Aker, S.; Kuhr, N.; Grabensee, B. & Ivens, K. (2007). Influence of cytokine genes polymorphisms on long-term outcome in renal transplantation. *Clinical transplantation,* Vol.21, No.5, pp. 615-21, ISSN 0902-0063

Campistol, J.M.; Inigo, P.; Larios, S.; Bescos, M. & Oppenheimer, F. (2001). Role of transforming growth factor-beta1 in the progression of chronic allograft nephropathy. *Nephrol.Dial.Transplant,* Vol.16 Suppl 1, No.0931-0509, pp. 114-6

Canossi, A.; Piazza, A.; Poggi, E.; Ozzella, G.; Di Rocco, M.; Papola, F.; Iaria, G. & Adorno, D. (2007). Renal Allograft Immune Response Is Influenced by Patient and Donor Cytokine Genotypes. *Transplant Proc.*, Vol.39, No.0041-1345; 6, pp. 1805-12

Cartwright, N.H.; Keen, L.J.; Demaine, A.G.; Hurlock, N.J.; McGonigle, R.J.; Rowe, P.A.; Shaw, J.F.; Szydlo, R.M. & Kaminski, E.R. (2001). A study of cytokine gene polymorphisms and protein secretion in renal transplantation. *Transpl.Immunol,* Vol.8, No.0966-3274; 4, pp. 237-44

Cartwright, N.H.; Demaine, A.G.; Hurlock, N.J.; McGonigle, R.J.; Rowe, P.A.; Shaw, J.F.; Szydlo, R.M. & Kaminski, E.R. (2000). Cytokine secretion in mixed lymphocyte culture: a prognostic indicator of renal allograft rejection in addition to HLA mismatching. *Transpl.Immunol,* Vol.8, No.0966-3274; 2, pp. 109-14

Chin, G.K.; Adams, C.L.; Carey, B.S.; Shaw, S.; Tse, W.Y. & Kaminski, E.R. (2008). The value of serum neopterin, interferon-gamma levels and interleukin-12B polymorphisms in predicting acute renal allograft rejection. *Clinical and experimental immunology,* Vol.152, No.2, pp. 239-44, ISSN 1365-2249

Cho, J.H.; Huh, S.; Kwon, T.G.; Choi, J.Y.; Hur, I.K.; Lee, E.Y.; Park, S.H.; Kim, Y.L. & Kim, C.D. (2008). Association of C-509T and T869C polymorphisms of transforming growth factor-beta1 gene with chronic allograft nephropathy and graft survival in Korean renal transplant recipients. *Transplantation proceedings,* Vol.40, No.7, pp. 2355-60, ISSN 0041-1345

Coppo, R.; Amore, A.; Chiesa, M.; Lombardo, F.; Cirina, P.; Andrulli, S.; Passerini, P.; Conti, G.; Peruzzi, L.; Giraudi, R.; Messina, M.; Segoloni, G. & Ponticelli, C. (2007). Serological and genetic factors in early recurrence of IgA nephropathy after renal transplantation. *Clinical transplantation,* Vol.21, No.6, pp. 728-37, ISSN 0902-0063

Crispim, J.C.; Wastowski, I.J.; Rassi, D.M.; Mendes-Junior Silva, C.T.; Bassi, C.; Castelli, E.C.; Costa, R.S.; Saber, L.T.; Silva, T.G. & Donadi, E.A. (2010). Interferon-gamma +874 polymorphism in the first intron of the human interferon-gamma gene and kidney allograft outcome. *Transplantation proceedings,* Vol.42, No.10, pp. 4505-8, ISSN 1873-2623

Derynck, R.; Jarrett, J.A.; Chen, E.Y.; Eaton, D.H.; Bell, J.R.; Assoian, R.K.; Roberts, A.B.; Sporn, M.B. & Goeddel, D.V. (1985). Human transforming growth factor-beta complementary DNA sequence and expression in normal and transformed cells. *Nature,* Vol.316, No.6030, pp. 701-5, ISSN 0028-0836

Dianzani, S. and Baron, S. (Eds.). (1996) Nonspecific Defenses. *Medical Microbiology.* Library of Congress Cataloging-in-Publication Data, Texas

Dinarello, C.A. (1997). Role of pro- and anti-inflammatory cytokines during inflammation: experimental and clinical findings. *Journal of Biological Regulators and Homeostatic Agents,* Vol.11, No.3, pp. 91-103, ISSN 0393-974X

Ding, L.; Linsley, P.S.; Huang, L.Y.; Germain, R.N. & Shevach, E.M. (1993). IL-10 inhibits macrophage costimulatory activity by selectively inhibiting the up-regulation of B7 expression. *Journal of immunology (Baltimore, Md.: 1950),* Vol.151, No.3, pp. 1224-34, ISSN 0022-1767

Dmitrienko, S.; Hoar, D.I.; Balshaw, R. & Keown, P.A. (2005). Immune response gene polymorphisms in renal transplant recipients. *Transplantation,* Vol.80, No.0041-1337; 12, pp. 1773-82

Dong, C.; Juedes, A.E.; Temann, U.A.; Shresta, S.; Allison, J.P.; Ruddle, N.H. & Flavell, R.A. (2001). ICOS co-stimulatory receptor is essential for T-cell activation and function. *Nature,* Vol.409, No.6816, pp. 97-101 , ISSN 0028-0836

Duffy, D.L. (2007). Genetic determinants of diabetes are similarly associated with other immune-mediated diseases. *Current opinion in allergy and clinical immunology,* Vol.7, No.6, pp. 468-74, ISSN 1528-4050

Elahi, M.M.; Asotra, K.; Matata, B.M. & Mastana, S.S. (2009). Tumor necrosis factor alpha -308 gene locus promoter polymorphism: an analysis of association with health and disease. *Biochimica et biophysica acta,* Vol.1792, No.3, pp. 163-72, ISSN 0006-3002

Gendzekhadze, K.; Rivas-Vetencourt, P. & Montano, R.F. (2006). Risk of adverse post-transplant events after kidney allograft transplantation as predicted by CTLA-4 +49 and TNF-alpha -308 single nucleotide polymorphisms: A preliminary study. *Transpl.Immunol.,* Vol.16, No.0966-3274; 3-4, pp. 194-9

George, S.; Turner, D.; Reynard, M.; Navarrete, C.; Rizvi, I.; Fernando, O.N.; Powis, S.H.; Moorhead, J.F. & Varghese, Z. (2001). Significance of cytokine gene polymorphism in renal transplantation. *Transplant.Proc.,* Vol.33, No.041-1345; 1-2, pp. 483-4

Gorgi, Y.; Sfar, I.; Abdallah, T.B.; Abderrahim, E.; Ayed, S.J.; Aouadi, H.; Bardi, R. & Ayed, K. (2006). Ctla-4 exon 1 (+49) and promoter (-318) gene polymorphisms in kidney transplantation. *Transplantation proceedings,* Vol.38, No.7, pp. 2303-5, ISSN 0041-1345

Grenda, R.; Prokurat, S.; Ciechanowicz, A.; Piatosa, B. & Kalicinski, P. (2009). Evaluation of the genetic background of standard-immunosuppressant-related toxicity in a cohort of 200 paediatric renal allograft recipients--a retrospective study. *Annals of Transplantation : Quarterly of the Polish Transplantation Society,* Vol.14, No.3, pp. 18-24, ISSN 1425-9524

Grinyo, J.; Vanrenterghem, Y.; Nashan, B.; Vincenti, F.; Ekberg, H.; Lindpaintner, K.; Rashford, M.; Nasmyth-Miller, C.; Voulgari, A.; Spleiss, O.; Truman, M. & Essioux, L. (2008). Association of four DNA polymorphisms with acute rejection after kidney transplantation. *Transplant international : official journal of the European Society for Organ Transplantation,* Vol.21, No.9, pp. 879-91, ISSN 0934-0874

Hahn, A.B.; Kasten-Jolly, J.C.; Constantino, D.M.; Graffunder, E.; Singh, T.P.; Shen, G.K. & Conti, D.J. (2001). TNF-alpha, IL-6, IFN-gamma, and IL-10 gene expression polymorphisms and the IL-4 receptor alpha-chain variant Q576R: effects on renal allograft outcome. *Transplantation,* Vol.72, No.0041-1337; 4, pp. 660-5

Haimila, K.; Einarsdottir, E.; Kauwe, A.D.; Koskinen, L.L.; Pan-Hammarström, Q.; Kaartinen, T.; Kurppa, K.; Ziberna, F.; Not, T.; Vatta, S.; Ventura, A.; Korponay-Szabo, I.R.; Adany, R.; Pocsai, Z.; Szeles, G.; Dukes, E.; Kaukinen, K.; Mäki, M.; Koskinen, S.; Partanen, J.; Hammarström, L. & Saavalainen, P. (2009a). The shared CTLA4-ICOS risk locus in celiac disease, IgA deficiency and common variable immunodeficiency. *Genes and immunity,* Vol.10, No.2, pp. 151-61, ISSN 1476-5470

Haimila, K.; Turpeinen, H.; Alakulppi, N.S.; Kyllönen, L.E.; Salmela, K.T. & Partanen, J. (2009b). Association of genetic variation in inducible costimulator gene with outcome of kidney transplantation. *Transplantation,* Vol.87, No.3, pp. 393-6, ISSN 1534-6080

Harper, K.; Balzano, C.; Rouvier, E.; Mattei, M.G.; Luciani, M.F. & Golstein, P. (1991). CTLA-4 and CD28 activated lymphocyte molecules are closely related in both mouse and human as to sequence, message expression, gene structure, and chromosomal location. *Journal of immunology (Baltimore, Md.: 1950),* Vol.147, No.3, pp. 1037-44, ISSN 0022-1767

Hattersley, A.T. and McCarthy, M.I. (2005). What makes a good genetic association study? *Lancet,* Vol.366, No.1474-547; 9493, pp. 1315-23

Hehlgans, T. and Pfeffer, K. (2005). The intriguing biology of the tumour necrosis factor/tumour necrosis factor receptor superfamily: players, rules and the games. *Immunology,* Vol.115, No.0019-2805; 1, pp. 1-20

Hidalgo, L.G. and Halloran, P.F. (2002). Role of IFN-gamma in allograft rejection. *Crit Rev Immunol,* Vol.22, No.1040-8401; 4, pp. 317-49

Hoffmann, S.; Park, J.; Jacobson, L.M.; Muehrer, R.J.; Lorentzen, D.; Kleiner, D.; Becker, Y.T.; Hullett, D.A.; Mannon, R.; Kirk, A.D. & Becker, B.N. (2004). Donor genomics influence graft events: the effect of donor polymorphisms on acute rejection and chronic allograft nephropathy. *Kidney.Int,* Vol.66, No.0085-2538; 4, pp. 1686-93

Hoffmann, T.W.; Halimi, J.M.; Buchler, M.; Velge-Roussel, F.; Goudeau, A.; Al Najjar, A.; Boulanger, M.D.; Houssaini, T.S.; Marliere, J.F.; Lebranchu, Y. & Baron, C. (2008). Association between a polymorphism in the IL-12p40 gene and cytomegalovirus reactivation after kidney transplantation. *Transplantation,* Vol.85, No.10, pp. 1406-11, ISSN 0041-1337

Holopainen, P.M. and Partanen, J.A. (2001). Technical note: linkage disequilibrium and disease-associated CTLA4 gene polymorphisms. *Journal of immunology (Baltimore, Md. : 1950),* Vol.167, No.0022-1767; 5, pp. 2457-8

Hueso, M.; Navarro, E.; Moreso, F.; Beltran-Sastre, V.; Ventura, F.; Grinyo, J.M. & Seron, D. (2006). Relationship Between Subclinical Rejection and Genotype, Renal Messenger RNA, and Plasma Protein Transforming Growth Factor-beta1 Levels. *Transplantation,* Vol.81, No.0041-1337; 10, pp. 1463-6

Hutchings, A.; Guay-Woodford, L.; Thomas, J.M.; Young, C.J.; Purcell, W.M.; Pravica, V.; Perrey, C.; Hutchinson, I.V. & Benfield, M.R. (2002). Association of cytokine single nucleotide polymorphisms with B7 costimulatory molecules in kidney allograft recipients. *Pediatr.Transplant.,* Vol.6, No.1397-3142; 1, pp. 69-77

Hutloff, A.; Dittrich, A.M.; Beier, K.C.; Eljaschewitsch, B.; Kraft, R.; Anagnostopoulos, I. & Kroczek, R.A. (1999). ICOS is an inducible T-cell co-stimulator structurally and functionally related to CD28. *Nature,* Vol.397, No.6716, pp. 263-6, ISSN 0028-0836

Israni, A.; Leduc, R.; Holmes, J.; Jacobson, P.A.; Lamba, V.; Guan, W.; Schladt, D.; Chen, J.; Matas, A.J.; Oetting, W.S. & DeKAF Investigators (2010). Single-nucleotide polymorphisms, acute rejection, and severity of tubulitis in kidney transplantation, accounting for center-to-center variation. *Transplantation,* Vol.90, No.12, pp. 1401-8, ISSN 1534-6080

Israni, A.K.; Li, N.; Cizman, B.B.; Snyder, J.; Abrams, J.; Joffe, M.; Rebbeck, T. & Feldman, H.I. (2008). Association of donor inflammation- and apoptosis-related genotypes and delayed allograft function after kidney transplantation. *American Journal of Kidney Diseases : The Official Journal of the National Kidney Foundation,* Vol.52, No.2, pp. 331-9, ISSN 1523-6838

Jacobson, P.A.; Schladt, D.; Oetting, W.S.; Leduc, R.; Guan, W.; Matas, A.J.; Lamba, V.; Mannon, R.B.; Julian, B.A.; Israni, A. & for the DeKAF investigators (2010). Genetic

Determinants of Mycophenolate-Related Anemia and Leukopenia After Transplantation. *Transplantation,* ISSN 1534-6080

Jin, Y. and Ruiz, P. (2008). Molecular genetic analysis of interleukin-1 promoter and receptor antagonist tandem repeat polymorphisms among HLA-identical renal transplant recipient and donor pairs. *Transplantation proceedings,* Vol.40, No.5, pp. 1329-32, ISSN 0041-1345

Kaartinen, T.; Lappalainen, J.; Haimila, K.; Autero, M. & Partanen, J. (2007). Genetic variation in ICOS regulates mRNA levels of ICOS and splicing isoforms of CTLA4. *Molecular immunology,* Vol.44, No.0161-5890; 7, pp. 1655-62

Kao, C.C.; Lian, J.D.; Chou, M.C.; Chang, H.R. & Yang, S.F. (2010). Tumor necrosis factor alpha promoter polymorphism in posttransplantation diabetes mellitus of renal transplant recipients. *Transplantation proceedings,* Vol.42, No.9, pp. 3559-61, ISSN 1873-2623

Khan, F.; Sar, A.; Gonul, I.; Benediktsson, H.; Doulla, J.; Yilmaz, S. & Berka, N. (2010). Graft inflammation and histologic indicators of kidney chronic allograft failure: low-expressing interleukin-10 genotypes cannot be ignored. *Transplantation,* Vol.90, No.6, pp. 630-8, ISSN 1534-6080

Kim, C.D.; Ryu, H.M.; Choi, J.Y.; Choi, H.J.; Choi, H.J.; Cho, J.H.; Park, S.H.; Won, D.I. & Kim, Y.L. (2008). Association of G-137C IL-18 promoter polymorphism with acute allograft rejection in renal transplant recipients. *Transplantation,* Vol.86, No.11, pp. 1610-4, ISSN 1534-6080

Kim, H.J.; Jeong, K.H.; Lee, S.H.; Moon, J.Y.; Lee, T.W.; Kang, S.W.; Park, S.J.; Kim, Y.H. & Chung, J.H. (2010). Polymorphisms of the CTLA4 gene and kidney transplant rejection in Korean patients. *Transplant immunology,* Vol.24, No.1, pp. 40-4, ISSN 1878-5492

Kocierz, M.; Siekiera, U.; Kolonko, A.; Karkoszka, H.; Chudek, J.; Cierpka, L. & Wiecek, A. (2011). -174G/C interleukin-6 gene polymorphism and the risk of transplanted kidney failure or graft loss during a 5-year follow-up period. *Tissue antigens,* Vol.77, No.4, pp. 283-90, ISSN 1399-0039; 0001-2815

Kolesar, L.; Novota, P.; Krasna, E.; Slavcev, A.; Viklicky, O.; Honsova, E. & Striz, I. (2007). Polymorphism of interleukin-18 promoter influences the onset of kidney graft function after transplantation. *Tissue antigens,* Vol.70, No.5, pp. 363-8, ISSN 0001-2815

Koss, K.; Satsangi, J.; Fanning, G.C.; Welsh, K.I. & Jewell, D.P. (2000). Cytokine (TNF alpha, LT alpha and IL-10) polymorphisms in inflammatory bowel diseases and normal controls: differential effects on production and allele frequencies. *Genes and immunity,* Vol.1, No.3, pp. 185-90, ISSN 1466-4879

Kozak, M.; Kurzawski, M.; Wajda, A.; Lapczuk, J.; Lipski, M.; Dziewanowski, K. & Drozdzik, M. (2011). TGF-beta1 gene polymorphism in renal transplant patients with and without gingival overgrowth. *Oral diseases,* ISSN 1601-0825

Krajewska, M.; Koscielska-Kasprzak, K.; Weyde, W.; Drulis-Fajdasz, D.; Madziarska, K.; Mazanowska, O.; Kusztal, M. & Klinger, M. (2009). Impact of donor-dependent genetic factors on long-term renal graft function. *Transplantation proceedings,* Vol.41, No.8, pp. 2978-80, ISSN 1873-2623

Krichen, H.; Sfar, I.; Hadj Kacem, H.; Bardi, R.; Jendoubi-Ayed, S.; Makhlouf, M.; Ben Romdhane, T.; Besseghair, F.; Aouadi, H.; Ben Abdallah, T.; Ayadi, H.; Ayed, K. &

Gorgi, Y. (2010). (AT) repeat in the 3' untranslated region of the CTLA-4 gene and susceptibility to acute allograft rejection in Tunisian renal transplantation. *Transplantation proceedings,* Vol.42, No.10, pp. 4314-7, ISSN 1873-2623

Krichen, H.; Sfar, I.; Jendoubi-Ayed, S.; Makhlouf, M.; Ben Rhomdhane, T.; Bardi, R.; Aouadi, H.; Ben Abdallah, T.; Ayed, K. & Gorgi, Y. (2009). Genetic polymorphisms of immunoregulatory proteins in acute renal allograft rejection. *Transplantation proceedings,* Vol.41, No.8, pp. 3305-7, ISSN 1873-2623

Kruger, B.; Walberer, A.; Farkas, S.; Tokmak, F.; Obed, A.; Schenker, P.; Henning, B.; Schlitt, H.J.; Kramer, B.K. & Banas, B. (2009). The impact of "high-producer" interleukin-6 haplotypes on cardiovascular morbidity and mortality in a kidney transplant population. *Transplantation proceedings,* Vol.41, No.6, pp. 2539-43, ISSN 1873-2623

Kusztal, M.; Koscielska-Kasprzak, K.; Drulis-Fajdasz, D.; Magott-Procelewska, M.; Patrzalek, D.; Janczak, D.; Chudoba, P. & Klinger, M. (2010). The influence of CTLA-4 gene polymorphism on long-term kidney allograft function in Caucasian recipients. *Transplant immunology,* Vol.23, No.3, pp. 121-4, ISSN 1878-5492

Kusztal, M.; Radwan-Oczko, M.; Koscielska-Kasprzak, K.; Boratynska, M.; Patrzalek, D. & Klinger, M. (2007). Possible association of CTLA-4 gene polymorphism with cyclosporine-induced gingival overgrowth in kidney transplant recipients. *Transplantation proceedings,* Vol.39, No.9, pp. 2763-5, ISSN 0041-1345

La Manna, G.; Cappuccilli, M.L.; Cianciolo, G.; Conte, D.; Comai, G.; Carretta, E.; Scolari, M.P. & Stefoni, S. (2010). Cardiovascular disease in kidney transplant recipients: the prognostic value of inflammatory cytokine genotypes. *Transplantation,* Vol.89, No.8, pp. 1001-8, ISSN 1534-6080

Lacha, J.; Hribova, P.; Kotsch, K.; Brabcova, I.; Bartosova, K.; Volk, H.D. & Vitko, S. (2005). Effect of cytokines and chemokines (TGF-beta, TNF-alpha, IL-6, IL-10, MCP-1, RANTES) gene polymorphisms in kidney recipients on posttransplantation outcome: influence of donor-recipient match. *Transplant.Proc,* Vol.37, No.0041-1345; 2, pp. 764-6

Lee, D.Y.; Song, S.B.; Moon, J.Y.; Jeong, K.H.; Park, S.J.; Kim, H.J.; Kang, S.W.; Lee, S.H.; Kim, Y.H.; Chung, J.H.; Ihm, C.G. & Lee, T.W. (2010). Association between interleukin-3 gene polymorphism and acute rejection after kidney transplantation. *Transplantation proceedings,* Vol.42, No.10, pp. 4501-4, ISSN 1873-2623

Lee, H.; Clark, B.; Gooi, H.C.; Stoves, J. & Newstead, C.G. (2004). Influence of recipient and donor IL-1alpha, IL-4, and TNFalpha genotypes on the incidence of acute renal allograft rejection. *J Clin.Pathol.,* Vol.57, No.0021-9746; 1, pp. 101-3

Ligeiro, D.; Sancho, M.R.; Papoila, A.; Barradinhas, A.M.; Almeida, A.; Calao, S.; Machado, D.; Nolasco, F.; Guerra, J.; Sampaio, M.J. & Trindade, H. (2004). Impact of donor and recipient cytokine genotypes on renal allograft outcome. *Transplant.Proc,* Vol.36, No.0041-1345; 4, pp. 827-9

Lin, M.T.; Storer, B.; Martin, P.J.; Tseng, L.H.; Gooley, T.; Chen, P.J. & Hansen, J.A. (2003). Relation of an interleukin-10 promoter polymorphism to graft-versus-host disease and survival after hematopoietic-cell transplantation. *The New England journal of medicine,* Vol.349, No.23, pp. 2201-10, ISSN 1533-4406

Ling, V.; Wu, P.W.; Finnerty, H.F.; Sharpe, A.H.; Gray, G.S. & Collins, M. (1999). Complete sequence determination of the mouse and human CTLA4 gene loci: cross-species

DNA sequence similarity beyond exon borders. *Genomics,* Vol.60, No.3, pp. 341-55, ISSN 0888-7543

Lobashevsky, A.L.; Manwaring, J.E.; Travis, M.M.; Nord, B.L.; Higgins, N.G.; Serov, Y.A.; Arnoff, T.S.; Hommel-Berrey, G.A.; Goggins, W.C.; Taber, T.E.; Carter CB, S.; Smith, D.S.; Wozniak, T.C.; O'Donnell, J.A. & Turrentine, M.W. (2009). Effect of desensitization in solid organ transplant recipients depends on some cytokines genes polymorphism. *Transplant immunology,* Vol.21, No.3, pp. 169-78, ISSN 1878-5492

Loucaidou, M.; Stitchbury, J.; Lee, J.; Borrows, R.; Marshall, S.E.; McLean, A.G.; Cairns, T.; Griffith, M.; Hakim, N.; Palmer, A.; Papalois, V.; Welsh, K. & Taube, D. (2005). Cytokine polymorphisms do not influence acute rejection in renal transplantation under tacrolimus-based immunosuppression. *Transplant.Proc,* Vol.37, No.0041-1345; 4, pp. 1760-1

Low, A.S.; Azmy, I.; Sharaf, N.; Cannings, C. & Wilson, A.G. (2002). Association between two tumour necrosis factor intronic polymorphisms and HLA alleles. *European journal of immunogenetics : official journal of the British Society for Histocompatibility and Immunogenetics,* Vol.29, No.1, pp. 31-4, ISSN 0960-7420

Manchanda, P.K.; Kumar, A.; Sharma, R.K.; Goel, H. & Mittal, R.D. (2008). Association of pro/anti-inflammatory cytokine gene variants in renal transplant patients with allograft outcome and cyclosporine immunosuppressant levels. *Biologics : targets & therapy,* Vol.2, No.4, pp. 875-84, ISSN 1177-5475

Manchanda, P.K. and Mittal, R.D. (2008). Analysis of cytokine gene polymorphisms in recipient's matched with living donors on acute rejection after renal transplantation. *Molecular and cellular biochemistry,* Vol.311, No.1-2, pp. 57-65, ISSN 0300-8177

Marshall, S.E.; McLaren, A.J.; McKinney, E.F.; Bird, T.G.; Haldar, N.A.; Bunce, M.; Morris, P.J. & Welsh, K.I. (2001). Donor cytokine genotype influences the development of acute rejection after renal transplantation. *Transplantation,* Vol.71, No.0041-1337; 3, pp. 469-76

Marshall, S.E.; McLaren, A.J.; Haldar, N.A.; Bunce, M.; Morris, P.J. & Welsh, K.I. (2000). The impact of recipient cytokine genotype on acute rejection after renal transplantation. *Transplantation,* Vol.70, No.0041-1337; 10, pp. 1485-91

Martin, J.; Worthington, J.; Harris, S. & Martin, S. (2009). The influence of class II transactivator and interleukin-6 polymorphisms on the production of antibodies to donor human leucocyte antigen mismatches in renal allograft recipients. *International journal of immunogenetics,* Vol.36, No.4, pp. 235-9, ISSN 1744-313X

Maury, C.P. and Teppo, A.M. (1987). Raised serum levels of cachectin/tumor necrosis factor alpha in renal allograft rejection. *The Journal of experimental medicine,* Vol.166, No.4, pp. 1132-7, ISSN 0022-1007

McAdam, A.J.; Greenwald, R.J.; Levin, M.A.; Chernova, T.; Malenkovich, N.; Ling, V.; Freeman, G.J. & Sharpe, A.H. (2001). ICOS is critical for CD40-mediated antibody class switching. *Nature,* Vol.409, No.6816, pp. 102-5, ISSN 0028-0836

McCarroll, S.A.; Bradner, J.E.; Turpeinen, H.; Volin, L.; Martin, P.J.; Chilewski, S.D.; Antin, J.H.; Lee, S.J.; Ruutu, T.; Storer, B.; Warren, E.H.; Zhang, B.; Zhao, L.P.; Ginsburg, D.; Soiffer, R.J.; Partanen, J.; Hansen, J.A.; Ritz, J.; Palotie, A. & Altshuler, D. (2009).

Donor-recipient mismatch for common gene deletion polymorphisms in graft-versus-host disease. *Nature genetics,* Vol.41, No.12, pp. 1341-4, ISSN 1546-1718

McDaniel, D.O.; Barber, W.H.; Nguyan, C.; Rhodes, S.W.; May, W.L.; McDaniel, L.S.; Vig, P.J.; Jemeson, L.L. & Butkus, D.E. (2003). Combined analysis of cytokine genotype polymorphism and the level of expression with allograft function in African-American renal transplant patients. *Transpl.Immunol,* Vol.11, No.0966-3274; 1, pp. 107-19

Meier-Kriesche, H.U.; Schold, J.D.; Srinivas, T.R. & Kaplan, B. (2004). Lack of improvement in renal allograft survival despite a marked decrease in acute rejection rates over the most recent era. *Am.J.Transplant,* Vol.4, No.1600-6135; 3, pp. 378-83

Mendoza-Carrera, F.; Ojeda-Duran, S.; Angulo, E.; Rivas, F.; Macias-Lopez, G.; Buen, E.P. & Leal, C. (2008). Influence of cytokine and intercellular adhesion molecule-1 gene polymorphisms on acute rejection in pediatric renal transplantation. *Pediatric transplantation,* Vol.12, No.7, pp. 755-61, ISSN 1399-3046

Mittal, R.D.; Srivastava, P.; Singh, V.; Jaiswal, P. & Kapoor, R. (2011). Association of Common Variants of Vascular Endothelial Growth Factor and Interleukin-18 Genes with Allograft Survival in Renal Transplant Recipients of North India. *DNA and cell biology,* ISSN 1557-7430

Muller-Steinhardt, M.; Fricke, L.; Muller, B.; Kirchner, H. & Hartel, C. (2002). The interleukin-6 -174promoter polymorphism is associated with long-term kidney allograft survival. *Hum.Immunol,* Vol.63, No.0198-8859; 10, pp. S13

Mytilineos, J.; Laux, G. & Opelz, G. (2004). Relevance of IL10, TGFbeta1, TNFalpha, and IL4Ralpha Gene Polymorphisms in Kidney Transplantation: A Collaborative Transplant Study Report. *Am J Transplant.,* Vol.4, No.1600-6135; 10, pp. 1684-90

Nikolova, P.N.; Ivanova, M.I.; Mihailova, S.M.; Myhailova, A.P.; Baltadjieva, D.N.; Simeonov, P.L.; Paskalev, E.K. & Naumova, E.J. (2008). Cytokine gene polymorphism in kidney transplantation - Impact of TGF-beta1, TNF-alpha and IL-6 on graft outcome. *Transpl.Immunol.,* Vol.18, No.0966-3274; 4, pp. 344-8

Omrani, M.D.; Mokhtari, M.R.; Bagheri, M. & Ahmadpoor, P. (2010). Association of interleukin-10, interferon-gamma, transforming growth factor-beta, and tumor necrosis factor-alpha gene polymorphisms with long-term kidney allograft survival. *Iranian journal of kidney diseases,* Vol.4, No.2, pp. 141-6, ISSN 1735-8582

Ozkaynak, E.; Gao, W.; Shemmeri, N.; Wang, C.; Gutierrez-Ramos, J.C.; Amaral, J.; Qin, S.; Rottman, J.B.; Coyle, A.J. & Hancock, W.W. (2001). Importance of ICOS-B7RP-1 costimulation in acute and chronic allograft rejection. *Nature immunology,* Vol.2, No.7, pp. 591-6, ISSN 1529-2908

Park, J.Y.; Park, M.H.; Park, H.; Ha, J.; Kim, S.J. & Ahn, C. (2004). TNF-alpha and TGF-beta1 gene polymorphisms and renal allograft rejection in Koreans. *Tissue antigens,* Vol.64, No.0001-2815; 6, pp. 660-6

Pawlik, A.; Domanski, L.; Rozanski, J.; Czerny, B.; Juzyszyn, Z.; Dutkiewicz, G.; Myslak, M.; Halasa, M.; Slojewski, M. & Dabrowska-Zamojcin, E. (2008). The association between cytokine gene polymorphisms and kidney allograft survival. *Ann Transplant,* Vol.13, No.1425-9524; 2, pp. 54-8

Pawlik, A.; Domanski, L.; Rozanski, J.; Florczak, M.; Dabrowska-Zamojcin, E.; Dutkiewicz, G. & Gawronska-Szklarz, B. (2005). IL-2 and TNF-alpha Promoter Polymorphisms in Patients With Acute Kidney Graft Rejection. *Transplant.Proc,* Vol.37, No.0041-1345; 5, pp. 2041-3

Pelletier, R.; Pravica, V.; Perrey, C.; Xia, D.; Ferguson, R.M.; Hutchinson, I. & Orosz, C. (2000). Evidence for a genetic predisposition towards acute rejection after kidney and simultaneous kidney-pancreas transplantation. *Transplantation,* Vol.70, No.0041-1337; 4, pp. 674-80

Plothow, A.; Bicalho, M.G.; Benvenutti, R. & Contieri, F.L. (2003). Interleukin-10 and acute rejection in renal transplantation. *Transplant.Proc.,* Vol.35, No.0041-1345; 4, pp. 1338-40

Poli, F.; Boschiero, L.; Giannoni, F.; Tonini, M.; Scalamogna, M.; Ancona, G. & Sirchia, G. (2000). Tumour necrosis factor-alpha gene polymorphism: implications in kidney transplantation. *Cytokine,* Vol.12, No.1043-4666; 12, pp. 1778-83

Poole, K.L.; Gibbs, P.J.; Evans, P.R.; Sadek, S.A. & Howell, W.M. (2001). Influence of patient and donor cytokine genotypes on renal allograft rejection: evidence from a single centre study. *Transpl.Immunol,* Vol.8, No.0966-3274; 4, pp. 259-65

Reviron, D.; Dussol, B.; Andre, M.; Brunet, P.; Mercier, P. & Berland, Y. (2001). TNF-alpha and IL-6 gene polymorphism and rejection in kidney transplantation recipients. *Transplant Proc,* Vol.33, No.0041-1345; 1-2, pp. 350-1

Ro, H.; Hwang, Y.H.; Kim, H.; Jeong, J.C.; Lee, H.; Doh, Y.S.; Park, H.C.; Oh, K.H.; Park, M.H.; Ha, J.; Yang, J. & Ahn, C. (2010). Association of Polymorphisms of Interleukin-8, CXCR1, CXCR2, and Selectin With Allograft Outcomes in Kidney Transplantation. *Transplantation,* ISSN 1534-6080

Rodrigo, E.; Sanchez-Velasco, P.; Ruiz, J.C.; Fernandez-Fresnedo, G.; Lopez-Hoyos, M.; Pinera, C.; Palomar, R.; Gomez-Alamillo, C.; Gonzalez-Cotorruelo, J.; Leyba-Cobian, F. & Arias, M. (2007). Cytokine polymorphisms and risk of infection after kidney transplantation. *Transplantation proceedings,* Vol.39, No.7, pp. 2219-21, ISSN 0041-1345

Rubtsov, Y.P. and Rudensky, A.Y. (2007). TGFbeta signalling in control of T-cell-mediated self-reactivity. *Nat.Rev.Immunol.,* Vol.7, No.1474-1733; 6, pp. 443-53

Sanchez-Velasco, P.; Rodrigo, E.; Fernandez-Fresnedo, G.; Ocejo-Vinyals, J.G.; Ruiz, J.C.; Arnau, A.; Leyva-Cobian, F. & Arias, M. (2010). Influence of interleukin-6 promoter polymorphism -174 g/c on kidney graft outcome. *Transplantation proceedings,* Vol.42, No.8, pp. 2854-5, ISSN 1873-2623

Sankaran, D.; Asderakis, A.; Ashraf, S.; Roberts, I.S.; Short, C.D.; Dyer, P.A.; Sinnott, P.J. & Hutchinson, I.V. (1999). Cytokine gene polymorphisms predict acute graft rejection following renal transplantation. *Kidney Int,* Vol.56, No.0085-2538; 1, pp. 281-8

Satoh, S.; Saito, M.; Inoue, K.; Miura, M.; Komatsuda, A. & Habuchi, T. (2007). Association of cytokine polymorphisms with subclinical progressive chronic allograft nephropathy in Japanese renal transplant recipients: preliminary study. *International journal of urology : official journal of the Japanese Urological Association,* Vol.14, No.11, pp. 990-4, ISSN 0919-8172

Singh, R.; Kesarwani, P.; Ahirwar, D.K.; Kapoor, R. & Mittal, R.D. (2009). Interleukin 8 -251T>A and Interferon gamma +874A>T polymorphism: potential predictors of allograft outcome in renal transplant recipients from north India. *Transplant immunology,* Vol.21, No.1, pp. 13-7, ISSN 1878-5492

Slavcheva, E.; Albanis, E.; Jiao, Q.; Tran, H.; Bodian, C.; Knight, R.; Milford, E.; Schiano, T.; Tomer, Y. & Murphy, B. (2001). Cytotoxic T-lymphocyte antigen 4 gene polymorphisms and susceptibility to acute allograft rejection. *Transplantation,* Vol.72, No.0041-1337; 5, pp. 935-40

Snanoudj, R.; de Preneuf, H.; Creput, C.; Arzouk, N.; Deroure, B.; Beaudreuil, S.; Durrbach, A. & Charpentier, B. (2006). Costimulation blockade and its possible future use in clinical transplantation. *Transplant international : official journal of the European Society for Organ Transplantation,* Vol.19, No.9, pp. 693-704 , ISSN 0934-0874

Swallow, M.M.; Wallin, J.J. & Sha, W.C. (1999). B7h, a novel costimulatory homolog of B7.1 and B7.2, is induced by TNFalpha. *Immunity,* Vol.11, No.4, pp. 423-32, ISSN 1074-7613

Thakkinstian, A.; Dmitrienko, S.; Gerbase-Delima, M.; McDaniel, D.O.; Inigo, P.; Chow, K.M.; McEvoy, M.; Ingsathit, A.; Trevillian, P.; Barber, W.H. & Attia, J. (2008). Association between cytokine gene polymorphisms and outcomes in renal transplantation: a meta-analysis of individual patient data. *Nephrology, dialysis, transplantation : official publication of the European Dialysis and Transplant Association - European Renal Association,* Vol.23, No.9, pp. 3017-23, ISSN 1460-2385

Thompson, C.B.; Lindsten, T.; Ledbetter, J.A.; Kunkel, S.L.; Young, H.A.; Emerson, S.G.; Leiden, J.M. & June, C.H. (1989). CD28 activation pathway regulates the production of multiple T-cell-derived lymphokines/cytokines. *Proceedings of the National Academy of Sciences of the United States of America,* Vol.86, No.4, pp. 1333-7, ISSN 0027-8424

Tinckam, K.; Rush, D.; Hutchinson, I.; Dembinski, I.; Pravica, V.; Jeffery, J. & Nickerson, P. (2005). The relative importance of cytokine gene polymorphisms in the development of early and late acute rejection and six-month renal allograft pathology. *Transplantation,* Vol.79, No.0041-1337; 7, pp. 836-41

Tivol, E.A.; Borriello, F.; Schweitzer, A.N.; Lynch, W.P.; Bluestone, J.A. & Sharpe, A.H. (1995). Loss of CTLA-4 leads to massive lymphoproliferation and fatal multiorgan tissue destruction, revealing a critical negative regulatory role of CTLA-4. *Immunity,* Vol.3, No.5, pp. 541-7, ISSN 1074-7613

Tsai, J.P.; Yang, S.F.; Wu, S.W.; Hung, T.W.; Tsai, H.C.; Lian, J.D. & Chang, H.R. (2011). Association between interleukin 23 receptor polymorphism and kidney transplant outcomes: A 10-year Taiwan cohort study. *Clinica chimica acta; international journal of clinical chemistry,* ISSN 1873-3492

Turner, M.S.; Timms, P.; Hafner, L.M. & Giffard, P.M. (1997). Identification and characterization of a basic cell surface-located protein from Lactobacillus fermentum BR11. *Journal of Bacteriology,* Vol.179, No.10, pp. 3310-6, ISSN 0021-9193

Uboldi de Capei, M.; Dametto, E.; Fasano, M.E.; Messina, M.; Pratico', L.; Rendine, S.; Segoloni, G. & Curtoni, E.S. (2004). Cytokines and chronic rejection: a study in kidney transplant long-term survivors. *Transplantation,* Vol.77, No.4, pp. 548-52, ISSN 0041-1337

Ueda, H.; Howson, J.M.; Esposito, L.; Heward, J.; Snook, H.; Chamberlain, G.; Rainbow, D.B.; Hunter, K.M.; Smith, A.N.; Di Genova, G.; Herr, M.H.; Dahlman, I.; Payne, F.; Smyth, D.; Lowe, C.; Twells, R.C.; Howlett, S.; Healy, B.; Nutland, S.; Rance, H.E.; Everett, V.; Smink, L.J.; Lam, A.C.; Cordell, H.J.; Walker, N.M.; Bordin, C.; Hulme, J.; Motzo, C.; Cucca, F.; Hess, J.F.; Metzker, M.L.; Rogers, J.; Gregory, S.; Allahabadia, A.; Nithiyananthan, R.; Tuomilehto-Wolf, E.; Tuomilehto, J.; Bingley, P.; Gillespie, K.M.; Undlien, D.E.; Ronningen, K.S.; Guja, C.; Ionescu-Tirgoviste, C.; Savage, D.A.; Maxwell, A.P.; Carson, D.J.; Patterson, C.C.; Franklyn, J.A.; Clayton,

D.G.; Peterson, L.B.; Wicker, L.S.; Todd, J.A. & Gough, S.C. (2003). Association of the T-cell regulatory gene CTLA4 with susceptibility to autoimmune disease. *Nature,* Vol.423, No.6939, pp. 506-11, ISSN 0028-0836

Vincenti, F. and Luggen, M. (2007). T cell costimulation: a rational target in the therapeutic armamentarium for autoimmune diseases and transplantation. *Annual Review of Medicine,* Vol.58, pp. 347-58, ISSN 0066-4219

Vincenti, F. (2005). Current use and future trends in induction therapy. *Saudi journal of kidney diseases and transplantation : an official publication of the Saudi Center for Organ Transplantation, Saudi Arabia,* Vol.16, No.4, pp. 506-13, ISSN 1319-2442

Viola, A. and Lanzavecchia, A. (1996). T cell activation determined by T cell receptor number and tunable thresholds. *Science (New York, N.Y.),* Vol.273, No.5271, pp. 104-6, ISSN 0036-8075

Waterhouse, P.; Penninger, J.M.; Timms, E.; Wakeham, A.; Shahinian, A.; Lee, K.P.; Thompson, C.B.; Griesser, H. & Mak, T.W. (1995). Lymphoproliferative disorders with early lethality in mice deficient in Ctla-4. *Science (New York, N.Y.),* Vol.270, No.5238, pp. 985-8, ISSN 0036-8075

Weimer, R.; Mytilineos, J.; Feustel, A.; Preiss, A.; Daniel, V.; Grimm, H.; Wiesel, M. & Opelz, G. (2003). Mycophenolate mofetil-based immunosuppression and cytokine genotypes: effects on monokine secretion and antigen presentation in long-term renal transplant recipients. *Transplantation,* Vol.75, No.0041-1337; 12, pp. 2090-9

Wilson, A.G.; Symons, J.A.; McDowell, T.L.; McDevitt, H.O. & Duff, G.W. (1997). Effects of a polymorphism in the human tumor necrosis factor alpha promoter on transcriptional activation. *Proc.Natl.Acad Sci U S.A.,* Vol.94, No.0027-8424; 7, pp. 3195-9

Wisniewski, A.; Kusztal, M.; Magott-Procelewska, M.; Klinger, M.; Jasek, M.; Luszczek, W.; Nowak, I.; Kosmaczewska, A.; Ciszak, L.; Frydecka, I.; Gorski, A. & Kusnierczyk, P. (2006). Possible association of cytotoxic T-lymphocyte antigen 4 gene promoter single nucleotide polymorphism with acute rejection of allogeneic kidney transplant. *Transplantation proceedings,* Vol.38, No.1, pp. 56-8, ISSN 0041-1345

Wramner, L.G.; Norrby, J.; Hahn-Zoric, M.; Ahlmen, J.; Borjesson, P.A.; Carlstrom, J.; Hyt÷nen, A.M.; Olausson, M.; Hanson, L. & Padyukov, L. (2004). Impaired Kidney Graft Survival is Associated with the TNF-alpha Genotype. *Transplantation,* Vol.78, No.0041-1337; 1, pp. 117-21

Yamada, A.; Salama, A.D. & Sayegh, M.H. (2002). The role of novel T cell costimulatory pathways in autoimmunity and transplantation. *Journal of the American Society of Nephrology : JASN,* Vol.13, No.2, pp. 559-75 , ISSN 1046-6673

Yates, P.J. and Nicholson, M.L. (2006). The aetiology and pathogenesis of chronic allograft nephropathy. *Transplant immunology,* Vol.16, No.3-4, pp. 148-57, ISSN 0966-3274

Yoshinaga, S.K.; Whoriskey, J.S.; Khare, S.D.; Sarmiento, U.; Guo, J.; Horan, T.; Shih, G.; Zhang, M.; Coccia, M.A.; Kohno, T.; Tafuri-Bladt, A.; Brankow, D.; Campbell, P.; Chang, D.; Chiu, L.; Dai, T.; Duncan, G.; Elliott, G.S.; Hui, A.; McCabe, S.M.; Scully, S.; Shahinian, A.; Shaklee, C.L.; Van, G.; Mak, T.W. & Senaldi, G. (1999). T-cell co-stimulation through B7RP-1 and ICOS. *Nature,* Vol.402, No.6763, pp. 827-32, ISSN 0028-0836

Zibar, L.; Wagner, J.; Pavlinic, D.; Galic, J.; Pasini, J.; Juras, K. & Barbic, J. (2011). The relationship between interferon-gamma gene polymorphism and acute kidney allograft rejection. *Scandinavian journal of immunology* ISSN 1365-3083

18

Sleep Disturbances Among Dialysis Patients

Gianluigi Gigli, Simone Lorenzut, Anna Serafini and Mariarosaria Valente
Sleep Disorder Center, Neurology and Neurorehabilitation,
University of Udine Medical School and University Hospital, Udine
Italy

1. Introduction

Sleep disturbances are extremely common among dialysis patients. Subjective sleep complaints are reported in up to 80% of patients and are characterized by difficulty in initiating and maintaining sleep, problems with restlessness, jerking legs, snoring, choking sensations and/or daytime sleepiness (Holley et al., 1992; Walker et al., 1995; Veiga et al., 1997). Epidemiological studies have found how sleep apnea syndrome (SAS), restless legs syndrome (RLS) and periodic limb movement disorder (PLMD) are much more prevalent than in the general population. These sleep problems appear to have significant negative effects on the quality of life as they are often cited as major sources of stress. Indeed, interviews of patients on hemodialysis and on peritoneal dialysis have found that sleep disturbances are one of the seven most distressing symptoms experienced (Eichel et al., 1986; Bass et al., 1999). Half of patients complaining of sleep disturbances feel that these problems affect their daily living and activity, and 21% consider that relief of this symptom would improve significantly their subjective quality of life (Parfrey et al., 1988; Iliescu et al., 2003).
In the following sections two major sleep disturbances associated with Insomnia, Restless Legs Syndrome and Sleep Apnea Syndrome, will be reviewed in detail.

2. Sleep disturbances among dialysis patients

2.1 Insomnia

Insomnia, one of the major causes of sleep disturbances, is defined by the presence of difficulty in falling asleep, frequent awakenings with difficulty in falling asleep again and early morning awakenings. In order to be considered an insomniac, these symptoms should be reported at least 3 times per week and the presence of resultant daytime dysfunction should be investigated in order to distinguish two levels of insomnia (level 1, without daytime dysfunction, and level 2, with daytime dysfunction) (Ohayon et al., 1996). Insomnia should be distinguished in primary and secondary insomnia. Secondary forms of insomnia can be the consequence of internal medical disturbances but also of other sleep disturbances such as RLS and SAS, which will be further reviewed in detail. Insomnia is primarily a clinical diagnosis and is most frequently diagnosed using data obtained from patient histories and sleep diaries. The prevalence estimates of insomnia vary because of differences in definition, diagnosis, population characteristics, and research methodologies. Its prevalence in the general population ranges from 4% to 64% (Ohayon et al., 2002, Chevalier et al., 1999).

The assessment of sleep disturbances can be done through sleep questionnaires (i.e. Pittsburgh Quality Index- PSQI) aimed to evaluate subjectively these disorders, or through polysomnographic measures, able to offer an objective analysis of sleep disturbances. The latter would also have a role in the diagnosis of SAS or periodic limbs movements and for the objective characterization of macro or micro alterations of sleep architecture in insomnia.
Many studies have been conducted up to now in order to assess the prevalence of sleep complaints among dialysis patients. Prevalence rates of subjective sleep complaints vary among studies due to the different methodological approaches (e.g. modalities of interview, type of questionnaires, definition of inclusion criteria, etc.) and sample sizes.
The prevalence of insomnia among dialysis patients is greater than the general population, rates up to 70% have been reported (Sabbatini et al., 2002; Iliescu et al., 2003; Merlino et al., 2006). The earliest study to have evaluated the prevalence of subjective sleep complaints among dialysis patients was conducted in 1982 (Strub et al., 1982). They found that 63% of patients reported sleep disturbances characterized by diminished, fragmented sleep and increased wake time after sleep onset. Similar data were found by a study of Holley et al. in which the most common complaints included trouble falling asleep (67%), nighttime awaking (80%), early morning awaking (72%), restless legs (83%), and jerking legs (28%). Daytime sleepiness was common and dialysis patients reported napping for periods averaging 1.1+1.3 h per day (Holley et al., 1992). After these pioneer studies many others have addressed on this topic and have found similar prevalence rates. A recent study from 20 Italian dialysis centers, showed the prevalence of insomnia, RLS, and symptoms suggestive of SAS to be 69.3%, 18%, and 27%, respectively (higher than in the general non-renal population) (Merlino et al., 2006).
Most of these studies have also looked for a correlation between sleep complaints and numerous demographic, clinical, and laboratory data. Sleep complaints seem to be more common in elderly patients on dialysis than in younger patients (Kutner et al., 2001; Walker et al., 1995). It has been reported that each decade of age increases the risk of insomnia (subclinical and clinical) by 239% and the risk of overt clinical insomnia by 51% (De Santo et al., 2005). The effect of gender on sleep quality is controversial. It has been found that male patients are more likely to have sleep complaints than female patients, even though women report using more sleep medications than men (Kutner et al., 2001; Walker et al., 1995). White patients have a higher prevalence of restless sleep than blacks (Walker et al., 1995). Positive relationship between subjective sleep complaints and caffeine intake and cigarette use has also been reported (Holley et al., 1992). Increased stress, anxiety, depression and worry, as observed also in the general population, are associated with poor subjective sleep quality in dialysis patients (Holley et al., 1992; Kutner et al., 2001; Parker et al., 1996). Depression seems to be the primary mental health problem in this group of patients. Dialysis patients with sleep disturbances have a prevalence of depression of 20% (Iliescu et al., 2003). The use of sleep ipnotic medications among dialysis patients is about 8-10% (De Santo et al., 2001; 2005).
Concerning laboratory data, one study has reported that improvement of anemia leads to amelioration of sleep quality, reduction of nighttime awakenings and reduction of sleep fragmentation. Thus, a more efficient sleep is obtained, leading to a decreased daytime somnolence (Ohayon et al., 1997). Other previous studies have shown how low levels of Hb are associated with a deteriorated sleep quality (Kusleikaite et al., 2005; Iliescu et al., 2003; Benz et al., 1999). However, this situation is controversial and is not confirmed by all studies. Other studies assessing an association between sleep disturbances in peritoneal

dialysis patients and Hb levels have failed to show such an association (Walker et al., 1995; Holley et al., 1992; Stepanski et al., 1995). No consistent relationships have been found between subjective sleep complaints and laboratory measures of renal failure (blood urea nitrogen-BUN, creatinine) and parameters of dialysis efficacy (Kt/V) (Puntriano et al., 1999; Holley et al., 1992; Walker et al., 1995). Only a small study by Millman et al., has reported a significant relationship between sleep apnea and azotemia (Millman et al., 1985).

A correlation between the type and the duration of dialysis has also been searched. No difference has been found between hemo (HD) and peritoneal dialysis (PD). Both of them, indeed, are associated with a high rate of poor sleep quality (Eryavus et al., 2008). A relationship with the dialysis vintage has been found. It appears that, the longer the dialysis vintage, the higher the prevalence of sleep disturbances. In an Italian study, those patients on dialysis who presented sleep disturbances had a double dialysis vintage when compared to those on dialysis who did not have sleep problems (De Santo et al., 2005). When analyzing the timing of dialysis shifts, a higher rate of insomnia has been reported among patients on the morning dialysis shift. In fact, compared to patients receiving their dialysis in the afternoon, subjects treated in the morning show a significantly higher risk of being affected by insomnia ($p<0.001$) (Merlino et al., 2006). However these results have not been confirmed. In fact, a later study by Eryavuz et al. has found a higher rate of insomnia among patients on the afternoon shift. Regarding dialysis duration, results seem to be controversial as well. Only some studies have reported an association between longer dialysis duration and insomnia (Sabbatini et al., 2001; Veiga et al., 1997). In particular, higher PSQI scores have been found among patients who have received HD for a long period of time. Whereas, a positive correlation has also been found with a premature discontinuation of dialysis.

Recently literature has focused the attention on inflammatory markers. It has been demonstrated indeed, how they can be increased in sleep disorders with normal renal function or in end stage renal disease (ESRD) patients. Subsequently persistent elevation of these markers is associated with many clinically important complications, including atherosclerosis and cardiovascular mortality. These findings, together with the finding of a poorer sleep quality independently linked to higher mortality rate among ESRD patients, has led to the search of an association between inflammatory markers in ESRD and poor sleep quality. A recent study has shown that higher systemic inflammation, as demonstrated by serum hsCRP and IL-1β levels, is associated with poorer sleep quality in stable HD patients. Other inflammatory markers, such as IL-6 and TNF-α, are also positively correlated with poorer sleep quality; even though these results did not reach statistical significance (Yen-Ling Chiu et al., 2009).

Polysomnographic studies of this population have found how sleep macrostructure can be altered. The earliest studies are reported in the late 1960s and early 1970s. These reports described sleep as being characterized by decreased total sleep time, irregular sleep cycles, and long periods of interspersed waking (Reichenmiller et al., 1971; Passouant et al., 1970). Recent studies have confirmed a sleep characterized by short duration and fragmentation with sleep efficiencies ranging between 66% and 85%, long periods of wake time after sleep onset (77±135 min), and frequent arousals (25±30/h of sleep) (Parker et al., 2003). The macrostructural analysis has shown an increase of Stage 1 and 2 and a decrease of slow wave sleep (SWS) and REM sleep (Wadhwa et al., 1992; Parker et al., 2003; Stepanski et al., 1995). Parker et al has conducted a polysomnographic study on HD patients and has observed that these patients have a total sleep time and sleep efficiency significantly reduced compared to the general population, while, in comparison with patients affected by

chronic kidney disease but not undergoing dialysis therapy, they have a significantly higher brief arousal index (Parker et al., 2005).
The presence of insomnia among dialysis patients has led to the hypothesis that kidney transplant, by restoring renal function and alleviating many uremic symptoms, might also reduce sleep complaints. A cross sectional study, has used the Athens Insomnia Scale to assess the prevalence of insomnia in a large sample of kidney transplant recipients compared with wait-listed dialysis patients and also a matched group obtained from a nationally representative sample of the Hungarian population. Authors found that the prevalence of insomnia was lower among kidney transplant patients than among those on dialysis (Novak et al., 2006).

2.2 Excessive Daytime Sleepiness

Excessive daytime sleepiness (EDS), the major daytime consequence of sleep disturbances, has also been assessed among dialysis patients. EDS is defined by the inability to stay awake and alert during the major waking periods of the day, resulting in unintended lapses into drowsiness or sleep. Prevalence of EDS can be assessed subjectively, by standardized questionnaires, or objectively, by Multi Sleep Latency Test (MSLT). Most studies prefer to use subjective scales. Prevalence of EDS in patients ongoing dialysis therapy varies between 12% and 67% (Mucsi et al 2004, Merlino et al 2006, Hanly et al, American Accademy of sleep medicine). This large variability may be explained by different sample size and cut-off scores to indicate pathological sleepiness.
Parker et al. showed that 32,6 % of hemodialyzed patients had MSLT score < 8 minute and 13% < 5 minutes. MSLT scores were negatively correlated with respiratory disturbances (P= 0,028) and brief arousals (p=0,009). Metabolic parameters and sleep apnea seemed to directly or indirectly influence daytime sleepiness (Parker et al. 2003). Hanly et al. reported that MSLT score was negatively correlated to blood urea nitrogen, a marker of renal function, (r= -0,58; p=0,008. These studies hypothesized some possible mechanisms able to explain the presence of EDS. First, dialyzed patients frequently receive multiple medications, some of which can have sedative effects. Second, sleep apnea and sleep fragmentation, typical among dialyzed patients, can be associated with EDS. Third, renal function might affect the ability to stay awake, due to uremic encephalopathy, elevations of parathyroid hormone and abnormalities in neurotransmitter synthesis. Fourth, inflammatory cytokines may be released following stimulation of neutrophiles by the dialyzing membrane, which may have sleep inducing properties.

2.3 Restless legs syndrome

Restless legs syndrome is a common neurological disorder that is characterized by an urge to move the legs (rarely also the arms) and peculiar unpleasant sensations deep in the legs. Sensations appear during periods of rest or inactivity , particularly in the evening and at the night , and are tipically relieved by movements. Prevalence of RLS in general population ranges between 3 and 5%; RLS may occur as an idiopathic form or secondary to other conditions; the main secondary forms are iron deficiency, pregnancy , use of drugs and kidney disease. The association has been described for other diseases, among them, for diabetes (Merlino et al., 2007; Lopes et al., 2005) and multiple sclerosis (Italian REMS Study Group). RLS secondary to end stage renal disease is one of the most important secondary forms. In the past most of the studies have analyzed only hemodialysis. However, recently there is an increasing interest on the pre-dialytic phase of kidney disease and on the peritoneal dialysis.

The prevalence of RLS in patients undergoing dialysis varies widely, from 12% to 57,4% (Takaki et al., 2003; Walker et al., 1995). This large variability is due to the heterogeneity of the study population and to the different criteria used to diagnose RLS. Pathophysiology of RLS in ESRD is still unclear. Some studies have suggested a possible role of anemia. In a study with 55 dialyzed patients, authors found RLS's symptoms in 40 % of patients and showed that RLS's patients had lower hemoglobin values compared to others dialyzed patients (P=0,03). Same authors subsequently demonstrated that symptoms in this group of patients improved with the correction of anemia with epoetin alfa (Roger et al., 1991). The role of calcium/phosphate in the pathogenesis of RLS has also been hypothesized. In a study with 136 dialyzed patients, with a prevalence of RLS of 23%, there were no significant differences between the two groups, except for intact parathyroid hormone (iPTH). Uremic patients with RLS showed a significantly lower iPTH (p< 0,01) concentration (Collado Seidel V et al., 1998). However, this hypothesis has not been confirmed by other studies. Successful renal transplantation has immediate dramatic effects on uremic RLS. In a study including 11 patients with a long term course of RLS symptoms, they all had a complete recovery within 1 to 21 days after a kidney transplantation. Whereas, among those patients who again became dependent on dialysis due to a chronic transplant failure, RLS symptoms reoccurred within a few days after restarting hemodialysis. (Wilkelmann et al., 2002). In 2005 Molnar et al showed that RLS's symptoms were less frequent in patients after kidney transplantation than in patients undergoing dialysis therapy. Thus, authors suggested that "uremic factors ", responsible for the higher prevalence of RLS in dialysis patients, are largely eliminated after a successful kidney transplantation (Molnar et al., 2005). Differently from transplantation, dialysis did not show any positive effect on RLS. Indeed, studies reported that frequency of dialysis session per week and dialysis dependency, are higher in uremic patients with RLS than in those without it (Gigli et al., 2004; Huiqi et al., 2000). Several observations have suggested an association between RLS and neuropathy, especially with involvement of small sensory fibers. In fact, abnormal hyperexcitability of spinal circuits in RLS could be induced not only by impaired descending dopaminergic modulation, but also by changes in the spinal cord itself (Paulus et al., 2007) or by abnormal inputs as found in peripheral nervous system (PNS) diseases (Gemignani et al., 2006). In general, prevalence estimates of RLS in neuropathy of any kind are extremely variable, ranging from 5.2% to 54% (Rutkove et al., 1996; Nineb et al., 2007). The occurrence of symptoms of burning feet suggested a prominent role of C fibers, assuming that receptors are hyperexcitable due to irritative changes in unmyelinated fibers conveying hot sense (Lacomis, 2002; Ochoa et al., 2005; Ørstavik et al., 2006). Alternatively, abnormal thermal sensations may be produced by impaired central integration of information from nociceptive and thermal channels, as suggested by paradoxical heat sensation produced by A-delta fiber deafferentation (Susser et al., 1999). In accordance with previous data suggesting that RLS occurs preferentially in sensory polyneuropathy of mild to moderate degree and/or in early phase (Iannaccone et al., 2000), patients with RLS had less severe changes in SAPs. This pathogenetical mechanism could explain, at least partially, the association between RLS and ESRD.

There is a lack of studies about prevalence of RLS in patients undergoing PD. Personal preliminary observations suggest that PD patients might have a lower prevalence of RLS than HD patients but higher than "pre-dialysed" patients, with characteristics which resemble more to those of idiopathic forms than of secondary forms. These aspects confirm the possible role of hemodialysis in causing RLS. RLS symptoms in dialysis are severe and have a negative impact on quality of life and increase the risk of mortality in this specific population. In particular, different studies have showed a correlation between RLS and an increased cardiovascular risk. In particular, periodic limb movements during sleep induce rises in blood pressure, which may play a role in the pathogenesis of cardiovascular diseases (Winkelman et al., 2008). Another possible mechanism is that sleep deprivation, tipically found in patients with severe forms of RLS, can increase inflammatory markers. A persistent and chronic increase of inflammatory markers can be associated with and increased cardio and cerebrovascular risk.

2.4 Sleep apnea syndrome

Sleep apnea syndrome (SAS) is characterized by disordered breathing during sleep, resulting in heavy snoring, repetitive apnea, restless sleep, fragmented sleep structure, morning headache, and daytime sleepiness. Often SAS is associated with personality and mood change such as depression. The following types of apnea can be distinguished: i- obstructive apnea ii- central apnea iii-mixed apnea. Obstructive sleep apnea syndrome is characterized by repetitive closures of the upper airways during sleep, usually at the pharyngeal level, which produce apneas, increasing respiratory effort against the collapsed airways inducing repetitive arousals. Central sleep apnea is characterized by unstable decrease or even absent regulatory motor activity of the respiratory centers in the central nervous system during sleep, leading to apneic episodes. Most central apneas occur at sleep onset. They are characterized by a cycle of decreased or absent respiratory effort or absent respiratory effort and are terminated by ongoing arousals. Apneic episodes lead to microarousals determining a fragmentation of sleep and the activation of sympathetic nervous system.

Studies have reported a high prevalence of SAS in patients with chronic kidney disease. Compared with the general population where the prevalence of SAS is estimated to be 2-4%, prevalence in the ESRD population appears to be 30% or more (Kuhlmann et al. 2000; Young et al. 1993; Kimmel et al. 1989). This is partly explained by the fact that the most common comorbid conditions of ESRD, such as atherosclerosis and diabetes, are also independently associated with ESRD. Among dialysis patients, central and obstructive sleep apnea are almost equally observed, whereas, in the general population the prevalence of obstructive sleep apnea is higher. A mechanism able to cause both destabilization of central ventilator and upper airway obstruction has been suggested. Indeed, central events could be due to metabolic acidosis that may change the apnea PCO2 threshold and consequently destabilize respiratory control. In addition, dialyzed patients show an accumulation of uremic toxins and endogenous opioids that may result in an unstable breathing pattern. Other factors that can worsen SAS in dialysis are: i- the central uremic neuropathy that might reduce airway muscle tone during sleep or destabilize respiratory control; ii- edema from fluid overload that tend to favor upper airway collapse; iii- elevated values of several cytokines (observed during dialysis) that can influence sleep (Vgontzas et al. 2000). Sleep apnea syndrome is frequent both in HD and in PD. In past studies, it was not found a significant difference between these two types of dialysis for sleep apnea. Studies have found that nocturnal peritoneal dialysis (NPD) seems to improve SAS. In a study, Tang et al. recruited 23 NPD patients and 23 Continuous ambulatory peritoneal dialysis (CAPD) patients. The prevalence of sleep apnea with AHI > 15 was 52 % for NPD and 91% for CAPD. Bioelectrical impedance analysis revealed that total body water (TBW) content was significantly lower during NPD

than CAPD (32,8 L vs 35,1 L; p< 0,004). Probably, the improvement of sleep apnea by NPD is due to the improved extracellular fluid control during sleep (Tang et al. 2006).
Similar to nocturnal haemodialysis, improved clearance of uremic toxins after successful kidney transplant would be expected to alleviate SAS, but the relationship between SAS and renal transplant can be viewed as a paradox. In fact, although renal transplant can potentially improve SAS in the dialysis population, the post-transplant state may add another risk for SAS, specifically by predisposing patients to the metabolic syndrome. The prevalence of SAS among renal transplant patients is comparable with the dialysis population: in a study with a population of 1037 kidney transplant patients and 175 patients wait-listed for transplant, 27% of transplant patients had a high risk of SAS that was comparable with 33% in the wait-listed group (Molnar et al. 2007). The possible mechanism that can cause SAS in renal transplant patients is that immunosuppressive therapy, particularly corticosteroids, has been associated with the cushingoid features such as weight gain, obesity, abnormal fat distribution and development of the metabolic syndrome. Brilakis et al. in a study in a population of 17 heart transplant recipients, found an average weight gain of 10,7 kg in 16 patients (Brilakis et al 2000) who were diagnosed with SAS. In another study on cardiac transplant patients, SAS was diagnosed in 36 of 45 patients (80%) studied with polisomnography. In patients with SAS, weight gain was greater that in patients without SAS (Javaheri et al. 2004).

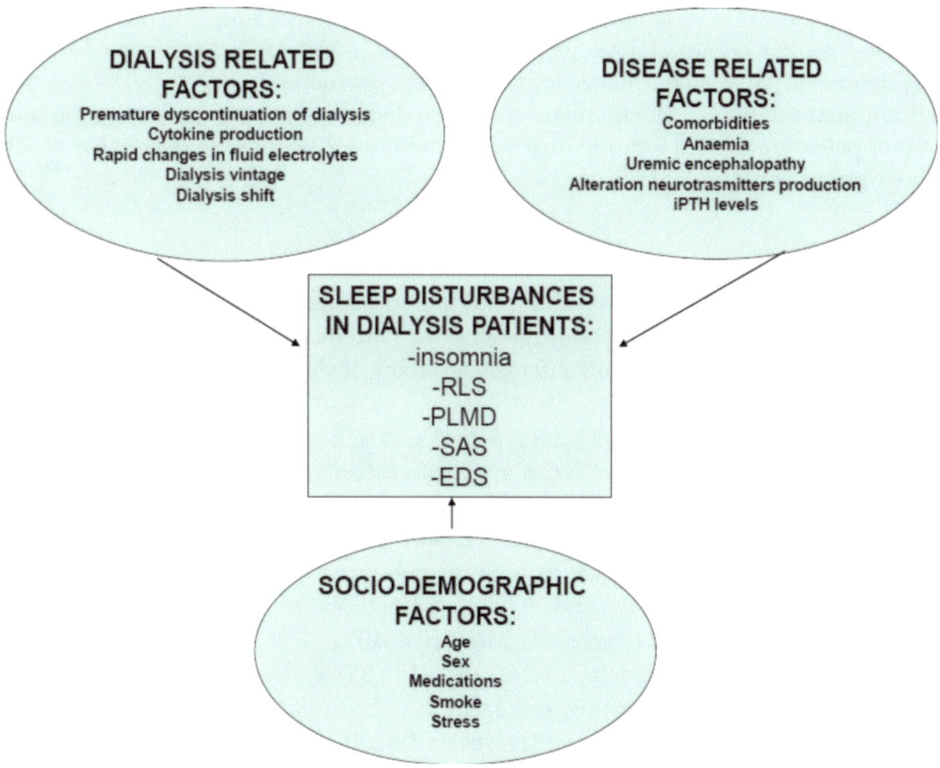

Figure. The possible causal relationships between the different sleep disturbances and the phatogenethical mechanisms is outlined. RLS: Restless Legs Syndrome; PLMD: Periodic Limbs Movement Disorder; SAS: Sleep apnea Syndrome; EDS: Excessive Daytime Sleepiness. Modified from Parker et al., 2003.

The clinical presentation of sleep apnea in ESRD patients is similar to that observed in patients without chronic renal failure, namely the presence of loud snoring and witnessed apneas during sleep, nocturnal awakenings, and excessive daytime sleepiness. However, some of these symptoms may be mistakenly attributed to Chronic renal failure (CRF) itself, or to comorbid condition. This has led to the under-diagnosis and under-treatment of sleep apnea in this specific population. The presence of untreated SAS in this population, can exacerbate the symptoms of CRF, contributing to daytime fatigue and sleepiness and, may exacerbate the cardiovascular complications of ESRD, which are the most important cause of death in this population of patients.

3. Conclusions

In conclusion, sleep disorders are very common among dialysis patients and the pathogenethical mechanism that have been hypothesized are various (see Figure). These disorders play an important role among dialysis patients affecting both the quality of life (sleep disturbances are referred as to one of the most important distressing symptoms) and the mortality risk. The increased mortality risk among dialysis patients affected by sleep disturbances has been demonstrated by many epidemiological studies. In addition, recent studies have also confirmed the association between sleep disturbances, such as RLS, and vascular diseases . These data confirm once more the role of sleep in contributing to the increased vascular risk in dialysis patients. However, more studies are needed in order to better define the pathogenetical mechanism of sleep disorders.
Nephrologists should became familiar with these disorders, promptly identify them in this group of patients and start a proper management in order to improve the quality of life and reduce the vascular risk.

4. References

American Accademy of Sleep Medicine (1999): Sleep related breathing disorders in adults: recommendations for syndrome definition and measurement techniques in clinical research. The report of an amarican academy of sleep medicine task force. *Sleep*; 22: 667-689.

Bass, EB; Jenckes, MW; Fink, NE; Cagney, KA; Wu, AW; Sadler, JH; Meyer, KB; Levey, AS & Powe, NR. (1999). Use of focus groups to identify concerns about dialysis. Choice Study. *Med Decis Making*; 19(3): 287±295.

Benz, RL.; Pressman, MR; Hovick, ET & Peterson, DD (1999). A preliminary study of the effects of correction of anemia with recombinant human erythropoietin therapy on sleep, sleep disorders, and daytime sleepiness in hemodialysis patients (The SLEEPO study). *Am J Kidney Dis* 34(6): 1089–1095.

Brilakis, ES; Olson, EJ; Mc Gregor, CG & Olson LJ (2000). Sleep apnea in renal transplant recipients: type, symptoms, risk factors, and respons to nasal continuous positive airway pressure. *J Heart Lung Transplant*. 19: 330-336.

Chevalier, H; Los, F; Boichut, D; Bianchi, M; Nutt, DJ; Hajak, G; Hetta, J; Hoffmann, G & Crowe, C (1999) Evaluation of severe insomnia in the general population: Results of a European multinational survey. *J Psychopharmacol* 13:S21-S24, (suppl 1).

Chiu, YL; Chuang, YF; Fang, KC; Liu, SK; Chen, HY; Yang, JY; Pai, MF; Peng, YS; Wu, KD & Tsai, TJ (2009). Higher systemic inflammation is associated with poorer sleep quality in stable haemodialysis patients. Nephrol Dial Transplant. Jan;24(1):247-51.

Collado-Seidel, V; Kohnen, R; Samtleben, W; Hillebrand, GF; Oertel, WH & Trenkwalder, C. (1998) Clinical and biochemical findings in uremic patients with and without restless legs syndrome. *Am J Kidney Dis* 31:324-328.

De Santo, RM; Lucidi, F; Violani, C & Di Iorio, BR (2005) Sleep disorders in hemodialyzed patients—the role of comorbidities. *Int J Artif Organs* 28:557–565.

De Santo, RM; Lucidi, F; Violani, C & Bertini, M (2001). Insomnia is associated with systolic hypertension in uremic patients on hemodialysis. *Int J Artif Organs* 24:853–862.

Eichel CJ (1986). Stress and coping in patients on CAPD compared to hemodialysis patients. *ANNA Journal*; 13(1): 9±13.

Eryavuz, N; Yuksel, S; Acarturk, G; Uslan, I; Demir, S; Demir, M & Sezer, MT (2008). Comparison of sleep quality between hemodialysis and peritoneal dialysis patients. Int Urol Nephrol. 2008;40(3):785-91. Epub Apr 22.

Gemignani, F; Brindani, F; Negrotti, A; Vitetta, F; Alfieri, S & Marbini A (2006) Restless legs syndrome and polyneuropathy. *Mov Disord* 21(8):1254–1257.

Gigli, GL; Adorati, M; Dolso, P; Piani, A; Valente, M; Brotini, S & Budai R (2004). Restless legs syndrome in end-stage renal disease. *Sleep Med* 5:309-315.

Hanly, PJ; Gabor, JY; Chan, G & Pierratos, A (2003). Daytime sleepiness in patients with CRF: impact of nocturnal hemodialysis. *Am J Kidney Disease*; 41: 403-10.

Holley, JL; Nespor, S & Rault, R (1992) A comparison of reported sleep disorders in patients on chronic hemodialysis and continuous peritoneal dialysis. *Am J Kidney Dis* 19(2):156–161.

Huiqi, Q; Shan, L & Minqcai Q (2000). Restless legs syndrome (RLS) in uremic patients is related to the frequency of hemodialysis sessions. *Nephron* 86:540.

Iannaccone, S; Quattrini, A; Sferrazza, B; Ferini-Strambi, L; Gemignani, F; Marbini, A & Terzano MG (2000). Charcot- Marie-Tooth disease type 2 with restless legs syndrome. *Neurology* 54:1013–1014.

Iliescu, EA; Coo, H; McMurray, MH; Meers, CL; Quinn, MM; Singer, MA & Hopman, WM (2003). Quality of sleep and health-related quality of life in haemodialysis patients. *Nephrol Dial Transplant* 18:126–132.

Italian REMS Study Group, Manconi, M; Ferini-Strambi, L; Filippi, M; Bonanni, E; Iudice, A; Murri, L; Gigli, GL; Fratticci, L; Merlino, G; Terzano, G; Granella, F; Parrino L, Silvestri, R; Aricò, I; Dattola, V; Russo, G; Luongo, C; Cicolin, A; Tribolo, A; Cavalla, P; Savarese, M; Trojano, M; Ottaviano, S; Cirignotta, F; Simioni, V; Salvi, F; Mondino, F; Perla, F; Chinaglia, G; Zuliani, C; Cesnik, E; Granieri, E; Placidi, F; Palmieri, MG; Manni, R; Terzaghi, M; Bergamaschi, R; Rocchi, R; Ulivelli, M; Bartalini, S; Ferri, R; Lo Fermo, S; Ubiali, E; Viscardi, M; Rottoli, M; Nobili, L; Protti, A; Ferrillo, F; Allena, M; Mancardi, G; Guarnieri, B & Londrillo, F (2008). Multicenter case-control study on restless legs syndrome in multiple sclerosis: the REMS study. *Sleep* 1;31(7):944-52.

Javaheri, S; Abraham, WT; Brown, C; Nishiyama, H; Giesting, R & Wagoner, LE (2004). Prevalence of obstructive sleep apneaand periodic limb movement in 45 subjects with heart transplantation. *Eur Heart J*. 25:260-266.

Kimmel, PL; Miller, G & Mendelson, WB (1989). Sleep apnea syndrome in chronic renal disease. *Am J Med*. 86:308-314.

Kuhlmann, U; Becker, HF; Birkhalm, M; Peter, JH; von Wichert, P; Schütterle, S & Lange H (2000). Sleep apnea in patients with end stage renal disease and objective results. *Clin Nephrol*; 53: 460-66.

Kusleikaite, N; Bumblyte, IA; Razukeviciene, L; Sedlickaite, D & Rinkunas, K (2005) Sleep disorders and quality of life in patients on hemodialysis. *Medicina (Kaunas)* 41(Suppl 1): 69–74

Kutner, NG; Bliwise, DL; Brogan, D & Zhang, R (2001). Race and restless sleep complaint in older chronic dialysis patients and nondialysis community controls. *J Gerontol B Psychol Sci Soc Sci*; 56(3): 170±175.

Young, T; Palta, M; Dempsey, J; Skatrud, J; Weber, S & Badr S (1993). The occurrence of sleep disoredered breathingamong middle aged adults. *N. Engl. J. Med*; 328: 1230-35.

Lacomis, D (2002). Small-fiber neuropathy. *Muscle Nerve*.Aug;26(2):173-88.

Lopes, LA; Lins Cde, M ; Adeodato, VG ; Quental, DP ; de Bruin, PF ; Montenegro, RM Jr & de Bruin VM (2005). Restless legs syndrome and quality of sleep in type 2 diabetes. *Diabetes Care* 28(11):2633-6.

Merlino, G; Lorenzut, S; Gigli, GL; Romano, G; Montanaro, D; Moro, A & Valente M (2010) A case control study on restless leg syndrome in nondialyzed patients with chronic renal failure. *Mov Dis; 25 (8): 1019-1025.*

Merlino, G; Fratticci, L; Valente, M; Del Giudice, A; Noacco, C; Dolso, P; Cancelli, I; Scalise, A & Gigli GL (2007). Association of restless legs syndrome in type 2 diabetes: a case-control study. *Sleep*. 30(7):866-71.

Merlino, G; Piani, A; Dolso, P; Adorati, M; Cancelli, I; Valente, M & Gigli GL (2006). Sleep disorders in patients with end stage renal disease undergoing dialysis therapy. *Nephrol Dial Transplant*; 21: 184-190.

Millman, RP; Kimmel, PL; Shore, ET & Wasserstein AG (1985). Sleep apnea in hemodialysis patients: the lack of testosterone effect on its pathogenesis. *Nephron* 40:407–410.

Molnar, AZ ; Novak, M ; Ambrus, C ; Szeifert, L; Kovacs, A; Pap, J; Remport, A & Mucsi I (2005). Restless Legs Syndrome in patients after renal transplantation. *Am J Kidney Dis* 45:388-396.

Molnar, MZ; Szentkiralyi, A; Lindner, A; Czira, ME; Szabo, A; Mucsi, I & Novak M (2007). High prevalence of patients with a high risk for obstructive sleep apnea syndrome after kidney transplantation association with declining renal function. Nephrol Dial Transplant. 22: 2686-2692.

Mucsi, I; Molnar, AZ; Ambrus; Szeifert, L; Kovacs, AZ; Zoller, R; Barótfi, S; Remport, A & Novak M (2005) Restless legs syndrome, insomnia and quality of life in patients on maintenance dialysis. *Nephrol Dial Transplant* 20:571-577.

Mucsi, I; Molnar, MZ; Rethelyi, J; Vamos, E; Csepanyi, G; Tompa, G; Barotfi, S; Marton, A & Novak M (2004). Sleep disorders and illness intrusiveness in patients on chronic dialysis. *Nephrol Dial Transplant*; 19: 1815-22.

Nineb, A ; Rosso, C ; Dumurgier, J ; Nordine, T ; Lefaucheur, JP & Créange A (2007). Restless legs syndrome is frequently overlooked in patients being evaluated for polyneuropathies. *Eur J Neurol*. 7 Jul;14(7):788-92.

Novak, M ; Molnar, MZ; Ambrus, C; Kovacs, AZ; Koczy, A; Remport, A; Szeifert, L; Szentkiralyi, A; Shapiro, CM; Kopp, MS & Mucsi, I. (2006) Chronic insomnia in kidney transplant recipients. *Am J Kidney Dis*. Apr;47(4):655-65.

Ochoa, JL; Campero, M; Serra, J & Bostock, H (2005). Hyperexcitable polymodal and insensitive nociceptors in painful human neuropathy. *Muscle Nerve* 32:459–472.

Ohayon MM (2002) Epidemiology of insomnia: What we know and what we still need to learn. *Sleep Med Rev* 6:97-111.

Ohayon, MM ; Caulet, M ; Philip, P ; Guilleminault, C & Priest, RG (1997). How sleep and mental disorders are related to complaints of daytime sleepiness. *Arch Intern Med*. 7 Dec 8-22;157(22):2645-52.

Ohayon M (1996). Epidemiological study on insomnia in the general population. *Sleep* 19:S7-S15, 6 (suppl 3).

Ørstavik, K; Namer, B; Schmidt, R; Schmelz, M; Hiliges, M; Weidner, C; Carr, RW; Handwerker, H; Jorum, E & Torebjork HE (2006). Abnormal function of C-fibers in patients with diabetic neuropathy. *J Neurosci* 26:11287–11294.

Parfrey, PS; Vavasour, HM; Henry, S; Bullock, M & Gault MH (1988). Clinical features and severity of nonspecific symptoms in dialysis patients. *Nephron*; 50(2): 121±128.

Parker, KP; Bliwise, DL; Bayley, JL & Rye DB (2003) Daytime sleepiness in stable hemodialysis patients. *Am J kidney Dis*. 41:394-402.

Parker, KP; Bliwise, DL; Bailey, JL & Rye DB (2005). Polysomnographic measures of nocturnal sleep in patients on chronic, intermittent daytime haemodialysis vs those with chronic kidney disease. *Nephrol Dial Transplant.*;20:1422-1428.

Passouant, P; Cadilhac, J; Baldy-Moulinier, M & Mion, C (1970). Night sleep in chronic uremics under extrarenal purification. *Electroencephalogr Clin Neurophysiol*. 29(5): 441±449.

Paulus, W; Dowling, P; Rijsman, R; Stiasny-Kolster, K & Trenkwalder, C. (2007) Update of the pathophysiology of the restless-legs-syndrome. *Mov Disord*. 22 Suppl 18:S431-9.

Puntriano, M (1999). The relationship between dialysis adequacies and sleep problems in hemodialysis patients. *Anna J*; 26(4): 405-407.

Reichenmiller, HE; Reinhard, U & Durr, F (1971). Sleep EEG and uraemia. *Electroencephalogr Clin Neurophysiol*; 30(3): 263±264.

Roger, SD; Harris, DC & Stewart, JH (1991). Possible relation between restless legs and anaemia in renal dialysis patients. *Lancet*;337:1551.

Rutkove, SB; Matheson, JK & Logigian EL (1996) Restless legs syndrome in patients with polyneuropathy. *Muscle Nerve*. 19(5):670–672.

Sabbatini, M; Minale, B; Crispo, A; Pisani, A; Ragosta, A; Esposito, R; Cesaro, A; Cianciaruso, B & Andreucci VE (2002). Insomnia in maintenance haemodialysis patients. *Nephrol Dial Transplant* 17:852-856.

Strub, B; Schneider-Helmert, D; Gnirss, F & Blumberg A (1982). Sleep disorders in patients with chronic renal insufficiency in long-term hemodialysis treatment. *Schweiz Med Wochenschr.* 112(23): 824±828.

Susser, E; Sprecher, E & Yarnitsky, D (1999). Paradoxical heat sensation in healthy subjects: peripherally conducted by Ad or C fibres? *Brain* 122:239–246.

Stepanski, E; Faber, M; Zorick, F; Basner, R & Roth T (1995) Sleep disorders in patients on continuous ambulatory peritoneal dialysis. J Am Soc Nephrol 6(2):192–197.

Takaki, J; Nishi, T; Nangaku, M; Shimoyama, H; Inada, T; Matsuyama, N; Kumano, H & Kuboki T (2003). Clinical and psychological aspects of restless legs syndrome in uremic patients on hemodialysis. *Am J Kidney Dis* 41:833-839.

Veiga, J; Goncalves, N & Gomes F (1997) Sleep disturbances in end-stage renal disease patients on hemodialysis. *Dial Transplant* 26:380–384.

Vgontzas AN, Papanicolaou DA, Bixler EO et al. (2000) J Clin Endocrinol Metab. 85: 1151-1158.

Wadhwa, NK & Mendelson, WB (1992). A comparison of sleep-disordered respiration in ESRD patients receiving hemodialysis and peritoneal dialysis. *Adv Perit Dial*; 8: 195-198.

Walker, SL; Fine, A & Kryger, MH (1995). Sleep complaints are common in dialysis unit. Am J Kidney Dis; 26:751 756.

Winkelman, JW; Shahar, E; Sharief, I & Gottlieb DJ (2008). Association of restless legs syndrome and cardiovascular disease in the Sleep Heart Health Study. *Neurology*;70: 35-42

Winkelman, J; Stautner, A; Samtleben, W & Trenkwalder C (2002). Long-term course of restless legs syndrome in dialysis patients after kidney transplantation. *Mov Disord* 17:1072-1076.

19

Bridging the 'Gap' in Developing Countries: At what Expense?

Chulananda DA Goonasekera
University of Peradeniya
Sri Lanka

1. Introduction

Experts from all continents have called for the emerging countries to start chronic kidney disease prevention and screening programs, develop end-stage renal disease registries and start or further strengthen transplantation programs through International as well as regional collaborations to acquire the information, technology, experience and skills necessary whilst acknowledging these goals are ambitious (Remuzzi, Perico, et al. 2010).

Transplantation is the optimal renal replacement therapy for children with end-stage renal disease. Compared with dialysis, successful transplantation in children and adolescents not only ameliorates uremic symptoms but also allows for significant improvement of delayed growth, sexual maturation, and psychosocial functioning. The child with a well-functioning kidney can enjoy a quality of life that cannot be achieved by dialysis therapy (Uchida 2010).

Although renal transplantation is an excellent option for the treatment of uremic children, it is more difficult compared to adults due to different etiologies often congenital, difficult surgical technique(van Heurn and deVries 2009), size match problems of the donor kidney and the post-operative hemodynamic effects due to poorly managed chronic renal failure and its effects upon growth and development. Most importantly, the lack of expertise, financial restraints and low-level national prioritization adds to the problem and prevents the establishment of fully-fledged pediatric renal transplant programs in developing countries (Bamgboye, 2009).

However, despite the negativism (Muthusethupathi & Shivakumar 1993), many medical personnel in developing countries have attempted to bridge the gap (Usta et al. 2008), often successfully and have developed pediatric kidney transplant programs (Badmus et al. 2005) (Kandus et al 2009). Doctors embarking on such programs would inevitably feel the punch as healthcare in developing countries are less funded than developed nations (0.8 to 4% vs. 10 to 15%, respectively), and must contend against approximately 1/3 of the population living below the poverty line ($1US/day), poor literacy (58% males/29% females), and less access to portable water and basic sanitation. Cultural and societal constraints combine with these economic obstacles. Donor shortage is a universal problem. Post-transplant infections are a major problem in developing countries, with 15% developing tuberculosis, 30% cytomegalovirus, and nearly 50% bacterial infections. The solutions may seem simplistic: alleviate poverty, educate the general population, and expand the transplant programs in the public sector hospitals where commerce is less likely to play a major role. This is not forthcoming as in most developing countries it is not the governments' priority. The SIUT model in Pakistan, funded by a community-government partnership is an exception to the rule and sustainable (Rizvi & Naqvi 1997). Over the last 15 years, it has operated by complete financial transparency, public audit and accountability. The scheme has proven effective and currently 110 transplants/year are performed, with free after care and immunosuppressive drugs. Confidence has been built in the community to attract strong donations of money, equipment and medicines (Rizvi et al. 2003).

According to the databases maintained by North American Pediatric Renal Transplant Co-operate Study (NAPRTCS) and the United States Renal Data System (USRDS) the 1, 2, and 5 year survival rates for primary live donor kidney transplantation (LDKT) were 98%, 97%, 95% respectively. The graft survival rate at 1 year and 7 years for primary LDKT were 92% and 74% respectively. According to the United Kingdom Transplant (UKT) report, the graft survival rate for all pediatric recipients during the 1 and 5 year were 79% and 68%, respectively. Developed centers attribute such excellent results to technical improvements in tissue typing and donor-recipient cross matching, modification of immune-suppression protocols and rigorous donor-recipient selection. (Porrett et al. 2009)

Despite many limitations, Sri Lanka embarked upon a pediatric kidney transplant programme in July 2004 amidst various adversities to offer some hope to children dying of ESRF. Most were transplanted pre-emptively as there was no established dialysis programme for children in Sri Lanka. Renal transplantation is considered pre-emptive if it occurs before the initiation of dialysis and it is not considered detrimental for graft survival compared to dialyzed children (Jung et al. 2010). In the literature, pre-emptive transplantation has been shown not only to reduce the costs of renal replacement therapy but also to avoid the long-term adverse effect of dialysis (Haberal et al 2009) and often involve a live donor that also appear to be slightly more advantageous compared to graft survival rates observed following deceased donor transplantation (Ng et al 2009). On the other hand pre-transplant dialysis modality, neither HD nor PD affects the outcome of renal transplantation (Caliskan et al. 2009).

Initiating a pediatric program in a developing country is more difficult (Rizvi et al. 2001). We experienced at the inception, due to lack of chronic renal failure (CRF) or dialysis programme for children, most children presenting late and displaying complications of CRF such as severe anemia, hyper-dynamic circulation, cardiomegaly, metabolic bone disease, growth stunting and poor nutritional state. A plasma urea level of 40 - 50 mmol/ litre (normal range 2.7 - 7.0 mmol/l) preoperatively was not an uncommon finding. Since pre-emptive transplantation was the only option, we noted at the initial stages of the programme that, most were not capable cardiovascularly to handle massive fluid and electrolyte shifts that occur during the immediate post transplant period. A polyuric-transplanted adult kidney would bring down the plasma urea to very low levels within 24-48 hours and this contributed to the onset of cerebral edema and convulsions. Inability to monitor plasma cyclosporin levels at short notice also contributed to the high incidence of seizures. Thus, elective mechanical ventilation postoperatively was useful until such time the postoperative polyuric phase was subsiding. Furthermore, the rapid onset pulmonary edema occurred 2-3 days after transplantation in a few cases. This was associated with a rapidly rising CVP, for example, from a stable 12cm of H_2O to 25cm H_2O despite accurate fluid balancing and appeared to be related to a rapid onset-myocardial weakness perhaps precipitated by precipitous electrolyte losses (e.g. $PO4^{3-}$)(Sakhaee, 2010) other than what was replaced i.e. Na+ and K+. These patients needed dobutamine as an inotrope to improve cardiac output and resolve pulmonary edema in addition to 1-2 doses of frusemide. Low calcium and low magnesium levels that may ensue due to polyuria could be a contributory factor.

Inadequate chronic renal failure (CRF) supportive care programme led to children presenting for transplantation have many co-morbid factors that made them vulnerable to higher peri-operative and anesthetic risks and difficulties in management. Limited laboratory, operating theatre and supplies of pharmaceutical agents, and the relatively inexperienced work force added to the shortcomings.

Expert inputs from multi disciplinary teams including pediatric nephrologists, transplant surgeons, and pediatric intensivists are imperative to provide optimum care in the peri-operative period for the transplant recipient. However, such expertise are hard to come by in the developing world and doctors involved in transplantation should be prepared to exceed their boundaries and provide the care necessary for these children irrespective of the time of the day.

For better outcomes in renal transplantation, it is necessary to optimize medical conditions associated with long-term renal impairment prior to surgery. In the developed world, a kidney transplant centre for children would be supported by many specialists, namely, transplant surgeons, pediatric nephrologists, dieticians, clinical pharmacists, social workers, dialysis teams, home care teams etc to achieve the above set goals. However, this is not feasible for a transplant centre in a developing country. Often the only specialist available would be a general surgeon with transplantation skills, general pediatrician with nephrology interest, and trained nurses. There may not be a social worker, pharmacist, dietician to assist holistic clinical management of the patient. Despite all these drawbacks, the outcomes of kidney transplantation i.e. the graft and patient survival can be similar in developing countries in the short-term, even in children (Wisaanuyotin & Jiravuttipong 2009) to that of established centers in the developed world, but at what expense? This chapter looks at this issue.

2. The pre-operative shortcomings

The pre-operative status of children admitted for renal transplantation in the context of nutritional status, body weight, hemoglobin, and blood urea is far from ideal due to poor management of ESRD resulting from the lack of facilities and inadequacies in dialysis and non-availability of dedicated chronic renal failure management programs. In an ideal centre, they would have their recipients at near normal physical status through aggressive nutritional programs despite being on dialysis.

In our centre, among 29 (20 male) children receiving kidney transplantation aged median 10 years (range 2-16),the mean (± SD) pre-transplant hemoglobin and blood urea were 9.36 ± 2.46g/dl and 21.97 ± 10.17 mmol/l respectively. Nearly a ⅔ (n=19) were on regular antihypertensive treatment. Of them, 1 patient (3.57%) had haemodialysis (HD), 7(25%) peritoneal dialysis (PD) and 3(10.71%) both prior to transplant. Seventeen (60.71%) were pre-emptive transplants. Preoperative blood transfusion to correct anemia was not attempted and it is also considered unimportant to improve outcomes (Aalten et al. 2009). The children in ESRF were cared for in the general pediatric ward, mostly assisted by parents or guardians. Supplementary funding came from external resources.

3. The operative difficulties

In established centers, the operative difficulties in pediatric transplantation are mainly urological (e.g. VUR 12.4%, ureteral stricture 5%, anastomotic leak 2%, ureteral necrosis 1%, and incrustative pyelitis 0.5%) and vascular (arterial stricture 7.2%, arterial thrombosis 2%, venous thrombosis 1%) (Irtan et al. 2010) . Donors aged less than six years were a risk factor of vascular complications leading to graft loss, whereas patients with PUV had more complications that are urological. Overall, patient and graft survival is 93.1% and 84% at 5-years, respectively. Surgical complications remain a major cause of graft loss (12%) and morbidity in children's kidney transplantation (38.9%).
Among the difficulties encountered during anesthesia, that also has an impact on postoperative care includes poor cardio-respiratory reserve due to cardiomegaly/myopathy (resulting from chronic anemia, uremia and hypertension) and pleural, pericardial effusions, anemia and liver dysfunction. Cardiac dysfunction and excessive bleeding were the commonest complications encountered under anesthesia during operation. It was not uncommon for some children with poor control of hypertension, cardiomyopathy with an EF of 35-40%, and body weight below 3rd centile to be operated.

4. A unique set of postoperative problems

In addition to providing good analgesia, the postoperative care of renal transplant recipients include establishment of hemodynamic stability, maintaining adequate perfusion of the newly transplanted kidney and prevention and treatment of complications resulting from fluid imbalance, electrolyte imbalance or myocardial weakness.
The post operative complications encountered in a poorly nourished child with established complications of ESRD such as anemia, osteodystrophy, hypertension, cardiac failure were markedly different to what was described in most published work that involves well prepared, adequately dialyzed and well nourished children who seek kidney transplantation in the developed world.

4.1 The poly-uric phase

During the immediate post transplant period the urine output via the transplanted kidney can reach 1-2 liters / hour. Managing this phenomenon in a child of 10 kg where the total blood volume is only 700 ml can be a daunting task requiring fluid balancing and replacement every 15 minutes. Thus, one patient needs constant attention of several nurses to keep the fluid and electrolytes in balance. Provision of a work force to cater for this need is not an easy task in this part of the world.
During the poly-uric phase, hypokalemia and hypophosphateamia (Sakhaee 2010) are common complications due to unrestrained loss of these electrolytes in urine. This can lead to severe myocardial weakness and arrhythmias. Appropriate cardiac support and anticipation of such problems are needed to be avoided to avert disaster. The potassium loss in the diuretic phase can lead to severe hypokalemia, unless replacement fluids are replenished with at least 5 mmol/liter of KCl.

4.2 Non functioning transplanted kidney

The transplanted kidney may not function as a result of well-recognized causes such as, (a) acute rejection (b) acute vascular thromboses and (c) acute tubular necrosis. However, we noted several extraneous factors contributing to a non functioning transplanted kidney. These include (a) high CVP (b) high intra abdominal pressure (c) obstructed or leaking ureter and (d) a relatively low systolic pressure that cannot provide adequate perfusion pressure for the transplanted kidney. It was also easy to overload these children, especially in whom the transplanted kidney did not work immediately postoperatively. Thus, careful restraint is also necessary in fluid management to avoid the need for urgent dialysis that is not promptly achievable in this part of the world.

4.3 Heart failure and pulmonary edema

This is usually seen 24-48 hours after transplantation during the latter part of the poly-uric phase. The onset of pulmonary oedema can be very rapid and florid (within a few minutes) and can occur even with meticulous fluid balancing. Thus, it is likely that an acquired myocardial weakness contributing to this complication, most probably due to electrolyte depletion especially phosphate. It should be noted that even in advanced centers, nearly 1/3rd of post transplant deaths are attributed to cardio-vascular events (Koshy et al 2009). However, some other centers that record a low mortality rate following pediatric renal transplantation observe a majority of deaths due to malignancies and infections but have no impact of cardiovascular disease (Allain-Launay et al. 2009). On the other hand careful follow-up studies have revealed that repolarization abnormalities shown on an electrocardiogram of pre-RT patients improved significantly after RT (QTc dispersion 50.8+/-37.3 to 37.4+/-11.9 msec, P=0.009) and left ventricular hypertrophy with increased LV mass index of pre-RT patients regressed remarkably after RT (LV mass index 120.9+/-40.5 to 69.2+/-14.5 g/m2, P<0.001). Still LV mass was significantly higher in RT patients than the controls (54.0+/-9.6 g/m2, P<0.001). Compared to the controls, the RT patients showed diastolic dysfunction (lower E/A ratio and higher isovolumic relaxation time) and lower myocardial performance (higher LV Tei index and weaker strain pattern)(Kim et al. 2009). Other investigators too have observed persistent diastolic dysfunction following kidney transplantation in children (Ten Harkel et al . 2009).

4.4 Convulsions

Although this would be commonly alluded to drug toxicity (e.g. cyclosporine), in our set up, this could result from rapid loss of urea through the poly-uric transplanted kidney leading to a reverse osmosis and cerebral edema. Thus, the need for mechanical ventilation especially in children who had high blood urea levels pre-operatively (e.g. over 30 mmol/l) is justifiable.

4.5 Bleeding diathesis

This often results from preoperative liver dysfunction (due to chronic congestion) and anti-platelet agents used for the prevention of acute vascular thrombosis. In chronically anemic patients, usually aspirin is avoided as the resulting bleed will not stop unless and until almost an exchange transfusion has occurred and the transfused platelets have taken effect. The need for leucocyte depleted blood to minimize the risk of sensitization, cryo precipitate and fresh frozen plasma in the management of this case scenario which is often an unbearable burden for our support services.

4.6 Hyperglycemia

Often a hyperglycemic state is noted, especially in children during the poly-uric phase. This is a direct result of the use of saline/dextrose solutions far exceeding the amounts the body can handle metabolically during the given time. The hyperglycemia noted in this post operative phase is not usually associated with a metabolic derangement as seen in, for example, in diabetic keto acidosis and it is often impossible to normalize glucose levels through insulin therapy during the ongoing replacement therapy with dextrose/saline. The use of, for example, 0.45% saline alone is also harmful due to its hypo tonicity. In our experience, this resultant hyperglycemia is relatively harmless and resolves spontaneously once the poly-uric phase is over.

4.7 Drug monitoring

It is not possible to monitor drug levels as much as one would like and more often than not an empirical dosage adjustment is carried out.

4.8 Sepsis

The mortality of pediatric renal transplant recipient is 4 to 4.5 % in the long term; and in 40-45% this mortality, is caused by infection.

4.9 Our experience

From among the 29 children receiving kidney transplantation in our centre over the last 6 years,, all children received a standard general anesthetic (Biriulina e al 2008), balanced using a low-flow inhalational isoflurane with non- invasive BP monitoring combined with internal jugular vein catheterization for CVP monitoring. The major component of infusion therapy was freshly frozen plasma and leukocyte depleted blood to correct anemia and operative blood loss.

In our cohort, all were admitted to the ICU for postoperative mechanical ventilation following transplantation. The need to maintain adult blood pressures in children to drive the transplanted adult kidney with added problems of splinted diaphragm and a large proportion of the cardiac output diverting through the adult transplanted kidney imposed further difficulties for the already strained cardiovascular system in children. Thus, most children needed post operative intensive care necessitating inotropes and mechanical ventilation support. In our cohort, the mean (±SD) duration of mechanical ventilation was 4.59 ± 2.77 days while the mean (±SD) ICU stay was 6.44 ± 3.35 days. Post operative ICU complications occurred in 85.71%.

Hypertension (53%), heart failure (32%) and convulsions (32%) were the commonest problems. Hyperglycemia (25%), bleeding diathesis (25%), temporary transplant kidney failure needing dialysis, acute exacerbation of asthma, low calcium, lung collapse, hypo-natremia, paralytic ileus, and cyclosporine toxicity were among the other complications. No ICU deaths of post renal transplant patients were reported.

We are only relieved that there were no patient or graft losses especially at this early phase of the program. This helped us build the much needed confidence of the public and that of colleagues. The experiences gained by the surgeon, nephrologists and anesthesiologist abroad in developed countries, contributed to this favorable outcome as they all functioned with a degree of anticipation for known complications and prevention. The nursing staff had no previous exposure but had learnt rapidly on the job using their intensive care skills to manage these cases.

It was not possible to make any statistically significant causal inferences with the present study as it comprised of a small number of cases and had relatively short duration of follow up. However, medical professionals develop the pattern of recognition necessary for infrequent clinical entities, through confrontation with real life demonstrations or lively papers best examples being case reports and case series. In this context, this paper would help those who are envisaging kidney transplant programmes in the developing world with limited resources.

5. Limitations

In a recent review, collating 16 reports of 300 pediatric transplants in the developing world found that recipients were older than 6 years and donors were living relatives in more than 94% of the series. Cyclosporine, azathioprin and steroids were the mainstay of immunosuppression and in many centers, the high costs of drugs resulted in noncompliance and discontinuation of immunosuppression. Therefore, acute rejection rates were high, more than 40% in half of the series. One-year and 5-year survival rates for grafts were 89-98% and 67-84% and for patients 88-98% and 65-90%, respectively. Major causes of graft loss were chronic rejection, acute rejection and infection and for the patients, it was infection. Growth analysis was not generally reported but when reported the deficit remains or gets worse. They concluded that high rejection and infection rates result in poor patient and graft survival (Rizvi et al 2009).

With increased awareness, improved resources, and more health professionals trained in the field, it is likely that the renal transplantation would be routine in Sri Lanka as in many other countries. Although it offers survival advantage to these children, it is a complex procedure and is not without complications. The financial implications of costly regular medications these children need is an intolerable blow to the affected families and hence we are working towards meeting these costs via charity.

Improving survival and quality of life for kidney transplant recipients in developing countries in the long-term is an awesome task. A recent review looking into factors affecting long-term outcome after renal transplantation in childhood, summarized in the table below would bring useful hints for the clinicians involved in caring for these children and adults in the developing world.

6. Conclusion

Kidney transplantation in the current context in a developing country may warrant a significant duration of postoperative ICU therapy in children. Since chronic dialysis also increases morbidity in these patients as it is associated with cardiovascular damage, impaired cognitive development and retardation of growth, pre-emptive kidney transplantation in children with ESRD, seems the treatment of choice in the developing world.

Minimizing the risk of chronic allograft nephropathy is invariably a major task during follow up. Appropriate titration of the immunosuppressive agents of the high-risk patients (such as in those with higher serum creatinine level) will be very important. Compliance can be improved by regular supervision and education of the patients and the parents and being empathetic towards their problems and needs, (especially those of the adolescent child) and also by minimizing the unnecessary hospital admissions and clinic visits, making the drug prescriptions as less complicated as possible and timely attending to the unwanted side effects of the drugs.

TRANSPLANT OUTCOME DETERMINANTS	WHAT IS ALREADY KNOWN
Factors influencing outcome	• Available resources affect patient selection, follow-up and drug regimens • Community attitudes influence treatment of high-risk patients such as neonates and children with handicaps • Some diagnoses are more common in particular ethnic backgrounds and patient and graft survival are affected by racial group • The outcome is generally superior for LD transplantation
Patient survival	• The mortality rate of children on the waiting list is 55 per 1000 at risk • The overall mortality rate, with a relative risk of death after transplantation is 12.7-times higher than that of the age-related general population
Overall patient survival	• Between 70% and 100% at 5 years • Between 75% to 95% at 10 years • Between 83% to 94% at 15 years • Between 54% to 86% at 20 years • 81% at 25-years.
Effect of recipient age	• Mortality twice as high in those < 5 years of age than in those 6 to 10 years old • 5-year survival rate of over 97% in under 6 year olds • 91% 10-year survival rate in those weighing <15 kg at transplantation • 87% 15-year survival rate in those <11 kg at transplantation
Effect of donor type	• Small benefit of LD on mortality at all ages up to 5 years after transplantation • The survival rate for recipients of LDs, 96.1% 5 years after transplantation • LD has a particular benefit for the very young child: 5-year patient survival rates for recipients less than 2 years old was 86% following LD and 70% following DD
Causes of death after transplantation	• Cardiovascular disease (CVD) 30-36% • Infection 24–56%

TRANSPLANT OUTCOME DETERMINANTS	WHAT IS ALREADY KNOWN
	• Malignancy 11-20% • Other important factors (a) non-concordance with medications, or treatment withdrawal (b) obesity
Comparison of mortality after transplantation with mortality on dialysis	• lifespan of a child on dialysis is 40–60 years less, with a transplant, 20–25 years less, than that of age- and race-matched general populations • Eighty percent of patients on HD, 83% of those on PD and 93% of those with a transplant survive 5 years • Mortality rates are seven-times higher in those who have been on dialysis for longer than they have had a transplant • Treatment with dialysis is associated with a risk more than four-times as high as for renal transplantation. • Most of the increased mortality in children on dialysis is due to CVD • Adolescents who had undergone pre-emptive transplantation have a better survival rate.
Effect of race	• Poorer outcomes for Afro-Americans than for the white population due to increased incidence of cardiovascular deaths by approximately 1.6 times. • Among black patients, cardiac deaths occurred in 11% of transplant recipients and 34% of dialysis patients, and, among white patients, 9% and 25%, respectively
Overall transplant survival	• Current projected half-life 10 years. • Given a median age at transplantation of 13 years, 50% of all current pediatric kidney recipients will need a second graft before the age of 25 years • Overall 5-year transplant survival varies between 44% to 95% • at 5 years, 23%–95% at 10 years, 35% at 15 years [8] and 21-36% at 20 years. • Graft survival of repeat transplants are slightly lower than first grafts. • When DDs were used, graft survival rates at 1, 3 and 5 years were 79%, 69%, and 62%, compared with 74%, 60%, and 47%, respectively, for the repeat transplants

TRANSPLANT OUTCOME DETERMINANTS	WHAT IS ALREADY KNOWN
	• For LDs, graft survival rates for 1,3 and 5 years were 91%, 83%, and 76% compared to 86%, 78%, and 72%, respectively, for repeat transplants.
Effect of recipient age	• Graft survival at 1 year and 5 years • 71% and 60% in those under the age of 2 years at transplantation, • 83% and 64% in those aged 3 to 12 years • 85% and 57% in those aged 13 to 21 years • In adolescents, as a group, have the worst graft survival rate of all ages
Effect of donor age	• Kidneys from deceased donors aged 11–17 years do best, with a 73% 5-year survival • Transplant survival of 55% after 5 years, for donors <6 years of age, and of 60% for donors over that age • 5-year graft survival rate from donors <1 year of age 60% and to 70% for donors aged 1 year to 5 years
Effect of donor type	• Living related donation (LD) benefit outcome, graft survival 75% - 85% at 10 years, compared to 46% for DDs • LRD is of particular benefit to the recipient under 2 years of age, 5-year graft survival 86% compared to 38% following DD
Effect of pre-emptive transplant	• Transplant survival better in patients receiving a pre-emptive transplant compared with those undergoing PD and HD. • Graft loss resulting from vascular thrombosis is more common in children who undergo PD than in those who on HD • Graft survival between those not on dialysis and those on dialysis of 82% and 69%, respectively, at 6 years • Waiting time on dialysis is an independent risk factor for failure of LRD transplants in adolescents
Recurrent diseases	• Diseases that recur after transplantation with a potential to affect outcome include FSGS, membranoproliferative glomerulonephritis

TRANSPLANT OUTCOME DETERMINANTS	WHAT IS ALREADY KNOWN
	(MPGN) and haemolytic uraemic syndrome (HUS) • Oxalate will continue to be deposited in the transplant if liver transplantation is not undertaken in patients with hyperoxaluria. • Nephrotic syndrome can recur in patients with congenital nephrotic syndrome, and anti-glomerular basement membrane (anti-GBM) nephritis in patients with Alport's syndrome, both due to the development of antibody to the 'missing' protein. • FSGS recurs in approximately 30% of transplants
Human leukocyte antigen matching	• Donor-specific HLA mismatching is a risk for poor outcome • Worst outcome has been observed for two HLA-DR mismatched grafts • 000 and favourably matched kidneys (100, 010, 110 HLA-A, -B, -DR mismatches) survived longest • Sensitised patients [panel reactive antibodies (PRA) > 40%]have a poorer outcome • Donor antigen-specific hyporeactivity correlates with better graft function
Immunosuppression	• The use of MMF in association with ciclosporin is associated with better outcome at 5 years than a similar regimen using AZA, transplant survival's being 90.7% for MMF and 68.5% for AZA patients. • Cumulative rejection-free survival was also better in the MMF group, at 51.2% versus 37.0% in AZA patients. • Tacrolimus is significantly more effective than ciclosporin in both preventing acute rejection and maintaining graft function, with a 4-year transplant survival rate of 86% and 69%, respectively
Concordance with therapeutic regimens	• Non-concordance with therapeutic regimens affects all ages, but particularly adolescence. • Non-concordance is the main contributor for late graft loss, accounting for 71% of cases, and was a particular problem in Afro-American recipients
Hypertension	• Very common after transplantation, and its

TRANSPLANT OUTCOME DETERMINANTS	WHAT IS ALREADY KNOWN
	incidence varies with time, ranging from 46%, 40%, and 66% of children at 1, 5, and 10 years, respectively. • Hypertension is a significant and independent predictor of poor long-term transplant function, regardless of the number of rejection episodes or transplant function at 1 year.
Bladder dynamics	• Transplantation into an abnormal urinary tract is associated with a high incidence of urological and infectious complications but no effect on patient survival or transplant outcome. • Careful surveillance of lower urinary tract function by urodynamic evaluation is essential before transplantation. • Reflux does not need to be corrected before transplantation, unless it is causing symptoms or infection .
Laparoscpic donor nephrectomy	• Despite longer warm ischaemia and cold ischaemia times in LDs, graft outcome does not seem to be affected.
Final height and incidence of obesity	• Improvements in pre-transplantation management, particularly nutrition, have led to a better height attainment at transplantation • Decline in steroid dosing as immunosuppression has a positive benefit on growth. Patients who received recombinant human growth hormone (rHGH) suggest that final height is better than for those not receiving it. • Obesity, defined by a body mass index (BMI) >95th centile, is increasing in the transplant population (12.4% after 1995 and 8% before 1995) and seems to be more common in girls.
Psychosocial outcome	• Psychosocial outcome seems to be better after transplantation than for patients on dialysis. • Employment: Several studies have revealed satisfactory employment levels., The range of occupations is broad, with a normal average working time each week. • Relationships: Successful relationships are reported 50% married

TRANSPLANT OUTCOME DETERMINANTS	WHAT IS ALREADY KNOWN
	• Physical morbidity: Co-morbidity was found in 40% of all patients: motor, hearing, or visual disabilities were found in 19%. Bone disease, headaches, itching, and tremors were the most reported disabling problems. Other complications included osteoporosis in 53% of patients, avascular bone necrosis in 13%, post-transplantation diabetes mellitus in 10%, and hypertension in 60%. • Education: Distribution of educational level was lower than national averages: 27.4% were at the lowest level versus 3% of the general population, 41.4% were at the middle level, 31.2% had reached the baccalaureate level, and 11% had followed a university course.
Independence	• 46% lived in their parents' home • 54% lived independently

Table 1. A summary of long-term outcome after renal transplantation in childhood (Rees 2009).

In spite of increase graft survival, mortality rates of renal transplant patients remain higher than the normal population. Cardio-vascular diseases, de-novo malignancy and infections are the commonest causes of death in the long run. Careful management of hypertension, left ventricular hypertrophy, dyslipidaemias and calcium and phosphate homeostasis, from the pre-transplant period, would help to reduce the cardio-vascular related deaths. Incidence of infections and malignancy can be reduced by the appropriate selection of the immune-suppressive drugs with timely tailoring off the dosages in patients, who are at lower risk for rejection.

Another important challenge ahead is to optimize the care given to the patient with chronic kidney disease or CRF. One of the main obstacles that prevent this is the late presentation of these patients. Increased awareness of the health personnel and the general public regarding identification of the patients with renal problems and appropriate management of them will invariably reduce the incidence of ESRF, and better care provided to the CRF patients will delay the progression to end stage and will also reduce the pre-operative co-morbidities.

In addition, the provision of regular medication, improving laboratory facilities, establishment of pediatric dialysis programmes and increasing the number of resource persons (pediatric transplant surgeons, pediatric nephrologists, pediatric anesthetists and trained paramedical personnel) are important goals to be achieved in the future, to assure successful ongoing transplant programs in the developing world.

7. Acknowledgements

The author especially acknowledge the contributions made by the nephrologists Abeysekara C K, Abegunawardena A, Abeysekara T, Wazil M, and the surgeons Fernando O, Buthpitiya

AG, Lamawansa MD for the sustenance of above pediatric kidney transplant program assisted by B Hevavithana (Radiologist), Dr N Ratnatunga (Pathologist) and all other hospital staff and Mr Mahes Salgado for assistance with the manuscript.

8. References

Aalten J. Bemelman FJ. van den Berg-Loonen EM. Claas FH. Christiaans MH. de Fijter JW. Hepkema BG. Hene RJ. van der Heide JJ. van Hooff JP. Lardy NM. Lems SP. Otten HG. Weimar W. Allebes WA. Hoitsma AJ. (2009 Aug) Pre-kidney-transplant blood transfusions do not improve transplantation outcome: a Dutch national study. Nephrology Dialysis Transplantation. 24(8):2559-66

Allain-Launay E. Roussey-Kesler G. Ranchin B. Guest G. Maisin A. Novo R. Andre JL. Cloarec S. Guyot C. (2009 Sep) Mortality in pediatric renal transplantation: a study of the French pediatric kidney database. Pediatric Transplantation. 13(6):725-30

Badmus TA. Arogundade FA. Sanusi AA. Akinsola WA. Adesunkanmi AR. Agbakwuru AO. Salako AB. Faponle AF. Oyebamiji EO. Adetiloye VA. Famurewa OC. Oladimeji BY. Fatoye FO (2005) Kidney transplantation in a developing economy: challenges and initial report of three cases at Ile Ife. . Central African Journal of Medicine. 51(9-10):102-6.

Bamgboye EL. (2009) Barriers to a functional renal transplant program in developing countries. Ethnicity & Disease. 19(1 Suppl 1):S1-56-9.

Biriulina NIu. Ushakova IA. Vabishchevich AV. (2008 Sep-Oct.) [Anesthetic maintenance of renal transplantation in children]. [Russian] Anesteziologiia i Reanimatologiia. (5):58-61

Caliskan Y. Yazici H. Gorgulu N. Yelken B. Emre T. Turkmen A. Yildiz A. Aysuna N. Bozfakioglu S. Sever MS.(2009 Feb) Effect of pre-transplant dialysis modality on kidney transplantation outcome. Peritoneal Dialysis International. 29 Suppl 2:S117-22.

Haberal M. Karakayali H. Sevmis S. Akbulut S. Colak T. Baskin E. Moray G. Torgay A. Arslan G. (2009 Sept) Preemptive living donor renal transplantation: a single-center experience. Transplantation Proceedings. 41(7):2764-7.

Irtan S. Maisin A. Baudouin V. Nivoche Y. Azoulay R. Jacqz-Aigrain E. El Ghoneimi A. Aigrain Y (2010 Jun) Renal transplantation in children: critical analysis of age related surgical complications. Pediatric Transplantation. 14(4):512-9.

Jung GO. Moon JI. Kim JM. Choi GS. Kwon CH. Cho JW. Kim SJ.(2007 Apr) Can preemptive kidney transplantation guarantee longer graft survival in living-donor kidney transplantation? Single-center study. Transplantation Proceedings. 42(3):766-74.

Kandus A. Arnol M. Bren AF.(2009 Aug) Survey of renal transplantation in Slovenia. Therapeutic Apheresis & Dialysis: Official Peer-Reviewed Journal of the International Society for Apheresis, the Japanese Society for Apheresis, the Japanese Society for Dialysis Therapy. 13(4):264-7

Kim GB. Kwon BS. Kang HG. Ha JW. Ha IS. Noh CI. Choi JY. Kim SJ. Yun YS. Bae EJ. (2009 Jun 15). Cardiac dysfunction after renal transplantation; incomplete resolution in pediatric population. Transplantation. 87(11):1737-43

Koshy SM. Guttmann A. Hebert D. Parkes RK. Logan AG (2009 Dec) Incidence and risk factors for cardiovascular events and death in pediatric renal transplant patients: a single center long-term outcome study. . Pediatric Transplantation. 13(8):1027-33

Muthusethupathi MA. Shivakumar S.(1993 Mar) Renal transplantation in India-problems and prospects. Journal of the Association of Physicians of India. 41(3):129.

Ng KH. Shrestha P. Aragon E. Lau YW. Yeo WS. Chan YH. Krishnan P. Yap HK.(2009 Apr) Nineteen-year experience of paediatric renal transplantation in Singapore. Annals of the Academy of Medicine, Singapore. 38(4):300-9.

Persy VP. Remuzzi G. Perico N. Benghanem Gharbi M. Adu D. Jha V. Rizvi A. Ben Ammar M. Fongoro S. De Broe ME. (2010) Prevention and transplantation in chronic kidney disease: what is achievable in emerging countries? Meeting report: Bamako meeting December 4-6, 2008. Nephron. 115(2):c122-32.

Porrett PM. Kamoun M. Parsons R. Bloom R. Goral S. Reese P. Grossman R. Baluarte J. Bleicher M. Doyle A. Markmann JF. Levine M. Barker C. Olthoff K. Naji A. Shaked A. Abt P.(2009) Kidney transplantation at the University of Pennsylvania: 1998-2008. . Clinical Transplants. :143-52.

Rees L. Long-term outcome after renal transplantation in childhood. [Review] 2009 Mar. Pediatric Nephrology. 24(3):475-84

Rizvi A. Naqvi A. Hussain Z. Hussain M. Hashmi A. Akhtar F. Zafar MN. Ahmed E. Sultan S. Aziz S. Shehzad A. Khalid R. . (2001 Feb-Mar) Why is it more difficult to transplant children? A perspective in developing countries. Transplantation Proceedings 33(1-2):1742-3,.

Rizvi SA. Naqvi SA (1997 Feb-Mar) Need for increasing transplant activity: a sustainable model for developing countries. Transplantation Proceedings. 29(1-2):1560-2

Rizvi SA. Naqvi SA. Hussain Z. Hashmi A. Akhtar F. Hussain M. Ahmed E. Zafar MN. Hafiz S. Muzaffar R. Jawad F.(2003 Feb) Renal transplantation in developing countries. [Review] Kidney International - Supplement. (83):S96-100.

Rizvi SA. Zafar MN. Lanewala AA. Naqvi SA. (2009 Oct) Challenges in pediatric renal transplantation in developing countries. [Review] Current Opinion in Organ Transplantation. 14(5):533-9

Sakhaee K. (2010 Feb) . Post-renal transplantation hypophosphatemia. [Review] Pediatric Nephrology. 25(2):213-20

Ten Harkel AD. Cransberg K. Van Osch-Gevers M. Nauta J.(2009 Jun). Diastolic dysfunction in paediatric patients on peritoneal dialysis and after renal transplantation. Nephrology Dialysis Transplantation. 24(6):1987-91

Uchida K. (2010 Sep) [Pediatric renal transplant in Japan]. [Review] [Japanese] Nippon Geka Gakkai Zasshi. Journal of Japan Surgical Society. 111(5):299-304.

Usta A. Shawish T. Mishra A. Ehtuish EF. Ajaj H. Milud N. Shebani A. Abdulmola T. Tejori U. (2008 Dec) Living related kidney transplantation in Libya: a single center experience. Transplantation Proceedings. 40(10):3428-33.

van Heurn E. de Vries EE (2009 May) Kidney transplantation and donation in children. [Review]. Pediatric Surgery International. 25(5):385-93.

Wisanuyotin S. Jiravuttipong A.(2009 Dec) Pediatric renal transplantation: a single-center experience in northeast Thailand. Journal of the Medical Association of Thailand. 92(12):1635-9.